Lyme Disease

An Evidence-based Approach

2nd Edition

_____

Lyme Disease

An Evidence-based Approach

2nd Edition

Edited by

John J. Halperin, MD

Overlook Medical Center, New Jersey, USA

and

Sidney Kimmel Medical College at Thomas Jefferson University, Philadelphia, USA

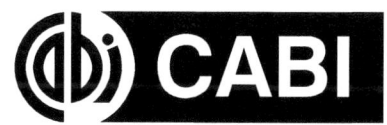

CABI is a trading name of CAB International

CABI	CABI
Nosworthy Way	745 Atlantic Avenue
Wallingford	8th Floor
Oxfordshire OX10 8DE	Boston, MA 02111
UK	USA
Tel: +44 (0)1491 832111	Tel: +1 (617)682-9015
Fax: +44 (0)1491 833508	E-mail: cabi-nao@cabi.org
E-mail: info@cabi.org	
Website: www.cabi.org	

© CAB International 2018. All rights reserved. No part of this publication may be reproduced in any form or by any means, electronically, mechanically, by photocopying, recording or otherwise, without the prior permission of the copyright owners.

A catalogue record for this book is available from the British Library, London, UK.

Library of Congress Cataloging-in-Publication Data

Names: Halperin, John J., editor. | C.A.B. International, publisher.
Title: Lyme disease : an evidence-based approach / edited by John J. Halperin.
Other titles: Lyme disease (Halperin)
Description: 2nd edition. | Wallingford, Oxfordshire, UK ; Boston, MA : CABI, [2018] | Includes bibliographical references and index.
Identifiers: LCCN 2017060811 (print) | LCCN 2017061260 (ebook) | ISBN 9781786392084 (pdf) | ISBN 9781786392091 (ePub) | ISBN 9781786392077 (hardback : alk. paper)
Subjects: | MESH: Lyme Disease
Classification: LCC RC155.5 (ebook) | LCC RC155.5 (print) | NLM WC 406 | DDC 616.9/246--dc23
LC record available at https://lccn.loc.gov/2017060811

ISBN-13: 9781786392077 (hbk)
   9781786392084 (PDF)
   9781786392091 (ePub)

Commissioning editor: Rachael Russell
Editorial assistant: Alexandra Lainsbury
Production editor: Tim Kapp

Typeset by SPi, Pondicherry, India
Printed and bound in the UK by CPI Group (UK) Ltd, Croydon, CR0 4YY

Contents

Contributors vii

Preface to First Edition ix

Preface to Second Edition xi

PART I: BIOLOGICAL SUBSTRATE

1. **Ticks: The Vectors of Lyme Disease** 1
   Robert P. Smith

2. **Biology of the Lyme Disease Agents: A Selective Survey of Clinical and Epidemiologic Relevance** 29
   Alan G. Barbour

3. ***Borreliella*: Interactions with the Host Immune System** 45
   Kirk Sperber and Raymond J. Dattwyler

4. **Diagnostic Testing for Lyme Disease** 58
   Paul G. Auwaerter

5. **Global Epidemiology of *Borreliella burgdorferi* Infections** 76
   Paul S. Mead

PART II: CLINICAL ASPECTS

6. **Antibiotic Therapy for Infection Caused by *Borrelia burgdorferi* Sensu Lato** 93
   Gary P. Wormser

7. **Lyme Borreliosis: The European Perspective** 105
   Franc Strle, Gerold Stanek and Klemen Strle

8. **Lyme Neuroborreliosis: A European Perspective** 124
   Rick Dersch

9	Medically Unexplained Symptoms and Lyme Neuroborreliosis – Not the Same: A Study in an Endemic Area of Norway *Erlend Roaldsnes, Randi Eikeland and Dag Berild*	139
10	**Erythema Migrans** *Robert B. Nadelman and Linden Hu*	142
11	**Lyme Carditis** *Jonathan R. Salik and David M. Dudzinski*	168
12	**The Musculoskeletal Manifestations of Lyme Disease (Infection with *Borrelia burgdorferi*)** *Leonard H. Sigal*	180
13	**Nervous System Involvement** *John J. Halperin*	202
14	**Lyme Disease in Children** *Eugene D. Shapiro*	216
15	**The Psychology of 'Post-Lyme Disease Syndrome' and 'Not Lyme'** *Afton L. Hassett and Leonard H. Sigal*	227
16	**Chronic Lyme Disease** *Adriana Marques*	247
17	**Lyme Disease: The Great Controversy** *John J. Halperin, Phillip Baker and Gary P. Wormser*	262
Index		279

Contributors

Paul G. Auwaerter, MD, MBA, Sherrilyn and Ken Fisher Professor of Medicine, Fisher Center for Environmental Infectious Diseases, Division of Infectious Diseases, Department of Medicine, Johns Hopkins University School of Medicine, 725 North Wolfe Street, Rm 231, Baltimore, MD 21205, USA. E-mail: pauwaert@jhmi.edu

Phillip J. Baker, PhD, Executive Director, American Lyme Disease Foundation, Lyme, CT 06371, USA.

Alan G. Barbour, MD, Professor of Medicine, Microbiology and Molecular Genetics, and Ecology and Evolutionary Biology, University of California Irvine, Irvine, CA 92697, USA. E-mail: abarbour@uci.edu

Dag Berild, MD, PhD, Professor of Infectious Diseases, Department of Infectious Diseases, Oslo University Hospital, Oslo University and Oslo Metropolitan University, Oslo, Norway. E-mail: dag.berild@medisin.uio.no

Raymond J. Dattwyler, MD, Professor of Microbiology/Immunology and Medicine, New York Medical College, Valhalla, NY 10595, USA. E-mail: raymond_dattwyler@nymc.edu

Rick Dersch, MD, Department of Neurology, Medical Center – University of Freiburg, Breisacher Str. 64, D-79106, Freiburg, Germany. E-mail: rick.dersch@uniklinik-freiburg.de

David M. Dudzinski, MD, JD, Director, Cardiac Intensive Care Unit, Division of Cardiology, Massachusetts General Hospital, Boston, MA 02114, USA. E-mail: ddudzinski@mgh.harvard.edu

Randi Eikeland, MD, PhD, Director of the National Advisory Unit for Tick-borne Diseases, Department of Neurology, Hospital of Southern Norway, Norway. E-mail: randi.eikeland@sshf.no

John J. Halperin, MD, Chair, Department of Neurosciences, Overlook Medical Center, 99 Beauvoir Avenue, Summit, NJ 07902, USA and Professor of Neurology and Medicine, Sidney Kimmel Medical College of Thomas Jefferson University, Philadelphia, PA, USA. E-mail: john.halperin@atlantichealth.org

Afton L. Hassett, PsyD, Associate Research Scientist, Chronic Pain and Fatigue Research Center, Department of Anesthesiology, University of Michigan, Ann Arbor, MI 48106, USA. E-mail: afton@med.umich.edu

Linden Hu, MD, Professor and Vice Dean for Research, Tufts University School of Medicine, 136 Harrison Ave, Boston, MA 02111, USA. E-mail: linden.hu@tufts.edu

Adriana Marques, MD, Laboratory of Clinical Immunology and Microbiology, National Institute of Allergy and Infectious Diseases, National Institutes of Health, 9000 Rockville Pike, Bethesda, MD 20892, USA. E-mail: amarques@niaid.nih.gov

Paul S. Mead, MD, MPH, Bacterial Diseases Branch, Division of Vector-borne Diseases, National Center for Emerging and Zoonotic Infectious Diseases, Centers for Disease Control and Prevention (CDC), 3156 Rampart Road, Ft Collins, CO 80521, USA. E-mail: pmead@cdc.gov

Robert B. Nadelman, Professor of Medicine, Department of Medicine, Division of Infectious Diseases, New York Medical College, Valhalla, NY, USA.

Erlend Roaldsnes, MD, Department of Acute Medicine, Oslo University Hospital, Kirkeveien 166, 0450, Oslo, Norway. E-mail: erlend.roaldsnes@gmail.com

Jonathan R. Salik, MD, Division of Cardiology, Massachusetts General Hospital, 55 Fruit St, Boston, MA 02114, USA. E-mail: jsalik@partners.org

Eugene D. Shapiro, MD, Professor of Pediatrics, of Epidemiology and of Investigative Medicine, Yale University, Department of Pediatrics, PO Box 208064, 333 Cedar Street, New Haven, CT 06520-8064, USA. E-mail: eugene.shapiro@yale.edu

Leonard H. Sigal, MD, FACP, FACR, Clinical Professor, Department of Medicine, Division of Rheumatology, RUTGERS – Robert Wood Johnson Medical School, PO Box 301, Stockbridge, MA 01262, USA. E-mail: lensigal@gmail.com

Robert P. Smith, MD, MPH, Director, Division of Infectious Disease, Maine Medical Center, Portland, ME, USA; and Director, Vector-borne Disease Laboratory, Maine Medical Center Research Institute, Portland, ME, USA; and Professor of Medicine, Tufts University School of Medicine, 81 Research Drive, Scarborough, ME 04074, USA. E-mail: smithr@mmc.org

Kirk Sperber, MD, Associate Professor of Medicine, New York Medical College, Valhalla, NY 10595, USA. E-mail: Kirk_Sperber@nymc.edu

Gerold Stanek, MD, Professor, Medical University of Vienna, Institute for Hygiene and Applied Immunology, Kinderspitalgasse 15, 1095 Vienna, Austria.

Franc Strle, MD, PhD, Professor of Infectious Diseases, Department of Infectious Diseases, University Medical Center Ljubljana, Japljeva 2, 1525 Ljubljana, Slovenia. E-mail: franc.strle@kclj.si

Klemen Strle, PhD, Assistant Professor of Medicine, Massachusetts General Hospital/Harvard Medical School, Room 8301 (CNY149), 55 Fruit St, Boston, MA 02114, USA. E-mail: kstrle@mgh.harvard.edu

Gary P. Wormser, MD, Chief, Division of Infectious Diseases, Vice Chairman, Department of Medicine, Medical Director and Founder of the Lyme Disease Diagnostic Center, Professor of Medicine, Microbiology and Immunology, and Pharmacology, New York Medical College, 40 Sunshine Cottage Rd, Valhalla, NY 10595, USA. E-mail: gwormser@nymc.edu

Preface to First Edition

Spirochetal infections somehow seem to take on larger-than-life roles. 'The French disease', a.k.a. syphilis, assumed almost mythic proportions. Initially brought back from the New World to the Old, perhaps as divine retribution for measles, smallpox and myriad other curses visited on North America's aboriginal populations by European conquerors, neurosyphilis affected so many historic personalities as to give it a legitimate claim as a moulder of history. Even early in the 20th century, a lack of understanding of the pathophysiology of many other diseases led to the attribution of all manner of disorders to this infection, often by default, because nobody could come up with a better explanation.

Early in the history of Lyme disease, many latched on to the syphilis parallel, asserting that this new spirochetosis, like its cousin, could masquerade as innumerable other ailments. However, the greatest similarity between the two has been the tendency to inappropriately attribute unrelated, but otherwise not readily explained, disorders to the unjustly accused spirochete.

The past decade or two has seen medicine move broadly and strongly toward the requirement for evidence-based support for its conclusions and actions. For those of us over a certain age, although this is certainly intellectually satisfying, it produces a distinct cognitive dissonance. When I was a resident, the truth was what the professors said and wrote in textbooks. The evidence basis at best consisted of case series and anecdotal observations. Unfortunately, even the most brilliant minds, individuals who led medicine for decades, were often proved wrong as new technologies – imaging, biochemical assays, DNA analysis or whatever – provided more powerful tools to answer questions.

The Lyme disease 'debate' is this tension writ large. On the one hand, there is a group, consisting largely of family practitioners and other primary care providers, who see large numbers of patients suffering with medically unexplained symptoms. They struggle (quite legitimately) to understand the causes of these patients' suffering, and draw on whatever technologies appear applicable – often accepting the test results uncritically. They then accept responsibility for treating these patients and actually try things! This earns them the sincere gratitude of patients who have been struggling both with chronic disabling symptoms and the inability of mainstream medicine to provide them with satisfying answers. Patients and treaters then provide each other with strong reinforcement.

In contrast, other physicians, often with more advanced specialty-oriented training, have adopted the more rigorous, scientific approach. This group looks critically at all efforts to understand, diagnose and treat this disorder, and would rather say 'I don't know' than make assertions felt not to be based on sound science. They demand that all conclusions, diagnostic approaches and treatments meet current standards of evidence-based medicine. This culture clash fuels the debate – a debate that, if it were based just on scientific evidence, would have disappeared long ago due to the totally one-sided nature of the observations.

However, the debate has not ended and many physicians in practice continue to see patients who are convinced that their symptoms are due to a chronic infection with *Borrelia burgdorferi*. Not only do these patients fear that they have a chronic, debilitating and difficult-to-treat infection, but they have been told that this infection will damage their nervous system and lead to inevitable irreparable brain damage. These frightened patients often come armed with reams of almost plausible-sounding material downloaded from the internet, and are only too happy to debate the contents with their physicians.

The goal of this book is to present the relevant evidence so that practicing physicians can better understand the arguments being made and use the best information available to help their patients. The intent is to cover the areas most often identified as 'controversial' and to provide perspective, clarifying the debate. It is the hope of all the authors that this will help calm some of the anxiety (among both physicians and patients) about this disorder, and allow physicians to provide their patients with the most appropriate treatment.

Before diving into the substance of the debate, it is essential that I acknowledge those who have made this work possible. First, I thank the patients who freely share not only their stories but also their insights and their fears, teaching me daily about the reality of their illnesses. Secondly, I am grateful to the numerous colleagues – many of whom graciously agreed to contribute to this volume – who have gone through the 'Lyme wars' with me over the years, educating me, debating with me, together contributing to the maturation of the knowledge base regarding this illness. Thirdly, I am forever grateful to the mentors of my formative years – the innumerable college and medical school faculty who taught me the importance of thinking critically and analytically about complex issues. At the apex of these were the three ultimate exemplars of what my son calls 'eminence-based medicine' – Raymond Adams, C. Miller Fisher and E.P. Richardson – three of the greats of 20th-century neurology, with whom I had the privilege of working. Long before there was evidence-based medicine, these giants made it crystal clear that truth would be found not in the pronouncements of the giants but in a meticulous analysis of the data.

I owe a very special thank you to the American Lyme Disease Foundation, which graciously provided funding to allow the publication of the colour illustrations in this volume. And finally, and most importantly, I thank my son, for being a never ending source of pride, joy, inquisitiveness and intellectual rigor, and my wonderful bride of three dozen years – who gamely puts up with my long hours, battle stories and innumerable imperfections, yet is always there as the supportive anchor of my universe, making it all possible.

John J. Halperin

Preface to Second Edition

It has been 7 years since the writing of the first edition of this book – 7 years that have seen significant advances in our understanding of the disorders collectively referred to as Lyme disease or Lyme borreliosis. In this update, each author has built on the solid foundation of the first edition, incorporating the meaningful advances in the field.

Several major changes deserve emphasis. The first comes from the world of microbiology. As detailed by Dr Barbour, new members of the borreliosis family have been identified – *Borrelia miyamotoi, B. mayonii, B. bavariensis* among others. As the family tree has expanded so too has our knowledge of these spirochetes' genomes – leading to the introduction of a new genus, *Borreliella* ('*Borrelia*-like'), subsuming the former *Borrelia burgdorferi* sensu lato, and distinguishing these from the relapsing fever-like pathogens, which retain the genus name *Borrelia*. Like most changes to a long-established order, this reclassification has not met with universal enthusiasm. In most of this volume the new names have been adopted. A few remain with the resistance – identifying them will be left as an exercise for the careful reader.

Diagnostics are improving. The two-tier testing paradigm, so important in standardizing diagnostics for more than two decades, may soon be updated, incorporating newer and simpler tests. Our epidemiology colleagues stirred the pot several years ago when they estimated how many patients are actually being diagnosed with and treated for Lyme disease in the USA, going beyond the precise case definitions used for epidemiologic purposes – and, as Dr. Mead discusses, estimating that ten times as many patients are being treated for Lyme disease as are reported as meeting case definitions. The alternative-fact universe immediately saw this as evidence of a longstanding cover-up. Those who see patients who have been diagnosed with Lyme disease saw it as evidence of overtesting, overtreatment (including retreating because the serology is positive after treatment) and of the self-evident fact that a symptomatic patient in the real world with a positive test would usually prefer to be treated with oral antibiotics for a likely but not absolutely certain infection. Importantly, evidence continues to accrue that simple oral antibiotic regimens are effective in most instances – including for most patients with neuroborreliosis. At the same time, there has been ever more evidence that prolonged treatment confers no added benefit while subjecting patients to considerable risk.

Several different perspectives are provided regarding 'post-treatment Lyme disease syndrome' (PTLDS). Whether these non-specific, highly prevalent symptoms are causally related to Lyme disease, or whether this reflects anchoring bias, remains to be resolved. Regardless, given the wide prevalence of these symptoms, and their substantial impact on quality of life in individuals experiencing them, gaining a better understanding of their pathophysiology clearly remains an important goal, whether or not they have any relationship to Lyme disease. Importantly, there are now abundant data that this state is not indicative of nervous system infection or inflammation.

One might have hoped that the 'great controversy' would have calmed down by now. Sadly, not so much. Proponents of the 'Lyme literate' perspective have become ever more convinced that they own the correct world view and have become adept at using the explosion of on-line for-profit 'journals' to assert that their conjectures are supported by published medical literature. Given the larger environment in which we live – where facts, logical reasoning and a solid basis in science are undervalued at best, it is hard to know how this will play out.

Once again, I am extremely grateful to my colleagues for contributing their time, knowledge and effort to provide their chapters. I particularly valued our debates over various fine points – I certainly learned a lot. Several new contributors graciously agreed to join the effort; to them a special thank you and welcome. Several from the first edition have retired; I wish them all the best.

I must single out Dr. Robert Nadelman for particular thanks, who, despite being severely ill, contributed importantly to the update of Chapter 10 on erythema migrans. Sadly, Dr Nadelman passed away in March 2018, as this volume was undergoing final preparation. In addition to being an astute clinician and scholarly clinical scientist, Rob was a truly honourable gentleman, and a good friend. He will be sorely missed.

As with everything we do in medicine and science this volume presents a perspective at a point in time. I do not pretend that what we describe is carved in stone. Our effort has been to summarize the best science available today. I'm sure 7 years from now much that is here will remain accurate; some, undoubtedly will fall by the wayside. Hopefully, more of the former.

As before, I am grateful to my mentors, my colleagues and my students, all of whom inspire a passion to sort fact from fiction, to advance our understanding of human biology and to help our patients. A special thank you to my colleagues on the Guideline Development and Dissemination Committee of the American Academy of Neurology, who continue to teach me about evidence-based medicine. I am particularly grateful to my patients for sharing their very personal stories and perspectives.

And most important of all, my undying gratitude to my bride of 43 years, for always putting up with my long hours and way too many meetings, to my wonderful son and daughter-in-law, and to the greatest invention ever – my two absolutely delightful grandchildren, who can put a smile on my face no matter what!

John J. Halperin

1 Ticks: The Vectors of Lyme Disease

Robert P. Smith[1,2]
[1]*Division of Infectious Disease, Maine Medical Center, Portland, ME, USA;*
[2]*Vector-borne Disease Laboratory, Maine Medical Center Research Institute, Scarborough, ME, USA*

1.1 Introduction

Lyme disease, human granulocytic anaplasmosis, babesiosis and a febrile illness caused by the relapsing fever group bacterium *Borrelia miyamotoi* are diseases transmitted in temperate zones around the northern hemisphere by *Ixodes* ticks. In Eurasia, the same ticks also transmit the viral agents of tick-borne encephalitis, while in North America they cause infection with a related flavivirus known as Powassan virus (lineage 2) or deer tick virus (Telford, 1997; Ebel *et al.*, 2000; Tavakoli *et al.*, 2009). Most disease transmission to humans in North America and Eurasia is due to bites from four species of ticks (*I. scapularis, I. pacificus, I. ricinus* and *I. persulcatus*) that are grouped in the *Ixodes ricinus* species complex (Keirans *et al.*, 1999).

These four species serve as bridge vectors of disease from ancient cycles in nature to humans. They are 'generalist species' that during their multi-year life cycles feed on diverse hosts that may include species of mammals, birds or reptiles. Their importance as vectors of human disease varies with the disease agent, species of tick, vertebrate host community, geographic region and local ecologic factors. As an example, *I. scapularis* (the black-legged tick, commonly known as the 'deer tick') is present throughout the eastern US from Florida to Maine (Dennis *et al.*, 1998; Diuk-Wasser, 2006) and the Midwestern US from Texas to Minnesota. It accounts for the majority of human bites by ticks in the north-east US (Falco and Fish, 1988; Rand *et al.*, 2007) where 10–30% of nymphs and 20–70% of adult *I. scapularis* ticks carry *Borreliella burgdorferi* (Feldman *et al.*, 2015). In the south-east US, however, juvenile *I. scapularis* ticks rarely parasitize humans (Felz *et al.*, 1996) and, due to differences in preferred hosts, are infected with the agent of Lyme disease <2% of the time (Oliver *et al.*, 2003; Rosen *et al.*, 2012). Tick questing behavior in southern sites differs from those in the north-east and Midwest, with the southern clade of *I. scapularis* nymphal ticks questing beneath rather than above the leaf litter (Arsnoe *et al.*, 2015; Ginsberg *et al.*, 2017). As a consequence of limited human contact and low infection rates, locally acquired Lyme disease in most southern states is a rare event, despite the wide range of the potential vector.

Lyme disease is transmitted by *I. scapularis* ticks in the eastern and Midwestern US and south-central and eastern Canada, and by *I. pacificus* (western black-legged tick) in the coastal Pacific states. *Ixodes ricinus*, the castor bean or sheep tick, causes Lyme disease in Europe and far-western Asia, and *I. persulcatus*, the taiga tick, is its vector in eastern Europe and central Asia (Fig. 1.1). In addition, other species of *Ixodes* ticks maintain Lyme disease in 'silent' enzootic cycles but do not serve as a vector of the disease to humans. For example, in the western US, *I. spinipalpis* is a vector of enzootic *B. burgdorferi*

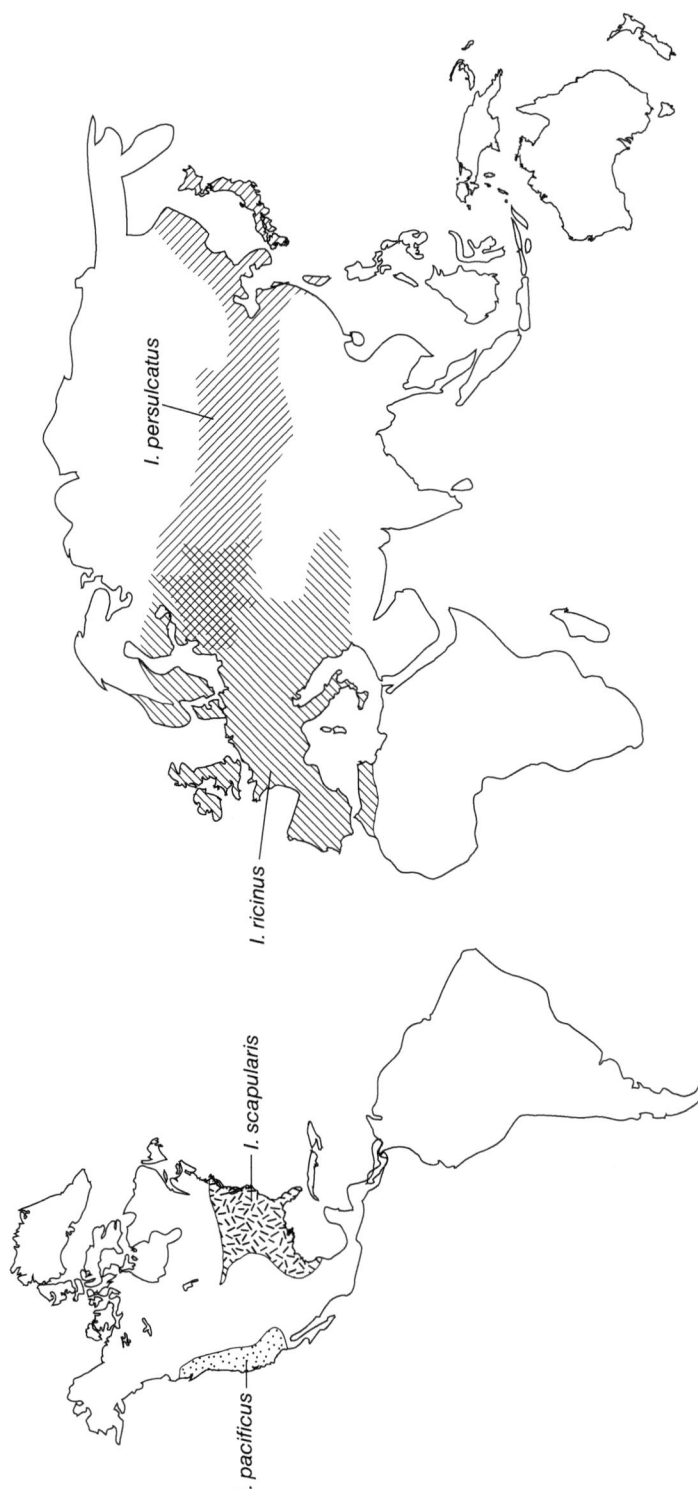

Fig. 1.1. The geographical distributions of the primary vectors of Lyme borreliosis spirochetes. (Designed by B. Kaye.)

infection in woodrats in regions where Lyme disease is not endemic due to absence of a human biting (or 'bridge') vector (Maupin *et al.*, 1994). The seabird tick, *I. uriae*, which is not a member of the *I. ricinus* group, maintains enzootic *Borreliella garinii* infection in colonies of puffins, auks and kittiwakes in both the northern and southern hemisphere (Olsen *et al.*, 1995). But humans are rarely in contact with this tick, and documented transmission of Lyme disease to humans by *I. uriae* bites has not been reported.

Although these enzootic cycles between ticks and their hosts are ancient, the emergence of Lyme disease over the past 50 years in both North America and Europe highlights changes in the range and abundance of these ticks, the environment we share with them and in the activities that put us at risk. Despite great strides in our understanding of these factors, efforts to control these ticks and to prevent transmission of the diseases they carry have not yet had a major impact when viewed on a large regional scale. Interventions at the small scale of an individual lot or neighborhood have had varying success. It is the purpose of this chapter to review the existing evidence for our current understanding of the evolution of these vectors, their means of dispersal and the reasons for range expansion, the mechanisms they use to transmit disease and the effectiveness of interventions to bring about their control.

1.2 Evolution and Historical Biogeography of *Ixodes* Ticks

Ticks and insects last shared a common ancestor 550 million years ago (Douzery *et al.*, 2004). Based on 16SrDNA phylogenies, hard ticks may have evolved during the radiation of bird taxa 50–100 million years ago (Black and Piesman, 1994). However, reconstruction of the evolutionary history of these invertebrates is based on a very limited fossil record (Klompen *et al.*, 1996; de la Fuente, 2003).

Phylogenetic analyses of existing *I. ricinus* complex ticks delineate more recent evolutionary history. Using 16S ribosomal DNA of 11 species, Xu *et al.* (2003) provided evidence for four distinct clades within the *I. ricinus* group. One clade includes *I. persulcatus*, *I. pacificus* and four other tick species, the second includes *I. ricinus*, and *I. scapularis* is in a third. The fourth clade consists of two tick species not known to parasitize humans. As natural hybridization of *I. ricinus* and *I. persulcatus* ticks has been reported from an area in Eurasia where they are sympatric, evolutionary species history may not denote absolute reproductive isolation (Kovalev *et al.*, 2016). Other ticks in these clades include several enzootic vectors that maintain 'silent cycles' of *Borreliella burgdorferi* (i.e. *I. minor* in the southern US), but do not parasitize humans (Xu *et al.*, 2003). Not all important tick vectors of enzootic *Borreliella* in nature are in the *I. ricinus* complex. For example, *I. hexagonus*, a major enzootic vector in Europe, is not closely related to ticks in the *I. ricinus* complex. That these vectors are not monophyletic is evidence that the ability to transmit and maintain borrelial spirochetes evolved multiple times.

Population genetics of North American *I. scapularis* ticks indicate a bottleneck occurring at the time of the Pleistocene Ice Age around 12,000 years ago. As per Humphrey *et al.* (2010), 'the mitochondria in both the Midwestern and northeastern *I. scapularis* populations are derived from a single colonizing tick that originated in refugia to the south of the ice sheet'. These studies, using 16S mitochondrial DNA, suggest that the Midwestern population is younger than the northeastern population, and both are more recent than southeastern populations, a conclusion also reached by others (Qiu *et al.*, 2002; Rosenthal and Spielman, 2004). The three tick populations have distinct haplotype frequencies, with low genetic variation between the Midwestern and northeastern population and more diversity present in the older southeastern group (Humphrey *et al.*, 2010; Gulia-Nuss *et al.*, 2016).

Spielman *et al.* (1979) described the northern population or clade of the black-legged or deer tick as a distinct species (i.e. *I. dammini*) based upon differences in nymphal tick morphology and questing behavior (with associated differences in human parasitism). Subsequent genetic analyses differed on the separate species status of *I. dammini*, with differences in mitochondrial DNA (Rich *et al.*, 1995; Caporale *et al.*, 1995; Norris *et al.*, 1996) but not nuclear ribosomal DNA (Wesson *et al.*, 1993; Norris *et al.*, 1996; McClain *et al.*, 2001) evident between northern and southern populations. After assimilation of conflicting evidence, including assortative mating studies (Oliver et al., 1993b), *I. dammini* was relegated as a junior synonym of *I. scapularis* (Wesson et al., 1993; Norris et al., 1996; Rosenthal and Spielman, 2004). Whether a separate species or not, the vectors of most cases of Lyme disease in the northeastern US derive from a common post-glacial founding population (Rosenthal and Spielman, 2004; Humphrey et al., 2010).

European colonization of North America resulted in near extirpation of white-tailed deer by the end of the 19th century, creating another bottleneck for *I. scapularis* tick populations (McCabe and McCabe, 1997; Piesman et al., 2002). The current emergence of Lyme disease in the northeastern US parallels the sharp increase in deer herd density and range (Spielman et al., 1993). Only a few remote or isolated refugia for deer remained in the northeastern US by the early 20th century (Spielman et al., 1993; McCabe and McCabe, 1997; Piesman et al., 2002). One such site, Naushon Island, located off the coast of Massachusetts, maintained a deer herd in a private hunting reserve, and museum collections document *I. scapularis* ticks from areas near this location in the 1920s (Spielman et al., 1993). Although *I. scapularis* was first described in the US in 1821 (Say, 1821), an authoritative review of *Ixodes* ticks (Cooley and Kohls, 1945) listed only 21 records of this tick, all in the southern US, while citing a report of one isolated population in Cape Cod, Massachusetts (Piesman et al. 2002). Nineteenth-century museum specimens of formalin-preserved mice from this area reveal the presence of *B. burgdorferi* DNA (Marshall et al., 1994). Return of deer herds, sometimes to overabundance, presumably led to the recent expansion of the range of *I. scapularis* in the northern US (Spielman et al., 1985, 1993; Piesman et al., 2002).

In Europe, where the erythema migrans rash of Lyme disease was first described nearly a century ago, it is unclear if post-Pleistocene population bottlenecks have occurred, as landscape features have been more stable, as has deer herd management (Zonneveld and Foreman, 1990). Nevertheless, deer herd densities are reported to have increased in many areas after World War II, parallel with increasing abundance of *I. ricinus* in some locations (Matuschka and Spielman, 1986; Rizzoli et al., 2009; Medlock et al., 2013).

Unlike *I. scapularis*, *I. ricinus* may be maintained in the absence of deer. This tick exists from coastal western Europe and Scandinavia to central Asia (50–60° longitude) and south to the Atlas Mountains of North Africa (Gern, 2002). Habitats encompass moist coniferous forests and grasslands as well as temperate deciduous forests (Gern, 2002). The ecological web supporting enzootic Lyme disease is also more complex in Eurasia, with at least three (and probably six) separate genospecies of *Borreliella* causing Lyme disease (Kurtenbach et al., 2002). Only limited data exist on the phylogenetics of different populations of *I. ricinus* and *I. persulcatus*, but one study of *I. ricinus* populations from throughout Europe demonstrated homogeneity with no evidence for phylogeographic structure (Casati et al., 2008).

It might be postulated that geographic evolutionary patterns in *I. scapularis* would be reflected in the pathogen as well, as evidence suggests that *B. burgdorferi* sensu strictu (ss), with the possible exception of one recently introduced subtype, has been present in North America for many thousands of years (Margos et al., 2008; Qiu et al., 2008; Gatewood Hoen et al., 2009a; Walter et al., 2017). Reflecting the evolutionary history of its vector, Brisson et al. (2010) noted a greater degree of overlap of *B. burgdorferi* ss subtypes within the northeast and Midwestern tick populations when compared to subtypes from the southeastern US. Others (i.e. Gatewood Hoen et al., 2009b; Walter et al., 2017) also document ancient phylogenetic relatedness of northeast and Midwestern US populations of *B. burgdorferi* ss, with evidence of more recent genetic divergence within each of these regions. Geographic distribution of *B. burgdorferi* ss subtypes suggests independent emergence in the northeast and Midwest from separate relict foci, but with more rapid expansion of *B. burgdorferi* ss in the northeast US (Gatewood Hoen et al., 2009a). Phylogenetics and migration rate analyses support ancient genomic diversity with extensive gene flow of *B. burgdorferi* ss across North America, likely facilitated by bird dispersal (Walter et al., 2017). A phylogeographic comparison of the diversity of tick 16S mitochondrial haplotypes of *I. scapularis* in northeast, Midwestern and southeast regions did not demonstrate similar patterns of genetic structure in populations of the vector ticks and populations of *B. burgdorferi* ss (Humphrey *et al.*, 2010). Similarly, Walter *et al.* (2017) found no genetic evidence of a geographic linkage of *I. scapularis* ticks and *B. burgdorferi* ss populations, consistent with active gene flow between regional bacterial but not tick populations.

1.3 Life Cycles of *I. ricinus* Complex Ticks

1.3.1 Vertebrate hosts

Although there is great complexity of tick–host associations in this group, representing differing ecologic communities and species histories, there are several features common to their life cycles. They are all 'three host ticks' that take a blood meal once in each stage or instar (i.e. larva, nymph, adult) on a vertebrate host before molting to the next stage (Keirans, 1999). Mated female ticks lay a single mass of eggs (n = 800–3000) that hatch months later. The entire life cycle typically lasts 2 years for *I. scapularis* (range 2–4 years) and 3 years for *I. pacificus*, *I. persulcatus* and *I. ricinus* (range 2–6) years. Subadult ticks generally parasitize rodents or small mammals, birds and reptiles, but will also feed on large mammals including deer. There may be marked geographical differences in host choice for these subadults, even within a species, depending upon the regional composition of the host community. For example, *I. scapularis* ticks in the southeastern US feed preferentially on lizards, whereas northern populations feed predominantly on small rodents (Piesman and Spielman, 1979; Spielman *et al.*, 1985; Oliver *et al.*, 1993a; 2003). This difference in host feeding results in the marked differences seen in tick infection by *B. burgdorferi* ss, *Anaplasma phagocytophilum* and *Babesia microti*, all of which are transmitted by infected rodents – but not reptiles – to *I. scapularis* ticks as they feed. On one island site with limited mammalian biodiversity (Nantucket Island, Massachusetts), Spielman *et al.* concluded that over 90% of larval and nymphal *I. scapularis* ticks fed on white-footed mice (Spielman *et al.*, 1985; Piesman, 2002). In Dutchess County, New York, however, while white-footed mice hosted most larval ticks, eastern chipmunks hosted threefold more nymphs than mice (Schmidt *et al.*, 1999). Recent blood meal molecular studies suggest a greater proportion of ticks may feed on non-rodent hosts than earlier studies demonstrate (Brisson *et al.*, 2008). It is unclear if fluctuations in rodent populations (i.e. mice) may also shift tick population host exposure to other mammals or birds, giving rise to temporal differences in pathogen prevalence in the same locale (Rand *et al.*, 1998; Schmidt *et al.*, 1999; Swei *et al.*, 2012). Limited host choice may not limit establishment of this tick. On Monhegan Island, Maine, where most mammal species including mice are absent, subadult ticks feeding on Norway rats (and all stages feeding on deer) alone maintained the tick population until deer were removed from the island (Smith *et al.*, 1993; Rand *et al.*, 2004a).

Adult ticks typically feed on medium sized or larger mammals to the exclusion of rodents and birds (Eisen and Lane, 2002). Deer are the predominant definitive host for *I. scapularis*, though adult ticks will feed on a variety of mammals, including ungulates, black bear, coyotes, raccoons, skunks, opossums, dogs, cats, livestock and humans (Piesman and Spielman, 1979; Fish and Dowler, 1989; Piesman, 2002). *Ixodes scapularis* tick populations are associated with areas with co-existing deer populations (Piesman and Spielman, 1979; Wilson *et al.*, 1985; 1990; Rand *et al.*, 2003; Werden *et al.*, 2014). Adventitious importation on birds may lead to occasional records of ticks from areas where a tick population is not established or maintained (Smith *et al.*, 1996; Ogden *et al.*, 2008).

Ixodes pacificus ticks parasitize over 100 vertebrate species (Castro and Wright, 2007). The primary hosts for subadult ticks are lizards (western fence lizard, southern alligator lizard), but many rodent and bird species are also parasitized (Eisen and Lane, 2002; Eisen *et al.*, 2004; Salkeld *et al.*, 2008; Newman *et al.*, 2015). Infestation of rodents increased, but did not surpass lizards in more moist habitats such as redwood/tanoak woodlands (Eisen *et al.*, 2004). Western gray squirrels are frequently parasitized by this tick in oak woodland habitats (Lane *et al.*, 2005; Salkeld *et al.*, 2008). Similar to *I. scapularis*, the primary hosts for adult ticks in northern California are deer (i.e. black-tailed), though they have been noted to feed on 29 mammal species (Westrom *et al.*, 1985; Castro and Wright, 2007). However, unlike the single vector cycle present in the northeastern US, sylvatic maintenance of enzootic *B. burgdorferi* in the western states involves not only *I. pacificus* but also *I. spinipalpis* and perhaps *I. jellisoni* (Brown et al., 2006). Of these three ticks, however, only *I. pacificus* is considered a bridge vector, transmitting infection to humans.

Life cycles for *I. ricinus* ticks are more variable reflecting the heterogeneity of the ecological situations in which they exist (Balashov, 1972; Gern and Humair, 2002). While they have been reported to feed on over 300 species of mammals and birds, subadult ticks preferentially feed on smaller mammals and birds, while adult ticks feed on larger mammals such as deer (Gray et al., 1992; TäLleklint and Jaenson, 1996). But unlike *I. scapularis*, deer do not appear to be essential to perpetuation of this tick. In a heavily grazed sheep farming environment with a paucity of other mammals, sheep were the predominant hosts of all stages of the tick (Ogden et al., 1997). On an island off Sweden lacking large mammals, the *I. ricinus* population is maintained almost entirely by feeding on hares (Jaenson and Talleklint, 1996). There is evidence of genetic structure of *I. ricinis* ticks removed from particular mammal, bird or reptile hosts, suggesting that while these *I. ricinis* ticks feed on many different types of vertebrate hosts, there may be evolution of genetic adaptations within this tick species to particular host types (Kempf et al., 2011).

The life history of *I. persulcatus*, which has a range in forests from the Far East to the Russian northwest, is similar in its diversity of hosts to that of *I. ricinus* (Balashov, 1972; Grigoryeva and Stanyukovich, 2016). However, while subadult *I. persulcatus* ticks may parasitize up to 50 species of small animals (Korenberg et al., 2002), there is a particular association of this tick with voles (*Clethrionomys* sp.) and shrews (*Sorex* sp.) across its range. Subadults may frequently also feed on chipmunks and red squirrels, and nymphs often feed on hooved animals (Korenberg et al., 2002). Birds are also frequently parasitized. Hares are notable because all three stages will feed on them, sometimes in large numbers (Korenberg et al., 2002). Adult ticks parasitize most larger mammals, whether wild or domestic. Korenberg and colleagues note that 'in the southern taiga forests of the eastern East European Plain, cattle are parasitized by 52% of adult *I. persulcatus* ticks, hares 34%, elks 4%, and red foxes 2%'. A different situation exists in the Far East, where 62% feed on cattle and 24% on red deer (Korenberg et al., 2002). In Japan, mice (*Apodemus* sp.), voles and shrews, along with birds, are frequently parasitized by *I. persulcatus*, while adult ticks primarily feed on sika deer and red foxes (Miyamoto and Matuzawa, 2002). In contrast to *I. scapularis* and *I. ricinus* ticks, only the adult stages of *I. persulcatus* commonly parasitize humans (Korenburg, 2001).

To what extent vertebrate host species diversity determines abundance of these ticks is an area of ongoing controversy. *Ixodes scapularis* abundance may be higher in some environments with less mammalian biodiversity, provided that *Peromyscus* mice are present (Allan and Keesing, 2003; Werden et al., 2014). Due to high larval tick mortality associated with feeding on some hosts (i.e. opossums, squirrels), their absence from the host community may increase tick abundance (Keesing et al., 2009). Increased feeding on competent reservoir hosts such as mice, chipmunks and shrews may lead not only to higher nymphal tick abundance, but to higher levels of nymphal and adult tick infection with *B. burgdorferi* (Logiudice et al., 2003; Brisson et al., 2008; Keesing et al., 2009; Werden et al., 2014). This occurrence is context-dependent however (Ogden and Tsao, 2009). For example, a comparison of nymphal infection rates in a species-poor island community to a mainland area in Connecticut revealed no difference, with higher tick abundance on the mainland site (States et al., 2014).

Given the diversity of hosts in any one site, and in different ecological settings, comprehensive field studies to determine host associations of these ticks are difficult and may require examination of many species of mammals and birds. Techniques for identification of prior hosts from remnant blood in ticks provide a means to quantify tick feeding history in a particular population, and to link this information to presence of pathogen infection in the vector (Humair et al., 2007). Using reverse line blots to target host mitochondrial DNA in ticks, researchers in Switzerland documented different host exposures in different populations of field-collected *I. ricinus* on north and south slopes of a single mountain (Cadenas et al., 2007). In an Irish research site, blood meal analysis revealed birds to be a major reservoir host for *I. ricinus* ticks (Pichon et al., 2005).

1.3.2 Questing behavior

These tick species all quest for hosts from vegetation, waiting for vibration, heat or other signals of the presence of a host as it passes (Balashov, 1972; Eisen and Lane 2002; Tomkins et al., 2014). This activity leads to a loss of energy and water, so ticks will descend to resorb water in the litter zone as needed. A requirement for *Ixodes* tick survival is access to microhabitats with high humidity (>80–85%) at ground level (Stafford, 1994).To varying degrees, all species of this group have evolved behaviors to limit water loss and maximize questing success (Balashov, 1972). Subadults of northern *I. scapularis* ticks (but not southern populations) often quest from the leaf litter or from low shrubs and grasses just above the ground, while adult ticks often quest 1 m or less from the ground in bushes and other forest understory (Spielman et al., 1985; Arsnoe et al., 2015; Ginsberg et al., 2017). Dessication stress is the proposed reason that southern subadult *I. scapularis* ticks quest below the leaf litter (Ginsberg et al., 2017). Questing behavior for *I. pacificus* ticks in northwest California is similar to that described for northern populations of *I. scapularis* (Lane et al., 2007). But unlike *I. scapularis* ticks, whose host seeking behavior varies with temperature and relative humidity (Clark, 1995; Vail and Smith, 1998; 2002), no such relationship has been observed in the diurnal behavior of *I. pacificus* nymphs (Lane et al., 2007). Prior experimental studies of adult *I. pacificus*, however, have documented a positive association between questing activity and relative humidity, and lower nymph densities at mean daily temperatures >23°C (Loye and Lane, 1988; Eisen et al., 2002). Similarly, questing by *I. ricinus* primarily depends upon relative humidity and solar radiation (Jensen, 2000). Questing behavior, and locomotor activities to move to a new site, may be decreased in dessicating environments (Balashov, 1972). Computer-assisted video tracking of *I. ricinus* ticks to measure locomotor activity under controlled climactic conditions documented regulation of this activity by water saturation deficit (Perret et al., 2003). Locomotor activity (i.e. movement from one site to another) was primarily nocturnal, serving also to reduce water loss. A similarly designed study of *I. scapularis* activity revealed diurnal locomotor activity only for autumn adults, with spring adults and nymphs exhibiting a unimodal pattern of activity peaking after dark (Madden and Madden, 2005). Interestingly, temperature changes exerted a more predictable response in activity than did daylight (Madden and Madden, 2005).

1.3.3 Phenology (seasonal cycle development)

While there are similarities in the life cycles of these ticks, there are differences in tick phenology (seasonal cycle development) that have an impact upon transmission of enzootic pathogens. The bimodal seasonal inversion of subadult stages of northeastern US populations of *I. scapularis*, with nymphal population peaks (May to July) preceding larval peaks (August to September), increases infection transmission to hosts prior to larval contact (Spielman et al., 1985; Daniels et al., 1989). Regardless of the time of feeding, female *I. scapularis* ticks produce eggs in late spring leading to larval appearance in late summer (Yuval and Spielman, 1990). Based on field studies using confined ticks in their natural microhabitats, survival of different stages of unfed ticks could be determined, and progression to the next developmental stage could be timed in fed ticks (Yuval and Spielmen, 1990). Adult *I. scapularis* ticks survived the winter, whether fed or not, but did not survive the following summer. Larvae that feed in September overwinter as nymphs, while later feeders overwinter as larvae. Unfed larvae survive less than 1 year. Fed nymphs molt to adults that appear in late autumn. Unfed nymphs may survive through two seasons, so that annual cohorts overlap (Yuval and Spielman, 1990). All stages of fed *I. scapularis* may enter diapause (dormancy), but only larvae and adults appear to survive the winter.

This phenology is less evident in *I. ricinus* populations, however, though bimodal population peaks (spring and autumn) are observed. Eggs laid before mid-July may hatch in August, but many do not hatch until the following spring (Gray, 1981; 1991). Randolph et al. (2002) developed a quantitative framework for seasonal population dynamics of *I. ricinus* ticks that predicted tick demographic processes using a temperature-dependent model and measurements of tick fat content. This framework is consistent with emergence of nymphs and adults in autumn followed by diapauses. Unfed ticks that feed in spring complete their development by autumn, along with the cohort of ticks that fed in the autumn. Although temperature differences may alter timing, the procession of a single cohort is maintained during these two periods.

No bimodality of population peaks was reported in northwest Russian populations of *I. persulcatus* (Grigoryeva and Stanyukovich, 2016). Metamorphosis between stages occurred from late June to early August, and lasted 30–50 days, so summer questing activity was low. The entire life cycle is 3 years, with each stage living 11–12 months. Winter survival of fed and unfed subadult ticks was high (>88%).

Ixodes pacificus ticks exhibit an extended life cycle with active host seeking limited to the cooler season in late winter and spring (Padgett and Lane, 2001). Although eggs were laid in late winter or early spring by fed females, larvae hatching in late summer remained in behavioral diapause until the next winter. Replete larvae molted in mid-summer, with nymphs also remaining in diapause until spring. Adults become active in late autumn and winter (Padgett and Lane, 2001). Based on these field studies in northwestern California, *I. pacificus* requires a minimum of 3 years to complete its life cycle (Padgett and Lane, 2001).

1.3.4 Ecological determinants of population dynamics

Models of tick population dynamics in *I. scapularis* attempt to provide insight into the drivers of tick abundance as well as determinants of *B. burgdorferi* infection (Mount et al., 1997; Dunn et al., 2013). Annual variation in precipitation, as a correlate for substrate moisture, and temperature, have been posited as determinants of black-legged tick population dynamics (Jones and Kitron, 2000; Eisen et al., 2016a), but have not predicted tick abundance over the span of 8–10 years in well-established areas (Ostfeld et al., 2006; Schulze et al., 2009). However, given the multiple variables involved, it is difficult to acquire adequate longitudinal data to provide robust conclusions. Assuming acceptable abiotic conditions (i.e. humidity, temperature), debate continues on the relative role of different host species communities (i.e. host species type, diversity, abundance) in determining tick population dynamics. Once again, it appears that the relative importance of these variables may differ in different ecological settings (Ogden and Tsao, 2009; Levi et al., 2012; Eisen et al., 2016a). Ostfeld et al. (2006) provided evidence that small rodent population surges in response to acorn mast production predicted subsequent increases in *I. scapularis* numbers in a research site in New York State, and that climate and deer density were not predictive. But others, working in habitats less dominated by oaks, have not observed a clear association of acorn mast and tick populations (Piesman and Spielman, 1979; Schulze and Jordan, 1996; Ginsberg et al., 2004; Werden et al., 2014).

Although the presence of a deer population is considered necessary for maintenance of *I. scapularis* populations, substantial variations in deer herd density, if already high, may not be associated with marked changes in questing tick populations, perhaps due to aggregation of adult ticks on remaining deer or on medium sized mammals (Jordan and Schulze, 2005; Ostfeld et al., 2006). However, in regions where deer populations are not already overabundant, deer herd density appears to be correlated with tick density (Wilson et al., 1985; 1990; Rand et al., 2003; Kilpatrick et al., 2014; Werden et al., 2014). In the rare event of complete removal of deer, the deer tick life cycle may be disrupted, with marked decline in tick numbers after 2–3 years (Wilson et al., 1988; Rand et al., 2004a). Limited data suggest that if a deer reduction threshold for associated reduction of *I. scapularis* tick abundance exists, it is at a low density, i.e. <5 deer/km^2 (Wilson et al., 1988; Rand et al., 2004a). However, field studies are limited and evidence to date that deer control lowers human Lyme disease incidence is fragmentary (Kugeler et al., 2015). Assertions that deer herd reduction to low (<5 deer/km^2) levels cannot lower Lyme disease risk are also unsupported and require additional study (Telford, 2017).

1.4 Range Expansion and Projected Effects of Climate Change

The rapid expansion of the range of *I. scapularis* into new areas throughout the northeastern US, and to a lesser extent, the upper Midwest and southern Canada, accounts, in part, for the remarkable rise of tick-borne disease attributable to this vector (Spielman et al., 1985; White et al., 1991; French et al., 1992; Chen et al., 2005; Rand et al., 2007; Hamer et al., 2010; Eisen et al., 2016b; Hahn et al., 2016). Although systematic surveys do not exist, reports of *I. scapularis* ticks (Cooley and Kohls, 1945) from the first half of the 20th century suggest that the tick was not frequently encountered by humans, whether as tick bite victims or academic collectors, and its range was largely limited to the southeastern US. Although widely distributed in the southeastern US, this tick is uncommonly found when vegetation is flagged, and rarely bites humans (Felz et al., 1996; Diuk-Wasser et al., 2006). In striking contrast to these observations, black-legged ticks are now the most abundant tick collected by flagging of vegetation in the northeastern and upper Midwest US (Diuk-Wasser et al., 2006). In endemic areas, they also may be the commonest tick parasitizing humans (Falco and Fish, 1988; Rand et al., 2007).

During the past four to five decades, *I. scapularis* ticks have become established, often with high population density, in suitable wooded or edge habitats throughout the northeastern and upper Midwest US (Dennis et al., 1998; Diuk-Wasser et al., 2006), and are newly emergent in bordering provinces of Canada (Ogden et al., 2008; 2010; Eisen et al., 2016b). In New York State and southern New England, *I. scapularis* distribution moved progressively from coastal areas to more inland sites over a decade or less (White et al., 1991; Chen et al., 2005). During a 10-year span, larval abundance on rodents increased 30-fold in Westchester County, New York (Falco et al., 1995). Passive and active surveillance studies in Maine (1988–2006), at the northeastern edge of the tick's current range, document initial recognition of the vector in the mid-1980s followed by range expansion along much of the coast and then to inland areas (Rand et al., 2007). In the northeastern US, cases of Lyme disease increased in incidence mirroring vector incursion and establishment, along with the appearance of anaplasmosis and, to a more geographically limited degree, babesiosis (Mather et al., 1996, p. 5; Chen et al., 2005; Kugeler et al., 2015; Walter et al., 2016).

It is likely that the parallel increase in deer herd densities in these areas during the past century provided the host availability to promote successful colonization of new areas (Spielman et al., 1985; 1993; Wilson et al., 1985; Piesman, 2002). While small rodent hosts such as *Peromyscus leucopus* are ubiquitous, deer, which are the major hosts for adult ticks, were scarce in much of the US at the start of the 20th century. By mid-century, overpopulation by deer had become an ecological problem in some areas (Leopold et al., 1947). In recent decades, deer herds have become superabundant in many coastal and some inland regions, with densities as high as 100 deer/km^2, well above the optimal carrying capacity of the environment (Warren, 1991). In general, dense *I. scapularis* populations are associated with dense deer herds (Piesman, 2002; Rand et al., 2003; Werden et al., 2014). Despite this general relationship, differences of scale for the range of vector populations, which may be aggregated in foci with particular habitat over a small range, and their definitive adult stage host, which range over a much larger area, may complicate precise comparisons of the population density of the two species (Kugeler et al., 2016).

Dispersal of ticks may occur within the range of deer (Madhav, 2004), but long-distance dispersal is facilitated by tick infestation of migratory songbirds (Anderson et al., 1986; Klich et al., 1996; Smith et al., 1996; Scott, 2001; Ogden et al., 2008; Loss et al., 2016). Between 1 and 2% of migrating birds carry *I. scapularis* ticks (predominantly nymphs) north during spring migration (Smith et al., 1996). Ticks aggregate on ground foraging species as they move from one stopover habitat to another. Several hundred miles may be covered between stops, and feeding ticks will likely be transported from one suitable habitat to another. Estimates of tick importation derived from ticks removed from migratory birds at an isolated island site are 165–457 adult ticks/ha/year, and it is expected that these ticks will be aggregated at bird resting sites (Elias et al., 2011). Although tick importation by birds provides a compelling explanation for the establishment of discontinuous tick populations on mainland and island sites, the introduction of enzootic Lyme disease by this means is more problematic, as trans-ovarial transmission of *Borreliella* is rare (Spielman et al., 1985). Nymphs dispersed by spring migrants will subsequently feed on deer or other non-reservoir hosts as adults. However, larvae infected by spirochetemic songbirds, or the birds themselves, could theoretically introduce B. burgdorferi to new sites, which is presumably the mechanism of enzootic introduction (Smith et al., 1996; Ginsberg et al., 2005; Ogden et al., 2008; 2010; Loss et al., 2016). *Ixodes pacificus* also feeds on birds, and has been removed from migratory songbirds (Morshed et al., 2005; Newman et al., 2015). This tick species, which has been reported from Baja Mexico to British Columbia, does not appear to have undergone range expansion in recent decades (Eisen et al., 2016b). No genetic structuring is apparent in *I. pacificus* populations, though an isolated montane population in Utah lacked the expected mitochondrial DNA polymorphism, consistent with a post-Pleistocene founder event (Kain et al., 1999).

Over 40 years ago, Hoogstraal and Kaiser (1965) documented dispersal of *I. ricinus* ticks during bird migration, and subsequent reports from other European sites document prevalence of these ticks as high as 20% on some ground foraging species during migration (Mehl, 1984; Comstedt et al., 2006; Dubska et al., 2009). Larvae more commonly infest migrating birds in autumn than spring (2.1% to 0.9% of birds examined), while nymphal infestation is similar in the two seasons (2%). Tick abundance on birds (2.1–2.6 ticks/bird) was 20–30× less than infestation of rodents (Comstedt et al., 2006). In contrast to these observations of bird dispersal of *I. ricinus*, few *I. persulcatus* ticks were on birds examined in Japan, where over 90% of ectoparasites on birds were *Hemophysalis* tick species (Ishiguro et al., 2000).

Models of range expansion and retraction of *I. scapularis* ticks with climate change predict continued expansion of the vector into upper Midwestern areas of the US and southern Canada during this century with associated decline of these ticks in the southern-most areas of the US (Brownstein et al., 2005b; Ogden et al., 2006; 2008; 2014; Eisen et al., 2016a; Hahn et al., 2016). Previous works using ticks in field enclosures and in climate controlled laboratory experiments document a consistent thermal requirement for successful egg laying and subsequent larval development (Lindsay et al., 1995; Ogden et al., 2004; Rand et al., 2004b). In addition to cumulative temperature, other abiotic factors (i.e. relative humidity, maximum summer and minimum winter temperatures) are important to tick survival (Eisen et al., 2016a; Hahn et al., 2016), as may be biotic factors such as habitat type or vegetation structure, host community and deer population density (Medlock et al., 2008; 2013; Eisen et al., 2016a; Hahn et al., 2016). In Europe, range expansion of *I. ricinus* to more northern latitudes and higher elevations is predicted with climate change (Lindgren et al., 2000; Gray et al., 2009; Dobson and Randolph, 2011; Medlock et al., 2013). *Ixodes ricinus* is already established in many northern areas of Europe, but there has been range expansion in Sweden since the 1980s, which is postulated to be related to increases in the number of degree days with temperatures needed for tick survival (Gray et al., 2009). Increases in altitudinal distribution of *I. ricinus* in recent decades has also been well documented (Gray et al., 2009). In addition to range expansion of a vector, there may be temperature-dependent changes in vector density and phenology that increase or decrease pathogen transmission, depending upon the seasonal synchrony of the tick life cycle (Randolph and Rogers, 2000). Socioeconomic or human activity change with warmer temperatures may be the most important variable determining human disease incidence. While recent increases in cases of tick-borne encephalitis in central Europe were postulated to be a consequence of warmer temperatures, Randolph et al. (2008) provided evidence that increased disease incidence could be better attributed to changes in human activities during the warm weather rather than changes in vector distribution, abundance or infection prevalence. In Italy, where an upsurge of tick-borne encephalitis cases was also noted, changes in forest structure and increased density of roe deer best predicted increased disease risk rather than changes in climate (Rizzoli et al., 2009). As noted by Gray et al. (2009), given the multiple environmental and human components involved, 'a complex chain of processes exists that makes the precise factors responsible for changes in disease incidence often difficult to determine'.

1.5 The Tick–Pathogen Interface

During the millennia of association between *I. ricinus* complex ticks and *Borreliella burgdorferi* sensu lato (as well as other *Borreliella*), this vector–pathogen interaction has been maintained in multiple ecologic settings throughout temperate areas around the northern hemisphere. In fact, a guild (or group of species that use a common resource) of different vertebrate pathogens (*B. burgdorferi, Anaplasma phagocytophilum, Babesia* spp., *Borrelia miyamotoi, Flavivirus* (i.e. tick-borne encephalitis virus and Powassan/deer tick virus) are transmitted by these ticks in both North America and Eurasia (Telford, 1997). Although elegant work delineates the orchestrated interaction between tick and *Borreliella* at times of vertebrate host feeding (Schwan *et al.*, 1995), little is known about other interactions between these pathogens and their invertebrate hosts.

The concept of vector competence for transmission of pathogenic agents to a particular host is sometimes incompletely understood. The presence of a known pathogen in a tick does not indicate that the tick is a vector of this agent. For example, other biting flies or ticks may ingest microbes from an infected reservoir host that exist passively in this insect or tick, but these microbes are not subsequently transmitted to another host. To be a vector for a particular pathogen requires not only that the tick feeds upon infectious vertebrates and acquires the pathogen through a blood meal, but that it maintains it through one or more life stages (trans-stadial passage) and then transmits it to a new host when feeding again. Vectors that transmit pathogens from enzootic cycles to humans are considered 'bridge vectors', though they may be of minor importance in maintaining the cycle in nature.

The long contact time of tick and host provides an opportunity for transmission of different disease agents that have evolved mechanisms to maximize successful infection of the new host during this interface. Tick adaptations to permit feeding on the host during this time may have an impact on pathogen transmission as well (Diuk-Wasser *et al.*, 2016; de la Fuente *et al.*, 2016; Gulia-Nuss *et al.*, 2016). In addition, tick infection by one pathogen may enhance transmission of a second pathogen, as has been demonstrated for *Babesia microti* infection of mice in the presence of *B. burgdorferi* (Dunn *et al.*, 2014).

Ixodes ricinus complex ticks, which may feed on a host for 2–10 days, evolved mechanisms to facilitate successful feeding, including an array of salivary proteins that provide anticoagulants (Salp 14 and its paralogues), anti-complement proteins (ISAC), anti-oxidants (Salp 25) and a number of other immune-modulating proteins (Das *et al.*, 2001; Ribeiro and Frachischetti, 2003; Narasimhan *et al.*, 2004; Ramamoorthi *et al.*, 2005; Gulia-Nuss *et al.*, 2016). One of these proteins (Salp 15) is of particular interest as it facilitates *B. burgdorferi* infection of the vertebrate host as well (Tyson *et al.*, 2007), and its homologues are found in other *I. ricinus* group ticks (Hovius *et al.*, 2008). Salp 15 decreases IL-12 and T-cell activation at the site of tick feeding where it binds a lectin receptor and CD4. It also binds outer-surface protein C (osp C), the surface protein of *B. burgdorferi* that is expressed at the time of tick feeding, with the effect of protecting the bacteria from antibody-mediated killing (Ramamoorthi *et al.*, 2005). *Borreliella burgdorferi* resides in the tick midgut, expressing a different outer-surface protein (osp A) until activated by onset of the blood meal (Schwan *et al.*, 1995). While in the tick midgut, *Borreliella* numbers are relatively low. The spirochete binds to another protein (TROSP-A), which binds the osp A surface protein (Pal *et al.*, 2004). The induction of osp C 36–48 h into a blood meal initiates rapid bacterial multiplication and transport via the hemocele to the salivary glands prior to eventual invasion of the host (Schwan *et al.*, 1995; Piesman *et al.*, 2003). This delayed inoculation time varies somewhat between *Ixodes* species, and coincides with the time required for infection of vertebrate host in animal models following tick attachment (Piesman, and Dolan, 2002).

During feeding, ticks ingest blood slowly at first while cuticular growth occurs in the tick midgut, with more rapid feeding at 12–36 h. Duration of feeding varies with stage and species, but ranges from 2–5 days for larvae to 6–11 days for adults (Balashov, 1972). Tick weight increases after repletion from 10–20× for larvae to up to 100-fold for adult females (Balashov, 1972; Eisen and Lane, 2002).

As the tick feeds, with its injection of saliva, some vertebrate hosts may develop antibodies to tick proteins, leading to the possibility of decreased feeding success with subsequent bites, as was demonstrated with *I. ricinus* in a rabbit model (Bowessidjaou *et al.*, 1977). These observations led to efforts to investigate the possibility of an 'anti-tick' vaccine that would interrupt tick feeding before transmission of pathogens could occur (Wikel et al., 1997; de la Fuente and Kocan, 2006; de la Fuente et al., 2016). Identification of a highly conserved protein from *I. scapularis* involved in modulation of tick feeding and reproduction (subolesin) led to successful preliminary studies demonstrating effectiveness in cDNA or recombinant protein immunization experiments (Almazan et al., 2005). Other approaches using immunogenic proteins are underway. However, natural hosts with frequent exposure to ticks (i.e. mice, other small rodents, deer) may not readily mount an immune response to the tick salivary proteins (Randolph, 1979).

The guild of pathogens common to ticks in the *I. ricinus* complex, while sharing the same vector, and in some cases the same reservoir hosts, are maintained in different enzootic cycles (Telford, 1997; Telford and Goehert, 2004; Brown et al., 2006; Diuk-Wasser et al., 2016). Co-infection by major human pathogens may occur in up to a quarter of *I. scapularis* ticks and 13% of *I. ricinus* ticks (Diuk-Wasser et al., 2016). An analysis of multiple infections (i.e. *Babesia microti*, *Anaplasma phagocyophilum*, *Bartonella* sp., cowpox virus) of field voles in Europe demonstrated interactions between some of these microbes in this rodent host (Telfer et al., 2010), and experimental evidence indicates presence of *B. burgdorferi* facilitates infection of mice by *B. microti* (Dunn et al., 2014; Diuk-Wasser et al., 2016). However, prevalence surveys document that tick co-infection occurs at frequencies reflecting the individual pathogen prevalence in samples of ticks from the same areas (Steiner et al., 2008; Barbour et al., 2009). *Borreliella burgdorferi* is generally more prevalent in *I. scapularis* ticks than *Anaplasma* or *Babesia* (Diuk-Wasser et al., 2016). In highly endemic areas for these pathogens, co-infection may be more prevalent, but even in the highest prevalence areas tick infection by *Babesia* or *Anaplasma* is usually 10% or less, whereas 40–60% of adult *I. scapularis* ticks host *B. burgdorferi*. Flavivirus infection of ticks appears less common. Like the viral agents of tick-borne encephalitis in Eurasia (Korenburg, 2001), the closely related flavivirus found in *I. scapularis* (Powassan virus lineage 2, or deer tick virus) is present in 1–4% ticks (Telford et al., 1997; Ebel et al., 2000). Unlike tick-borne encephalitis viruses, however, the deer tick virus has been implicated in only a few human cases of encephalitis (Tavakoli et al., 2009; Cavanaugh et al., 2017).

Ixodes ricinus ticks may also be infected with *B. burgdorferi* sensu lato, *Anaplasma phagocytophilum* and *Babesia* (i.e. *Babesia divergens*, *Babesia microti*, *Babesia EU1*), with varying prevalence in different habitats and geographic areas (Wielenga, 2006; Brown et al., 2008; Gray et al., 2009; Lommano et al., 2012). However, *I. ricinus* tick infection prevalence with *Babesia* sp. in Eurasia is low (1–2%), and human cases of babesiosis are rare (Becker et al., 2009; Gray et al., 2009; Lommano et al., 2012).While *I. ricinus* ticks may serve as a bridge vector for anaplasmosis and babesiosis to humans in Europe, other ticks (i.e. *Ixodes trianguloceps*) may be more important for maintaining enzootic transmission (Brown et al., 2008). Both *I. ricinus* and *I. persulcatus* are the vectors of tick-borne encephalitis to humans over large regions of Eurasia, though geographic distribution of infected ticks is highly focal (Randolph and Rogers, 2000). *Ixodes persulcatus* ticks may also be co-infected with *B. burgdorferi* and *A. phagocytophilum*, but little is known of their role as vectors of *Babesia* sp. (Masuzawa et al., 2008). In 1995, Fukunaga reported the presence of a relapsing fever group spirochete in *I. persulcatus* (Fukunaga, 1995). Named after Dr K. Miyamotoi, *Borrelia miyamotoi* was subsequently confirmed to be present in other tick species, including *I. ricinus*, *I. scapularis*, and *I. pacificus* (Scoles et al., 2001; Richter et al., 2003; Mun et al., 2006; Padgett et al., 2014; Sato et al., 2014). This agent has been implicated as a cause of febrile illness, including a relapsing fever presentation, and, in several immune-compromised patients, meningoencephalitis (Platanov, 2011; Gugliotta et al., 2013). In *I. scapularis* nymphs from 11 northern states, prevalence of infection with *B. miyamotoi* averages 10-fold less (0.2 vs. 0.02) than *B. burgdorferi*. Cultures of *P. leucopus* skin and blood revealed higher densities in mouse skin than blood for *B. burgdorferi*, but the reverse was true for *B. miyamotoi*, where bacterial densities were higher in blood (Barbour et al., 2009).

In addition to known pathogens, these ticks carry other microbes of interest (Benson et al., 2004). Rickettsia are generally considered endosymbionts rather than pathogens in ticks of the

I. ricinus species complex because despite their high prevalence they have not been associated with known human disease (Steiner *et al.*, 2008). However, *I. ricinus* harbors one species, *Rickettsia helvetica*, which has been associated with human disease in a small number of cases (Fournier *et al.*, 2000; Sprong *et al.*, 2009). In addition, the presence of another rickettsial pathogen, 'Candidatus Neoehrlichia mikurensis', in as many as 6% of *I. ricinus* ticks is of interest (Lommano *et al.*, 2012). The microbial ecology of these ticks also includes a diversity of bacteria, the composition of which changes with the stage of the tick and with engorgement (Benson *et al.*, 2004; Moreno *et al.*, 2006).

1.6 The Tick–Human Interface and Vector Control Strategies

Risk of tick-borne disease, and Lyme disease in particular, depends upon the density of the vector ticks coupled with the prevalence of infection of the ticks, or entomologic risk index, and also upon human activities and behaviors that lead to contact with infected ticks (Mather *et al.*, 1996; Hayes and Piesman, 2007; Connally *et al.*, 2009). For Lyme disease, density of nymphal ticks, which is the stage responsible for most human infections, is typically measured by drag sampling (or 'flagging') of vegetation (Daniels *et al.*, 2000). This provides a measure of host seeking ticks that might parasitize humans, but may not always correlate directly with nymphal populations as assessed on hosts (Schulze *et al.*, 2009). Nymphal tick populations may fluctuate several fold from year to year, and Lyme disease cases correlate with these fluctuations (Stafford *et al.*, 1998; Falco *et al.*, 1999; Ostfeld *et al.*, 2006). In the northeastern US, Lyme disease risk is considered primarily peridomestic, with individual exposure due to outdoor activities in habitats conducive to *I. scapularis* (Maupin *et al.*, 1991). While the entomologic risk index correlated with Lyme disease case rate when using data on the scale of towns, it did not correlate with human cases on the scale of individual residences in an endemic area (Mather *et al.*, 1996; Connally *et al.*, 2006; 2009), presumably because human behavior ultimately determines exposure to ticks in an area where ticks are prevalent.

In studies of human outdoor activities in the northeastern US, it is often difficult to identify specific high risk behaviors (Eisen and Dolan, 2016). However, exposure to the western black-legged tick, which is less clearly peridomestic, was strongly correlated with prolonged contact on or near fallen logs on forest trails or collecting firewood in forested areas during the spring or summer (Lane *et al.*, 2004; Eisen *et al.*, 2016a). In Europe, rural residence and outdoor recreational activities and forestry work are risk factors for *I. ricinus* exposures, though the recreational activities involving risk may include both urban parks and rural forested settings (Matuschka *et al.*, 1996; O'Connell *et al.*, 1998; Gray, 1998; Lauterbach *et al.*, 2013).

Mapping geographic areas or ecological areas for risk of contact to *I. scapularis* ticks permits more targeted public education regarding protective measures. Habitat type and landscape features predict *I. scapularis* distribution at the large scale of a state or region (i.e. 'north central US' or 'middle Atlantic region'), and density of these ticks is associated with particular habitat types and landscape patterns at scales as fine as individual yards. On a large scale, using geographic information system analysis, populations of *I. scapularis* in the middle Atlantic region are positively associated with proximity to forest edge, sandy soils, vegetative cover and a moderate distance to water (Bunnell *et al.*, 2003), and in the upper Midwest, to deciduous, dry to mesic forests and sandy or loam soil types overlying sedimentary rock (Guerra *et al.*, 2002). On a smaller scale, landscape features such as forest fragmentation (forest patch size <2 ha vs. 2–8 ha) were associated with high nymphal tick densities (and, inconsistently, with entomologic risk), but did not predict Lyme disease cases (Cromley *et al.*, 1998; Allan and Keesing, 2003; Keesing *et al.*, 2010; Brownstein *et al.*, 2005a; Zolnik *et al.*, 2015). Other models support the association of particular landscape features with lower Lyme disease risk. Ecotone or 'edge' areas are important landscape features with regard to tick-borne illness, not because they present the highest entomologic risk habitat, but because of high levels of human use (Maupin *et al.*, 1991; Horobrik *et al.*, 2007). Although Lyme disease transmission is less clearly associated with peridomestic exposure in the western US, geographic information system modeling of higher risk wooded habitats for *I. pacificus* exposure in Mendocino County, California correlated with Lyme disease incidence at the scale of residential zip codes (Eisen *et al.*, 2004).

Landscape design or modification may provide one mechanism for prevention of Lyme disease, either by decreasing human–tick contact or by lowering entomologic risk (Jackson *et al.*, 2006; Lauterbach *et al.*, 2013). Vegetation structure such as high shrub habitats rather than grassy or low shrub habitats, and wooded areas with understory rather than open areas appear most conducive to black-legged tick presence (Ginsberg and Ewing, 1989; Adler *et al.*, 1992; Lubelczyk *et al.*, 2004). Particular shrubs appear to be associated with dense tick populations in some areas. For example, in New England, invasive plants such as Japanese barberry, which occurs in areas with heavy deer browse, are associated with high densities of all three stages of *I. scapularis* ticks (Lubelczyk *et al.*, 2004; Elias *et al.*, 2006; Williams *et al.*, 2009). Removal of barberry lowered tick density in these areas (Williams *et al.*, 2009). Though a study of invasive multiflora rose demonstrated similar associations with *I. scapularis* ticks with this species, uninvaded forests had higher tick populations, which correlated with more leaf litter (Adalsteinsson *et al.*, 2016).

Landscape design measures to lower human exposure to questing ticks might include placement of wood chip or other barriers to tick movement between lawns and shrubby or wooded areas (Piesman, 2006a; Dolan *et al.*, 2009), or simple removal of shrub vegetation from a heavily used part of the yard to create more open areas. As these ticks are sensitive to dessication, increased exposure to sun by removal of brush and leaf litter has lowered tick density (Schulze *et al.*, 1995). In general, black-legged ticks are absent from or occur in low density on maintained lawns, fields or grasslands, as well some forested habitats such as northern coniferous forests with little understory (Guerra *et al.*, 2002; Lubelczyk *et al.*, 2004; Brownstein *et al.*, 2005b). Despite these observations, tick population correlations with particular habitats may vary by stage and year within study areas, and are also determined by other abiotic and biotic variables that may fluctuate such as humidity of microhabitat, temperature, host prevalence and host movement (Ostfeld *et al.*, 2006; Schulze *et al.*, 2009). Developing consistent approaches to testing the predictive value of these different factors that will be applicable in different ecological settings remains a challenge (Killilea *et al.*, 2008; Eisen and Dolan, 2016).

In addition to the landscape modifications described above, vector control to reduce human risk of exposure to ticks may include application of acaricides to lawns or to tick hosts, biological tick control (i.e. fungal or bacterial tick control) and deer herd reduction. Spraying of acaricides (bifenthrin, carbaryl, cyfluthrin, deltamethrin) in early spring on lawns and/or their perimeters lowers nymph tick populations by 68–100% (Stafford, 1991; Curran *et al.*, 1993; Schulze *et al.*, 2000). However, a large controlled trial of standard lawn acaricide application versus a water substitute did not demonstrate a lower risk of Lyme disease among residents with the treated lawns (Hinckley *et al.*, 2016). In addition to a lack of data demonstrating efficacy in lowering cases of Lyme disease, the cost of acaricide application and concerns regarding pesticide impacts on non-target species have limited public acceptance of these interventions (Piesman, 2006b). The use of acaricides derived from botanicals provides another approach that is under study (Dolan *et al.*, 2009; Bharadwaj and Stafford, 2012; Elias *et al.*, 2013; Bissinger *et al.*, 2014). Innovative methods to target acaricides to ticks feeding on hosts (i.e. mice, deer) have had variable success when used as the sole intervention, but may provide a component to integrated tick management strategies. Providing mice with cotton-based nesting material that contains permethrin has been effective in some environments and not in others, presumably due to differences in the tick host communities (Daniels *et al.*, 1991; Deblinger, 1991; Stafford, 1992). A 3-year trial of mouse 'bait boxes' (Maxforce TMS) designed to use topical fipronil to kill subadult ticks feeding on rodents demonstrated reduction of mouse nymphal and larval tick infestations by 68% and 84%, and questing nymphs by 50% (Dolan *et al.*, 2004). An integrated tick management study that incorporated the initial use of these boxes and an application of a barrier acaricide (deltamethrin) followed by continued use of a deer targeted topical acaricide ('4-Posters') demonstrated control of host seeking nymphs and larvae (85.9% and 89%) over 2 years (Schulze *et al.*,

2008). Even the development of these protected, host-targeted acaricides has caused concern regarding pesticide use, however, and interfered with their more general application.

Biological control of *I. scapularis* began in the 1930s with introduction of a parasitoid wasp in an unsuccessful attempt to control tick numbers, but more recent efforts have focused on entomopathogenic fungi (Mather *et al.*, 1987; Zhioua *et al.*, 1997; Bharadwaj *et al.*, 2012). Field trials of the native soil fungus (*Metarhizium anisopliae*) in nest boxes showed limited effectiveness on questing nymphs (Hornbostel *et al.*, 2005), but the fungus has a lethal effect on *I. scapularis* and evaluations in other settings are ongoing.

As deer herd density is correlated with *I. scapularis* density in some settings (Wilson *et al.*, 1984; 1988; Rand *et al.*, 2003; Kilpatrick *et al.*, 2014; Werden *et al.*, 2014), deer exclusion or deer herd control is of interest as a means to decrease entomologic risk and human Lyme disease. Several deer reduction or exclusion studies demonstrate associated declines in host seeking nymphal ticks (Wilson *et al.*, 1984; 1988; Deblinger *et al.*, 1993; Daniels *et al.*, 1993; Daniels and Fish, 1995; Stafford *et al.*, 2003; Kilpatrick *et al.*, 2014). On two island sites where deer were either extirpated or nearly extirpated, *I. scapularis* density declined markedly, to the point of tick extirpation at one site (Wilson *et al.*, 1988; Rand *et al.*, 2004a). However, in areas with dense deer populations, deer reduction may not significantly lower entomologic risk (Schulze *et al.*, 2005). Declines in entomologic risk in these areas may require reductions of herd density to levels that are difficult to achieve and sustain (Wilson *et al.*, 1984; 1988; Deblinger *et al.*, 1993; Rand *et al.*, 2004b). Successful control of deer population to limit density to four deer/km^2 has been achieved in large rural areas (>160 km^2) with controlled hunts, but is labor intensive and must be continued on an annual basis (McDonald *et al.*, 2007). To date, evidence of the effectiveness of deer control for prevention of Lyme disease in highly endemic mainland sites is lacking and awaits further study (Kugeler *et al.*, 2016). Alternatives may include deer exclosure with fencing, but the minimum size of exclosure needed to provide protection is not known (Piesman, 2006b; Connally *et al.*, 2009). In those areas where deer herd densities are not already high, and Lyme disease not yet endemic, it is possible that limitation of deer herd size might delay or preclude colonization by *I. scapularis*, but the threshold of deer herd density necessary for establishment of *I. scapularis* and enzootic *B. burgdorferi* is not known.

Contact with ticks may also be prevented by personal measures such as avoidance of high tick density areas and the use of tick repellents on skin (i.e. diethyltoluamide (DEET) or picaridin) or clothing (permethrin) (Faulde *et al.*, 2015). Educational programs to increase knowledge regarding the use of repellents and avoidance of high density areas demonstrate good knowledge levels but inconsistent application (Shadick *et al.*, 1997; Malouin *et al.*, 2003; Gould *et al.*, 2008). Based upon a case-controlled study of personal protective measures, protective clothing and use of tick repellents both appeared to confer a degree of protection (Vasques, 2008). In one controlled trial of an innovative education program for prevention of tick exposure, a decrease in tick-borne illness was demonstrated during the following 2 months (Daltroy *et al.*, 2007).

'Tick checks' (daily visual inspection for ticks) to prevent disease after tick exposure has a sound biological basis (Sood *et al.*, 1997; Piesman and Dolan, 2002; Eisen and Dolan, 2016). In a retrospective case-controlled study in Connecticut, tick checks within 36 h of exposure, and bathing within 2 h of yard exposure were associated with Lyme disease prevention (Connally *et al.*, 2009). Transmission of Lyme disease by *I. scapularis* requires at least 36 h once attachment has occurred, at which time the blood meal stimulates replication of *B. burgdorferi* and its migration from the tick midgut to the salivary glands prior to infecting a host (Piesman and Dolan, 2002). Risk of infection increases exponentially after 48–72 h of attachment to the host. Therefore, removal of attached ticks in this interval prevents infection (Sood, 1997). If an *I. scapularis* tick is already engorged, and removed within 72 h of its discovery, Lyme disease risk may be reduced from an average of 3.2% to 0.4% by treatment of the tick bite victim with a single (200 mg) dose of doxycyline, but this strategy is not currently approved for use in children under 8 years of age or pregnant women (Nadelman *et al.*, 2001) (see Chapter 7).

New concepts for prevention of tick-borne illness from *I. scapularis* include vaccination of rodent hosts against *B. burgdorferi* infection, a strategy that achieved modest success in a proof of principle field trial (Tsao et al., 2004; Gomes-Solecki et al., 2006). Challenges with this strategy include differences in reservoir host importance to enzootic maintenance of disease in different host communities, and methods of delivery to rodent populations (Brisson et al., 2008). Vaccines to limit tick feeding ('anti-tick vaccines') on wildlife represent another strategy. These vaccines might employ antigens related to salivary proteins ('exposed antigens') or other 'concealed antigens', or a combination of them designed to immunize hosts to tick proteins. While this concept has been successfully tested with laboratory rodents, it may be more difficult to apply in natural hosts, who may fail to mount an immune response to repeated bites by ticks (Randolph, 1979; de la Fuente and Kocan, 2006). However, if successful, and sustained over a number of years, interruption of local tick life cycles appears feasible (Mount, 1997). A human 'anti-tick' vaccine might be a simpler approach. However, while interrupted tick feeding might prevent infection with *B. burgdorferi*, it is less clear that it would provide protection against other tick-borne pathogens with shorter times required for disease transmission (i.e. flavivirus).

While developing new approaches to prevention of tick-borne diseases, additional evaluation of combinations of methods already developed, and tailored for particular communities where risk of tick-borne illness is high, may show benefit (Piesman, 2006b; Eisen and Dolan, 2016). A logistic challenge for projects that integrate tested methods of vector control with interventions designed to limit tick–human contact is the demonstration not only of decreased entomologic risk indices, but also of a measurable effect on the local incidence of Lyme disease and other tick-borne illnesses. Given the difficulties of achieving adequate population size in a community trial to prove an impact on human disease incidence, it may be necessary to develop methods to better link entomologic risk index reduction to predicted effects on human disease.

References

Adalsteinsson, S.A., D'Amico, V., Shriver, W.G., Brisson, D. and Buler, J. (2016) Scale-dependent effects of nonnative plant invasion on host-seeking tick abundance. *Ecosphere* 7(e01317), 1–9.

Adler, G.H., Telford, S.R., Wilson, M.L. and Spielman, A. (1992) Vegetation structure influences the burden of immature *Ixodes dammini* on its main host, *Peromyscus leucopus*. *Parasitology* 105, 105–110.

Allan, B.F. and Keesing, F.O. (2003) Effect of forest fragmentation on Lyme disease risk. *Conservation Biology* 17, 267–272.

Almazan, C., Blas-Machado, U., Kocan, K.M. et al. (2005) Characterization of three *Ixodes scapularis* cDNAs protective against tick infestations. *Vaccine* 23, 4403–4416.

Anderson, J.F., Johnson, R.C., Magnerelli, L.A. and Hyde, F.W. (1986) Involvement of birds in the epidemiology of the Lyme disease agent *Borrelia burgdorferi*. *Infection and Immunity* 51, 394–396.

Arsnoe, I.M., Hickling, G.J., Ginsberg, H.S., McElreath, R. and Tsao, J. (2015) Different populations of blacklegged tick nymphs exhibit differences in questing behavior that have implications for human Lyme disease risk. *PLoS One* 10(5), e0127450. DOI: 10.1371/journal.pone.0127450

Balashov, Y.S. (1972) Bloodsucking ticks (Ixodoidea): vectors of diseases of man and animals. *Miscellaneous Publications of the Entomological Society of America* 8, 161–376.

Barbour, A.G., Bunikis, J., Travinsky, B., Gatewood Hoen, A., Diuk-Wasser, M.A., Fish, D. and Tsao, J.I. (2009) Niche partitioning of *Borrelia burgdorferi* and *Borrelia miyamotoi* in the same tick vector and mammalian reservoir species. *The American Journal of Tropical Medicine and Hygiene* 81, 1120–1131.

Becker, C.A.M., Bouju-Albert, A., Jouglin, M., Chauvin, A. and Malandrin, L. (2009) Natural transmission of zoonotic *Babesia* spp. by *Ixodes ricinus* ticks. *Emerging Infectious Diseases* 15, 320–322. DOI: 10.3201/eid1502.081247

Benson, M.J., Gawronski, J.D., Eveleigh, D.E. and Benson, D.R. (2004) Intracellular symbionts and other bacteria associated with deer ticks (*Ixodes scapularis*) from Nantucket and Wellfleet, Cape Cod, Massachusetts. *Applied and Environmental Microbiology* 70, 616–620.

Bharadwaj, A. and Stafford, K.C. (2012) Susceptibility of *Ixodes scapularis* to *Metarhizium brunneum* F52 using three exposure assays in the laboratory. *Journal of Economic Entomology* 10, 222–231.

Bharadwaj, A., Stafford, K.C. and Behle, R.W. (2012) Efficacy and environmental persistence of nootkatone for the control of the blacklegged tick in residential landscapes. *Journal of Medical Entomology* 49, 1035–1044.

Bissinger, B.W., Schmidt, J.P., Owens, J.J., Mitchell, A.S.M. and Kennedy, M.K. (2014) Activity of plant-based repellent, TT-4302 against the ticks *Amblyomma americanum, Dermacentor variabilis, Ixodes scapularis*, and *Rhipicephalus sanguineous*. *Experimental and Applied Acarology* 62, 105–113.

Black, W.C. IV and Piesman, J. (1994) Phylogeny of hard- and soft-tick taxa (Acari: Ixodidae) based on mitochondrial 16S r DNA sequences. *Proceedings of the National Academy of Sciences of the USA* 91, 10034–10038.

Bowessidjaou, J., Brossard, M. and Aeschlimann, A. (1977) Effects and duration of resistance acquired by rabbits on feeding and egg laying in *Ixodes ricinus* L. *Experientia* 33, 528–530.

Brisson, D., Dykhuizen, D.E. and Ostfeld, R.S. (2008) Conspicuous impacts of inconspicuous hosts on the Lyme disease epidemic. *Proceedings of the Royal Society B* 275, 227–235.

Brisson, D., Vandermause, M.F., Meece, J.K., Reed, K. and Dykhuizen, D.E. (2010) Evolution of north-eastern and midwestern *Borrelia burgdorferi*, United States. *Emerging Infectious Disease* 16, 911–917.

Brown, R.N., Peot, M.A. and Lane, R.S. (2006) Sylvatic maintenance of *Borrelia burgdorferi* (Spirochaetales) in northern California: untangling the web of transmission. *Journal of Medical Entomology* 43, 743–751.

Brown, K.J., Lambin, X., Telford, G.R., Ogden, N.H., Telfer, S.T., Woldehiwet, Z. and Birtles, R.J. (2008) Relative importance of *Ixodes ricinus* and *Ixodes trianguliceps* as vectors for *Anaplasma phagocytophilum* and *Babesia microti* in field vole (*Microtus agrestis*) populations. *Applied and Environmental Microbiology* 74, 7118–7125.

Brownstein, J.S., Skelly, D.K., Holford, T.R. and Fish, D. (2005a) Forest fragmentation predicts local heterogeneity of Lyme disease risk. *Oecologia* 146, 469–475.

Brownstein, J.S., Holford, T.R. and Fish, D. (2005b) Effect of climate change on Lyme disease risk in North America. *EcoHealth* 2, 38–46.

Bunnell, J.E., Price, S.D., Das, A., Shields, T.M. and Glass, G.E. (2003) Geographic information systems and spatial analysis of adult *Ixodes scapularis* (Acari: Ixodidae) in the Middle Atlantic region of the USA. *Journal of Medical Entomology* 40, 570–576.

Cadenas, F.M., Rais, O., Humair, P.-F., Douet, V., Moret, J. and Gern, L. (2007) Identification of host blood-meal source and *Borrelia burgdorferi* sensu lato in field-collected *Ixodes ricinus* ticks in Chaumont (Switzerland). *Journal of Medical Entomology* 44, 1109–1117.

Caporale, D.A., Rich, S.M., Spielman, A., Telford, S. and Kocher, T.D. (1995) Discriminating between *Ixodes* ticks by means of mitochondrial DNA sequences. *Molecular Phylogenetics and Evolution* 4, 361–365.

Casati, S., Bernasconi, M.V. and Gern, L. (2008) Assessment of intraspecific mtDNA variability of European *Ixodes ricinus* sensu stricto (Acari: Ixodidae). *Infection, Genetics and Evolution* 2008(8), 152–158.

Castro, M.B. and Wright, S.A. (2007) Vertebrate hosts of *Ixodes pacificus* (Acari: Ixodidae) in California. *Journal of Vector Ecology* 32, 140–149.

Cavanaugh, C.E., Muscat, P.L., Telford, S.R., Goethert, H., Pendelbury, W., Elias, S.P., Lubelczyk, C.B. and Smith, R.P. (2017) Fatal deer tick virus infection in Maine. *Clinical Infectious Diseases* 65(6), 1043–1046.

Chen, H.D., White, D.J., Caraco, T.B. and Stratton, H.H. (2005) Epidemic and spatial dynamics of Lyme disease in New York State, 1990–2000. *Journal of Medical Entomology* 42, 899–908.

Clark, D.D. (1995) Lower temperature limits for activity of several Ixodid ticks (Acari: Ixodidae): effects of body size and rate of temperature change. *Journal of Medical Entomology* 32, 449–452.

Comstedt, P., Bergstom, S., Olsen, B., Garpmo, U., Marjavaara, L., Mejlon, H., Barbour, A. and Bunikis, J. (2006) Migratory passerine birds as reservoirs of Lyme borreliosis in Europe. *Emerging Infectious Diseases* 12, 1087–1095.

Connally, N.P., Ginsberg, H.S. and Mather, T.N. (2006) Assessing peridomestic entomologic factors as predictors for Lyme disease. *Journal of Vector Ecology* 31, 364–370.

Connally, N.P., Durante, A.J., Yousey-Hindes, K.M., Meek, J., Nelson, R.S. and Heimer, R. (2009) Peridomestic Lyme disease prevention: results of a population based case-control study. *American Journal of Preventive Medicine* 37(3), 201–206.

Cooley, R.A. and Kohls, G.M. (1945) The genus *Ixodes* in North America. *National Institute of Environmental Health Sciences* 184, 1–246.

Cromley, E.K., Cartter, M.L., Mrozinski, R.D. and Ertel, S.H. (1998) Residential setting as a risk factor for Lyme disease in a hyperendemic region. *American Journal of Epidemiology* 147, 472–477.

Curran, K.L., Fish, D. and Piesman, J. (1993) Reduction of nymphal *Ixodes dammini* (Acari: Ixodidae) in a residential suburban landscape. *Journal of Medical Entomology* 30, 107–113.

Daltroy, L.H., Phillips, C., Lew, R., Wright, E., Shadick, N.A. and Liang, M.H. (2007) A controlled trial of a novel primary prevention program for Lyme disease and other tick-borne illnesses. *Health Education and Behavior* 34, 531–542.

Daniels, T.J. and Fish, D. (1995) Effect of deer exclusion on the abundance of immature *I. scapularis* (Acari: Ixodidae) parasitizing small and medium-sized rodents. *Journal of Medical Entomology* 32, 5–11.

Daniels, T.J., Fish, D. and Falco, R.C. (1989) Seasonal activity and survival of adult *I. dammini* (Acari: Ixodidae) in southern New York state. *Journal of Medical Entomology* 26, 610–614.

Daniels, T.J., Fish, D. and Falcon, R.C. (1991) Evaluation of a host-targeted acaricide for decreasing Lyme disease risk in southern New York State. *Journal of Medical Entomology* 28, 537–543.

Daniels, T.J., Fish, D. and Schwartz, I. (1993) Reduced abundance of *Ixodes scapularis* (Acari: Ixodidae) and Lyme disease risk by deer exclusion. *Journal of Medical Entomology* 30, 1043–1049.

Daniels, T.J., Falco, R.C. and Fish, D. (2000) Estimating population size and drag sampling efficiency for the blacklegged tick (Acari: Ixodidae). *Journal of Medical Entomology* 37, 357–363.

Das, S., Banerjee, G., DePonte, K., Marcantonia, N., Kantor, F.S. and Fikrig, E. (2001) Salp25D, and *Ixodes scapularis* antioxidant, is 1 of 14 immunodominant antigens in engorged tick saliva. *Journal of Infectious Diseases* 184, 1056–1064.

Deblinger, R.D. and Rimmer, D.W. (1991) Efficacy of a permethrin based acaricide to reduce the abundance of *Ixodes dammini* (Acari: Ixodidae). *Journal of Medical Entomology* 38, 708–711.

Deblinger, R.D., Wilson, M.L., Rimmer, D.W. and Spielman, A. (1993) Reduced abundance of immature *I. dammini* (Acari: Ixodidae) following incremental removal of deer. *Journal of Medical Entomology* 30, 144–150.

de la Fuente, J. (2003) The fossil record and origin of ticks (Acari: Parasitiformes: Ixodida). *Experimental and Applied Acarology* 29, 331–344.

de la Fuente, J. and Kocan, K.M. (2006) Strategies for development of vaccines for control of ixodid tick species. *Parasite Immunology* 28, 275–283.

de la Fuente, J., Villar, M., Cabezas-Cruz, A. *et al.* (2016) Tick-host-pathogen interactions: conflict and co-operation. *PLoS Pathogens* 12(4), e1005488. DOI:10.1371/journal.ppat.1005488

Dennis, D.T., Nakomoto, T.S., Victor, J.C., Paul, W.S. and Piesman, J. (1998) Reported distribution of *I. scapularis* and *I. pacificus* (Acari: Ixodidae) in the United States. *Journal of Medical Entomology* 35, 629–638.

Diuk-Wasser, M.A., Gatewood, A.G., Cortinas, M.R., Yaremych-Hamer, S., Tsao, J., Kitron, U., Hickling, G., Brownstein, J.S., Walker, E., Piesman, J. and Fish, D. (2006) Spatiotemporal patterns of host-seeking *Ixodes scapularis* nymphs (Acari: Ixodidae) in the United States. *Journal of Medical Entomology* 43, 166–176.

Diuk-Wasser, M., Gatewood Hoen, A., Cislo, P. *et al.* (2012) Human risk of infection with *Borrelia burgdorferi*, the Lyme disease agent, in the eastern United States. *The American Journal of Tropical Medicine and Hygiene* 86, 320–327.

Diuk-Wasser, M.A., Vanneir, E. and Krause, P.J. (2016) Coinfection by *Ixodes* tick-borne pathogens: ecological, epidemiological, and clinical consequences. *Trends in Parasitology* 32, 30–42.

Dobson, A.D.M. and Randolph, S.W. (2011) Modelling effects of recent climate change, host density and acaracide treatment on population dynamics of *Ixodes ricinus* ticks in the UK. *Journal of Applied Ecology* 48, 1029–1037.

Dolan, M.C., Maupin, G.O., Schneider, B.S., Denatale, C., Hamon, N., Cole, C., Zeidner, N.S. and Stafford, K.C. III (2004) Control of immature *Ixodes scapularis* (Acari: Ixodidae) on rodent reservoirs of *Borrelia burgdorferi* in a residential community of southeastern Connecticut. *Journal of Medical Entomology* 41, 1043–1054.

Dolan, M.C., Jordan, R.A., Schulze, T.L., Schulze, C.J., Manning, M.C., Buffolo, D., Schmidt, J.P., Piesman, J. and Karches, J.J. (2009) Ability of two natural products, nootkatone and carvacrol, to suppress *Ixodes scapularis* and *Amblyomma americanum* (Acari: Ixodidae) in a Lyme disease endemic area of New Jersey. *Journal of Medical Entomology* 102, 2316–2324.

Douzery, E.J.P., Snell, E.A., Bapteste, E., Delsuc, F. and Philippe, H. (2004) The timing of eukaryotic evolution: does a relaxed molecular clock reconcile proteins and fossils? *Proceedings of the National Academy of Sciences of the USA* 101, 15386–15391.

Dubska, L., Literak, I., Kocianova, E., Targelova, V. and Sychra, O. (2009) Differential role of passerine birds in distribution of Borrelia spirochetes, based on data from ticks collected from birds during postbreeding migration period in Central Europe. *Applied and Environmental Microbiology* 75, 596–602.

Dunn, J.M., Davis, S., Stacey, A. and Diuk-Wasser, M.A. (2013) A simple model for the establishment of tick-borne pathogens of *Ixodes scapularis*: a global sensitivity analysis of Ro. *Journal of Theoretical Biology* 335, 213–221.

Dunn, J.M., Krause, P.J., Davis, E. et al. (2014) *Borrelia burgdorferi* promotes the establishment of *Babesia microti* in the northeastern United States. *PLoS ONE* 9(12), e115494; DOI: 10.1371/journal.pone.0115494

Ebel, G.D., Campbell, E.N., Goethert, H.K., Spielman, A. and Telford, S.R. III (2000) Enzootic transmission of deer tick virus in New England and Wisconsin sites. *American Journal of Tropical Medicine and Hygiene* 63, 36–42.

Eisen, L. and Lane, R.S. (2002) Vectors of *Borrelia burgdorferi* sensu lato. In: Gray, J.S., Kahl, O., Lane, R.S. and Stanek, G. (eds) *Lyme Borreliosis*. CAB International, Wallingford, UK.

Eisen, L. and Dolan, M. (2016) Evidence for personal protective measures to reduce human contact with blacklegged ticks and for environmentally based control methods to suppress host-seeking blacklegged ticks and reduce infection with Lyme disease spirochetes in tick vectors and rodent vectors. *Journal of Medical Entomology* 53(5), 1063–1092.

Eisen, L., Eisen, R.J. and Lane, R.S. (2002) Seasonal activity patterns of *Ixodes pacificus* nymphs in relation to climatic conditions. *Medical and Veterinary Entomology* 16, 235–244.

Eisen, R.J., Eisen, L. and Lane, R.S. (2004) Habitat-related variation in infestation of lizards and rodents with *Ixodes* ticks in dense woodlands in Mendocino County, California. *Experimental Applied Parasitology* 33, 215–233.

Eisen, R.J., Eisen, L., Odgen, N.H. and Beard, C.H. (2016a) Linkages of weather and climate with *Ixodes pacificus* and *Ixodes scapularis* (Acari: Ixodidae) enzootic transmission of *Borrelia burgdorferi* and Lyme disease in North America. *Journal of Medical Entomology* 53(2), 250–261.

Eisen, R.J., Eisen, L. and Beard, C.H. (2016b) County scale distribution of *Ixodes scapularis* and *Ixodes pacificus* in the continental United States. *Journal of Medical Entomology* 53(2), 349–386.

Elias, S.P., Lubelczyk, C.B., Rand, P.W., Lacombe, E.H., Holman, M.S. and Smith Jr, R.P. (2006) Deer browse resistant exotic-invasive understory: an indicator of elevated human risk of exposure to *Ixodes scapularis* (Acari: Ixodidae) in southern Maine coastal woodlands. *Journal of Medical Entomology* 43, 1142–1152.

Elias, S.P., Smith Jr, R.P., Morris, S.R., Rand, P.W., Lubelczyk, C.B. and Lacombe, E.H. (2011) Density of *Ixodes scapularis* Say on Monhegan Island after complete deer removal: a question of avian importation? *Journal of Vector Ecology* 36, 1–13.

Elias, S.P., Lubelczyk, C.B., Rand, P.W., Staples, J.K., St. Amand, T.W., Stubbs, C.S., Lacombe, E.H., Smith, L.B. and Smith, R.P. (2013) Effect of a botanical acaricide on *Ixodes scapularis* (Acari: Ixodidae) and non-target arthropods. *Journal of Medical Entomology* 50, 126–136.

Falco, R.C. and Fish, D. (1988) Ticks parasitizing humans in a Lyme disease endemic area in southern New York State. *American Journal of Epidemiology* 128, 1146–1152.

Falco, R.C., Daniels, T.J. and Fish, D. (1995) Increase in abundance of immature *Ixodes scapularis* (Acari: Ixodidae) in an emergent Lyme disease endemic area. *Journal of Medical Entomology* 32, 522–526.

Falco, R.C., McKenna, D.F., Daniels, T.J., Nadelman, R.B., Nowakowski, J., Fish, D. and Wormser, G.P. (1999) Temporal relation between *I. scapularis* abundance and risk of Lyme disease associated with erythema migrans. *American Journal of Epidemiology* 149, 771–776.

Faulde, M.K., Rutenfranz, M., Keth, A., Hepke, J., Rogge, M. and Gorner, A. (2015) Pilot study assessing the effectiveness of factory-treated, long-lasting permethrin-impregnated clothing for the prevention of tick bites during occupational tick exposure in highly infested military training areas, Germany. *Parasitology Research* 114, 671–678.

Feldman, K.A., Connally, N.P., Hojgaard, A., Jones, E.H., White, J.L. and Hinckley, A.F. (2015) Abundance and infection rates of *Ixodes scapularis* nymphs collected from residential properties in Lyme disease-endemic areas in Connecticut, Maryland, New York. *Journal of Vector Ecology* 40(1), 198–201.

Felz, M., Durden, L.A. and Oliver Jr, J.H. (1996) Ticks parasitizing humans in Georgia and South Carolina. *Journal of Parasitology* 82, 505–508.

Fish, D. and Dowler, R.C. (1989) Host associations of ticks parasitizing medium sized mammals in a Lyme disease endemic area of southern New York. *Journal of Medical Entomology* 26, 200–204.

Fournier, P.E., Grunnenberger, F., Jaulhac, B., Gastinger, G. and Raoult, D. (2000) Evidence of *Rickettsia helvetica* infection in humans, eastern France. *Emerging Infectious Diseases* 6, 389–392.

French, J.B., Schell, W.L., Kazmierczak, J.J. and Davis, J.P. (1992) Changes in population density and distribution of *Ixodes dammini* (Acari: Ixodidae) in Wisconsin during the 1980s. *Journal of Medical Entomology* 29, 723–728.

Fukunaga, M., Takahashi, Y., Tsurata, Y., Matsushita, O., Ralph, D., McClelland, M. and Nakao, M. (1995) Genetic and phenotype analysis of *Borrelia miyamotoi* sp. nov., isolated from the ixodid tick *Ixodes persulcatus*, the vector of Lyme disease in Japan. *International Journal of Systematic Bacteriology* 45, 804–810.

Gatewood Hoen, A., Margos, G., Bent, S.J., Diuk-Wasser, M.A., Barbour, A., Kurtenbach, K. and Fish, D. (2009a) Phylogeography of *Borrelia burgdorferi* in the eastern United States reflects multiple independent Lyme disease emergence events. *Proceedings of the National Academy of Sciences of the USA* 106, 15013–15018.

Gatewood Hoen, A.G., Liebman, K.A., Vourc'h, G., Bunikis, J., Hamer, S.A., Corinas, R., Melton, F., Cislo, P., Kitron, U., Tsao, J., Barbour, A.G., Fish, D. and Diuk-Wasser, M.A. (2009b) Climate and seasonality are predictors of *Borrelia burgdorferi* genotype distribution. *Applied and Environmental Microbiology* 75, 2476–2483.

Gern, L. and Humair, P.-F. (2002) Ecology of *Borrelia burgdorferi* sensu lato in Europe. In: Gray, J.S., Kahl, O., Lane, R.S. and Stanek, G. (eds) *Lyme Borreliosis*. CAB International, Wallingford, UK.

Ginsberg, H.S. and Ewing, C.P. (1989) Habitat distribution of *Ixodes dammini* (Acari: Ixodidae) and Lyme disease spirochetes on Fire Island, New York. *Journal of Medical Entomology* 26, 183–189.

Ginsberg, H.S., Zhioua, E., Mitra, S. *et al*. (2004) Woodland type and spatial distribution of nymphal *Ixodes scapularis* (Acari: Ixodidae). *Environmental Entomology* 33, 1266–1273.

Ginsberg, H.S., Buckley, P.A., Balmforth, M.G., Zhioua, E., Mitra, S. and Buckley, F.G. (2005) Reservoir competence of native North American birds for the Lyme disease spirochete, *Borrelia burgdorferi*. *Journal of Medical Entomology* 42, 445–449.

Ginsberg, H.S., Albert, M., Acevedo, L., Dyer, M.C., Arsnoe, I.M., Tsao, J.I., Mather, T.N. and LeBrun, R.A. (2017) Environmental factors affecting the survival of immature *Ixodes scapularis* and implications for geographical distribution of Lyme disease: the climate-behavior hypothesis. *PLoS ONE* 12, e0168723. DOI: 1371/journal.pone.0168723

Gomes-Solecki, M.J., Brisson, D.R. and Dattwyler, R.J. (2006) Oral vaccine that breaks transmission cycle in Lyme disease spirochetes can be delivered via bait. *Vaccine* 24, 4440–4449.

Gould, L.H., Nelson, R.S., Griffith, K.S., Hayes, E.B., Piesman, J., Mead, P.S. and Cartter, M.L. (2008) Knowledge, attitudes, and behaviors regarding Lyme disease prevention among Connecticut residents, 1999–2004. *Vector Borne and Zoonotic Diseases* 8, 769–776.

Gray, J.S. (1981) The fecundity of *Ixodes ricinus* and the mortality of its developmental stages under field conditions. *Bulletin of Entomological Research* 71, 533–542.

Gray, J.S. (1991) The development and seasonal activity of *I. ricinus*: a vector of Lyme borreliosis. *Review of Medical and Veterinary Entomology* 79, 323–333.

Gray, J.S. (1998) The ecology of ticks transmitting Lyme borreliosis. *Experimental & Applied Acarology* 22(5), 249–258.

Gray, J.S., Kahl, O., Janetzki, G. and Stein, J. (1992) Studies on the ecology of Lyme disease in a deer forest in County Galway Ireland. *Journal of Medical Entomology* 29, 915–920.

Gray, J.S., Dautel, H., Estrada-Pena, A. *et al.* (2009) Effects of climate change on ticks and tick-borne diseases in Europe. *Interdisciplinary Perspectives on Infectious Diseases* 593232. DOI: 10.1155/2009/593232

Grigoryeva, L.A. and Stanyukovich, A.G. (2016) Life cycle of the taiga tick *Ixodes persulcatus* (Acari: Ixodidae) in north-west Russia. *Experimental and Applied Acarology* 69, 347–357.

Guerra, M., Walker, E., Jones, C., Paskewitz, S., Cortinas, M.R., Stancil, A., Beck, L., Bobo, M. and Kitron, U. (2002) Predicting the risk of Lyme disease: habitat suitability for *Ixodes scapularis* in the north central United States. *Emerging Infectious Diseases* 8(3), 289–296.

Gugliotta, J.L., Goethert, H., Berardi, V.P. and Telford, S.R. (2013) Meningoencephalitis from *Borrelia miyamotoi* in an immunecompromised patient. *New England Journal of Medicine* 368, 240–245.

Gulia-Nuss, M., Nuss, A.B., Meyer, J.M. *et al*. (2016) Genomic insights into the *Ixodes scapularis* tick vector of Lyme disease. *Nature Communications* 7, 10507. DOI:10.1038/ncomms10507

Hahn, M., Jarnevich, C.S., Monaghan, A.J. and Eisen, R.J. (2016) Modeling the geographic distribution of *Ixodes scapularis* and *Ixodes pacificus* (Acari: Ixodidae) in the contiguous United States. *Journal of Medical Entomology* 53(5), 1176–1191.

Hamer, S.A., Tsao, J.I., Walker, E.D. and Hickling, G.J. (2010) Invasion of the Lyme disease vector *Ixodes scapularis*:implications for *Borrelia burgdorferi* endemnicity. *EcoHealth* 7, 47–63.

Hayes, E.B. and Piesman, J. (2007) How can we prevent Lyme disease? *New England Journal of Medicine* 348, 2420–2430.

Hinckley, A.F., Meek, J.I., Ray, J.A., Niesobecki, S.A., Connally, N.P., Feldman, K.A., Jones, E.H., Backenson, P.B., White, J.L., Lukacik, G., Kay, A.B., Miranda, W.P. and Mead, P.S. (2016) Effectiveness of residential acaricides to prevent Lyme and other tick-borne diseases in humans. *The Journal of Infectious Diseases* 214, 182–188.

Hoogstraal, H. and Kaiser, M.W. (1965) Ticks from European-Asiatic birds migrating through Egypt into Africa. *Science* 133, 277–278.

Hornbostel, V.L., Ostfeld, R.S. and Benjamin, M.A. (2005) Effectiveness of *Metarhizium anisopliae* (Deuteromycetes) against *Ixodes scapularis* (Acari: Ixodidae) engorging on *Peromyscus leucopus*. *Journal of Vector Ecology* 30, 91–101.

Horobrik, V., Keesing, F. and Ostfeld, R.S. (2007) Abundance and *Borrelia burgdorferi* – infection prevalence of nymphal *Ixodes scapularis* ticks along forest-field edges. *Ecosystem Health* 3, 262–268.

Hovius, J.W., Schuijt, T.J., de Groot, K.A., Roelofs, J.J.T.H., Oei, G.A., Marquart, J.A., de Beer, R., van Veer, C., van der Poll, T., Ramamoorthi, N., Fikrig, E. and van Dam, A.P. (2008) Preferential protection of *Borrelia burgdorferi* sensu strictu by a Salp 15 homologue in *Ixodes ricinus* saliva. *Journal of Vector Ecology* 198, 1189–1197.

Humair, P.-F., Douet, V., Cadenas, F.M., Schouls, L.M., Van de Pol, I. and Gern, L. (2007) Molecular identification of bloodmeal source in *Ixodes ricinus* ticks using 12S rDNA as a genetic marker. *Journal of Medical Entomology* 44, 869–880.

Humphrey, P.T., Caporale, D.A. and Brisson, D. (2010) Uncoordinated phylogeography of *Borrelia burgdorferi* and its tick vector, *Ixodes scapularis*. *Evolution* 64(9), 2653–2663.

Ishiguro, F., Takada, N., Masuzawa, T. and Fukui, T. (2000) Prevalence of Lyme disease *Borrelia* spp. in ticks from migratory birds on the Japanese mainland. *Applied and Environmental Microbiology* 66, 982–986.

Jackson, L.E., Hilborn, E.D. and Thomas, J.C. (2006) Towards landscape design guidelines for reducing Lyme disease risk. *International Journal of Epidemiology* 35, 315–322.

Jaenson, T.G.T. and Talleklint, L. (1996) Lyme borreliosis spirochetes in *Ixodes ricinus* and the varying hare on isolated islands in the Baltic Sea. *Journal of Medical Entomology* 33, 339–343.

Jensen, P.M. (2000) Host seeking activity of *Ixodes ricinus* ticks based on daily flagging samples. *Experimental and Applied Acarology* 24, 695–708.

Jones, C.J. and Kitron, U. (2000) Populations of *Ixodes scapularis* (Acari: Ixodidae) are modulated by drought at a Lyme disease endemic focus in Illinois. *Journal of Medical Entomology* 37, 408–415.

Jordan, R.A. and Schulze, T.L. (2005) Deer browsing and the distribution of *Ixodes scapularis* (Acari: Ixodidae) in central New Jersey forests. *Journal of Medical Entomology* 34, 801–806.

Kain, D.E., Sperling, F.A.H., Daly, H.V. and Lane, R.S. (1999) Mitochondrial DNA sequence variation in *Ixodes pacificus* (Acari: Ixodidae). *Heredity* 83, 378–386.

Keesing, F., Brunner, J., Duerr, S., Killilea, M., LoGiudice, K., Schmidt, K., Vuong, H. and Ostfeld, R.S. (2009) Hosts as ecological traps for the vector of Lyme disease. *Proceedings of the Royal Society B* 276, 3911–3919.

Keesing, F., Belden, L.K., Daszak, P., Dobson, A., Harvell, C.D. et al. (2010) Impacts of biodiversity on the emergence and transmission of infectious diseases. *Nature* 468(7324), 647–652.

Keirans, J.E., Needham, G.R. and Oliver Jr, J.H. (1999) The *Ixodes (Ixodes) ricinus* complex worldwide: diagnosis of the species in the complex, hosts, and distribution. In: Needham, G.R., Mitchell, R., Horn, D.J. and Welbourn, W.C. (eds) *Acarology IX: Symposia*. Ohio Biological Survey, Columbus, Ohio, pp. 341–347.

Kempf, F., De Meeus, T., Vaumourin, E. et al. (2011) Host races of *Ixodes ricinus*, the European vector of Lyme borreliosis. *Infection, Genetics and Evolution* 11, 2043–2048.

Killilea, M.E., Swei, A., Lane, R.S., Briggs, C.J. and Ostfeld, R.S. (2008) Spatial dynamics of Lyme disease: a review. *Ecosystem Health* 5, 167–195.

Kilpatrick, H.J., Labonte, A.M. and Stafford, K.C. (2014) The relationship between deer density, tick abundance and human cases of Lyme disease in a residential community. *Journal of Medical Entomology* 51, 777–784.

Klich, M., Lankester, M.W. and Wu, K.W. (1996) Spring migratory birds (Aves) extend the northern occurrence of blacklegged tick (Acari: Ixodidae). *Journal of Medical Entomology* 33, 581–585.

Klompen, J.S.H., Black, W.C., Kierans, J.E. and Oliver Jr, J.H. (1996) Evolution of ticks. *Annual Review of Entomology* 41, 141–161.

Korenburg, E., Gorban, L.Y., Kovalevskii, Y.V., Frizen, V.I. and Karavanov, A.S. (2001) Risk for human tick-borne encephalitis, borreliosis, and double infection in the pre-Ural region of Russia. *Emerging Infectious Diseases* 7, 459–462.

Korenburg, E.I., Gorelova, N.B. and Kovaleskii, Y.V. (2002) Ecology of *Borrelia burgdorferi* sensu lato in Russia. In: Gray, J.S., Kahl, O., Lane, R.S. and Stanek, G. (eds) *Lyme Borreliosis*. CAB International, Wallingford, UK.

Kovalev, S.Y., Golovjova, I.V. and Mukacheva, T.A. (2016) Natural hybridization between *Ixodes ricinus* and *Ixodes persulcatus* ticks evidenced by genetic methods. *Ticks and Tick-borne Diseases* 7, 113–118.

Kugeler, K.J., Farley, G.M., Forrester, J.D. and Mead, P.S. (2015) Geographic distribution and expansion of human Lyme disease, United States. *Emerging Infectious Diseases* 21(8), 1455–1457.

Kugeler, K.J., Jordan, R.A., Schulze, T.L., Griffith, K.S. and Mead, P.S. (2016) Will culling white-tailed deer prevent Lyme disease? *Zoonoses and Public Health* 63, 337–345.

Kurtenbach, K., Schafer, S.M., de Michelis, S., Etti, S. and Sewell, H.-S. (2002) *Borrelia burgdorferi* sensu lato in the vertebrate host. In: Gray, J.S., Kahl, O., Lane, R.S. and Stanek, G. (eds) *Lyme Borreliosis*. CAB International, Wallingford, UK.

Lane, R.S., Steinlein, D.B. and Mun, J. (2004) Human behaviors elevating exposure to *Ixodes pacificus* (Acari: Ixodidae) nymphs and their associated bacterial agents in a hardwood forest. *Journal of Medical Entomology* 41, 239–248.

Lane, R.S., Mun, J., Eisen, R.J. and Eisen, L. (2005) Western gray squirrel (Rodentia: Sciuridae): a primary reservoir host of *Borrelia burgdorferi* in California oak woodlands? *Journal of Medical Entomology* 42, 388–396.

Lane, R.S., Mun, J., Peribanez, M.A. and Stubbs, H.A. (2007) Host-seeking behavior of *Ixodes pacificus* (Acari: Ixodidae) nymphs in relation to environmental parameters in dense-woodland and woodland-grass habitats. *Journal of Vector Ecology* 32, 342–357.

Lauterbach, R., Wells, K., O'Hara, R.B., Kalko, E.K. and Renner, S.C. (2013) Variable strength of forest stand attributes and weather conditions on the questing activity of *Ixodes ricinus* ticks over years in managed forests. *PLoS One* 8(1), e55365. DOI:10.137/journal.pone.0055365

Leopold, A., Sowls, L.K. and Spencer, D.L. (1947) A survey of over-populated deer ranges in the United States. *Journal of Wildlife Management* 11, 162–177.

Levi, T., Kilpatrick, A.M., Mangel, M. and Wilmers, C. (2012) Deer, predators, and the emergence of Lyme disease. *PNAS* 109, 10942–10947.

Lindgren, E., Talleklint, L. and Polfeldt, T. (2000) Impact of climate change on the northern latitude limit and population density of the disease transmitting European tick, *Ixodes ricinus*. *Environmental Health Perspectives* 108, 119–123.

Lindsay, L.R., Barker, I.K., Surgeoner, G.A., McEwen, S.A., Gillespie, T.J. and Robinson, J.T. (1995) Survival and development of *Ixodes scapularis* (Acari: Ixodidae) under various climatic conditions in Ontario Canada. *Journal of Medical Entomology* 32, 143–152.

Logiudice, K., Ostfeld, R.S., Schmidt, K.A. and Keesing, F. (2003) The ecology of infectious disease: effects of host diversity and community composition on Lyme disease risk. *Proceedings of the National Academy of Sciences of the USA* 100, 567–571.

Lommano, E., Bertaiola, L., Dupasquier, C. and Gern, L. (2012) Infections and coinfections in questing *Ixodes ricinus* ticks by emerging zoonotic pathogens in western Switzerland. *Applied and Environmental Microbiology* 78, 4606–4612.

Loss, S.R., Noden, B.H., Hamer, G.L. and Hamer, S.A. (2016) A quantitative synthesis of the role of birds in carrying ticks and tick-borne pathogens in North America. *Oecologia* 183, 947–959.

Loye, J.E. and Lane, R.S. (1988) Questing behavior of *Ixodes pacificus* (Acari: Ixodidae) in relation to meterological and seasonal factors. *Journal of Medical Entomology* 25, 391–398.

Lubelczyk, C.B., Elias, S.P., Rand, P.W., Holman, M.S., Lacombe, E.H. and Smith Jr, R.P. (2004) Habitat associations of *Ixodes scapularis* (Acari: Ixodidae) in Maine. *Environmental Entomology* 33, 900–906.

Madden, S.G. and Madden, R.C. (2005) Seasonality in diurnal locomotory patterns of adult blacklegged ticks (Acari: Ixodidae). *Journal of Medical Entomology* 42, 582–588.

Madhav, N.K., Brownstein, J.S., Tsao, J.I. and Fish, D. (2004) A dispersal model for range expansion of blacklegged tick (Acari: Ixodidae). *Journal of Medical Entomology* 41, 842–845.

Malouin, R., Winch, P., Leontsnini, E., Glass, G., Simon, D., Hayes, E.B. and Schwartz, B.S. (2003) Longitudinal evaluation of an educational intervention for preventing tick bites in an area with endemic Lyme disease in Baltimore County, Maryland. *American Journal of Epidemiology* 157, 1039–1051.

Margos, G., Gatewood, A.G., Aanensen, D.M. *et al.* (2008) MLST of housekeeping genes captures geographic population structure of a European origin of *Borrelia burgdorferi*. *Proceedings of the National Academy of Sciences of the USA* 105, 8730–8735.

Marshall, W.F. III, Telford, S.R. III, Rys, P.M., Rutledge, R.J., Mathiesen, D., Malawista, S.E., Spielman, A. and Persing, D.H. (1994) Detection of *Borrelia burgdorferi* DNA in museum specimens of *Peromyscus leucopus*. *Journal of Infectious Diseases* 170, 1027–1032.

Masuzawa, T., Kharitonenkov, I.G., Okamoto, Y., Fukui, T. and Ohashi, N. (2008) Prevalence of *Anaplasma phagocytophilum* and its coinfection with *Borrelia afzelii* in *Ixodes ricinus* and *Ixodes persulcatus* ticks inhabiting Tver Province (Russia) – a sympatric region for both tick species. *Journal of Medical Microbiology* 57, 986–991.

Mather, T.N., Piesman, J. and Spielman, A. (1987) Absence of spirochaetes (*Borrelia burgdorferi*) and spiroplasmas (*Babesia microti*) in deer ticks (*Ixodes dammini*) parasitized by chalcid wasps. *Medical Vet Entomology* 1, 3–8.

Mather, T.N., Nicholson, M.C., Donnelly, E.F. and Matyas, B.T. (1996) Entomologic index for human risk of Lyme disease. *American Journal of Epidemiology* 144, 1066–1099.

Matuschka, F.R. and Spielman, A. (1986) The emergence of Lyme disease in a changing environment in North America and Central Europe. *Experimental and Applied Acarology* 2, 337–353.

Matuschka, F.R., Endepols, S., Richter, D., Ohlenbusch, A., Eiffert, H. and Spielman, A. (1996) Risk of urban Lyme disease enhanced by presence of rats. *Journal of Infectious Diseases* 174, 1108–1111.

Maupin, G.O., Fish, D., Zultowski, J., Compos, E.G. and Piesman, J. (1991) Landscape ecology of Lyme disease in a residential area of Westchester County New York. *American Journal of Epidemiology* 133, 1105–1113.

Maupin, G.O., Gage, K.L., Piesman, J., Montenieri, J., Sviat, S.L., VanderLanden, L., Happ, C.M., Dolan, M. and Johnson, B. (1994) Discovery of an enzootic cycle of *Borrelia burgdorferi* in *Neotoma mexicana* and *Ixodes spinipalpis* from Northern Colorado, an area where Lyme disease is nonendemic. *Journal of Infectious Diseases* 170, 636–643.

McCabe, T.R. and McCabe, R.E. (1997) Recounting whitetails past. In: McShea, W.J., Underwood, H.B. and Rappole, J.H. (eds) *The Science of Overabundance*. Smithsonian Books, Washington, DC, pp. 11–26.

McClain, D.K., Li, J. and Oliver, J.H. (2001) Interspecific and geographical variation in the sequence of rDNA expansion segment *D3* of *Ixodes* ticks (Acari: Ixodidae). *Heredity* 86, 234–242.

McDonald, J.E., Clark, D.E. and Woytek, W.A. (2007) Reduction and maintenance of a white-tailed deer herd in central Massachusetts. *Journal of Wildlife Management* 71, 1585–1593.

Medlock, J.M., Pietzsch, M.E., Rice, N.V.P., Jones, L., Kerrod, E., Avenell, D., Los, S., Ratcliffe, N., Leach, S. and Butt, T. (2008) Investigation of the ecological and environmental determinants for the presence of questing *Ixodes ricinus* (Acari:Ixodidae) on Gower, South Wales. *Journal of Medical Entomology* 45(2), 314–325.

Medlock, J.M., Hansford, K.M., Bormane, A. *et al.* (2013) Driving forces for changes in geographical distribution of *Ixodes ricinus* ticks in Europe. *Parasites and Vectors* 6, 1.

Mehl, R., Michaelsen, J. and Lid, G. (1984) Ticks (Acari, Ixodides) on migratory birds in Norway. *Fauna Norvegica Series B* 31, 46–58.

Miyamoto, K. and Masuzawa, T. (2002) Ecology of *Borrelia burgdorferi* senso lato in Japan and East Asia. In: Gray, J.S., Kahl, O., Lane, R.S. and Stanek, G. (eds) *Lyme Borreliosis*. CAB International, Wallingford, UK.

Moreno, C.X., Moy, F., Daniels, T.J., Godfrey, H.P. and Cabello, F.C. (2006) Molecular analysis of microbial communities identified in developmental stages of *Ixodes scapularis* ticks from Westchester and Dutchess Counties, New York. *Environmental Microbiology* 8, 761–772.

Morshed, M.G., Scott, J.D., Fernando, K., Beati, L., Mazerolle, D.F., Geddes, G. and Durden, L.A. (2005) Migratory songbirds disperse ticks across Canada, and first isolation of the Lyme disease spirochete, *Borrelia burgdorferi*, from the avian tick, *Ixodes auritulus*. *Journal of Parasitology* 91, 780–790.

Mount, G.A., Haile, D.G. and Daniel, E. (1997) Simulation of management strategies for the blacklegged tick (Acari: Ixodidae) and the Lyme disease spirochete, *Borrelia burgdorferi*. *Journal of Medical Entomology* 34, 461–484.

Mun, J., Eisen, R.J., Eisen, L. and Lane, R.S. (2006) Detection of a *Borrelia miyamotoi* sensu lato relapsing fever group spirochete from *Ixodes pacificus* in California. *Journal of Medical Entomology* 43, 120–123.

Nadelman, R.B., Nowakowski, J., Fish, D., Falco, R.C., Freeman, K., McKenna, D., Welch, P., Marcus, R., Aguero-Rosenfeld, M.E., Dennis, D.T. and Wormser, G.P. (2001) Prophylaxis with single-dose doxycycline for the prevention of Lyme disease after an *Ixodes scapularis* tick bite. *New England Journal of Medicine* 345, 79–84.

Narasimhan, S., Montgomery, R.R., DePonte, K. *et al*. (2004) Disruption of *Ixodes scapularis* anticoagulation by using RNA interference. *Proceedings of the National Academy of Science of the USA* 101, 1141–1146.

Newman, E.A., Eisen, L., Eisen, R.J., Fedoriva, N., Hasty, J.M., Vaughn, C. and Lane, R.S. (2015) *Borrelia burgdorferi* sensu lato spirochetes in wild birds in northwestern California: associations with ecological factors, bird behavior, and tick infestation. *PloS One* 10(2), e0118146. DOI:10:1371/journal.pone.0118146

Norris, D.E., Klompen, J.S.H., Kierans, J.E. and Black, W.C. (1996) Population genetics of *I. scapularis* (Acari: Ixodidae) based on the mitochondrial 16s and 12s genes. *Journal of Medical Entomology* 33, 78–83.

O'Connell, S., Granstrom, M., Gray, J.S. and Stanek, G. (1998) Epidemiology of European Lyme borreliosis. *Zent fur Bakteriol* 287, 229–240.

Ogden, N.H. and Tsao, J.I. (2009) Biodiversity and Lyme disease: dilution or amplification. *Epidemics* 1, 196–206.

Ogden, N.H., Nuttall, P.A. and Randolph, S.E. (1997) Natural Lyme disease cycles maintained via sheep by co-feeding ticks. *Parasitology* 115, 591–599.

Ogden, N.H., Lindsay, L.R., Beauchamp, G., Charron, D., Maarouf, A., O'Callaghan, C.J., Waltner-Toews, D. and Barker, I.K. (2004) Investigation of relationships between temperature and developmental rates of tick *Ixodes scapularis* (Acari: Ixodidae) in the laboratory and the field. *Journal of Medical Entomology* 41, 622–633.

Ogden, N.H., Maarouf, A., Barker, I.K., Bigras-Poulin, M., Lindsay, L.R., Morshed, M.G., O'Callaghan, C.J., Ramay, F., Waltner-Toews, D. and Charron, D.F. (2006) Climate change and the potential for range expansion of the Lyme disease vector *Ixodes scapularis* in Canada. *International Journal for Parasitology* 36, 63–70.

Ogden, N.H., Lindsay, L.R., Hanincova, K., Barker, I.K., Bigras-Poulin, M., Charron, D.F., Heagy, A., Francis, C.M., O'Callaghan, C.J., Schwartz, I. and Thompson, R.A. (2008) Role of migratory birds in introduction and range expansion of *Ixodes scapularis* ticks and of *Borrelia burgdorferi* and *Anaplasma phagocytophilum* in Canada. *Applied and Environmental Microbiology* 74, 1780–1790.

Ogden, N.H., Bouchard, C., Kurtenbach, K., Margos, G., Lindsay, L.R., Trudel, L., Nguon, S. and Milord, F. (2010) Active and passive surveillance and phylogenetic analysis of *Borrelia burgdorferi* elucidate the process of Lyme disease risk emergence in Canada. *Environmental Health Perspectives* 118, 909–914.

Ogden, N.H., Radojevic, M., Wu, X., Duvvvuri, V.R. and Leighton, P. (2014) Estimated effects of projected climate change on the basic reproductive number of the Lyme disease vector *Ixodes scapularis*. *Environmental Health Perspectives* 122, 631–638.

Oliver Jr, J.H., Cummins, G.A. and Joiner, M.S. (1993a) Immature *I. scapularis* (Acari: Ixodidae) parasitizing lizards from the southeast USA. *Journal of Parasitology* 79, 684–689.

Oliver Jr, J.H., Owsley, M.R., Hutcheson, H.J., James, A.M., Chen, C., Irby, W.S., Dotson, E.M. and McLain, D.K. (1993b) Conspecificity of the ticks *I. scapularis* and *I. dammini* (Acari: Ixodidae). *Journal of Medical Entomology* 30, 54–63.

Oliver Jr, J.H., Lin, T., Gao, L., Clark, K.L., Banks, C.W., Durden, L.A., James, A.M. and Chandler Jr, F.W. (2003) An enzootic transmission cycle of Lyme borreliosis spirochetes in the southeastern United States. *Proceedings of the National Academy of Science of the USA* 100, 11642–11645.

Olsen, B., Duff, D.C., Jaenson, T.G., Gykfe, A., Bibbedahi, H. and Bergstrom, S. (1995) Transhemispheric exchange of Lyme disease spirochetes by seabirds. *Journal of Clinical Microbiology* 33, 3270–3274.

Ostfeld, R.S., Canham, C.D., Oggenfuss, K., Winchecombe, R.J. and Keesing, F. (2006) Climate, deer, rodents and acorns as determinants of variation of Lyme disease risk. *PLoS Biology* 4(e145), 001–011.

Padgett, K.A. and Lane, R.S. (2001) Life cycle of *Ixodes pacificus* (Acari: Ixodidae): timing of developmental processes under field and laboratory conditions. *Journal of Medical Entomology* 38, 684–693.

Padgett, K., Bonilla, D., Kjemtrup, A., Vilcins, I.-M., Hardstone Yoshimizu, M., Hui, L., Sola, M., Quintana, M. and Kramer, V. (2014) Large scale spatial risk and comparative prevalence of *Borrelia miyamotoi* and *Borrelia burgdorferi* sensu lato in *Ixodes pacificus*. *PLoS One* 9(10), e110853.

Pal, U., Yang, X., Chen, M. et al. (2004) Osp C facilitates *Borrelia burgdorferi* invasion of *Ixodes scapularis* salivary glands. *Journal of Clinical Investigation* 113, 220–230.

Perret, J.-L., Guerin, P.M., Diehl, P.A., Vlimant, M. and Gern, L. (2003) Darkness induces mobility, and saturation deficit limits questing duration, in the tick *Ixodes ricinus*. *Journal of Experimental Biology* 206, 1809–1815.

Pichon, B., Rogers, M., Egan, D. and Gray, J. (2005) Blood-meal analysis for the identification of reservoir hosts of tick-borne pathogens in Ireland. *Vector Borne and Zoonotic Diseases* 5, 172–180.

Piesman, J. (2002) Ecology of *Borrelia burgdorferi* sensu lato in North America. In: Gray, J.S., Kahl, O., Lane, R.S. and Stanek, G. (eds) *Lyme Borreliosis*. CAB International, Wallingford, UK.

Piesman, J. (2006a) Response of nymphal *Ixodes scapularis*, the primary tick vector of Lyme disease spirochetes in North America, to barriers derived from wood products or related home and garden items. *Journal of Vector Ecology* 31, 412–417.

Piesman, J. (2006b) Strategies for reducing risk of Lyme borreliosis in North America. *International Journal of Medical Microbiology* 296(S1), 17–22.

Piesman, J. and Dolan, M. (2002) Protection against Lyme disease spirochete transmission provided by prompt removal of nymphal *Ixodes scapularis* (Acari: Ixodidae). *Journal of Medical Entomology* 39(3), 509–512.

Piesman, J. and Spielman, A. (1979) Host associations and seasonal abundance of immature *Ixodes dammini* in southeastern Massachusetts. *Annals of the Entomological Society of America* 72, 829–832.

Piesman, J., Zeidner, N.S. and Schneider, B.S. (2003) Dynamic changes in *Borrelia burgdorferi* populations in *Ixodes scapularis* (Acari: Ixodidae) during transmission studies at the mRNA level. *Vector Borne and Zoonotic Diseases* 3, 125–132.

Platonov, A.E., Karan, L.S., Kolyasnikova, N.M. et al. (2011) Human relapsing fever spirochete *Borrelia miyamotoi*, Russia. *Emerging Infectious Diseases* 17, 1816–1823.

Qiu, W.O.G., Dykhuizen, D.E., Acosta, M.S. and Luft, B.J. (2002) Geographic uniformity of the Lyme disease spirochete (*Borrelia burgdorferi*) and its shared history with the tick vector (*Ixodes scapularis*) in the northeastern United States. *Genetics* 160, 833–849.

Qiu, W.-G., Bruno, J.F., McCrain, W.D., Xu, Y., Livey, I., Schriefer, M.E. and Luft, B.J. (2008) Wide distribution of a high-virulence *Borrelia burgdorferi* clone in Europe and North America. *Emerging Infectious Diseases* 14, 1097–1103.

Ramamoorthi, N., Narasimhan, S. and Pal, U. et al. (2005) The Lyme disease agent exploits a tick protein to infect the mammalian host. *Nature* 436, 573–577.

Rand, P.W., Lacombe, E.H., Smith, R.P. Jr and Ficker, J. (1998) Participation of birds (Aves) in the emergence of Lyme disease in southern Maine. *Journal of Medical Entomology* 35, 270–276.

Rand, P.W., Lubleczyk, C., Lavigne, G.R., Elias, S., Holman, M.S., Lacombe, E.H. and Smith Jr, R.P. (2003) Deer density and the abundance of *Ixodes scapularis* (Acari: Ixodidae). *Journal of Medical Entomology* 40, 179–184.

Rand, P.W., Lubelczyk, C., Holman, M.S., Lacombe, E.H. and Smith Jr, R.P. (2004a) Abundance of *Ixodes scapularis* (Acari:Ixodidae) after the complete removal of deer from an isolated offshore island, endemic for Lyme disease. *Journal of Medical Entomology* 41, 779–784.

Rand, P.W., Holman, M.S., Lubelczyk, C., Lacombe, E.H., Degaetano, A.T. and Smith Jr, R.P. (2004b) Thermal accumulation and early development of *Ixodes scapularis*. *Journal of Vector Ecology* 29, 164–176.

Rand, P.W., Lacombe, E.H., Dearborn, R., Cahill, B., Elias, S., Lubelczyk, C.B., Beckett, G.A. and Smith Jr, R.P. (2007) Passive surveillance in Maine, an area emergent for tick-borne diseases. *Journal of Medical Entomology* 44, 1118–1129.

Randolph, S.E. (1979) Population regulation in ticks: the role of acquired resistance in natural and unnatural hosts. *Parasitology* 79, 141–156.

Randolph, S.E. and Rogers, D.J. (2000) Fragile transmission cycles of tick-borne encephalitis virus may be disrupted by predicted climate change. *Proceedings of the Royal Society B: Biological Sciences* 267, 1741–1744.

Randolph, S.E., Green, R.M., Hoodless, A.N. and Peacey, M.F. (2002) An empirical quantitative framework for the seasonal population dynamics of the tick *Ixodes ricinus*. *International Journal for Parasitology* 32, 979–989.

Randolph, S., Asokliene, L., Avsic-Zupanc, T., Bormane, A., Burri, C., Gern, L., Golovljova, I., Hubalek, Z., Knap, N., Kondrusik, M., Kupca, A., Pejoch, M., Vasilenko, V. and Zygutiene, M. (2008) Variable spikes in tick-borne encephalitis incidence in 2006 independent of variable tick abundance but related to weather. *Parasites and Vectors* 1(44), 1–18. DOI: 10.1186/1756-3305-1-44

Ribeiro, J.M. and Frachischetti, I.B.M. (2003) Role or arthropod saliva in blood feeding: sialome and post-sialome perspectives. *Annual Review of Entomology* 48, 73–78.

Rich, S.M., Caporale, D.A., Telford, S.R. III, Kocher, T.D., Hartl, D.L. and Spielman, A. (1995) Distribution of the *Ixodes ricinus*-like ticks of eastern North America. *Proceedings of the National Academy of Science of the USA* 92, 6284–6288.

Richter, D., Schlee, D.B. and Matuschka, F.-R. (2003) Relapsing fever-like spirochetes infecting European vector tick of Lyme disease agent. *Emerging Infectious Diseases* 9, 697–701.

Rizzoli, A., Hauffe, H.C., Tagliapietra, M., Neteler, M. and Rosa, R. (2009) Forest structure and roe deer abundance predict tick-borne encephalitis risk in Italy. *PloS ONE* 4, e4336. DOI: 10.1371/journal.pone.0004336

Rosen, M.S., Hamer, S., Gerhardt, R., Jones, C., Muller, L., Scott, M. and Hickling, G. (2012) *Borrelia burgdorferi* not detected in widespread *Ixodes scapularis* (Acari: Ixodidae) collected from white tailed deer in Tennessee. *Journal of Medical Entomology* 49(6), 1473–1481.

Rosenthal, B.M. and Spielman, A. (2004) Reduced variation among northern deer tick populations at an autosomal microsatellite locus. *Journal of Vector Ecology* 29, 227–235.

Salkeld, D., Leonhard, S., Girard, Y., Hanh, N., Mun, J., Padgett, K. and Lane, R.S. (2008) Identifying the reservoir hosts of the Lyme disease spirochete *Borrelia burgdorferi* in California: the role of the western gray squirrel (*Sciurus griseus*). *American Journal of Tropical Medicine and Hygiene* 79(4), 535–540.

Sato, K., Takano, A., Konnai, S., Nakao, M., Ito, T., Koyama, K., Kaneko, M., Ohnishi, M. and Kawabata, H. (2014) Human infections with *Borrelia miyamotoi* Japan. *Emerging Infectious Diseases* 20, 1391–1393.

Say, T. (1821) An account of the arachnides of the United States. *Journal of the Academy of Natural Sciences of Philadelphia* 2, 59–82.

Schmidt, K.A., Ostfeld, R.S. and Schauber, E.M. (1999) Infestation of *Peromyscus leucopus* and *Tamias striatus* by *Ixodes scapularis* (Acari: Ixodidae) in relation to the abundance of hosts and parasites. *Journal of Medical Entomology* 36, 749–757.

Schulze, T.L. and Jordan, R.A. (1996) Seasonal and long-term variation in abundance of adult *Ixodes scapularis* (Acari: Ixodidae) in different coastal plain habitats in New Jersey. *Journal of Medical Entomology* 33, 963–970.

Schulze, T.L., Jordan, R.A. and Hung, R.W. (1995) Suppression of subadult *Ixodes scapularis* (Acari: Ixodidae) ticks following removal of leaf litter. *Journal of Medical Entomology* 23, 396–399.

Schulze, T.L., Jordan, R.A. and Hung, R.W. (2000) Effects of granular carbaryl application on sympatric populations of *Ixodes scapularis* and *Amblyomma americanum* (Acari: Ixodidae) nymphs. *Journal of Medical Entomology* 37, 121–125.

Schulze, T.L., Jordan, R.A. and Schulze, C.J. (2005) Host associations of *Ixodes scapularis* (Acari: Ixodidae) in residential and natural settings in Lyme disease-endemic area in New Jersey. *Journal of Medical Entomology* 42, 966–973.

Schulze, T.L., Jordan, R.A., Dolan, M.C., Dietrich, G., Healy, S. and Piesman, J. (2008) Ability of a 4-poster passive topical treatment devices for deer to sustain low population levels of *Ixodes scapularis* (Acari: Ixodidae) after integrated tick management in a residential community. *Journal of Medical Entomology* 45(5), 899–904.

Schulze, T.L., Jordan, R.A., Schulze, C.J. and Hung, R.W. (2009) Precipitation and temperature as predictors of local abundance of *Ixodes scapularis* (Acari: Ixodidae) nymphs. *Journal of Medical Entomology* 46, 1025–1029.

Schwan, T.G., Piesman, J., Golde, W.T., Dolan, M.C. and Rosa, P.A. (1995) Induction of an outer surface protein on *Borrelia burgdorferi* during tick feeding. *Proceedings of the National Academy of Sciences of the USA* 92, 2909–2913.

Scoles, G.A., Papero, M., Beati, L. and Fish, D. (2001) A relapsing fever group spirochete transmitted by *Ixodes scapularis* ticks. *Vector Borne and Zoonotic Diseases* 1, 21–34.

Scott, J.D., Fernando, K., Banerjee, S.N., Durden, L.A., Byrne, S.K., Banerjee, M., Mann, R.B. and Morshed, M.G. (2001) Birds disperse ixodid (Acari: Ixodidae) and *Borrelia burgdorferi* infected ticks in Canada. *Journal of Medical Entomology* 38, 493–500.

Shadick, N.A., Daltroy, L.H., Phillips, C.B., Liang, U.S. and Liang, M.H. (1997) Determinants of tick-avoidance behaviors in an endemic area for Lyme disease. *American Journal of Preventive Medicine* 13, 265–270.

Smith Jr, R.P., Rand, P.W., Lacombe, E.H., Telford, S.R. III, Rich, S.M., Piesman, J. and Spielman, A. (1993) Norway rats as reservoir hosts for Lyme disease spirochetes on Monhegan Is, ME. *Journal of Infectious Diseases* 168, 687–691.

Smith Jr, R.P., Rand, P.W., Lacombe, E.H., Morris, S.R., Holmes, D.W. and Caporale, D.A. (1996) Role of bird migration in the long-distance dispersal of *Ixodes dammini*, the vector of Lyme disease. *Journal of Infectious Diseases* 174, 221–224.

Sood, S.K., Salzman, M.B., Johnson, B.J.B., Happ, C.M., Feig, K., Carmody, L., Rubin, L.G., Hilton, E. and Piesman, J. (1997) Duration of tick attachment as a predictor of the risk of Lyme disease in an area in which Lyme disease is endemic. *Journal of Infectious Diseases* 175, 996–999.

Spielman, A., Clifford, C.M., Piesman, J. and Corwin, M.D. (1979) Human babesiosis on Nantucket Island, USA: description of the vector, *Ixodes (Ixodes) dammini*, n. sp. (Acarina: Ixodidae). *Journal of Medical Entomology* 15, 218–234.

Spielman, A., Wilson, M.L., Levine, J.F. and Piesman, J. (1985) Ecology of *Ixodes dammini*-borne human babesiosis and Lyme disease. *Annual Review of Entomology* 30, 439–460.

Spielman, A., Telford, S.R. III and Pollak, R.J. (1993) The origins and course of the recent outbreak of Lyme disease. In: Ginsberg, H.S. (eds) *Ecology and Environmental Management of Lyme Disease*. Rutgers University Press, New Brunswick, New Jersey, USA, pp. 83–96.

Sprong, H., Wielinga, P.R., Fonville, M., Reusken, C., Brandenburg, A.H., Borgsteede, F., Gaasenbeek, C. and van der Giessen, J.W.B. (2009) *Ixodes ricinus* ticks are reservoir hosts for *Rickettsia helvetica* and potentially carry flea-borne *Rickettsia* species. *Parasites and Vectors* 2, 41–50. DOI: 10.1186/1756-3305-2-41

Stafford, K.C. III (1991) Effectiveness of carbaryl applications for the control of *Ixodes dammini* in an endemic residential area. *Journal of Medical Entomology* 28, 32–36.

Stafford, K.C. III (1992) Third-year evaluation of host targeted permethrin and control of *Ixodes dammini* (Acari: Ixodidae) in southeastern Connecticut. *Journal of Medical Entomology* 29, 717–720.

Stafford, K.C. III (1994) Survival of immature *Ixodes scapularis* (Acari: Ixodidae) at different relative humidities. *Journal of Medical Entomology* 31, 310–314.

Stafford, K.C. III, Cartter, M.L., Magnarelli, L.A., Ertel, S. and Mshar, P.A. (1998) Temporal correlation between tick abundance and prevalence and increasing incidence of Lyme disease. *Journal of Clinical Microbiology* 36, 1240–1246.

Stafford, K.C. III, DiNicola, A.J. and Kilpatrick, H.J. (2003) Reduced abundance of *Ixodes scapularis* (Acari: Ixodidae) and tick parasitoid *Ixodiphagus hookeri* (Heminoptera: Encrytidae) with reduction of white-tailed deer. *Journal of Medical Entomology* 40, 642–652.

States, S.L., Brinkerhoff, R.J., Carpi, G., Steeves, T.K., Folsom-O'Keefe, C., DeVeaux, M. and Duik-Wasser, M.A. (2014) Lyme disease risk not amplified in a species-poor vertebrate community: similar *Borrelia burgdorferi* tick infection prevalence and Osp C genotype frequencies. *Infection, Genetics and Evolution* 27, 566–577.

Steiner, F.E., Pinger, R.R., Vann, C.N., Grindle, N., Civitello, D., Clay, K. and Fuqua, C. (2008) Infection and co-infection rates of *Anaplasma phagocytophilum* variants, *Babesia* spp., *Borrelia burgdorferi*, and the rickettsial symbiont in *Ixodes scapularis* (Acari: Ixodidae) from sites in Indiana, Maine, Pennsylvania, and Wisconsin. *Journal of Medical Entomology* 45, 289–297.

Swei, A., Briggs, C.J., Lane, R.S. and Ostfeld, R.S. (2012) Impacts of an introduced forest pathogen on the risk of Lyme disease in California. *Vector Borne and Zoonotic Diseases* 12, 623–631.

TäLleklint, L. and Jaenson, T.G.T. (1996) Relationship Between *Ixodes ricinus* Density and Prevalence of Infection with Borrelia-Like Spirochetes and Density of Infected Ticks. *Journal of Medical Entomology* 33(5), 805–811.

Tavakoli, N.P., Wang, H., Dupuis, M., Hull, R., Ebel, G.D., Gilmore, E.J. and Faust, P.L. (2009) Fatal case of deer tick virus encephalitis. *New England Journal of Medicine* 360(20), 2099–2107.

Telfer, S., Lambin, X., Birtles, R., Beldomenico, P., Burthe, S., Paterson, S. and Begon, M. (2010) Species interactions in a parasite community drive infection risk in a wildlife population. *Science* 330, 243–246.

Telford, S.R. III (2017) Deer reduction is a cornerstone of integrated deer tick management. *Journal of Integrated Pest Management* 8(1), 251–255.

Telford, S.R. III and Goethert, H.K. (2004) Emerging tick-borne infections: rediscovered and better characterized, or truly new? *Parasitology* 129, S1–S27.

Telford, S.R., Armstrong, P.M., Katavolos, P., Foppa, I., Olmeda Garcia, S.A., Wilson, M.L. and Spielman, A. (1997) A new tick-borne encephalitis-like virus infecting New England deer ticks, *Ixodes dammini*. *Emerging Infectious Diseases* 3, 165–170.

Tomkins, J., Augier, J. and Hazel, W. (2014) Towards an evolutionary understanding of questing behavior in the tick *Ixodes ricinus*. *PLoS Pathogens* 9(10), 3110028.

Tsao, J.I., Wootton, J.T., Bunikkis, J., Luna, M.G., Fish, D. and Barbour, A.G. (2004) An ecological approach to preventing human infection: vaccinating wild mouse reservoirs intervenes in the Lyme disease cycle. *Proceedings of the National Academy of Sciences of the USA* 101, 18159–18164.

Tyson, K., Elkins, C., Patterson, H., Fikrig, E. and de Silva, A. (2007) Biochemical and functional characterization of Salp20, an *Ixodes scapularis* tick salivary protein that inhibits the complement pathway. *Insect Molecular Biology* 16, 469–479.

Vail, S.G. and Smith, G. (1998) Air temperature and relative humidity effects on behavioral activity of blacklegged tick (Acari: Ixodidae) nymphs in New Jersey. *Journal of Medical Entomology* 35(6), 1025–1028.

Vail, S.G. and Smith, G. (2002) Vertical movement and posture of blacklegged ticks (Acari: Ixodidae) nymphs as a function of temperature and relative humidity in laboratory experiments. *Journal of Medical Entomology* 39, 842–846.

Vasques, M., Muehlenbein, C., Cartter, M., Hayes, E.B., Ertel, S. and Shapiro, E.D. (2008) Effectiveness of personal protective measures to prevent Lyme disease. *Emerging Infectious Diseases* 14, 210–216.

Walter, K.S., Pepin, K.M., Webb, C.T., Gaff, H.D., Krause, P.K., Pitzer, V.E. and Diuk-Wasser, M.A. (2016) Invasion of two tick-borne diseases across New England: harnessing human surveillance data to capture underlying ecological invasion process. *Proceedings of the Royal Society B* 283, 20160834.

Walter, K.S., Carpi, G., Caccone, A. and Diuk-Wasser, M. (2017) Genomic insights into the ancient spread of Lyme disease across North America. *Nature, Ecology, Evolution* 1, 1569–1576.

Warren, R.J. (1991) Ecological justification for controlling deer populations in eastern national parks. *Transactions of the North American Wildlife and Natural Resources Conference* 56, 56–66.

Werden, L., Barker, I.K., Bowman, J., Gonzales, E.K., Leighton, P., Lindsay, L.R. and Jardine, C. (2014) Geography, deer, and host biodiversity shape the pattern of Lyme disease emergence in the thousand islands archipelago of Ontario Canada. *PLoS One* 9, e85640.

Wesson, D.M., McLain, D.K., Oliver, J.H., Piesman, J. and Collins, F.H. (1993) Investigation of the validity of the species status of *Ixodes dammini* (Acari: Ixodidae) using rDNA. *Proceedings of the National Academy of Sciences of the USA* 90, 10221–10225.

Westrom, D.R., Lane, R.S. and Anderson, J.R. (1985) *I. pacificus* population dynamics and distribution of Columbian black-tailed deer (*Odocoileus hemionus*). *Journal of Medical Entomology* 22, 507–511.

White, D.J., Chang, J.H.G., Benach, J.L., Bosler, E.M., Meldrum, S.C., Means, R.G., Debbie, J.G., Birkhead, G.S. and Morse, D.L. (1991) The geographical spread and temporal increase of the Lyme disease epidemic. *Journal of the American Medical Association* 266, 1230–1236.

Wielenga, P.R., Gaasenbeek, C., Fonville, M., de Boer, A., de Vries, A., Dimmers, W., Jagers, G.A.O., Schouls, L.M., Borgsteede, F. and van der Giessen, J.W.B. (2006) Longitudinal analysis of tick densities and *Borrelia*, *Anaplasma*, and *Ehrlichia* infections of *Ixodes ricinus* ticks in different habitat areas in the Netherlands. *Applied and Environmental Microbiology* 72, 7594–7601.

Wikel, S.K., Ramachandra, R.N., Bergman, D.K. *et al.* (1997) Infestation with pathogen free nymphs of the tick I*xodes scapularis* induces host resistance to transmission of *Borrelia burgdorferi* by ticks. *Infection and Immunity* 65, 335–338.

Williams, S.C., Ward, J.S., Worthley, T.E. and Stafford, K.C. III (2009) Managing Japanese barberry (Ranunculales: Berberidaceae) infestations reduces blacklegged tick (Acari: Ixodidae) abundance and infection prevalence with *Borrelia burgdorferi* (Spirochaetales: Spirochaetaceae). *Environmental Entomology* 38, 977–984.

Wilson, M.L., Levine, J.F. and Spielman, A. (1984) Effect of deer reduction on abundance of the deer tick. *Yale Journal of Biology and Medicine* 57, 697–705.

Wilson, M.L., Adler, G.H. and Spielman, A. (1985) Correlation between deer abundance and that of the deer tick *Ixodes dammini* (Acari: Ixodidae). *Annals of the Entomological Society of America* 78, 172–176.

Wilson, M.L., Telford, S.R., Piesman, J. and Spielman, A. (1988) Reduced abundance of immature *Ixodes dammini* (Acari: Ixodidae) following the elimination of deer. *Journal of Medical Entomology* 25, 224–228.

Wilson, M.L., Ducey, A.M., Litwin, T.S., Gavin, T.A. and Spielman, A. (1990) Microgeographic distribution of immature *Ixodes dammini* (Acari: Ixodidae) correlated with that of deer. *Medical and Veterinary Entomology* 4, 151–160.

Xu, G., Fang, Q.Q., Kierans, J.E. and Durden, L.A. (2003) Molecular phylogenetic analyses indicate that the *Ixodes ricinus* complex is a paraphyletic group. *Journal of Parasitology* 89, 442–457.

Yuval, B. and Spielman, A. (1990) Duration and regulation of the developmental cycle of *Ixodes dammini*. *Journal of Medical Entomology* 27, 196–201.

Zhioua, E., Browning, M., Johnson, P.W., Ginsberg, H.S. and Lebrun, R.A. (1997) Pathogenicity of the entomopathogenic fungus *Metarhizium anisopliae* (Deuteromycetes) to *Ixodes scapularis* (Acari: Ixodidae). *Journal of Parasitology* 83, 815–818.

Zolnik, C.P., Falco, R.C., Sergios-Orestis, K. and Daniels, T. (2015) No observed effect of landscape fragmentation on pathogen infection prevalence in blacklegged ticks (*Ixodes scapularis*) in the northeastern United States. *PloS One* 10(10), e0139473.

Zonneveld, I. and Foreman, R. (1990) *Changing Landscapes: An Ecological Perspective*. Springer, New York.

2 Biology of the Lyme Disease Agents: A Selective Survey of Clinical and Epidemiologic Relevance

Alan G. Barbour
University of California Irvine School of Medicine, Irvine, California, USA

2.1 Introduction

Since the book's last edition, knowledge of the biology and genetics of the agents of Lyme disease (or Lyme borreliosis) has further advanced. The genome sequences of several more strains and species have been added to the handful available before. A multitude of studies in which this or that gene has been knocked-out have revealed individual gene functions in animal models. Even a modestly ambitious survey of what is known now about the roles of 100 or so genes of the Lyme disease agents would greatly exceed the chapter's allotted space. Many of these genes and their products are known to be contributors to infectiousness, growth in the host or evasion of immunity (reviewed in Petzke and Schwartz, 2015; Caine and Coburn, 2016). But the impact of many of these basic science advances on improving the diagnosis and treatment of Lyme disease has been limited to this point. So, rather than attempt a broad but inevitably superficial overview, this chapter focuses on certain aspects that are more relevant in 2017 and the foreseeable future for clinical practice and the epidemiology of Lyme disease among human populations. The format is 'Q & As', with emphasis on controversies, such as whether some bacteria can carry on their mischief in the face of otherwise effective antibiotic treatments and immune responses (Barbour, 2012).

The other prefatory note regards the change in the taxonomy or classification of Lyme disease agents. The same advances in genome sequencing that provided complete genomes of several additional Lyme disease agents also deepened our understanding of other spirochetes and inferences about their evolutionary trajectories. As is occurring throughout biology, these new data justify reassessments of family or phylogenetic relationships. These take into account biological features, like morphology and host associations, as well as genome sequences.

The Lyme disease agents have hitherto been categorized under the umbrella term '*Borrelia burgdorferi* sensu lato'. This expediently served to distinguish them from other *Borrelia* species, such as the several species that cause relapsing fever. This chapter recognizes the distinctiveness of this group by accepting the assignment of '*Borrelia burgdorferi* sensu lato' species to the new genus *Borreliella* ('Borrelia-like') (Adeolu and Gupta, 2014; Barbour *et al.*, 2017; Barbour, 2018). The relapsing fever agents and sister species, including *Borrelia miyamotoi* (Krause *et al.*, 2015), retain the genus name *Borrelia* because of their historical priority, in this case by several decades. The Lyme disease agents were previously relegated to the very diverse family *Spirochetaceae*, which includes the agent of syphilis, *Treponema pallidum*, as well as termite symbionts and free-living spirochetes in alkaline ponds. But now the two genera of *Borrelia* and *Borreliella* constitute their own family: *Borreliaceae*.

A transition is underway, as textbooks, diagnostic codes, manuals, etc. undergo routine updates and revisions. During this transition '*Borrelia*' or '*Borreliella*', as alternative genus names for Lyme disease agents, will validly co-exist, as in this book. A species may be denoted as *Borreliella (Borrelia) burgdorferi*, for example, to provide a link to the prior taxonomy. In most contexts, including this chapter, the original Lyme disease species ('*Borrelia burgdorferi* sensu stricto' according to the former terminology) is still abbreviated as '*B. burgdorferi*', and similarly for other species. The medical term 'borreliosis' also still applies, since it derives from the family name *Borreliaceae*.

2.2 How is *B. burgdorferi* Different from Other Bacteria?

The spirochetes that cause Lyme disease are motile, spiral bacteria that are only distantly related to gram-negative and gram-positive pathogens. The cells have two cellular membranes like gram-negative bacteria, but their flagella, the organelles of motility, are uniquely located between the inner and outer membrane, rather than on the surface. *Borreliella* spp. cells are 10–30 μm in length and 0.2–0.3 μm in width. Their narrowness accounts for the inability to see Gram-stained spirochetes by standard light microscopy. A silver stain or the binding of fluorescein- or enzyme-conjugated antibodies is required for visualization of the cells in smears or tissue sections.

Spirochetes divide by transverse fission once they have grown lengthwise to a certain length. The two ends appear identical. In liquid media and in the blood under phase or dark field microscopy they display three modes of movement: forward, backward and, after a varying interval, a sudden contraction into a ball. After relaxation to an extended form again the spirochete continues on, more likely than not, in another direction until the next contraction. *Borreliella* species in particular also can get tangled up inadvertently or by design into small and large aggregates (Barbour, 1984). This phenomenon is considered under the question about 'biofilms' that follows.

Whether there are alternative stages or phases, such as endospores, of *B. burgdorferi* is discussed under the question about 'cysts' and 'round forms' that follows.

The genomes of *B. burgdorferi* and the other five species of Lyme disease agents each comprise a single linear chromosome of approximately 920 kb, and 20 or so linear and circular plasmids totaling another 400–500 kb (Casjens *et al.*, 2000). The largest plasmid is about 60 kb and the smallest observed is about 9 kb. Some of the genes of the plasmids have a recognizable function on the basis of their homologies with replication and partition genes of the plasmids of other kinds of bacteria. Some others, as described below, encode important antigens or virulence factors that are unique to either the genus or family. But most of the putative products of open reading frames of their plasmids are of unknown function.

The *B. burgdorferi* chromosome is less than a quarter the size of the *Escherichia coli* chromosome. The genetic content of the chromosome, plus a handful of plasmid-borne genes, is sufficient for growth outside of cells in both vertebrates and ticks, but the cells' limited biosynthetic capabilities restrict the environments in which they can grow. *Borreliella burgdorferi* and other Lyme disease agents obtain from their host more complex nutrients, such as long-chain fatty acids, nucleosides, amino acids or peptides, and vitamins. One notable growth requirement is N-acetylglucosamine, a key constituent of the cell wall's peptidoglycan (Barbour, 1986). As a consequence of these dependencies, these microorganisms have no capacity for surviving outside their animal habitats in nature or complex media in the laboratory.

The combined genetic content of the chromosome and plasmids confers a potential capability of producing about 1500 proteins. Some of the open reading frames either are pseudogenes, i.e. degraded gene sequences, or lack promoters for expression. Probably less than 1000 are ever expressed, and among those only 200 or so are produced in sufficient amounts (and are immunogenic enough) to elicit an immune response in infected humans, natural reservoir hosts or laboratory mice (Barbour *et al.*, 2008). Ten of these proteins are commonly enough recognized by antibodies in sera from patients with Lyme disease to be the specific criteria for interpreting

Western blots (immunoblots) of whole cell lysates. These include flagellin (the major structural protein of flagella, with an apparent size by electrophoresis of 41 kDa), as well as certain heat shock proteins (e.g. a 60kDa protein), an inner membrane protein of 39 kDa, an integral outer membrane protein of 66 kDa, and proteins with apparent sizes 58 kDa and 93 kDa of unknown function.

In addition, a unique feature of *B. burgdorferi* and other Lyme disease species is the large number of nucleotide sequences that it contains for lipoproteins with covalently-linked fatty acids at their N-terminal ends. Plasmid-encoded antigens include surface-exposed lipoproteins outer-surface protein (Osp) A (31 kDa), OspB (34 kDa), OspC (~23 kDa), the decorin-binding proteins (Dbp) A and B (18 kDa) and the VlsE protein (~35 kDa). The spirochete up-regulates or down-regulates expression of some of these proteins at different times in its life cycle, presumably to suit each environment, as described below, and under pressure from the immune response of the mammalian host (Schwan and Piesman, 2002). Not all of the proteins are expressed in cultured organisms. For example, VlsE, a major immunogen, is poorly expressed in culture, and, consequently, is produced as a recombinant protein in *E. coli* for its use for diagnostic assays.

OspA and OspB proteins are expressed in the tick and also abundantly under the usual conditions for *in vitro* cultivation in broth medium. With the exception of patients with late-stage pauciarticular arthritis, seropositive individuals with *B. burgdorferi* infection seldom have detectable antibodies to these proteins. At least one reference laboratory includes antibodies to OspA and OspB in their set of proteins for interpretation of Western blot bands of whole cell lysates, but in my experience the high concentration of these acidic proteins on the membranes leads to false-positive bands at 31 kDa and/or 34 kDa.

The *Borrelia* species that cause relapsing fever, including infection by *Ixodes* tick-borne *Borrelia miyamotoi* (Krause et al., 2015), have sufficient sequence similarity for some proteinaceous antigens of *B. burgdorferi* and other Lyme disease species for there to be antigenic cross-reactivity in whole cell-based immunoassays and some assays based on single recombinant proteins, including VlsE (and its 'C6 peptide'), which is homologous to immunodominant antigens of *Borrelia* species.

2.3 Briefly, How Does *B. burgdorferi* Infect a Human and Other Mammals?

Infection begins in the skin at the site of the tick bite. Unlike the relapsing fever agents, which usually are already in the salivary glands of the tick before it begins to feed, the Lyme disease agents at that point are still in the tick's intestine. In that environment, the spirochetes are producing the outer membrane lipoproteins OspA, OspB and OspD, as well as other proteins. OspA functions as an adhesin for the tick's intestinal epithelium. Before transmission can occur, the spirochetes have to penetrate the intestinal wall into the hemolymph, which functions as blood within the cavity containing the different organs and encased by the hard exoskeleton. This migration is stimulated by the incoming blood in the intestine as the tick feeds over the next few days. The combination of blood components, a change in pH in the intestine and the elevation in the temperature of the embedded tick in the animal skin also provide the initial signals that lead to changes in the expression of many proteins. Some proteins, such as OspA, are down-regulated, while others, such as OspC, are up-regulated (reviewed in Schwan and Piesman, 2002; Zückert, 2013). By the time the spirochetes enter the pool of blood and tissue fluid that has been excavated in the skin by the mouth parts of the tick, most spirochetes are no longer expressing OspA, expressing OspC instead. Besides the direct evidence of this, we can infer this from the following observations: (i) While the prevalence of antibodies to OspC is high in rodent reservoirs in areas where infection of natural hosts is very common, animals with serological or polymerase chain reaction (PCR) evidence of infection rarely have antibodies to OspA (Bunikis et al., 2004b). (ii) There is considerable diversity among OspC proteins representing different strains of *B. burgdorferi*, an indication of positive selection by adaptive immune systems (Barbour and Travinsky, 2010). In contrast, there are so few differences between the OspA proteins of different strains of *B. burgdorferi* (Bunikis et al., 2004a) that a single type was sufficient as the basis for a human vaccine in successful field trials in the United States (reviewed in Poland, 2011).

Borreliella species do not produce potent exotoxins or invasion-enhancing enzymes, but cause infection by migrating through the skin and other tissues, disseminating in the blood to other organs, adhering to host cells, and evading innate and adaptive immunity. Although Lyme disease spirochetes do not produce lipid A-containing lipopolysaccharide, they do produce lipoproteins that are ligands for toll-like receptors on mononuclear blood cells and other cells (Hirschfeld *et al.*, 1999). Binding to these receptors can lead to release of pro-inflammatory cytokines with effects qualitatively similar to responses to endotoxin.

2.4 Can *B. burgdorferi* Grow Inside Mammalian Cells?

Not to any meaningful extent. Some small proportion of a population may enter non-phagocytic cells, like fibroblasts (Klempner *et al.*, 1993) and umbilical cells (Ma *et al.*, 1991) under tissue culture conditions. There may even be long-term intracellular viability of the spirochetes in cultivated mammalian cells (Wu *et al.*, 2011), but there is little or no growth of spirochete populations within the cells themselves and no cytopathic effect (Livengood and Gilmore, 2006). If there are some intracellular spirochetes *in vivo*, tetracyclines and macrolide antibiotics would be expected to have an effect on bacteria inside the cells.

Facing professional phagocytes, like neutrophils or macrophages, *B. burgdorferi* cells are engulfed and killed with or without opsonization (Benach *et al.*, 1984; Rittig *et al.*, 1992; Montgomery *et al.*, 1993). *Borreliella burgdorferi* and other Lyme disease agents are catalase-negative (Johnson *et al.*, 1984), and on this basis are susceptible to the oxygen radicals produced by phagocytes (Modolell *et al.*, 1994).

2.5 What Species Cause Lyme Disease?

Three *Borreliella* species cause more than 95% of the cases of Lyme disease in the world: *B. burgdorferi*, *B. afzelii* and *B. garinii* (Stanek and Reiter, 2011). The clusters of strains constituting each of the three species had separate evolutionary histories since the last common ancestor (Fig. 2.1). *Borreliella garinii* displays more genetic diversity than either *B. burgdorferi* or *B. afzelii*. These three species produce both localized and disseminated infections in humans and experimental animal models. Other species have been isolated from human cases, but these instances are uncommon to rare. In the uncommon category are *B. mayonii* (Pritt *et al.*, 2016) and *B. bavariensis* (Margos *et al.*, 2013), both of which can cause disseminated infections. *Borreliella bavariensis* was formerly a strain within the species *B. garinii*. In the rare category are *B. speilmanii* and *B. lusitaniae*, both of which appear to be limited to the skin of humans. These species can also be characterized by their geographic distributions, some of which overlap. (See also Chapter 5 by Mead for epidemiology.)

In northeastern and north-central United States, as well as bordering regions of Canada, *B. burgdorferi* is by far the major cause of Lyme disease in humans. The organism is transmitted by *Ixodes scapularis*, the black-legged tick, or more colloquially in the northeast, the 'deer tick'. In northern California, and some other coastal and foothill regions of far-western North America, including Canada, human cases of Lyme disease are associated with exposure to *Ixodes pacificus*, the western black-legged tick. There is a wide variation in the prevalence of *B. burgdorferi* infection of these tick species, depending on the area. But overall the prevalence of infection in vectors is about 10-fold lower in the far west than in the northeastern United States (Hoen *et al.*, 2009; Padgett *et al.*, 2014).

The only other species that has been established as a cause of Lyme disease in North America is *B. mayonii*, which is transmitted by *I. scapularis* ticks in north-central United States (Pritt *et al.*, 2016). *Borrelia mayonii* has not been observed in *I. pacificus* ticks or *I. scapularis* ticks in the northeast. *Borreliella garinii* has been identified in Canada (Fig. 2.1) but only in ticks adapted to seabird colonies in Newfoundland and Labrador (Ogden *et al.*, 2015).

While *I. scapularis* ticks are found focally throughout the south-eastern US, they are rarely infected with *B. burgdorferi*, and the distinguishing behavior of this southern form of the

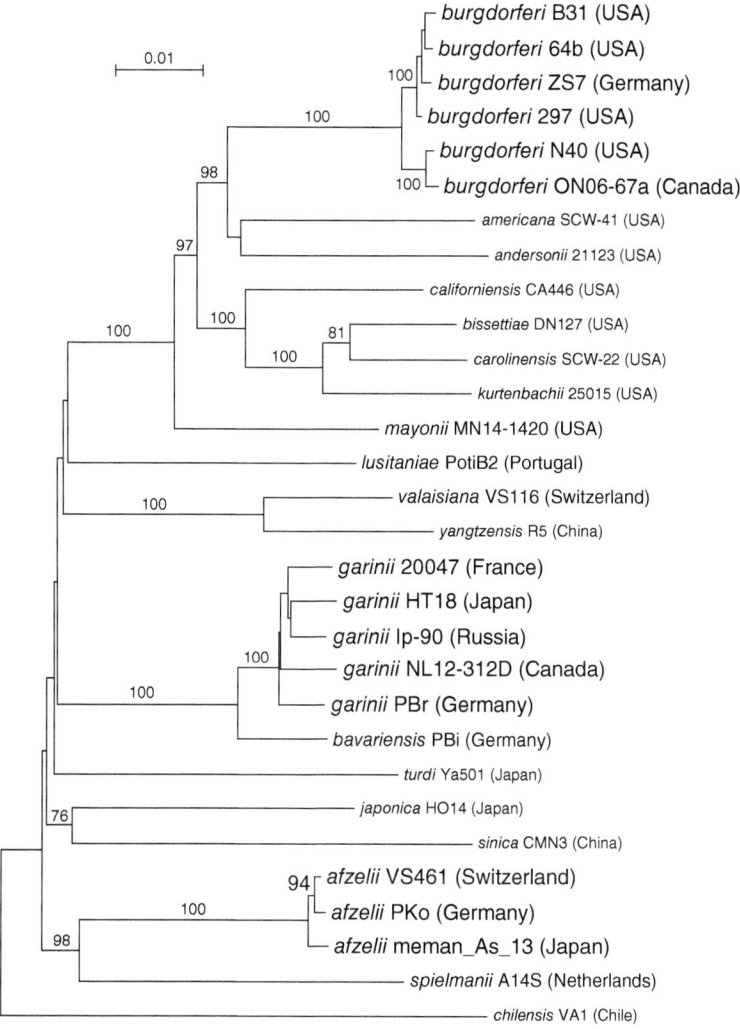

Fig. 2.1. Genetic distance phylogram of selected species and strains of *Borreliella*. Codon-aligned partial DNA sequences of eight housekeeping genes of the Multi-locus Sequence Typing set (*nifS, clpA, rplB, pyrG, recG, clpX, pepX* and *uvrA*) were concatenated. The evolutionary model for the neighbor-joining tree was Kimura 2-parameter, and there were 1000 bootstrap iterations. Representative strains are provided for *B. burgdorferi, B. afzelii* and *B. garinii*. There are three sizes of the font. The largest font indicates the most commonly documented agents of Lyme disease. The medium-sized font indicates species that have been infrequently or rarely isolated from humans in North America or Eurasia. The smallest font indicates species that have not been convincingly associated with human disease. The sequences used in the analysis can be found at http://pubmlst.net/borrelia by entering the species and strain identities. DNA distance is indicated by the bar.

tick species seldom puts people at risk of bites (Diuk-Wasser et al., 2012). *Borreliella burgdorferi* has been reported in ticks in Texas and northeastern Mexico (Feria-Arroyo et al., 2014), but there is evidence that this finding was the consequence of laboratory contamination (Norris et al., 2014).

Borreliella burgdorferi also occurs in Europe west of the Ural Mountains in Russia and is transmitted by *I. ricinus*, the sheep tick. But the more common Lyme disease agents in temperate regions of Eurasia, extending from Ireland and Norway in the west to the Pacific Coast and

Japan in the east, are *B. afzelii* and *B. garinii*. These are transmitted by *I. persulcatus*, the taiga tick, or *I. ricinus*, depending on the geographic area (Stanek *et al.*, 2012). *Borreliella burgdorferi* has not been documented in Asia, and *B. afzelii* has not been found in North America. Strains of *B. burgdorferi* in Europe and North America are closely related (Fig. 2.1), but they are distinguishable at the gene locus level (Bunikis *et al.*, 2004a). There is no evidence that *B. burgdorferi* was introduced into North America from Europe in colonial or modern times (Hoen *et al.*, 2009). *Borreliella bavariensis* clusters with *B. garinii* (Fig. 2.1), but the latter species resembles *B. afzelii* in its use of rodents as reservoirs rather than birds (Margos *et al.*, 2013), the preferred reservoir for *B. garinii* (Kurtenbach *et al.*, 2006).

2.6 What About All Those Other *Borreliella* Species?

Figure 2.1 shows several species besides the common (e.g. *B. burgdorferi*) and less common (e.g. *B. spielmanii*) agents of Lyme disease. The number of *Borreliella* species with either valid names or candidate names has increased, at an accelerating pace, from one in 1983 to 19 as of late 2017, with more in the pipeline. However, the majority of the *Borreliella* species are not associated with human disease. One of the downsides of the widespread and shortsighted use of '*Borrelia burgdorferi* sensu lato' to cover new species as they are named is the risk of misinterpretation of them as disease agents, simply from association with the name *B. burgdorferi*. Under this misconception, the risk of Lyme disease in a region may be overestimated by the lay public and some medical practitioners.

The infectiousness and pathogenicity for humans of any of the non-Lyme disease *Borreliella* species discussed here cannot be excluded, but there have been few attempts at experimental infections in laboratory animals or serosurveys with species-specific antigens that might provide insights into that.

The species of no or very low risk for humans have life cycles comprising an *Ixodes* species tick and one or more vertebrate hosts for these ticks, as do *B. burgdorferi*, *B. afzelii* and *B. garinii*. But these species do not cause human disease, either because they are not inherently infectious for humans or, more likely, the behaviors of their tick vectors rarely put humans in harm's way (See Chapter 1 on tick associations). At last count the species in North Amercia that have not been associated with human disease are *B. americana*, *B. andersoni*, *B. bissettiae* (formerly '*B. bissettii*'), *B. californiensis*, *B. carolinensis* and *B. kurtenbachii*. Distributions of some of these, such as *B. andersoni* and *B. bissettiae*, overlap with *B. burgdorferi* to some extent, while others largely do not.

In southern California we and others have identified *B. americana* in very low frequencies in *I. pacificus* ticks, which are endemic (Lane *et al.*, 2013; Barbour *et al.*, 2018). But there is no convincing evidence to date of a sustained presence of *B. burgdorferi* ('sensu stricto') in this populous region, where, anecdotally at least, diagnoses of locally acquired Lyme disease are more frequent than would be expected.

Elsewhere there are reports of identification of DNA sequences of some of these species in PCR amplification products from human specimens. But they have either been unconvincing on their own merits or unreplicated. One such report is the amplification of what was identified as *B. bissettiae* DNA from long-stored serum samples from individuals in northern California (Girard *et al.*, 2011). The same article also reported on amplification of *B. burgdorferi* DNA from other samples. But most of the reported DNA sequences were identical to a gene sequence of the common lab strain, B31, so contamination cannot be excluded as an explanation. A '*B. bissettii*-like' organism was reportedly isolated from a resident in south-eastern US with an 'undefined disorder' and 'symptoms not typical of Lyme disease' (Rudenko *et al.*, 2016). Apparent shortcomings in this reported study have been pointed out (Wormser *et al.*, 2017).

In Eurasia the species that have yet to be documented as human pathogens are *B. sinica*, *B. tanaka*, *B. turdi* and *B. yangtzensis*. The only *Borreliella* species documented outside of North America or Eurasia are (i) some strains of *B. garinii* and *B. bavariensis* that have an association with migrating seabirds and *Ixodes uriae* ticks of their remote sub-Arctic and sub-Antarctic nests (Olsen *et al.*, 1995); and (ii) *B. chilensis*, which was isolated from *Ixodes stilesi* ticks in South America (Ivanova *et al.*, 2014).

2.7 Are There Differences Between Species in the Manifestations of Infection?

As Fig. 2.1 illustrates there is considerable genetic diversity represented among the three major human pathogens. It is not surprising then that the Lyme disease species differ in their life cycles and ecologies, and in the types of infection they cause in humans. *Borreliella burgdorferi* and *B. afzelii* are mainly associated with rodents as reservoirs, whereas *B. garinii* is mainly associated with birds (Kurtenbach *et al.*, 2006). This pattern of reservoir hosts for these spirochetes is attributed in part to the relative susceptibility of specific host complement lysis.

Biologic differences have also been observed among the three predominant species of Lyme disease agents in the laboratory. In an *in vitro* study that included representatives of the three species, *B. burgdorferi* stimulated macrophages to secrete higher levels of cytokines and chemokines than did *B. afzelii* or *B. garinii* (Strle *et al.*, 2009).

These biologic differences likely account for some of the differences in clinical manifestations in patients in Europe compared with North America. As an example, although all three species have been recovered from various sites in patients (e.g. skin, blood and cerebrospinal fluid), infection with *B. afzelii* is associated with a lower risk of neurologic disease than infection with either *B. garinii* or *B. burgdorferi* (Steere *et al.*, 2004).

Borreliella mayonii infection of humans in the north-central US has featured higher densities of spirochetes in the blood during the phase of intravascular dissemination (Pritt *et al.*, 2016). The numbers of *B. mayonii* in the blood are not as high as observed during relapsing fever, but there may be enough spirochetes for them to be visualized in blood smears.

2.8 How Are Different Strains of *B. burgdorferi* Distinguished from One Another?

After there was more than one isolate of *B. burgdorferi*, microbiologists began to note differences among them (reviewed in Barbour and Cook, 2018). Initially this was in their protein profiles by gel electrophoresis or their reactivities with monoclonal antibodies. These protein-based methods were eventually supplanted by DNA-based approaches, mainly after the implementation of PCR, which allowed for specific amplification of genetic loci. One of the more informative early genotyping procedures was differing restriction fragment lengths of the intergenic spacer between the 16S and 23S ribosomal RNA genes (Liveris *et al.*, 1995). The identified genotypes are referred to as 'ribosomal RNA intergenic spacer types' or RSTs, and *B. burgdorferi* strains can be categorized into one of the three types: RST1, RST2 and RST3.

While this genotyping scheme still appears in some current publications, the more common genotyping methods now are the actual DNA sequences of the PCR products, not just the lengths of their restriction fragments. The sequence equivalent for the RST locus is the 'intergenic spacer' or IGS (Bunikis *et al.*, 2004a). Two other common sequence-based genotyping methods are the polymorphic *ospC* gene, which is encoded by one of the plasmids, and Multilocus Sequence Typing or MLST of a set of eight 'housekeeping' genes, i.e. conserved chromosomal genes, usually for an enzyme (Maiden *et al.*, 1998). The combination of the IGS and *ospC* sequences provides for a two-locus genotype that is as discriminatory as eight-locus MLST and at a lower cost (Bunikis *et al.*, 2004a). As the cost for whole-genome sequencing declines, that is becoming the preferred genotyping procedure for the characterization of novel strains and may eventually become a routine genotyping procedure.

In Lyme disease-endemic regions of North America, there are usually 10–15 genetically distinct strains of *B. burgdorferi* circulating among wildlife and ticks in a given area (Girard *et al.*, 2009; Hoen *et al.*, 2009). There are some strains, such as B31, the first isolate of *B. burgdorferi*, that occur in the US in all three regions where the microbe is endemic: the northeast, north-central region and far west. Other strains have more limited distributions (e.g. occurring in the north-central region but not in the northeast or the far west) (Barbour and Travinsky, 2010). A similar situation characterizes populations of *B. afzelii* and *B. garinii* in Europe (Bunikis *et al.*, 2004a).

The mix of strains in a given area is determined in part by frequency-dependent selection by adaptive immune responses of reservoir host animals over time. However, there may also be strain differences that reflect specific host associations, such as different patterns of susceptibility to complement of various vertebrate species. Susceptibility of *B. burgdorferi* to the non-immune bactericidal effects of the lizards' serum is one of the explanations for the lower prevalence of *B. burgdorferi* in *Ixodes* ticks in the far-western and southeastern United States. Lizards are common hosts for *I. pacificus* and *I. scapularis* ticks in these respective regions (Lane and Quistad, 1998). If an infected tick feeds on a lizard, the blood meal has a sterilizing action.

2.9 Does it Make a Difference What Strain of *B. burgdorferi* a Person is Infected With?

Some strains of *B. burgdorferi* are associated with a higher frequency of disseminated infection in humans and other mammals (Seinost et al., 1999; Wang et al., 2002; Wormser et al., 2008). RST1 genotype strains have been associated with more severe early disease and more frequent antibiotic-refractory Lyme arthritis (Jones et al., 2009) and with greater inflammation (Strle et al., 2011). Among *B. burgdorferi* strains, representative ones from the US generally elicit higher levels of cytokines and chemokines associated with innate and Th1-adaptive immune responses than a selection of strains from Europe (Cerar et al., 2016).

Whether infection with a more invasive strain calls for a longer duration of antibiotic treatment or for greater attention to post-treatment symptoms is not known. If identification of the genotype of the infecting strain provides added value for patient management, this can be achieved directly by PCR of DNA extracted from blood or skin biopsy samples. It is also possible for OspC type-specific antibody responses to be detected (Baum et al., 2013). In the absence of isolation of the bacterium or genotyping by sequence of PCR fragments, arrays of recombinant OspC could serve to identify the strain a patient has been infected with.

2.10 Why Are Isolates in Culture of *B. burgdorferi* or Other Species from Patients Infrequent?

For the great majority of bacterial infections health care workers encounter, the agent of the infection is isolatable in culture by routine, decades-old procedures. Think of the *E. coli* in the urine or *Staphylococcus aureus* in the blood or abscess aspirate. While it is true that cultivation of some pathogens is being replaced in clinical and public health laboratories by nucleic acid amplification tests, like PCR, e.g. for *Neisseria gonorrhoeae*, the 'gold standard' remains cultivation. This is also still the benchmark for *B. burgdorferi* and the other Lyme disease agents. But outside of research and specialized reference laboratories with a particular interest and expertise in Lyme disease, this diagnostic procedure is seldom performed. When it is, the isolation rate in cases of early infection is about 80% from the skin and about 50% from the blood (Liveris et al., 2002; O'Rourke et al., 2013).

With their limited biosynthetic capabilities, *B. burgdorferi* and other Lyme disease species require a complex medium for growth *in vitro* under microaerophilic conditions with elevated amounts of carbon dioxide and a temperature range of 33–37°C. Under the best of circumstances, growth is slow, with generation times of 6 h or longer.

Two types of media formulations are mainly used. The first, BSK II (Barbour, 1984), is a modification of the medium used for the first isolation of *B. burgdorferi* (Stoenner, 1974; Burgdorfer et al., 1982). The second, MKP medium (Preac-Mursic et al., 1986), is similar in composition and is used more often in Europe. Both begin with a commercial tissue culture medium comprising electrolytes, amino acids, nucleosides, vitamins and other simple growth factors. To this is added N-acetylglucosamine, a source of peptides, bovine serum albumin and serum, usually rabbit. The source of albumin is very important. It and the serum provide long-chain fatty acids among other nutrients. Gelatin, or some other thickening agent, provides enough viscosity to the broth for the spirochetes to be unrestrained in their motility.

In a comparison of BSK II with MKP in growth of organisms from skin biopsies of erythema migrans, BSK II was more successful than MKP (Ružić-Sabljić et al., 2006). A commercial version of BSK II, 'BSK-H', has some differences from the original formulation. In a similar comparison with MKP for recoveries from skin biopsies, the BSK-H medium was inferior (Ružić-Sabljić et al., 2014). PCR is generally more sensitive than either culture method in detecting Lyme disease spirochetes in blood or in skin biopsies.

Challenging the performance of these two established methods is the published report of Sapi et al., which claims a success rate of 94% in the identification of spirochetes in blood samples from individuals with the diagnosis of Lyme disease (Sapi et al., 2013). This method is also the basis of a laboratory test, which is neither cleared nor approved by the US Food and Drug Administration, offered at this writing by a commercial laboratory for around US$600 to $1000 each, depending on the options chosen.

The published method begins with BSK-H as a 'starter culture'. This is subsequently transferred to a second formulation that includes collagen-coated slides, which serve as a solid matrix for spirochetes to adhere. This long-term culture is maintained for up to 3–4 months. Spirochetes on the slides after fixation are identified with either a conjugated polyclonal antibody, which would likely bind to Borrelia spp. as well as Borreliella spp. cells, or with a monoclonal antibody raised against B. burgdorferi but of uncertain specificity. In the long-term cultures the purported spirochetes have atypical morphologies. In the published report there was no mention of an irrelevant conjugated polyclonal antiserum as a negative control. DNA extracts of cultures were also subject to nested PCR for the gene for cytidine triphosphate (CTP) synthase. There was no description of blinding of either the samples (patients vs. controls) or the operators of the procedure.

The validity of this report's claims has been questioned (Johnson et al., 2014). The authors of this critique point out that with few exceptions the DNA sequences that were deposited were identical or highly similar to either the standard lab strain of B. burgdorferi, B31, or a B. garinii strain from Japan. Both of these strains were included among the reference strains used in the development of the method, thus raising the possibility of laboratory contamination during the nested PCR assays. The critique also points out that there was little description of the cases, the durations of their illnesses and whether they had ever received antibiotics for Lyme disease.

2.11 What Are These 'Cysts' and 'Round Forms' and Are These an Explanation for Long-lasting Symptoms Even After Standard Antibiotic Treatment?

Under adverse conditions, spirochetes may turn into spherical and other atypical morphologic forms. For several decades investigators have noted that the loosely attached outer membrane separates from underlying cell structures when spirochetes are placed in hypotonic or hypertonic solutions (Lofgren and Soule, 1945b; Umemoto and Namikawa, 1980). Large outpouchings of the outer membrane, or blebs, are also seen when specific antibody and a complement source are incubated with a relapsing fever Borrelia species (Kemp et al., 1933), when cells are frozen and thawed (Lofgren and Soule, 1945a), at extremes of pH and heat for the spirochetes (Murgia and Cinco, 2004), when cells are exposed to some antibiotics (Barbour et al., 1982; Dever et al., 1993) and in aged cultures (Aristowsky and Höltzer, 1924). Similar morphologic variants among other bacterial species, typically after exposure to cell wall active antibiotics, have been called 'L-forms' (Domingue and Woody, 1997).

Claims about the clinical significance of these morphologic variants of spirochetes under adverse conditions are not new. A view that these morphologic variants of relapsing fever and syphilis represented a different stage in the life cycles was prevalent in the first half of the 20th century. Round forms or spirochetes with large blebs were called 'cysts' or 'gemmae' (reviewed in Barbour and Hayes, 1986). Some investigators noted enclosed dense inclusions, called 'granules' (DeLamater et al., 1951). The involuting mature spirochete was thought to produce small granules that were non-vegetative under adverse conditions but that in a more conducive environment would metamorphose into a full-length, vegetative spirochete again.

Why does this still merit attention? One reason is that these 'cysts' are claimed to be susceptible to metronidazole (Brorson and Brorson, 1999), in contrast to the usual form (i.e. helical, motile, dividing cells), which are known not to be susceptible to this antibiotic (Johnson et al., 1984; Caol et al., 2017). Not surprisingly, spherical 'cysts' form when the cells in medium are suspended at a 1:100 dilution in water, an extreme hypotonic condition not encountered by B. burgdorferi and other Lyme disease species outside the laboratory. The assessment of the effect of metronidazole, which was still in relatively high concentrations by pharmacodynamic standards, was by microscopic examination for a further morphologic effect and not by conventional measures of antibiotic effect *in vitro*, such as the frequency of killing of viable cells. If any reversion was noted, it was to 'immobile spirochetes' of undocumented viability (Brorson and Brorson, 1999).

In another paper reporting *in vitro* efficacy of metronidazole, as well as the related antiparasitic drug tinidazole, the cysts are called 'round bodies' (Sapi et al., 2011). The round bodies were said to be 'metabolically inactive', but the conditions for producing the round bodies by 'novel culture conditions' were not explicit. Doxycycline treatment was said to increase round bodies, while metronidazole and tinidazole decreased them.

While there may be differential effects of metranidozole and related compounds on growing populations versus stressed, aged populations *in vitro*, follow-up studies of the possible clinical significance of these effects in animal models of infections, let alone in a controlled clinical trial of humans, have not been reported. That has not stopped continuing recommendations for treatment of patients with the diagnosis of Lyme disease with metronidazole or tinidazole, for example the website for *The Treat Lyme Book* (Ross, 2014).

2.12 Are Some *B. burgdorferi* Cells in a Population Not Affected by Antibiotics and Are These What Are Called 'Persisters'?

A 'persister', in its stricter, current meaning in microbiology is a bacterial cell that survives exposure to an antibiotic at a concentration that adversely affects or kills a much greater number of cells in the same clonal population. This is a general phenomenon among bacteria of many types and certainly not limited to *B. burgdorferi* and other Lyme disease agents (Maisonneuve and Gerdes, 2014). The survival of a small proportion of the bacterial population in the face of an antibiotic is parsimoniously predicted by a theoretical model that links chemical reaction kinetics to bacterial population biology (Abel Zur Wiesch et al., 2015). Other well-known phenomena predicted by such models are post-antibiotic growth suppression and density-dependent antibiotic effects. One need not invoke genotypic or epigenetic change to account for the occurrence of some survivors with any bacterium, including *B. burgdorferi*.

The concept of 'persistence' is also more broadly applied for bacterial cells or residua, often in a different morphology, that continue to exert pathologic consequences after standard antibiotic therapy or an ongoing, otherwise effective immune response (Domingue and Woody, 1997). Persistence in this broader sense may also include residual bacterial proteins, membrane vesicles or DNA, in the absence of any remaining viable cells (Bockenstedt et al., 2012; Hodzic et al., 2014). The standard for viability is cells that are documented to be multiplying in a host, infectious in an animal model known to be susceptible and/or cultivable in a medium known to support growth of the microbe's population.

The narrower concern here, though, is with *in vitro* events – the survival of some spirochetes after exposure to an antibiotic. While the 'cysts' and 'round bodies' considered above and the 'biofilms' considered below can be imagined as contributing to the sum total of persistence, either in a culture tube or in a patient, the question at hand is the extent to which antibiotic susceptibility results are predictive of clinical outcomes.

The types of *in vitro* susceptibility studies that have demonstrated good correlation with *in vivo* experimental models and human clinical trials have these characteristics: (i) the cells are growing, i.e. not in stationary phase or directly from frozen stocks, in the starting inoculum; (ii) the inoculum density is at least 100-fold below the expected peak density; (iii) the degradation of an antibiotic, e.g. ampicillin, over time in the broth medium during incubation is recognized and compensated for; (iv) growth is measured by direct cell counts as well as by indirect measures, such as pH indicator change and transmittance; and (v) for assessments of viability either motile cells are enumerated or, preferably, colony counts on solid media are carried out. Many of the papers that report unexpected resistances or the necessity for certain antibiotic combinations for achieving desired effects lack one or more of these characteristics.

Even when there is discordance between *in vitro* and *in vivo* findings, this may be attributable to something other than true resistance or persistence on phenotypic or stochastic grounds. An example of this is the following. My colleagues and I demonstrated that vancomycin was bactericidal for *B. burgdorferi in vitro* and that the combination of penicillin and vancomycin was synergistic (Dever *et al.*, 1993). The morphologic effects, which included large blebs and cyst-like forms, of vancomycin on the growing spirochetes were indistinguishable from those of penicillin. In these and other studies in which we carried out time-kill studies, the criterion for the minimum bactericidal concentration was at least 99.9% killing. However, when we studied vancomycin as well as ceftriaxone in a mouse model, we found that vancomycin, in contrast to ceftriaxone, was not effective at eradicating cultivable spirochetes from immunodeficient mice with either *B. burgdorferi* or the relapsing fever agent *Borrelia turicatae*, if it was begun 7 days after the start of the infection (Kazragis *et al.*, 1996). This failure was attributable to persistence of viable spirochetes in the brain, a body site poorly accessed by vancomycin. This is a property of the antibiotic and unrelated to the bacterial species.

2.13 Does *B. burgdorferi* Form Biofilms That Shield the Bacteria from Antibiotics and Immunity?

The 2017 *Oxford English Dictionary* definition of a biofilm is a 'thin but robust layer of mucilage adhering to a solid surface, containing the community of bacteria and other microorganisms that generated it'. In other words, the biofilm is the consequence of the envelopment of a cell or mass of cells by an actively secreted substance, an extracellular polymeric matrix, usually a polysaccharide, sometimes a protein. Biofilms produce fouling of ship hulls and accretions in oil pipelines, as well as problems for infected hosts (Flemming *et al.*, 2016). Note the requirement for the bacteria to 'generate' the extracellular embedding substance. By this definition, do Lyme disease agents produce biofilms in mammals? I do not think so.

Some (but not all) strains of *B. burgdorferi* certainly form large macroscopic aggregates while growing in culture under stationary conditions (Fig. 2.2), first reported three decades ago (Barbour, 1984; Bundoc and Barbour, 1989). We did not note in these or other studies anything like extracellular material in which the spirochetes were enmeshed, let alone produced by them. The appearance of these aggregates is more akin to the pasta on a plate than to the impenetrable plate itself, so aggregation – even if it occurs in some tissues in host animals – does not imply exclusion of antibiotics from the center of the aggregate.

The most comprehensive study of what were called biofilms of *B. burgdorferi* was that of

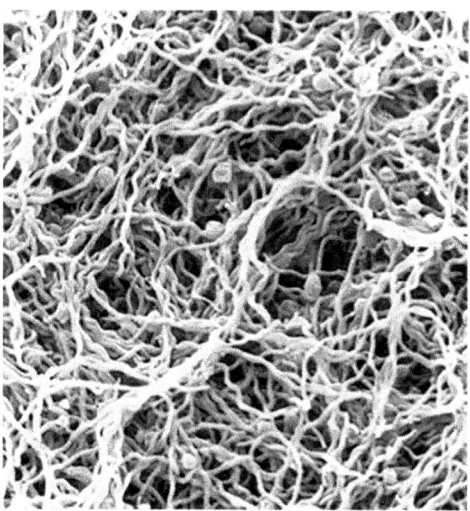

Fig. 2.2. Scanning electron photomicrograph of aggregate of *Borreliella (Borrelia) burgdorferi* strain 50-2 growing in BSK II broth medium. The aggregate was fixed in glutaraldehyde, post-fixed in osmium tetroxide, dehydrated in ethanol, critically point dried in carbon dioxide and sputter coated with gold. The small spherical extrusions on some cells are outer membrane blebs.

Sapi *et al.* (2012). This study interpreted a staining pattern of bacteria growing on a collagen-coated surface as extracellular 'sulfate and non-sulfated/carboxylated substrates, predominantly composed of alginate and calcium and extracellular DNA'. But, other than an anti-alginate polyclonal serum to back up the claim, the authors did not include a biochemical analysis to verify this interpretation. There was no conclusive evidence presented that this material was produced by the spirochetes and not deposited on the cells from the culture medium. There is also no evidence from the annotations of *Borreliella* genomes that there are pathways for the synthesis and export of alginate or other extracellular polysaccharides, such as produced by *Pseudomonas aeruginosa* in the lungs of individuals with cystic fibrosis (Flemming *et al.*, 2016).

References

Abel Zur Wiesch, P., Abel, S., Gkotzis, S., Ocampo, P., Engelstadter, J., Hinkley, T., Magnus, C., Waldor, M.K., Udekwu, K. and Cohen, T. (2015) Classic reaction kinetics can explain complex patterns of antibiotic action. *Science Translational Medicine* 7, 287ra73.

Adeolu, M. and Gupta, R.S. (2014) A phylogenomic and molecular marker based proposal for the division of the genus *Borrelia* into two genera: the emended genus *Borrelia* containing only the members of the relapsing fever *Borrelia*, and the genus *Borreliella* gen. nov. containing the members of the Lyme disease Borrelia (*Borrelia burgdorferi* sensu lato complex). *Antonie Van Leeuwenhoek* 105, 1049–1072.

Aristowsky, W.M. and Höltzer, R. (1924) Bemerkungen zur Morphologie der Spirochaeta obermeieri. *Cent. f. Bakt.* 91, 175–181.

Barbour, A.G. (1984) Isolation and cultivation of Lyme disease spirochetes. *Yale Journal of Biology and Medicine* 57, 521–525.

Barbour, A.G. (1986) Cultivation of *Borrelia*: a historical overview. *Zentralbl Bakteriol Mikrobiol Hyg [A]* 263, 11–14.

Barbour, A.G. (2012) Remains of infection. *Journal of Clinical Investigation* 122, 2344.

Barbour, A.G. (2018) Family *Borreliaceae*. In: Paster, B. (ed.) *Bergey's Manual of Systematics of Archaea and Bacteria*. John Wiley & Sons, Hoboken, New Jersey, USA.

Barbour, A.G. and Hayes, S.F. (1986) Biology of *Borrelia* species. *Microbiological Reviews* 50, 381–400.

Barbour, A.G. and Travinsky, B. (2010) Evolution and distribution of the *ospC* gene, a transferable serotype determinant of *Borrelia burgdorferi*. *MBio* 1, e00153–10.

Barbour, A.G. and Cook, V.J. (2018) Genotyping strains of Lyme disease agents directly from ticks, blood, or tissue. In: Pal, U. and Buyuktanir, O. (eds) *Borrelia burgdorferi: Methods and Protocols*. Springer, New York.

Barbour, A.G., Todd, W.J. and Stoenner, H.G. (1982) Action of penicillin on *Borrelia hermsii*. *Antimicrobial Agents Chemotherapy* 21, 823–829.

Barbour, A.G., Jasinskas, A., Kayala, M.A., Davies, D.H., Steere, A.C., Baldi, P. and Felgner, P.L. (2008) A genome-wide proteome array reveals a limited set of immunogens in natural infections of humans and white-footed mice with *Borrelia burgdorferi*. *Infection and Immunity* 76, 3374–3389.

Barbour, A.G., Adeolu, M. and Gupta, R.S. (in prep.) Division of the genus *Borrelia* into two genera (corresponding to Lyme disease and relapsing fever groups) reflects their genetic and phenotypic distinctiveness and will lead to a better understanding of these two groups of microbes (Margos *et al.* (2016) There is inadequate evidence to support the division of the genus *Borrelia*. *International Journal of Systematic and Evolutionary Microbiology* DOI:10.1099/ijsem.0.001717). *International Journal of Systematic and Evolutionary Microbiology* DOI:10.1099/ijsem.0.001815

Barbour, A.G., Brao, K., Hue, F. and Cook, V.J. (in prep.) A survey of *Ixodes pacificus* ticks of Southern California for Borreliaceae species. Manuscript in preparation.

Baum, E., Randall, A.Z., Zeller, M. and Barbour, A.G. (2013) Inferring epitopes of a polymorphic antigen amidst broadly cross-reactive antibodies using protein microarrays: a study of OspC proteins of *Borrelia burgdorferi*. *PLoS One* 8, e67445.

Benach, J.L., Habicht, G.S., Gocinski, B.L. and Coleman, J.L. (1984) Phagocytic cell responses to *in vivo* and *in vitro* exposure to the Lyme disease spirochete. *Yale Journal of Biology and Medicine* 57, 599–605.

Bockenstedt, L.K., Gonzalez, D.G., Haberman, A.M. and Belperron, A.A. (2012) Spirochete antigens persist near cartilage after murine Lyme borreliosis therapy. *Journal of Clinical Investigation* 122, 2652–2660.

Brorson, Ø. and Brorson, S.H. (1999) An *in vitro* study of the susceptibility of mobile and cystic forms of *Borrelia burgdorferi* to metronidazole. *Apmis* 107, 566–576.

Bundoc, V.G. and Barbour, A.G. (1989) Clonal polymorphisms of outer membrane protein OspB of *Borrelia burgdorferi*. *Infection and Immunity* 57, 2733–2741.

Bunikis, J., Garpmo, U., Tsao, J., Berglund, J., Fish, D. and Barbour, A.G. (2004a) Sequence typing reveals extensive strain diversity of the Lyme borreliosis agents *Borrelia burgdorferi* in North America and *Borrelia afzelii* in Europe. *Microbiology* 150, 1741–1755.

Bunikis, J., Tsao, J., Luke, C.J., Luna, M.G., Fish, D. and Barbour, A.G. (2004b) *Borrelia burgdorferi* infection in a natural population of *Peromyscus leucopus* mice: a longitudinal study in an area where Lyme borreliosis is highly endemic. *Journal of Infectious Diseases* 189, 1515–1523.

Burgdorfer, W., Barbour, A.G., Hayes, S.F., Benach, J.L., Grunwaldt, E. and Davis, J.P. (1982) Lyme disease – a tick-borne spirochetosis? *Science* 216, 1317–1319.

Caine, J.A. and Coburn, J. (2016) Multifunctional and redundant roles of *Borrelia burgdorferi* outer surface proteins in tissue adhesion, colonization, and complement evasion. *Frontiers in Immunology* 7, 442.

Caol, S., Divers, T., Crisman, M. and Chang, Y.F. (2017) *In vitro* susceptibility of *Borrelia burgdorferi* isolates to three antibiotics commonly used for treating equine Lyme disease. *BMC Veterinary Research* 13, 293.

Casjens, S., Palmer, N., Van Vugt, R., Huang, W.M., Stevenson, B., Rosa, P., Lathigra, R., Sutton, G., Peterson, J., Dodson, R.J., Haft, D., Hickey, E., Gwinn, M., White, O. and Fraser, C.M. (2000) A bacterial genome in flux: the twelve linear and nine circular extrachromosomal DNAs in an infectious isolate of the Lyme disease spirochete *Borrelia burgdorferi*. *Molecular Microbiology* 35, 490–516.

Cerar, T., Strle, F., Stupica, D., Ružić-Sabljić, E., Mchugh, G., Steere, A.C. and Strle, K. (2016) Differences in genotype, clinical features, and inflammatory potential of *Borrelia burgdorferi* sensu stricto strains from Europe and the United States. *Emerging Infectious Diseases* 22, 818–827.

DeLamater, E.D., Haanes, M., Wiggall, R.H. and Pillsbury, D.M. (1951) Studies on the life cycle of spirochetes. VIII. Summary and comparison of observations on various organisms. *Journal of Investigative Dermatology* 16, 231–256.

Dever, L.L., Jorgensen, J.H. and Barbour, A.G. (1993) *In vitro* activity of vancomycin against the spirochete *Borrelia burgdorferi*. *Antimicrobial Agents Chemotherapy* 37, 1115–1121.

Diuk-Wasser, M.A., Hoen, A.G., Cislo, P., Brinkerhoff, R., Hamer, S.A., Rowland, M., Cortinas, R., Vourc'h, G., Melton, F., Hickling, G.J., Tsao, J.I., Bunikis, J., Barbour, A.G., Kitron, U., Piesman, J. and Fish, D. (2012) Human risk of infection with *Borrelia burgdorferi*, the Lyme disease agent, in eastern United States. *American Journal of Tropical Medicine and Hygiene* 86, 320–327.

Domingue, G.J. Sr and Woody, H.B. (1997) Bacterial persistence and expression of disease. *Clinical Microbiology Reviews* 10, 320–344.

Feria-Arroyo, T.P., Castro-Arellano, I., Gordillo-Perez, G., Cavazos, A.L., Vargas-Sandoval, M., Grover, A., Torres, J., Medina, R.F., De Leon, A.A. and Esteve-Gassent, M.D. (2014) Implications of climate change on the distribution of the tick vector *Ixodes scapularis* and risk for Lyme disease in the Texas-Mexico transboundary region. *Parasites and Vectors* 7, 199.

Flemming, H.C., Wingender, J., Szewzyk, U., Steinberg, P., Rice, S.A. and Kjelleberg, S. (2016) Biofilms: an emergent form of bacterial life. *Nature Reviews Microbiology* 14, 563–575.

Girard, Y.A., Fedorova, N. and Lane, R.S. (2011) Genetic diversity of *Borrelia burgdorferi* and detection of *B. bissettii*-like DNA in serum of north-coastal California residents. *Journal of Clinical Microbiology* 49, 945–954.

Girard, Y.A., Travinsky, B., Schotthoefer, A., Fedorova, N., Eisen, R.J., Eisen, L., Barbour, A.G. and Lane, R.S. (2009) Population structure of the Lyme borreliosis spirochete *Borrelia burgdorferi* in the western black-legged tick (*Ixodes pacificus*) in Northern California. *Applied and Environmental Microbiology* 75, 7243–7252.

Hirschfeld, M., Kirschning, C.J., Schwandner, R., Wesche, H., Weis, J.H., Wooten, R.M. and Weis, J.J. (1999) Cutting edge: inflammatory signaling by *Borrelia burgdorferi* lipoproteins is mediated by toll-like receptor 2. *Journal of Immunology* 163, 2382–2386.

Hodzic, E., Imai, D., Feng, S. and Barthold, S.W. (2014) Resurgence of persisting non-cultivable *Borrelia burgdorferi* following antibiotic treatment in mice. *PLoS One* 9, e86767.

Hoen, A.G., Margos, G., Bent, S.J., Diuk-Wasser, M.A., Barbour, A., Kurtenbach, K. and Fish, D. (2009) Phylogeography of *Borrelia burgdorferi* in the eastern United States reflects multiple independent

Lyme disease emergence events. *Proceedings of the National Academy of Sciences of the USA* 106, 15013–15018.

Ivanova, L.B., Tomova, A., González-Acuña, D., Murúa, R., Moreno, C.X., Hernández, C., Cabello, J., Cabello, C., Daniels, T.J., Godfrey, H.P. and Cabello, F.C. (2014) *Borrelia chilensis*, a new member of the *Borrelia burgdorferi* sensu lato complex that extends the range of this genospecies in the southern hemisphere. *Environmental Microbiology* 16, 1069–1080.

Johnson, B.J., Pilgard, M.A. and Russell, T.M. (2014) Assessment of new culture method for detection of Borrelia species from serum of Lyme disease patients. *Journal of Clinical Microbiology* 52, 721–724.

Johnson, R.C., Hyde, F.W. and Rumpel, C.M. (1984) Taxonomy of the Lyme disease spirochetes. *Yale Journal of Biology and Medicine* 57, 529–537.

Jones, K.L., Mchugh, G.A., Glickstein, L.J. and Steere, A.C. (2009) Analysis of *Borrelia burgdorferi* genotypes in patients with Lyme arthritis: high frequency of ribosomal RNA intergenic spacer type 1 strains in antibiotic-refractory arthritis. *Arthritis and Rheumatism* 60, 2174–2182.

Kazragis, R.J., Dever, L.L., Jorgensen, J.H. and Barbour, A.G. (1996) *In vivo* activities of ceftriaxone and vancomycin against *Borrelia* spp. in the mouse brain and other sites. *Antimicrobial Agents Chemotherapy* 40, 2632–2636.

Kemp, H.A., Moursund, W.H. and Wright, H.E. (1933) Relapsing fever in Texas. *American Journal of Tropical Medicine and Hygiene* s1–s13, 425–435.

Klempner, M.S., Noring, R. and Rogers, R.A. (1993) Invasion of human skin fibroblasts by the Lyme disease spirochete, *Borrelia burgdorferi*. *Journal of Infectious Diseases* 167, 1074–1081.

Krause, P.J., Fish, D., Narasimhan, S. and Barbour, A.G. (2015) *Borrelia miyamotoi* infection in nature and in humans. *Clinical Microbiology and Infection* 21, 631–639.

Kurtenbach, K., Hanincova, K., Tsao, J.I., Margos, G., Fish, D. and Ogden, N.H. (2006) Fundamental processes in the evolutionary ecology of Lyme borreliosis. *Nature Reviews Microbiology* 4, 660–669.

Lane, R.S. and Quistad, G.B. (1998) Borreliacidal factor in the blood of the western fence lizard (*Sceloporus occidentalis*). *Journal of Parasitology* 84, 29–34.

Lane, R.S., Fedorova, N., Kleinjan, J.E. and Maxwell, M. (2013) Eco-epidemiological factors contributing to the low risk of human exposure to ixodid tick-borne borreliae in southern California, USA. *Ticks and Tick-borne Diseases* 4, 377–385.

Livengood, J.A. and Gilmore, R.D., Jr. (2006) Invasion of human neuronal and glial cells by an infectious strain of *Borrelia burgdorferi*. *Microbes and Infection* 8, 2832–2840.

Liveris, D., Gazumyan, A. and Schwartz, I. (1995) Molecular typing of *Borrelia burgdorferi* sensu lato by PCR-restriction fragment length polymorphism analysis. *Journal of Clinical Microbiology* 33, 589–595.

Liveris, D., Wang, G., Girao, G., Byrne, D.W., Nowakowski, J., Mckenna, D., Nadelman, R., Wormser, G.P. and Schwartz, I. (2002) Quantitative detection of *Borrelia burgdorferi* in 2-millimeter skin samples of erythema migrans lesions: correlation of results with clinical and laboratory findings. *Journal of Clinical Microbiology* 40, 1249–1253.

Lofgren, R. and Soule, M.H. (1945a) The effect of low temperature on the spirochetes of relapsing fever; the structure and motility of *Spirochaeta novyi*. *Journal of Bacteriology* 50, 313–321.

Lofgren, R. and Soule, M.H. (1945b) The structure of *Spirochaeta novyi* as revealed by the electron microscope. *Journal of Bacteriology* 50, 679–690.

Ma, Y., Sturrock, A. and Weis, J.J. (1991) Intracellular localization of *Borrelia burgdorferi* within human endothelial cells. *Infection and Immunity* 59, 671–678.

Maiden, M.C., Bygraves, J.A., Feil, E., Morelli, G., Russell, J.E., Urwin, R., Zhang, Q., Zhou, J., Zurth, K., Caugant, D.A., Feavers, I.M., Achtman, M. and Spratt, B.G. (1998) Multilocus sequence typing: a portable approach to the identification of clones within populations of pathogenic microorganisms. *Proceedings of the National Academy of Sciences of the USA* 95, 3140–3145.

Maisonneuve, E. and Gerdes, K. (2014) Molecular mechanisms underlying bacterial persisters. *Cell* 157, 539–548.

Margos, G., Wilske, B., Sing, A., Hizo-Teufel, C., Cao, W.-C., Chu, C., Scholz, H., Straubinger, R.K. and Fingerle, V. (2013) *Borrelia bavariensis* sp. nov. is widely distributed in Europe and Asia. *International Journal of Systematic and Evolutionary Microbiology* 63, 4284–4288.

Modolell, M., Schaible, U.E., Rittig, M. and Simon, M.M. (1994) Killing of *Borrelia burgdorferi* by macrophages is dependent on oxygen radicals and nitric oxide and can be enhanced by antibodies to outer surface proteins of the spirochete. *Immunology Letters* 40, 139–146.

Montgomery, R.R., Nathanson, M.H. and Malawista, S.E. (1993) The fate of *Borrelia burgdorferi*, the agent for Lyme disease, in mouse macrophages. Destruction, survival, recovery. *Journal of Immunology* 150, 909–915.

Murgia, R. and Cinco, M. (2004) Induction of cystic forms by different stress conditions in *Borrelia burgdorferi*. *Apmis* 112, 57–62.

Norris, S.J., Barbour, A.G., Fish, D. and Diuk-Wasser, M.A. (2014) Analysis of the intergenic sequences provided by Feria-Arroyo *et al.* does not support the claim of high *Borrelia burgdorferi* tick infection rates in Texas and northeastern Mexico. *Parasites and Vectors* 7, 467.

O'Rourke, M., Traweger, A., Lusa, L., Stupica, D., Maraspin, V., Barrett, P.N., Strle, F. and Livey, I. (2013) Quantitative detection of *Borrelia burgdorferi* sensu lato in erythema migrans skin lesions using internally controlled duplex real time PCR. *PLoS One* 8, e63968.

Ogden, N.H., Feil, E.J., Leighton, P.A., Lindsay, L.R., Margos, G., Mechai, S., Michel, P. and Moriarty, T.J. (2015) Evolutionary aspects of emerging Lyme disease in Canada. *Applied and Environmental Microbiology* 81, 7350–7359.

Olsen, B., Duffy, D.C., Jaenson, T.G., Gylfe, A., Bonnedahl, J. and Bergstrom, S. (1995) Transhemispheric exchange of Lyme disease spirochetes by seabirds. *Journal of Clinical Microbiology* 33, 3270–3274.

Padgett, K., Bonilla, D., Kjemtrup, A., Vilcins, I.M., Yoshimizu, M.H., Hui, L., Sola, M., Quintana, M. and Kramer, V. (2014) Large scale spatial risk and comparative prevalence of *Borrelia miyamotoi* and *Borrelia burgdorferi* sensu lato in *Ixodes pacificus*. *PLoS One* 9, e110853.

Petzke, M. and Schwartz, I. (2015) *Borrelia burgdorferi* pathogenesis and the immune response. *Clinics in Laboratory Medicine* 35, 745–764.

Poland, G.A. (2011) Vaccines against Lyme disease: what happened and what lessons can we learn? *Clinical Infectious Diseases* 52 Suppl 3, s253–s258.

Preac-Mursic, V., Wilske, B. and Schierz, G. (1986) European *Borrelia burgdorferi* isolated from humans and ticks culture conditions and antibiotic susceptibility. *Zentralbl Bakteriol Mikrobiol Hyg [A]* 263, 112–118.

Pritt, B.S., Respicio-Kingry, L.B., Sloan, L.M., Schriefer, M.E., Replogle, A.J., Bjork, J., Liu, G., Kingry, L.C., Mead, P.S., Neitzel, D.F., Schiffman, E., Hoang Johnson, D.K., Davis, J.P., Paskewitz, S.M., Boxrud, D., Deedon, A., Lee, X., Miller, T.K., Feist, M.A., Steward, C.R., Theel, E.S., Patel, R., Irish, C.L. and Petersen, J.M. (2016) *Borrelia mayonii* sp. nov., a member of the *Borrelia burgdorferi* sensu lato complex, detected in patients and ticks in the upper midwestern United States. *International Journal of Systematic and Evolutionary Microbiology* 66, 4878–4880.

Rittig, M.G., Krause, A., Haupl, T., Schaible, U.E., Modolell, M., Kramer, M.D., Lutjen-Drecoll, E., Simon, M.M. and Burmester, G.R. (1992) Coiling phagocytosis is the preferential phagocytic mechanism for *Borrelia burgdorferi*. *Infection and Immunity* 60, 4205–4212.

Ross, M. (2014) *A Lyme Disease Antibiotic Guide* [Online]. The Treat Lyme Book. Available at: www.treatlyme.net/treat-lyme-book/lyme-disease-antibiotic-guide/ (accessed 24 October 2017).

Rudenko, N., Golovchenko, M., Vancova, M., Clark, K., Grubhoffer, L. and Oliver, J.H., Jr (2016) Isolation of live *Borrelia burgdorferi* sensu lato spirochaetes from patients with undefined disorders and symptoms not typical for Lyme borreliosis. *Clinical Microbiology and Infection* 22(267), e9–15.

Ružić-Sabljić, E., Lotric-Furlan, S., Maraspin, V., Cimperman, J., Logar, M., Jurca, T. and Strle, F. (2006) Comparison of isolation rate of *Borrelia burgdorferi* sensu lato in MKP and BSK-II medium. *International Journal of Medical Microbiology* 296(Suppl 40), 267–273.

Ružić-Sabljić, E., Maraspin, V., Cimperman, J., Strle, F., Lotric-Furlan, S., Stupica, D. and Cerar, T. (2014) Comparison of isolation rate of *Borrelia burgdorferi* sensu lato in two different culture media, MKP and BSK-H. *Clinical Microbiology and Infection* 20, 636–641.

Sapi, E., Bastian, S.L., Mpoy, C.M., Scott, S., Rattelle, A., Pabbati, N., Poruri, A., Burugu, D., Theophilus, P.A., Pham, T.V., Datar, A., Dhaliwal, N.K., Macdonald, A., Rossi, M.J., Sinha, S.K. and Luecke, D.F. (2012) Characterization of biofilm formation by *Borrelia burgdorferi in vitro*. *PLoS One* 7, e48277.

Sapi, E., Kaur, N., Anyanwu, S., Luecke, D.F., Datar, A., Patel, S., Rossi, M. and Stricker, R.B. (2011) Evaluation of *in-vitro* antibiotic susceptibility of different morphological forms of *Borrelia burgdorferi*. *Infection and Drug Resistance* 4, 97–113.

Sapi, E., Pabbati, N., Datar, A., Davies, E.M., Rattelle, A. and Kuo, B.A. (2013) Improved culture conditions for the growth and detection of *Borrelia* from human serum. *International Journal of Medical Sciences* 10, 362–376.

Schwan, T.G. and Piesman, J. (2002) Vector interactions and molecular adaptations of Lyme disease and relapsing fever spirochetes associated with transmission by ticks. *Emerging Infectious Diseases* 8, 115–121.

Seinost, G., Dykhuizen, D.E., Dattwyler, R.J., Golde, W.T., Dunn, J.J., Wang, I.N., Wormser, G.P., Schriefer, M.E. and Luft, B.J. (1999) Four clones of *Borrelia burgdorferi* sensu stricto cause invasive infection in humans. *Infection and Immunity* 67, 3518–3524.

Stanek, G. and Reiter, M. (2011) The expanding Lyme Borrelia complex – clinical significance of genomic species? *Clinical Microbiology and Infection* 17, 487–493.

Stanek, G., Wormser, G.P., Gray, J. and Strle, F. (2012) Lyme borreliosis. *Lancet* 379, 461–473.

Steere, A.C., Coburn, J. and Glickstein, L. (2004) The emergence of Lyme disease. *Journal of Clinical Investigation* 113, 1093–1101.

Stoenner, H.G. (1974) Biology of *Borrelia hermsii* in Kelly medium. *Journal of Applied Microbiology* 28, 540–543.

Strle, K., Drouin, E.E., Shen, S., El Khoury, J., Mchugh, G., Ružić-Sabljić, E., Strle, F. and Steere, A.C. (2009) *Borrelia burgdorferi* stimulates macrophages to secrete higher levels of cytokines and chemokines than *Borrelia afzelii* or *Borrelia garinii*. *Journal of Infectious Diseases* 200, 1936–1943.

Strle, K., Jones, K.L., Drouin, E.E., Li, X. and Steere, A.C. (2011) *Borrelia burgdorferi* RST1 (OspC type A) genotype is associated with greater inflammation and more severe Lyme disease. *American Journal of Pathology* 178, 2726–2739.

Umemoto, T. and Namikawa, I. (1980) Electron microscopy of the spherical body of oral spirochetes *in vitro*. Further studies. *Medical Microbiology and Immunology* 24, 321–334.

Wang, G., Ojaimi, C., Wu, H., Saksenberg, V., Iyer, R., Liveris, D., Mcclain, S.A., Wormser, G.P. and Schwartz, I. (2002) Disease severity in a murine model of Lyme borreliosis is associated with the genotype of the infecting *Borrelia burgdorferi* sensu stricto strain. *Journal of Infectious Diseases* 186, 782–791.

Wormser, G.P., Brisson, D., Liveris, D., Hanincova, K., Sandigursky, S., Nowakowski, J., Nadelman, R.B., Ludin, S. and Schwartz, I. (2008) *Borrelia burgdorferi* genotype predicts the capacity for hematogenous dissemination during early Lyme disease. *Journal of Infectious Diseases* 198, 1358–1364.

Wormser, G.P., Shapiro, E.D. and Strle, F. (2017) Studies that report unexpected positive blood cultures for Lyme borrelia – are they valid? *Diagnostic Microbiology and Infectious Disease* 89, 178–181.

Wu, J., Weening, E.H., Faske, J.B., Hook, M. and Skare, J.T. (2011) Invasion of eukaryotic cells by *Borrelia burgdorferi* requires beta(1) integrins and Src kinase activity. *Infection and Immunity* 79, 1338–1348.

Zückert, W.R. (2013) A call to order at the spirochaetal host-pathogen interface. *Molecular Microbiology* 89, 207–211.

3 *Borreliella*: Interactions with the Host Immune System

Kirk Sperber and Raymond J. Dattwyler
New York Medical College, Valhalla, New York, USA

Lyme disease (LD) is the most common vector-borne infectious disease in North America and Europe (Stanek *et al.*, 2012). It is caused by infection with pathogenic members of the *Borrelia burgdorferi* sensu lato family (Bb) (Hu, 2012). Clinically, it is a progressive disease with a wide array of clinical manifestations. Early diagnosis and treatment is important to prevent progression (Halperin, 2012). About one third of those cases reported to the Centers for Disease Control and Prevention (CDC) represent late disease – neurological, cardiac or arthritic disease (www.cdc.gov/lyme/stats/humanCases.html). Timely antibiotic treatment of 2–3 weeks' duration is extremely effective in limiting the risk of progression (Wormser *et al.*, 2006).

The CDC estimates that there are 300,000 LD cases per year in the United States, with over 3 million LD serologies performed (www.cdc.gov/lyme/stats/humanCases.html). The number of cases and serologies ordered is increasing. Unlike most bacterial diseases where the presence of the pathogen can be defined microbiologically by direct observation, culture or polymerase chain reaction (PCR), LD is defined indirectly (Hinckley *et al.*, 2014). Erythema migrans (EM) is the classic marker of early infection, and in endemic areas, its presence is considered virtually diagnostic (Berger 1993; Nadelman *et al.*, 1996). However, not all patients infected with Bb develop EM and, even if present, it is variable in appearance and may not be recognized. It also may be fleeting and may be gone by the time a patient seeks medical attention (Stanek and Strle, 2003). Even if every patient with EM were appropriately diagnosed, the approximately 10–20% who do not develop EM – 30–60,000 people per year – need reliable laboratory diagnostics.

The infection evolves from early localized to early disseminated to late disease (Marques, 2008). The early localized form of LD starts after the tick bite and is associated with the characteristic EM skin lesion (Steere *et al.*, 2004). The early disseminated disease occurs weeks after the tick bite and is caused by bacteria that have disseminated hematogenously (Marques, 2010). Multiple skin EM lesions and extracutaneous manifestations, including acute carditis and neurologic manifestations can be present at this stage (Coyle and Schutzer, 2002). The late stage of the disease occurs months to years after the initial infection and can present as arthritis, late neuroborreliosis or acrodermatitis chronica atrophicans (Shapiro, 2014). Antibiotic treatment regimens are based on the stage or manifestation of the infection, although there are currently no established biomarkers to stage the disease (Wormser *et al.*, 2006).

Although antibiotic therapy is highly effective in the majority of cases, approximately 10% of Lyme arthritis patients develop antibiotic refractory arthritis (Steere, 2001). In this condition, the joint inflammation is not responsive to additional antibiotics, but it often responds to immunomodulatory medications like hydroxychloroquine

© CAB International 2018. *Lyme Disease: An Evidence-based Approach*, Second Edition (ed. J.J. Halperin)

(Steere et al., 1987). A small minority of patients experience persistent fatigue, and/or difficulties with concentration and memory after the antibiotic treatment even though there is no evidence of ongoing infection (Feder et al., 2007). This syndrome is termed post-treatment LD syndrome and can be associated with impairment of quality of life (Baker, 2008). The following is a brief review of the interaction of Bb with the host immune system and an update regarding how this relates to newer humoral and cellular diagnostic assays.

Interaction of Bb with the Host Immune System

The cell envelope of Bb is unusual – unlike most proteobacteria, it has no lipopolysaccharide (LPS) but rather contains large amounts of lipoproteins (Takayama et al., 1987). The expression of Bb lipoprotein varies under varying environmental conditions and Bb displays a wide array of different surface antigens depending on its location (Zhang et al., 1997). Some lipoproteins are expressed exclusively in either the mammalian host or the tick vector (Iyer et al., 2015). The ability of Bb to modify the antigenic nature of its surface by expressing different lipoproteins helps the bacteria evade the host immune system but also presents challenges in developing diagnostic assays. The bacteria can also inhibit the action of complement, which increases infectivity. The evasion of complement function by Bb is one of the best studied interactions between Bb and the host immune system (Kurternbach et al., 2002).

The susceptibility of different Bb strains to complement-mediating killing varies. Several investigators have demonstrated that Bb strains can bind complement regulatory factor H or factor H-like protein-1 and inhibit bacterial lysis (Kraiczy and Stevenson, 2013). Bb strains produce factor H-binding proteins that interfere with complement-mediated cell lysis by promoting inactivation of C3b (Kraiczy et al., 2001). For example, Bb strain B31 produces five different factor H-binding proteins (Kraiczy et al., 2003). Factor H-binding proteins are classified based on function and include complement regulator acquiring surface protein (CRASP) or genetic locus. CRASP-1 (CspA; BBA68) is a 29-kDa surface-exposed lipoprotein that binds factor H and factor H-like proteins (Hartmann et al., 2006). Inactivation of CRASP-1 in a complement-resistant strain renders Bb susceptible to complement lysis. CRASP-1 is expressed by Bb in the tick and is repressed during mammalian infection (Miller et al., 2003).

CRASP-2 (CspZ) is a 23-kDa lipoprotein that binds factor H and factor H-like protein-1 (Hovis et al., 2006). It is expressed during mammalian infection and at very low levels in ticks. Unlike CRASP-1, deletion of CRASP-2 does not affect complement sensitivity and the bacteria are as susceptible as the wild-type strain to undergoing cell lysis (Hellwage et al., 2001). CRASP-3, -4 and -5 are also referred to as ErpP, ErpC and ErpA/N, respectively; ErpP is encoded by bbn38, and ErpA is encoded by three separate loci on cp32-1, cp32-5 and cp32-8 (bbp38, bbl39). These proteins have high affinities for factor H (Bykowski et al., 2007). Other surface lipoproteins of Bb, OspE/OspF/Elp also bind factor H/factor H-like protein 1 (FHL-1) inhibiting complement function (Petzke and Schwartz, 2015). Most members of the OspE/OspF/Elp families are expressed during mammalian infection and to a lesser extent during tick colonization (Rahman et al., 2016). The overlapping functions of these proteins make gene inactivation studies difficult. The roles of CRASP-3, -4 and -5 in infectivity and pathogenesis are uncertain.

The innate immune system provides an immediate response to the presence of a pathogen or altered self-protein and initiates a protective or inflammatory response (Rahman et al., 2016). Most times this response is sufficient to control pathogenic organisms. However, if the innate response fails, the adaptive response is required to eliminate pathogens. In addition to complement, the innate immune responses include specialized leukocytes including natural killer (NK) cells, macrophages and dendritic cells (Gardiner and Mills, 2016). These cells express toll like receptors (TLRs), and intracellular sensors which are pattern recognition receptors (PRRs) that recognize pathogen-associated molecular patterns (PAMPs) expressed by invading microorganisms (Ma et al., 1994). The TLRs are membrane-bound proteins present on the cell surface or within endosomal compartments and are important to detect Bb PAMPs. Bb expresses lipoproteins that trigger responses through TLR2 but, unlike gram-negative bacteria, Bb does not contain LPS and does not induce responses through TLR4 (Ma et al., 1994).

The majority of the lipoproteins, including OspA and OspC, are immunostimulatory due to the presence of a tripalmitoyl-S-glyceryl-cysteine (Pam3Cys) modification (Brandt et al., 1990; Radolf et al., 1991). The interaction of Pam-3Cys-modified B burgdorferi lipoproteins by TLR2 results in the nuclear translocation of nuclear factor-kB (NF-kB) with the synthesis of TNF, IL-6, IL-8 and adhesion factors (E-selectin, vascular cell adhesion molecule 1 and intracellular adhesion molecule 1) (Wooten et al., 1996; Ebnet et al., 1997). Activation of TLR2 by surface-exposed spirochetal lipoproteins is the primary pathway responsible for the induction of Borrelia-elicited cytokine production and innate immunity (Lien et al., 1999; Wooten et al., 2002). There are other immunostimulatory proteins expressed by Bb. A TLR2-independent, but MyD88-dependent mechanism has been described in experiments demonstrating that TLR-2 knock-out mice infected with Bb have increased inflammation in some infected tissues despite being unable to control spirochete burdens (Wang et al., 2004). Data from different groups have demonstrated that PAMPs, PRRs and multiple signaling pathways contribute to the innate immune response to Bb in both humans and murine model systems (Moore et al., 2007; Berende et al., 2010; Miller et al., 2010).

Nucleic acid recognition by intracellular TLR receptors contributes to cytokine production by human innate immune cells in response to Bb infection. Activation of endosomal TLR-dependent signaling pathways by bacterial nucleic acid up-regulates the production of IFN-α and IFN-β by human dendritic cells and monocytes (Moore et al., 2007; Cruz et al., 2008). Different intracellular TLRs including TLR7, TLR8 and TLR 9 can recognize Bb nucleic acid. TLR7- and TLR9- recognize unmethylated Bb CpG moieties and induce the production of IFN-α by human plasmacytoid dendritic cells (Chuang et al., 2002). Synergy in signaling with TLR8 and TLR 2 has been demonstrated to be necessary for the optimal production of TNF-α, IL-6, IL-10 and IL-1β by monocytes and macrophages (Cervantes et al., 2013).

The roles of Type I IFNs in antiviral defenses and autoimmune diseases are well known, however, the role of IFN in bacterial infections is less well defined. Some studies have demonstrated that type III interferon is secreted through TLR-7 and TLR-9 signaling by human dendritic cells after bacterial infections (Petzke et al., 2009). The role of type III IFN in the immunopathogenesis of Bb infection has not been well established. Interestingly, investigators have shown that differential production of both IFN-α and type III IFNs varies depending on the virulence of the Bb genotype (Love et al., 2014). Bb strains that disseminate from skin lesions induce higher levels of IFN-α compared to strains that are less virulent (Krupna-Gaylord et al., 2014).

Over 80% of patients develop EM skin lesions at the tick bite site within 1 month (Wormser, 2006). EM is a localized immunologically mediated inflammatory response caused by spirochete replication and subsequent migration of the bacteria through the skin (Wormser, 2006). There is a paucity of studies on the immunopathogenesis of the EM. One study from central Europe investigated 42 patients with primary EM associated with B. afzelii, and found a perivascular infiltrate of mononuclear cells composed predominantly of macrophages, T cells and B cells, with a smaller number of plasma cells. In situ hybridization studies found that IFN-γ and IL-10 are the predominant cytokines expressed in these lesions. In patients with disseminated disease, TNF-α, IL-1β and IL-6 are observed (Mullegger et al., 2000). In another study by the same group, EM patients infected with B. afzelii were found to have up-regulation of T cell-active chemokines, including CXCL9 and CXCL10, with low level mRNA levels for the neutrophil chemoattractant CXCL1 and the dendritic cell chemoattractant CCL20 (Mullegger et al., 2007).

A third study compared cytokine expression in EM lesions from B. afzelii-infected patients with skin biopsy culture-confirmed Bb United States patients (Jones et al., 2008). Bb induced higher mRNA levels for chemoattractants for neutrophils (CXCL1), macrophages (CCL3 and CCL4) and CD4+ T cells (CXCL9, CXCL10, CXCL11). There was also increased mRNA expression for IL-1β, TNF-α, IL-10 and TGF-β. Bb-infected patients had more symptoms and had faster expanding lesions compared with B. afzelii-infected patients (Jones et al., 2008). The authors of the study suggested that the decreased cytokine production observed in B. afzelii-infected patients could explain the observation that *B. afzelii* disseminates less frequently than Bb but is more likely to persist in the skin (Stanek and Strle, 2003).

It is uncertain whether or not the magnitude of the local immune response contributes to spirochetal containment or dissemination. In order to address this, a study was performed involving 21 United States patients with localized or disseminated Bb infection based on a single EM lesion or multiple EM lesions. Skin biopsies were taken from the periphery of EM lesions and characterized for cytokine production and immunophenotype utilizing flow cytometry and demonstrated increased numbers of CD4+ and CD8+ T cells, monocytes/macrophage, plasmacytoid and monocytoid dendritic cells, and neutrophils. Innate immune cells expressed activation markers. IL-6 and IFN-γ were the predominant cytokines found.

Higher levels of both of these pro-inflammatory cytokines, and significantly lower levels of anti-inflammatory IL-10, were present in the EM biopsies of patients with a single lesion compared with patients with multiple EM lesions (Salazar et al., 2003). This result suggests that a strong local IFN-γ-driven pro-inflammatory cytokine response during the early stages of infection contributes to host protection. In contrast, and consistent with *ex vivo* studies using human cells, a potentially pathogen-promoting effect of type I IFN was implicated by the detection of significantly higher levels of IFN-α in biopsies of patients with multiple EM lesions. Other studies investigating vector–host interactions further support the correlation between inflammatory responses and spirochete dissemination (Haile et al., 2006; Berner et al., 2015).

Ixodes scapularis tick saliva immunomodulatory properties have been extensively investigated (Kazimirova and Stibraniova, 2013; Wikel, 2013). Both saliva and salivary proteins have been found to induce an anti-inflammatory response suppressing multiple dendritic cell functions, including CD4+ T cell proliferation and differentiation, spirochete phagocytosis and cytokine production in response to stimulation by *Borrelia* or TLR agonists (Lieskovska and Kopecky, 2012; Lieskovska et al., 2015). Tick saliva and a tick salivary cysteine protease inhibitor (sialostatin L2) interfered with type I IFN signaling via the JAK/STAT transcription pathway in mouse dendritic cells, resulting in reduced expression of two IFN-stimulated genes, interferon regulatory factor-7 and interferon gamma-inducible protein-10 (Lieskovska and Kopecky, 2012; Lieskovska et al., 2015). Co-inoculation of Bb with *I. scapularis* salivary gland lysate resulted in significantly higher spirochete burdens in the target tissues of needle-infected mice (Zeidner et al., 2002). The immunosuppressive effects of tick saliva could be partially overcome by intraperitoneal administration of pro-inflammatory cytokines (IFN-γ, TNF-α or IL-2, alone or in combination) for 10 days following a tick infection with Bb; up to 95% protection was achieved as determined by measuring the presence of spirochetes or spirochetal DNA in ear tissues (Zeidner et al., 1996). Similarly, spirochete burdens in infected tissues were reduced following the neutralization of two Th-2 cytokines, IL-4 and IL-5, in mice before transmission of Bb through tick feeding (Zeidner et al., 2008).

Human Antibody Response to *B. burgdorferi*

The adaptive immune response to infection with *B. burgdorferi* includes Ab responses to different bacterial proteins and glycolipids as noted above. An understanding of the humoral response to *Borrelia* antigens is important because the basis for the laboratory diagnosis of Lyme borreliosis is dependent on serologic assays (Johnson, 2011). Current serodiagnostics of Bb infection are largely based on studies carried out in the mid-1980s (CDC, 1995). Most contemporary Bb serodiagnostic assays still use whole cultured Bb or proteins derived from cultured Bb as antigen targets (CDC/ASTPHLD, 1994). Whole Bb or mixes of Bb proteins have the advantage of having multiple epitope targets, including conformational epitopes, but the disadvantage that some epitopes are cross-reactive with similar epitopes of other bacterial species (Wormser et al., 1999). Peptide-based diagnostics that contain one or two specific Bb epitopes, excluding cross-reactive epitopes, may provide an attractive alternative to currently available whole-protein assays (Nowakowski et al., 2001). Although peptides only contain linear epitopes and not conformational epitopes, the net gain of limiting the cross-reactive epitopes found in all whole proteins potentially far outweighs any effects from the loss of conformational epitopes (Liang et al., 2004).

The host immune response to *B burgdorferi* infection follows the usual pattern – IgM responses develop first, followed by IgG. Within 1–2 weeks following the onset of infection, IgM antibodies against *B burgdorferi* antigens can be measured in infected individuals. The earliest responses are to the 41-kDa flagellin B (FlaB) and OspC (25 kDa) with responses to a number of additional antigens, such as VlsE, fibronectin-binding protein (BBK32), FlaA (37 kDa), BmpA (39 kDa) and decorin-binding protein A (DbpA), developing later as the infection progresses (Craft et al., 1986; Coleman and Benach, 1987; Engstrom et al., 1995; Bacon et al., 2003; Nowalk et al., 2006).

VlsE and its IR6 region are among the best studied antigens in this latter group. Although the C6 enzyme linked immunosorbent assay (ELISA) based on the IR6 antigen was suggested as a possible single tier assay, it is not sufficiently specific. Additional drawbacks in using the IR6 peptide as the sole antigen include that VlsE is not expressed in the tick and is only expressed in the mammalian host after infection is established (Das et al., 1997; Hefty et al., 2001; Bykowski et al., 2006). The genes coding for VlsE are not induced until several days post-infection (Lahdenne et al., 2003; Alghaferi et al., 2005). Thus, in comparison to FlaB, OspC and other antigens expressed in the feeding tick, there is a delay in IR6 being available to the immune system. Lahdenne et al. (Engstrom et al., 1995) found that only 29/75 (39%) of patients with EM for 7–14 days had IgG antibodies to the IR6 peptide antigen, while 65/75 (87%) of these patients had IgG antibodies to one or more variants of BBK32, an antigen expressed in the feeding tick. Further complicating the use of the IR6 peptide to detect antibodies in early infection is that IR6 does not bind IgM very well. Embers et al. (2007) found that in a group of 37 patients with early LD, only one developed significant levels of IgM against IR6; the other 36 failed to develop levels greater than the healthy controls. In a study comparing the development of anti-VlsE IgM responses to the OspC peptide, pepC10, the sensitivity of the pepC10 ELISA was approximately 10 times greater in patients who presented within 1 week after the onset of EM (Mathiesen et al., 1998). These studies highlight the reasons why IR6-based assays cannot be relied on to accurately identify patients during the critical first weeks of infection. An additional issue with the IR6 peptide is that, like most bacterial antigens, the IR6 region of Bb is variable and, although it contains a relatively conserved epitope, there are sequence differences both between genospecies and within genospecies (Gomes-Solecki et al., 2007).

It has been possible to map the key proteins of Bb, identifying specific linear epitopes from OspC type K (Earnhart et al., 2005), OspC type A (Earnhart et al., 2005), FliLB (Barbour et al., 2008), DbpA (Roberts et al., 1998), DbpB (Pal et al., 2008), BmpA (Pal et al., 2008), OppA-II (Signorino et al., 2014), BBG33 (Arnaboldi and Dattwyler, 2015), LA-7 (Kraiczy et al., 2004), RecA (Liveris et al., 2004), ErpP (Brangulis et al., 2015), Bbk32 (Lahdenne et al., 2006), OspF (Wagner et al., 2013), p35 (Fikrig et al., 1997), CRASP2 (Kraiczy et al., 2004), p93 (Chandra et al., 2011) and p66 (Arnaboldi and Dattwyler, 2015). This allows for the development of seroassays with antigen targets composed of specific epitopes. It is problematic to have only one or two epitope targets in a sero-assay because the immune response to an individual epitope can vary between individuals. It has been demonstrated that resistance to variability (noise) in a test increases as the number of antigen targets increases (Bunikis and Barbour, 2002). Thus, while the efficacy of a single-peptide-based serological assay is limited by both antigenic variation and the variability inherent in the human immune response, a multi-peptide assay containing specific epitopes from several different Bb antigens significantly reduces these effects, maintaining superior specificity and sensitivity. Embers et al. proposed that an assay based on a combination of OppA2, DbpA, OspC, OspA and the C6 peptide would have the potential for detecting LD at all stages (Embers et al., 2016). Combining multiple peptides allows for the creation of a sensitive assay that offers the ability to independently analyze each antigen.

A multiplex assay utilizing peptides containing specific epitopes and select recombinant Bb antigens for the detection of anti-Bb antibodies offers the possibility of significantly improving sensitivity and specificity compared to current

LD serodiagnostics. A pilot study identified sensitive and specific antigen targets. Assays using peptides comprising epitopes from Erp and p35 proteins coupled to an IR6-like epitope were sensitive and as specific as the current two tier method (Lahey et al., 2015). Erp and p35 proteins are expressed by Bb very early in the course of infection and are important in the pathogenesis of LD. Members of the Erp protein family, OspE and F, bind both complement inhibitor factor H and plasminogen, allowing Bb to evade complement-mediated killing, bind host endothelium through plasminogen receptors and gain surface protease activity as noted above (Fikrig et al., 2000; Brissette et al., 2009). The p35 protein binds fibronectin, enabling Bb to attach to the extracellular matrix of the host (Probert et al., 1998; Strother et al., 2007). This supports the hypothesis that peptides derived from early-expressed virulence proteins have significant diagnostic utility.

Cellular Assays to Detect Infection with Bb

As part of the adaptive immune response, Bb-specific CD4+ and CD8+ T cells are generated that play a role in protection. Evidence of the importance of T cells has been demonstrated by the increased severity of disease in severe combined deficient (SCID) mice infected with Bb (Strother et al., 2007). It has been further suggested that NK T cells play a role in LD since a diacylglycerol glycolipid derived from Bb triggers a CD1d-dependent NK response (Katchar et al., 2013). Mice that are NK deficient are more susceptible to infection than wild-type mice with more joint damage (Katchar et al., 2013). A study by Kubes and colleagues suggests that iNKT cells are stimulated by Bb to limit the bacterial infection (Zajonc and Girardi, 2015). It had been previously demonstrated by this group that iNKT cells are activated by liver macrophages to induce an anti-Bb immune response. However, in iNKT cell-deficient mice infected with Bb, the bacteria accumulate in joints. In the liver, iNKT cells were located in blood vessels in contrast to iNKT cells that were found in knee joints and were present near the surface of the knee joint. It was further demonstrated that blocking CD1d had no effect on Bb killing, but interfering with granzymes eliminated Bb killing in the knee. The authors suggested that the reduced frequency of iNKT cells in human joints compared with in mice could explain why Bb infection leads to Lyme arthritis in humans, but not in rodents (Zajonc and Girardi, 2015).

Patients first develop signs or symptoms approximately a week after initial introduction of Bb into the skin by the feeding tick (Hinckley et al., 2014). Initial T and B cell activation occurs during this interval between the onset of infection and clinical manifestations. T cell responses have distinct kinetics compared to serum antibody responses (Dattwyler et al., 1988). Most notably, T cells are typically activated shortly after infection and, in contrast to IgG antibody-producing cells that remain elevated for years, the population of activated T cells wanes rapidly, coincident with clearance of the pathogen (Zoschke et al., 1991). In addition, T cell activation is primarily mediated through recognition of linear peptide epitopes presented in the context of MHC molecules on the surface of APCs; this also presents opportunities to establish a high specificity assay by excluding non-specific 'cross-reactive' epitopes (Nurmi et al., 1988; Shanafelt et al., 1992). It is therefore reasonable to hypothesize that a test that accurately monitors T cell activation specific for unique *Borrelia* spp. epitopes could be sensitive and discriminate active LD from past exposure. Moreover, the success of the QuantiFERON assay for *Mycobacterium tuberculosis* infection (Grinsdale et al., 2016), which accurately monitors T cell activation indirectly by measuring IFN-γ levels in blood plasma, provides additional compelling evidence that a T cell-based diagnostic assay for LD is feasible.

T cells that are specific for Bb are activated at the onset of infection. Activated T cells produce cytokines that have multiple functions including the maturation of Bb-specific B cells (Lasky et al., 2016). After the infection subsides the T cell response is diminished, resulting in reduced pro-inflammatory cytokine production with a marked reduction of activated T cells. An assay that can monitor activated T cells could be of utility and as an adjunct to Bb serology. The assay that determines the presence of activated T cells may be more accurate and provide better evidence of active infection compared to humoral responses.

Initial studies aimed at following anti-Bb T cell responses in patients with LD provided mixed results (Benach et al., 1988). These studies were not conclusive because they measured T cell proliferation to detect the presence of active infection. Unfortunately, a lack of specificity is a major drawback for this type of study. In addition, IFN-γ is commonly produced during Bb infection, which is well known to suppress T cell proliferation, reducing the utility of proliferation as a means to establish an active infection (Leguern, 2011). Other assays evaluating different aspects of T cell proliferation including antigen-induced cytokine release could provide a more accurate method to monitor T cell activation. Investigators have demonstrated the utility of such an approach. For example, it has been demonstrated that the IFN-γ produced by the peripheral blood mononuclear cells can provide useful information to confirm the presence of neurological LD (Forsberg et al., 1995; Widhe et al., 2005). There is also laboratory confirmation that this approach is valid. Bb antigens have been shown to induce IFN-γ *in vitro*. Decorin-binding protein A, outer-surface protein C (OspC), p100 or vmp-like sequence lipoprotein E induce IFN-γ production from T cells from LD patients following stimulation (Jin et al., 2013).

Our group evaluated the utility of a test measuring T cell immunity during LD (Callister et al., 2015). This test utilized QuantiFERON® technology that was developed to detect *Mycobacterium tuberculosis* infection by measuring the presence of IFN-γ from early LD patients. This assay included a 16-h incubation with *Borrelia* antigens p66, decorin-binding protein B (DbpB), OspC and flagellin (41 kDa) with whole blood of LD patients followed by detection of IFN-γ in the culture supernatant (Callister et al., 2015). Antibody testing is not helpful for assessing response to treatment since antibodies persist even though the spirochetes have been eliminated by antibiotic therapy. The lack of sensitivity during early infection and the persistence of positive serology despite the successful resolution of infection are problematic. The arthralgia and myalgia commonly observed in LD patients frequently are attributed to active infections even though the infection has been successfully treated with antibiotics.

In our study, there was considerable IFN-γ production after incubating early LD patient whole blood with *Borrelia* species peptides (Callister et al., 2015). Sixty-nine percent of the patients synthesized significant amounts of IFN-γ, in line with other studies that have demonstrated IFN-γ production during Bb infection (Kowalski et al., 2010). In our study, IFN-γ was produced from both CD4+ and CD8+ T cells (Callister et al., 2015). There was no correlation between IFN-γ levels with either the presence of single or multiple EM or the clinical severity of the infection (Callister et al., 2015). The IFN-γ release assay was more sensitive than the C6 ELISA (69% vs. 59%, respectively) and much more sensitive than Western blotting (17%) for the diagnosis of early disease (Callister et al., 2015). Subgroup analysis of the results comparing the C6 ELISA and the IFN-γ release assay gave different results although the overall sensitivity was almost the same (Callister et al., 2015). Eleven patients were positive for anti-C6 antibodies or only IFN-γ (Callister et al., 2015). A complementary approach yielded better results. A combination of the C6 and IFN-γ release assays increased the sensitivity of diagnosing early LD to 83% (24 of 29) (Callister et al., 2015).

Antibody responses for LD as assayed by the C6 assay and Western blotting can persist and even increase in titer despite successful antimicrobial therapy (Kowalski et al., 2010). This is in sharp contrast to the secretion of IFN-γ, which declines with successful therapy. It has been demonstrated by Kowalski et al. (2010) that antibiotic therapy (doxycycline) almost never fails to resolve early LD. This finding is consonant with other investigations pointing out the ineffectiveness of serology to determine the success of antibiotic treatment. In our study, levels of IFN-γ declined with doxycycline treatment and were absent in almost all (78%) of the patients with early LD within 2 months after the course of antibiotics was completed (Callister et al., 2015). Our study demonstrates the potential of measuring IFN-γ secretion after stimulation with *Borrelia* species antigens for a more accurate and sensitive test to make a laboratory diagnosis of early LD. Another corollary of our findings is the short-lived cytokine response to Bb antigens after effective antibiotic therapy of the infection.

Conclusion

Bb has complex interactions with its host, allowing it to evade detection and destruction by both the humoral and cellular components of the immune system. The anti-Bb response can be exploited to develop new and more accurate diagnostic testing allowing for earlier treatment of this infection. The evaluation of novel diagnostic markers on a multiplex antigen panel and in a T cell proliferative assay aimed at improving the immunologic detection of Bb in early LD patients provides a foundation for the development of the next generation of assays for the laboratory diagnosis of LD – in particular to aid the clinician in diagnosing and treating early LD. Our studies have shown that the 10-antigen panel and the T cell proliferative assay are more sensitive to detect early LD than the C6 assay and Western blotting. Our findings require validation in larger cohorts and in patients infected with *Borrelia* genospecies from other parts of the world (Asia and Europe). The 10-antigen panel and the T cell proliferation assay should provide a more accurate and sensitive methodology to detect LD.

References

Alghaferi, M.Y., Anderson, J.M., Park, J., Auwaerter, P.G., Aucott, J.N., Norris, D.E. and Dumler, J.S. (2005) *Borrelia burgdorferi* ospC heterogeneity among human and murine isolates from a defined region of northern Maryland and southern Pennsylvania: lack of correlation with invasive and noninvasive genotypes. *Journal of Clinical Microbiology* 43(4), 1879–1884.

Arnaboldi, P.M. and Dattwyler, R.J. (2015) Cross-reactive epitopes in *Borrelia burgdorferi* p66. *Clinical and Vaccine Immunology* 22(7), 840–843.

Bacon, R.M., Biggerstaff, B.J., Schriefer, M.E., Gilmore, R.D., Philipp, M.T., Steere, A.C., Wormser, G.P., Marques, A.R. and Johnson, B.J.B. (2003) Serodiagnosis of lyme disease by kinetic enzyme-linked immunosorbent assay using recombinant VlsE1 or peptide antigens of *Borrelia burgdorferi* compared with 2-tiered testing using whole-cell lysates. *Journal of Infectious Diseases* 187, 1187–1199.

Baker, P.J. (2008) Perspectives on "chronic Lyme disease." *American Journal of Medicine* 121, 562–564.

Barbour, A.G., Jasinskas, A., Kayala, M.A., Davies, D.H., Steere, A.C., Baldi, P. and Felgner, P.L. (2008) A genome-wide proteome array reveals a limited set of immunogens in natural infections of humans and white-footed mice with *Borrelia burgdorferi*. *Infection and Immunity* 76(8), 3374–3389.

Benach, J.L., Coleman, J.L., Garcia-Moreno, J.C. and Deponte, P.C. (1988) Biological activity of *Borrelia burgdorferi*. *Annals of the New York Academy of Science* 9339, 115–125.

Berende, A., Oosting, M., Kullberg, B.J., Netea, M.G. and Joosten, L.A.B. (2010) Activation of innate host defense mechanisms by *Borrelia*. *European Cytokine Network* 21, 7–18.

Berger, B.W. (1993) Lyme disease. *Seminars in Dermatology* 12(4), 357–362.

Berner, A., Bachmann, M., Pfeilschifter, J., Kraiczy, P. and Mühl, H. (2015) Interferon-α curbs production of interleukin-22 by human peripheral blood mononuclear cells exposed to live *Borrelia burgdorferi*. *Journal of Cellular and Molecular Medicine* 19(10), 2507–2511.

Brandt, M.E., Riley, B.S., Radolf, J.D. *et al.* (1990) Immunogenic integral membrane proteins of *Borrelia burgdorferi* are lipoproteins. *Infection and Immunity* 58, 573–577.

Brangulis, K., Petrovskis, I., Kazaks, A., Akopjana, I. and Tars, K. (2015) Crystal structures of the Erp protein family members *ErpP* and *ErpC* from *Borrelia burgdorferi* reveal the reason for different affinities for complement regulator factor H. *Biochimica et Biophysica Acta* 1854(5), 349–355.

Brissette, C.A., Haupt, K., Barthel, D., Cooley, A.E., Bowman, A., Skerka, C., Wallich, R., Zipfel, P.F., Kraiczy, P. and Stevenson, B. (2009) *Borrelia burgdorferi* infection-associated surface proteins ErpP, ErpA, and ErpC bind human plasminogen. *Infection and Immunity* 77, 300–306.

Bunikis, J. and Barbour, A.G. (2002) Laboratory testing for suspected Lyme disease. *Medical Clinics of North America* 86(2), 311–340.

Bykowski, T., Babb, K., von Lackum, K., Riley, S.P., Norris, S.J. and Stevenson, B. (2006) Transcriptional regulation of the *Borrelia burgdorferi* antigenically variable VlsE surface protein. *Journal of Bacteriology* 188, 4879–4889.

Bykowski, T., Woodman, M.E., Cooley, A.E. *et al.* (2007) Coordinated expression of *Borrelia burgdorferi* regulator-acquiring proteins during the Lyme disease spirochete's mammal-tick infection cycle. *Infection and Immunity* 75, 4227–4236.

Callister, S.M., Jobe, D.A., Stuparic-Stancic, A., Miyamasu, M., Boyle, J., Dattwyler, R.J. and Arnaboldi, P.M. (2015) Detection of IFN-γ secretion by T cells collected before and after successful treatment of early Lyme disease. *Clinical Infectious Diseases* 62, 1235–1241.

CDC/ASTPHLD (1994) *Proceedings of the Second National Conference on Serologic Diagnosis of Lyme Disease*. CDC/ASTPHLD, Dearborn, Michigan.

Centers for Disease Control and Prevention (CDC) (1995) Recommendations for test performance and interpretation from the Second National Conference on Serologic Diagnosis of Lyme Disease. *Morbidity and Mortality Weekly Report* 44, 590–591.

Cervantes, J.L., La Vake, C.J., Weinerman, B. *et al.* (2013) Human TLR8 is activated upon recognition of *Borrelia burgdorferi* RNA in the phagosome of human monocytes. *Journal of Leukocyte Biology* 94, 1231–1241.

Chandra, A., Wormser, G.P., Marques, A.R., Latov, N. and Alaedini, A. (2011) Anti-*Borrelia burgdorferi* antibody profile in post-Lyme disease syndrome. *Clinical and Vaccine Immunology* 18(5), 767–771.

Chuang, T.H., Lee, J., Kline, L. *et al.* (2002) Toll-like receptor 9 mediates CpG-DNA signaling. *Journal of Leukocyte Biology* 71, 538–544.

Coleman, J.L. and Benach, J.L. (1987) Isolation of antigenic components from the Lyme disease spirochete: their role in early diagnosis. *The Journal of Infectious Diseases* 155(4), 756–765.

Coyle, P.K. and Schutzer, S.E. (2002) Neurologic aspects of Lyme disease. *Medical Clinics of North America* 86(2), 261–284.

Craft, J.E., Fischer, D.K., Shimamoto, G.T. and Steere, A.C. (1986) Antigens of *Borrelia burgdorferi* recognized during Lyme disease. Appearance of a new immunoglobulin M response and expansion of the immunoglobulin G response late in the illness. *Journal of Clinical Investigation* 78(4), 934–939.

Cruz, A.R., Moore, M.W., La Vake, C.J. *et al.* (2008) Phagocytosis of *Borrelia burgdorferi*, the Lyme disease spirochete, potentiates innate immune activation and induces apoptosis in human monocytes. *Infection and Immunity* 76, 56–70.

Das, S., Barthold, S.W., Giles, S.S., Montgomery, R.R., Telford, S.R. III and Fikrig, E. (1997) Temporal pattern of *Borrelia burgdorferi* p21 expression in ticks and the mammalian host. *Journal of Clinical Investigation* 99(5), 987–995.

Dattwyler, R.J., Volkman, D.J., Halperin, J.J., Luft, B.J., Thomas, J. and Golightly, M.G. (1988) Specific immune responses in Lyme borreliosis. Characterization of T cell and B cell responses to *Borrelia burgdorferi*. *Annals of the New York Academy of Sciences* 539, 93–102.

Earnhart, C.G., Buckles, E.L., Dumler, J.S. and Marconi, R.T. (2005) Demonstration of diversity in invasive human lyme disease isolates and identification of previously uncharacterized epitopes that define the specificity of the OspC murine antibody response. *Infection and Immunity* 273(12), 7869–7877.

Ebnet, K., Brown, K.D., Siebenlist, U.K. *et al.* (1997) *Borrelia burgdorferi* activates nuclear factor-kappa B and is a potent inducer of chemokine and adhesion molecule gene expression in endothelial cells and fibroblasts. *Journal of Immunology* 158, 3285–3292.

Embers, M.E., Jacobs, M.B., Johnson, B.J. and Philipp, M.T. (2007) Dominant epitopes of the C6 diagnostic peptide of *Borrelia burgdorferi* are largely inaccessible to antibody on the parent VlsE molecule. *Clinical and Vaccine Immunology* 14, 931–936.

Embers, M.E., Hasenkampf, N.R., Barnes, M.B., Didier, E.S., Philipp, M.T. and Tardo, A.C. (2016) Five-antigen fluorescent bead-based assay for diagnosis of Lyme disease. *Clinical and Vaccine Immunology* 23, 294–303.

Engstrom, S.M., Shoop, E. and Johnson, R.C. (1995) Immunoblot interpretation criteria for serodiagnosis of early Lyme disease. *Journal of Clinical Microbiology* 33(2), 419–427.

Feder, H.M. Jr, Johnson, B.J., O'Connell, S. *et al.* (2007) A critical appraisal of 'chronic Lyme disease'. *New England Journal of Medicine* 357, 1422–1430.

Fikrig, E., Barthold, S.W., Sun, W., Feng, W., Telford, S.R. III and Flavell, R. (1997) *Borrelia burgdorferi* P35 and P37 proteins, expressed *in vivo*, elicit protective immunity. *Immunity* 6, 531–539.

Fikrig, E., Feng, W., Barthold, S.W., Telford, S.R. III and Flavell, R.A. (2000) Arthropod- and host-specific *Borrelia burgdorferi* bbk32 expression and the inhibition of spirochete transmission. *Journal of Immunology* 164, 5344–5351.

Forsberg, P., Ernerudh, J., Ekerfelt, C., Roberg, M., Vrethem, M. and Bergstrom, S. (1995) The outer surface proteins of Lyme disease *Borrelia* spirochetes stimulate T cells to secrete interferon-gamma (IFNγ): diagnostic and pathogenic implications. *Clinical and Experimental Immunology* 101, 453–460.

Gardiner, C.M. and Mills, K.H. (2016) The cells that mediate innate immune memory and their functional significance in inflammatory and infectious diseases. *Seminars in Immunology* 28, 343–350.

Gomes-Solecki, M.J., Meirelles, L., Glass, J. and Dattwyler, R.J. (2007) Epitope length, genospecies dependency, and serum panel effect in the IR6 enzyme-linked immunosorbent assay for detection of antibodies to *Borrelia burgdorferi*. *Clinical and Vaccine Immunology* 14, 875–879.

Grinsdale, J.A., Islam, S., Tran, O.C., Ho, C.S., Kawamura, L.M. and Higashi, J.M. (2016) Interferon-gamma release assays and pediatric public health tuberculosis screening: the San Francisco program experience 2005 to 2008. *Journal of the Pediatric Infectious Diseases Society* 5, 122–130.

Haile, W.B., Coleman, J.L. and Benach, J.L. (2006) Reciprocal upregulation of urokinase plasminogen activator and its inhibitor, PAI-2, by *Borrelia burgdorferi* affects bacterial penetration and host-inflammatory response. *Cellular Microbiology* 8(8), 1349–1360.

Halperin, J.J. (2012) Lyme disease: a multisystem infection that affects the nervous system. *Continuum* 18 (6 Infectious Disease), 1338–1350.

Hartmann, K., Corvey, C., Skerka, C. et al. (2006) Functional characterization of BbCRASP-2, a distinct outer membrane protein of *Borrelia burgdorferi* that binds to host complement regulators factor H and FHL. *Molecular Microbiology* 61, 1220–1236.

Hefty, P.S., Jolliff, S.E., Caimano, M.J., Wikel, S.K., Radolf, J.D. and Akins, D.R. (2001) Regulation of OspE-related, OspF-related, and Elp lipoproteins of *Borrelia burgdorferi* strain 297 by mammalian host-specific signals. *Infection and Immunity* 69(6), 3618–3627.

Hellwage, J., Meri, T. and Heikkila, T. (2001) The complement regulator factor H binds to the surface protein OspE of *Borrelia burgdorferi*. *Journal of Biological Chemistry* 276, 8427–8435.

Hinckley, A.F., Connally, N.P., Meek, J.I., Johnson, B.J., Kemperman, M.M., Feldman, K.A., White, J.L. and Mead, P.S. (2014) Lyme disease testing by large commercial laboratories in the United States. *Clinical Infectious Diseases* 59, 676–681.

Hovis, K.M., Tran, E., Sundy, C.M., Buckles, E., McDowell, J.V. and Marconi, R.T. (2006) Selective binding of *Borrelia burgdorferi* OspE paralogs to factor H and serum proteins from diverse animals: possible expansion of the role of OspE in Lyme disease pathogenesis. *Infection and Immunity* 74(3), 1967–1972.

Hu, L. (2012) In the clinic: Lyme disease. *Annals of Internal Medicine* 157, ITC2-m2-ITC2-16.

Iyer, R., Caiminao, M.J., Luthra, A. et al. (2015) Stage-specific global alterations in the transcriptomes of Lyme disease spirochetes during the tick feeding and following mammalian host adaption. *Molecular Microbiology* 85, 509–538.

Jin, C., Roen, D.R., Lehmann, P.V. and Kellermann, G.H. (2013) An enhanced ELISPOT assay for sensitive detection of antigen-specific T cell responses to *Borrelia burgdorferi*. *Cells* 13, 607–620.

Johnson, B.J. (2011) Laboratory diagnostic testing for *Borrelia burgdorferi* infection. In Halperin, J.J. (ed.) *Lyme Disease: An Evidence-based Approach*. CAB International, Wallingford, UK, pp. 73–88.

Jones, K.L., Muellegger, R.R., Means, T.K. et al. (2008) Higher mRNA levels of chemokines and cytokines associated with macrophage activation in erythema migrans skin lesions in patients from the United States than in patients from Austria with Lyme borreliosis. *Clinical Infectious Diseases* 46, 85–92.

Katchar, K., Drouin, E.E. and Steere, A.C. (2013) Natural killer cells and natural killer T cells in Lyme arthritis. *Arthritis Research and Therapy* 15, R183.

Kazimirova, M. and Stibraniova, I. (2013) Tick salivary compounds: their role in modulation of host defences and pathogen transmission. *Frontiers in Cellular and Infection Microbiology* 3, 43.

Kowalski, T.J., Tata, S., Berth, W., Mathiason, M.A. and Agger, W.A. (2010) Antibiotic treatment duration and long-term outcomes of patients with early Lyme disease from a Lyme disease-hyperendemic area. *Clinical Infectious Diseases* 50, 512–520.

Kraiczy, P. and Stevenson, B. (2013) Complement regulator-acquiring surface proteins of *Borrelia burgdorferi* structure, function, and regulation of gene expression. *Ticks and Tick-borne Diseases* 4, 26–34.

Kraiczy, P., Skerka, P., Brade, V. and Zipfel, P.F. (2001) Further characterization of complement regulator-acquiring surface proteins of *Borrelia burgdoferi*. *Infection and Immunity* 69, 7800–7809.

Kraiczy, P., Hellwage, J., Skerka, C. et al. (2003) Complement resistance of *Borrelia burgdorferi* correlates with the expression of BbCRASP-1, a novel linear plasmid-encoded surface protein that interacts with human factor H and FHL-1 and is unrelated to Erp proteins. *Journal of Biological Chemistry* 279, 2421–2419.

Kraiczy, P., Hartmann, K., Hellwage, J., Skerka, C., Kirschfink, M., Brade, V., Zipfel, P.F., Wallich, R. and Stevenson, B. (2004) Immunological characterization of the complement regulator factor H-binding CRASP and Erp proteins of *Borrelia burgdorferi*. *International Journal of Medical Microbiology* 293 Suppl 37, 152–157.

Krupna-Gaylord, M.A., Liveris, D., Love, A.C. et al. (2014) Induction of type I and type III interferons by *Borrelia burgdorferi* correlates with pathogenesis and requires linear plasmid 36. *PLoS One* 9, e100174.

Kurternbach, K., DeMichelis, S., Etti, S. et al. (2002) Host association of *Borrelia burgdorferi* sensu lato – the key role of host complement. *Trends in Microbiology* 10, 74–79.

Lahdenne, P., Panelius, J., Saxen, H., Heikkila, T., Sillanpaa, H., Peltomaa, M., Arnez, M., Huppertz, H.I. and Seppala, I.J. (2003) Improved serodiagnosis of erythema migrans using novel recombinant borrelial BBK32 antigens. *Journal of Medical Microbiology* 52, 563–567.

Lahdenne, P., Sarvas, H., Kajanus, R., Eholuoto, M., Sillanpää, H. and Seppälä, I. (2006) Antigenicity of borrelial protein *BBK32* fragments in early Lyme borreliosis. *Journal of Medical Microbiology* 55(11), 1499–1504.

Lahey, L.J., Panas, M.W., Mao, R., Delanoy, M., Flanagan, J.J., Binder, S.R., Rebman, A.W., Montoya, J.G., Soloski, M.J., Steere, A.C., Dattwyler, R.J., Arnaboldi, P.M., Aucott, J.N. and Robinson, W.H. (2015) Development of a multiantigen panel for improved detection of *Borrelia burgdorferi* infection in early Lyme disease. *Journal of Clinical Microbiology* 53(12), 3834–3841.

Lasky, C.E., Pratt, C.L., Hilliard, K.A., Jones, J.L. and Brown, C.R. (2016) T cells exacerbate Lyme borreliosis in TLR2-deficient mice. *Frontiers in Immunology* 3(7), 468.

Leguern, C. (2011) Regulatory T cells for tolerance therapy: revisiting the concept. *Critical Reviews in Immunology* 31, 189–207.

Liang, F.T., Yan, J., Mbow, M.L., Sviat, S.L. Gilmore, R.D., Mamula, M. and Fikrig, E. (2004) *Borrelia burgdorferi* changes its surface antigenic expression in response to host immune responses. *Infection and Immunity* 72, 5759–5767.

Lien, E., Sellati, T.J., Yoshimura, A. *et al.* (1999) Toll-like receptor 2 functions as a pattern recognition receptor for diverse bacterial products. *Journal of Biological Chemistry* 274, 33419–33425.

Lieskovska, J. and Kopecky, J. (2012) Tick saliva suppresses IFN signalling in dendritic cells upon *Borrelia afzelii* infection. *Parasite Immunology* 34, 32–39.

Lieskovska, J., Palenikova, J., Sirmarova, J. *et al.* (2015) Tick salivary cystatin sialostatin L2 suppresses IFN responses in mouse dendritic cells. *Parasite Immunology* 37, 70–78.

Liveris, D., Mulay, V. and Schwartz, I. (2004) Functional properties of *Borrelia burgdorferi* recA. *Journal of Bacteriology* 186(8), 2275–2280.

Love, A.C., Schwartz, I. and Petzke, M.M. (2014) *Borrelia burgdorferi* RNA induces type I and III interferons via Toll-like receptor 7 and contributes to production of NF-kB dependent cytokines. *Infection and Immunity* 82, 2405–2416.

Ma, Y., Seiler, K.P., Tat, K.F., Yang, L., Woods, M. and Weis, J.J. (1994) Outer surface lipoproteins of *Borrelia burgdorferi* stimulate nitric oxide production by the cytokine-inducible pathway. *Infection and Immunity* 62, 3663–3671.

Marques, A. (2008) Chronic Lyme disease: a review. *Infectious Disease Clinics of North America* 22, 341–360.

Marques, A.R. (2010) Lyme disease: a review. *Current Allergy and Asthma Reports* 10, 13–20.

Mathiesen, M.J., Christiansen, M., Hansen, K., Holm, A., Asbrink, E. and Theisen, M. (1998) Peptide-based OspC enzyme-linked immunosorbent assay for serodiagnosis of Lyme borreliosis. *Journal of Clinical Microbiology* 12, 3474–3479.

Miller, J.C., Maylor-Hagen, H., Ma, Y., Weis, J.H. and Weis, J.J. (2010) The Lyme disease spirochete *Borrelia burgdorferi* utilizes multiple ligands, including RNA, for interferon regulatory factor 3-dependent induction of type I interferon-responsive genes. *Infection and Immunity* 78, 3144–3153.

Miller, J.C., von Lackum, K., Babb, K. *et al.* (2003) Temporal analysis of *Borrelia burgdorferi* Erp expression throughout the mammalial–tick infectious cycle. *Infection and Immunity* 71, 6943–6952.

Moore, M.W., Cruz, A.R., LaVake, C.J. *et al.* (2007) Phagocytosis of *Borrelia burgdorferi* and *Treponema pallidum* potentiates innate immune activation and induces gamma interferon production. *Infection and Immunity* 75, 2046–2062.

Mullegger, R.R., McHugh, G., Ruthazer, R. *et al.* (2000) Differential expression of cytokine mRNA in skin specimens from patients with erythema migrans or acrodermatitis chronica atrophicans. *Journal of Investigative Dermatology* 115, 1115–1123.

Mullegger, R.R., Means, T.K., Shin, J.J. *et al.* (2007) Chemokine signatures in the skin disorders of Lyme borreliosis in Europe: predominance of CXCL9 and CXCL10 in erythema migrans and acrodermatitis and CXCL13 in lymphocytoma. *Infection and Immunity* 75, 4621–4628.

Nadelman, R.B., Nowakowski, J., Forseter, G. *et al.* (1996) The clinical spectrum of early Lyme borreliosis in patients with culture-confirmed erythema migrans. *American Journal of Medicine* 100, 502–508.

Nowakowski, J., Schwartz, I., Liveris, D., Wang, G., Aguero-Rosenfeld, M.E., Girao, G., McKenna, D., Nadelman, R.B., Cavaliere, L.F., Wormser, G.P. and Lyme Disease Study Group (2001) Laboratory diagnostic techniques for patients with early Lyme disease associated with erythema migrans: a comparison of different techniques. *Clinical Infectious Diseases* 33, 2023–2027.

Nowalk, A.J., Gilmore Jr, R.D. and Carroll, J.A. (2006) Serologic proteome analysis of *Borrelia burgdorferi* membrane-associated proteins. *Infection and Immunity* 74, 3864–3873.

Nurmi, L., McKernan, L., Blank, K.J., Spitanly, G.L. and Muraslo, D.M. (1988) Inhibition of macrophage induced antigen specific T cell proliferation by IFN-gamma. *Cell* 114, 432–439.

Pal, U., Wang, P., Bao, F., Yang, X., Samanta, S., Schoen, R., Wormser, G.P., Schwartz, I. and Fikrig, E. (2008) *Borrelia burgdorferi* basic membrane proteins A and B participate in the genesis of Lyme arthritis. *Journal of Experimental Medicine* 205(1), 133–141.

Petzke, M. and Schwartz, I. (2015) *Borrelia burgdorferi* pathogenesis and the immune response. *Clinical Chemistry and Laboratory Medicine* 35, 745–764.

Petzke, M.M., Brooks, A., Krupna, M.A. et al. (2009) Recognition of *Borrelia burgdorferi*, the Lyme disease spirochete, by TLR7 and TLR9 induces a type I IFN response by human immune cells. *Journal of Immunology* 183, 5279–5292.

Probert, W.S. and Johnson, B.J. (1998) Identification of a 47 kDa fibronectin-binding protein expressed by *Borrelia burgdorferi* isolate B31. *Molecular Microbiology* 30, 1003–1015.

Radolf, J.D., Norgard, M.V., Brandt, M.E. et al. (1991) Lipoproteins of *Borrelia burgdorferi* and *Treponema pallidum* activate cachectin/tumor necrosis factor synthesis. Analysis using a CAT reporter construct. *Journal of Immunology* 147, 1968–1974.

Rahman, S., Shering, M., Ogden, N.H., Lindsay, R. and Badawi, A. (2016) Toll-like receptor cascade and gene polymorphism in host-pathogen interaction in Lyme disease. *Journal of Inflammation Research* 9, 91–102.

Roberts, W.C., Mullikin, B.A., Lathigra, R. and Hanson, M.S. (1998) Molecular analysis of sequence heterogeneity among genes encoding decorin binding proteins A and B of *Borrelia burgdorferi* sensu lato. *Infection and Immunity* 66(11), 5275–5285.

Salazar, J.C., Pope, C.D., Sellati, T.J. et al. (2003) Coevolution of markers of innate and adaptive immunity in skin and peripheral blood of patients with erythema migrans. *Journal of Immunology* 171, 2660–2670.

Shanafelt, M.C., Anzola, J., Soderberg, C., Yssel, H., Turck, C.W. and Peltz, C.W. (1992) Epitopes on the outer surface protein A of *Borrelia burgdorferi* recognized by antibodies and T cells of patients with Lyme disease. *Journal of Immunology* 48, 218–224.

Shapiro, E.D. (2014) Clinical practice. Lyme disease. *New England Journal of Medicine* 370, 1724–1731.

Signorino, G., Arnaboldi, P.M., Petzke, M.M. and Dattwyler, R.J. (2014) Identification of OppA2 linear epitopes as serodiagnostic markers for Lyme disease. *Clinical and Vaccine Immunology* 21(5), 704–711.

Stanek, G. and Strle, F. (2003) Lyme borreliosis. *Lancet* 362, 1639–1647.

Stanek, G., Wormser, G.P., Gray, J. and Strle, F. (2012) Lyme borreliosis. *Lancet* 379, 461–473.

Steere, A.C. (2001) Lyme disease. *New England Journal of Medicine* 345, 115–125.

Steere, A.C., Schoen, R.T. and Taylor, E. (1987) The clinical evolution of Lyme arthritis. *Annals of Internal Medicine* 107, 725–731.

Steere, A.C., Coburn, J. and Glickstein, L. (2004) The emergence of Lyme disease. *Journal of Clinical Investigation* 113, 1093–1101.

Strother, K.O., Hodzic, E., Barthold, S.W. and de Silva, A.M. (2007) Infection of mice with Lyme disease spirochetes constitutively producing outer surface proteins A and B. *Infection and Immunity* 75, 2786–2794.

Takayama, K., Rothenberg, R.J. and Barbour, A.G. (1987) Absence of lipopolysaccharide in the Lyme spirochete genomes. *Infection and Immunity* 55, 2311–2313.

Wagner, B., Goodman, L.B., Rollins, A. and Freer, H.S. (2013) Antibodies to OspC, *OspF* and C6 antigens as indicators for infection with *Borrelia burgdorferi* in horses. *Equine Veterinary Journal* 45(5), 533–537.

Wang, G., Ma, Y., Buyuk, A. et al. (2004) Impaired host defense to infection and Toll-like receptor 2-independent killing of *Borrelia burgdorferi* clinical isolates in TLR2-deficient C3H/HeJ mice. *FEMS Microbiology Letters* 231, 219–225.

Widhe, M., Skogman, B.H., Jarefors, S., Eknefelt, M., Eneström, G., Nordwall, M., Ekerfelt, C., Croner, S., Bergström, S., Forsberg, P. and Ernerudh, J. (2005) Up-regulation of Borrelia-specific IL-4- and IFN-gamma-secreting cells in cerebrospinal fluid from children with Lyme neuroborreliosis. *International Immunology* 17, 1283–1291.

Wikel, S. (2013) Ticks and tick-borne pathogens at the cutaneous interface: host defenses, tick countermeasures, and a suitable environment for pathogen establishment. *Frontiers in Microbiology* 4, 337.

Wooten, R.M., Modur, V.R., McIntyre, T.M. et al. (1996) *Borrelia burgdorferi* outer membrane protein A induces nuclear translocation of nuclear factor-kappa B and inflammatory activation in human endothelial cells. *Journal of Immunology* 157, 4584–4590.

Wooten, R.M., Ma, Y., Yoder, R.A. *et al.* (2002) Toll-like receptor 2 is required for innate, but not acquired, host defense to *Borrelia burgdorferi*. *Journal of Immunology* 168, 348–355.

Wormser, G.P. (2006) Clinical practice. Early Lyme disease. *New England Journal of Medicine* 354, 2794–2801.

Wormser, G.P., Dattwyler, R.J., Shapiro, E.D. *et al.* (2006) The clinical assessment, treatment, and prevention of lyme disease, human granulocytic anaplasmosis, and babesiosis: clinical practice guidelines by the Infectious Diseases Society of America. *Clinical Infectious Diseases* 43, 1089–1134.

Wormser, G.P., Aguero-Rosenfeld, M.E. and Nadelman, R.B. (1999) Lyme disease serology: problems and opportunities. *Journal of the American Medical Association* 282, 79–80.

Zajonc, D.M. and Girardi, E. (2015) Recognition of microbial glycolipids by natural killer T cells. *Frontiers in Immunology* 4(6), 400.

Zeidner, N., Dreitz, M., Belasco, D. *et al.* (1996) Suppression of acute *Ixodes scapularis* induced *Borrelia burgdorferi* infection using tumor necrosis factor-alpha, interleukin-2, and interferon-gamma. *Journal of Infectious Diseases* 173, 187–195.

Zeidner, N.S., Schneider, B.S., Nuncio, M.S. *et al.* (2002) Coinoculation of *Borrelia* spp. with tick salivary gland lysate enhances spirochete load in mice and is tick species specific. *Journal of Parasitology* 88, 1276–1278.

Zeidner, N.S., Schneider, B.S., Rutherford, J.S. *et al.* (2008) Suppression of Th2 cytokines reduces tick-transmitted *Borrelia burgdorferi* load in mice. *Journal of Parasitology* 94, 767–769.

Zhang, J.R., Hardham, J.M., Barbour, A.G. *et al.* (1997) Antigenic Variation in Lyme disease borreliae by promiscuous recombination of VMP-like sequence cassettes. *Cell* 89, 275–285.

Zoschke, D.C., Archibald, A.S. and Defosse, D.L. (1991) Lymphoproliferative responses to *Borrelia burgdorferi* in Lyme disease. *Annals of Internal Medicine* 114, 285–289.

4 Diagnostic Testing for Lyme Disease

Paul G. Auwaerter
Johns Hopkins University School of Medicine, Baltimore, Maryland, USA

4.1 Introduction

While Lyme disease is a bacterial infection transmitted by a tick vector, the inherent fastidiousness of the causative *Borreliella burgdorferi* organism does not lend itself to recovery with traditional, widely available culture methods. The most common presentation of Lyme disease is a characteristic rash, erythema migrans (EM). Studies have found this spirochetal organism in the bloodstream in 40–75% or more of untreated adults with early Lyme disease, but only by sophisticated research laboratory methods (Liveris *et al.*, 2011, 2012). Despite this potential spirochetemia, molecular tests such as the polymerase chain reaction (PCR) have been less sensitive than anticipated likely due to transient presence of spirochetes or relative paucibacillary state. Therefore, PCR or other direct detection techniques have not been adopted as the primary diagnostic method (Wormser *et al.*, 2001, 2005; Aguero-Rosenfeld *et al.*, 2005; Liveris *et al.*, 2012). Clinicians evaluating a patient with an epidemiologic risk for this tick-borne infection but lacking the characteristic EM need to rely upon indirect methods to secure a clinical diagnosis of Lyme disease with serological testing the mainstay for nearly four decades.

Though by no means unique to *B. burgdorferi*, serology-based testing does come with inherent limitations that make it imperative for anyone ordering these tests to have a sufficient understanding of their proper utility. For infections routinely identified using serology such as syphilis, *Brucella*, *Coxiella* (Q fever) and infectious mononucleosis among others, diagnostic error and misinterpretation of such tests are common. For example, problematic interpretations of syphilis testing date to the 1930s and 1940s at the dawn of such testing (Moore and Eagle, 1941). Despite such early calls for standardization and ease of interpretation, serologic testing remains prone to fundamental misunderstandings. For Lyme disease, these difficulties are compounded by substantial conflicting information available on the internet, in lower quality medical journals and even certified continuing medical education that may lead either patient or healthcare provider astray (Cooper and Feder, 2004; Aucott *et al.*, 2012; Kwit *et al.*, 2017).

Some essential knowledge provides a helpful background before discussing specific laboratory testing for *B. burgdorferi* infection. Lyme disease is a vector-borne infection transmitted by the bite of infected *Ixodes ricinus* complex ticks. In the United States, this is mostly due to *I. scapularis* (black-legged tick) in the northeast, mid-Atlantic and upper Midwest regions while *I. pacificus* (western black-legged tick) occasionally transmits, mostly in northern California and the Pacific north-west. While *B. burgdorferi* sensu latu group has over 20 genospecies, *B. burgdorferi* sensu stricto solely accounts for Lyme disease in the US (Radolf *et al.*, 2012). In Europe and

Asia, *B. burgdorferi* sensu stricto causes only a small minority of infections; tick-transmitted *B. afzelii* and *B. garinii* are more frequently identified as the cause of Lyme borreliosis, the more commonly employed term outside of North America (Stanek *et al*., 2012).

When infection produces clinical symptoms, Lyme disease may be placed into certain stages: early localized (EM), early disseminated and late disease presentations. If a clinical diagnosis is not secured by the presence or the reliable history of EM, then serology is the only standardized, widely available method of laboratory testing existing in the United States. It is also the only method approved by the Food and Drug Administration (FDA). For early disease, EM typically manifests 7 to 14 days after successful transmission from an infected tick. The humoral immune response is not yet engaged sufficiently for detection of *B. burgdorferi*-specific antibodies until later. Studies of patients with EM have reported that approximately 50% are seronegative at initial presentation (Aguero-Rosenfeld *et al*., 1993; Nowakowski *et al*., 2001). For this reason, patients with an EM lesion in an appropriate epidemiological context may be given a Lyme disease diagnosis with laboratory testing discouraged (Wormser *et al*., 2006). As antibodies are generated, sensitivity improves, especially more than 14 days after acquisition of infection. Though acute and convalescent serologies can be performed, they are not routinely recommended for patients presenting with a characteristic rash – instead, these are reserved for scenarios when potentially atypical rashes are under consideration.

Methods other than FDA-approved serology include a number of both direct and indirect methods for detection of *B. burgdorferi*. Some have been used as part of research or have been developed in academic centers but are not routinely available for most clinical use. Increasingly, so-called Lyme specialty laboratories offer Lyme-related laboratory-developed tests (LDTs) that some practitioners order to evaluate for tick-borne diseases.

Clinicians need to be aware that though performed in a Clinical Laboratory Improvement Amendments (CLIA)-approved test site, these LDTs do not require review or approval by the FDA and therefore are infrequently clinically validated. Often, these 'in-house' or 'home-brew' tests may be promoted as superior to FDA-approved Lyme disease testing. Warnings from the Centers for Disease Control and Prevention (CDC) and others repeatedly advise against their use due to non-standard testing methods and interpretative criteria that lead to more positive results than testing done in laboratories using validated methods (CDC, 2005; Nelson *et al*., 2014). As one example, a study using blood from healthy patients submitted to an alternative testing center found the extraordinary rate of 58% false positive tests using non-rigorously validated criteria to interpret *B. burgdorferi* immunoblots (Fallon *et al*., 2014).

Healthcare providers who specialize in 'chronic Lyme disease' may use such tests, and patients often believe they are better than standardized and validated assays. The purported methods offered include: *B. burgdorferi* urine antigen capture assays, immunofluorescence or other staining of cells looking for cell wall-deficient or cystic forms, lymphocyte transformation assays, T cell stimulation assays, CD57 (natural killer (NK) cell) depletion, abnormal complement levels, proprietary blood culture systems, molecular testing, genomic/plasmid DNA analysis, alternative interpretation of immunoblots, urine reverse Western blots and immunoblots of cerebrospinal or synovial fluids as examples (Auwaerter *et al*., 2011; Barclay *et al*., 2012; Lantos *et al*., 2014). None of these should be used as evidence for authentic Lyme disease, especially from laboratories who advertise that they offer special and superior results.

Lastly, all diagnostic tests have a potential range of positive and negative predictive values based on the patient and the circumstances under consideration. For example, studies in non-endemic regions for *B. burgdorferi* have concluded that a patient with a positive Lyme serologic test living in North Carolina without travel outside the state is unlikely to have genuine Lyme disease, similar to what seropositive results represented from natives of tropical Papua New Guinea (Burkot *et al*., 1997; Lantos *et al*., 2015). Indeed, most cases in low-incidence regions are related to travel in high-incidence regions (Forrester *et al*., 2015).

Moreover, patients lacking objective evidence of Lyme disease but rather only having non-specific symptoms such as fatigue, pain or subjective neurocognitive dysfunction would have a low chance that a positive result would reflect active infection (Lightfoot et al., 1993; Markowicz et al., 2015). This has led to longstanding warnings against testing in such patients as treating positive tests with antibiotics would likely be ineffective or cause harm (Seltzer and Shapiro, 1996; Tugwell et al., 1997; Klempner et al., 2013). While a 20% pretest probability for ordering Lyme disease testing has been advocated to lessen false positive scenarios, such a threshold is difficult to precisely assess for many clinicians (Tugwell et al., 1997). Concerned patients and clinicians may be fearful of missing a diagnosis such as Lyme disease. This is no doubt partly why a large number of Lyme serologic tests are performed annually – likely more than 3.4 million according to one study using 2008 data from large US commercial laboratories – leading to concerns about both overtesting and lax reporting (Hinckley et al., 2014; Kwit et al., 2017).

4.2 Historical Background

First described in the 1970s as Lyme arthritis, the response to penicillin favored suspicions that Lyme disease was an infectious disease. The discovery of the spirochete *B. burgdorferi* came later when William Burgdorfer identified the organism from an infected tick causing EM in a patient living on Shelter Island, New York (Burgdorfer et al., 1982). Following this discovery, some diagnostic strategies emerged. Early difficulties with direct detection by culture, PCR and other methods led to reliance on indirect methods of assessing human antibody responses. These early serological tests lacked either standardization or good concordance with actual Lyme disease, leading to considerable problems with false positive more than false negative results (Hedberg et al., 1987; Bakken et al., 1992; 1997). Critics of testing for Lyme disease often misleadingly cite this early literature using first generation tests.

Calls for a standardized approach to serology as well as better specificity led to a 1994 conference of experts from the United States and Canada including representatives from the FDA, National Institutes of Health (NIH), Council of State and Territorial Epidemiologists, Association of Public Health Laboratories and the Clinical Laboratory Standards Institute (CDC, 1995). Upon evaluation of considerable data, this group decided that no single test could meet expectations. This diagnostic work group decided on a two-tiered serologic approach to enhance both sensitivity and specificity.

The two-tier algorithm employed a first-tier screening test with a very sensitive enzyme immunoassay (EIA). If this first tier was positive or fell in an equivocal range, testing continued as a reflex to a highly specific Western immunoblot to confirm the presence of specific anti-*B. burgdorferi* antibodies. This scheme (Fig. 4.1) has remained the standard and the most widely used method to support the diagnosis of Lyme disease in the absence of EM (CDC, 1995; Wormser et al., 2006; Shapiro, 2014; Sanchez et al., 2016; Dessau et al., 2018). An unfortunate misconception frequently stated in the lay press, by critics and elsewhere is that the two-tier testing strategy was meant only for surveillance purposes and epidemiologic case definition rather than clinical care. Although these testing methods were adopted in part for public health case criteria, they were developed and validated for diagnosis of Lyme disease in clinical practice (CDC, 1995; Shapiro, 2014; Sanchez et al., 2016).

4.3 Two-tiered Serology for *B. burgdorferi*

4.3.1 First tier

The first tier of the standardized two-tiered serologic test for *B. burgdorferi* is a screening test by sensitive EIA or immunofluorescence (IFA) methods. Nowadays typically an EIA, this method examines blood for the presence of class-specific IgM and IgG (together or separately) antibodies. IFA is now rarely employed as it requires skilled technical, microscopic expertise, whereas automated methodologies make EIA the modern customary choice (Cutler and Wright, 1989). If results fall below the threshold, then the first tier is reported as negative, and the test overall is considered negative with no need to perform immunoblotting. If sufficiently in the positive or equivocal range, then the second tier is performed. The first tier does quantitate antibody

Two-tiered testing for Lyme disease, United States[1]

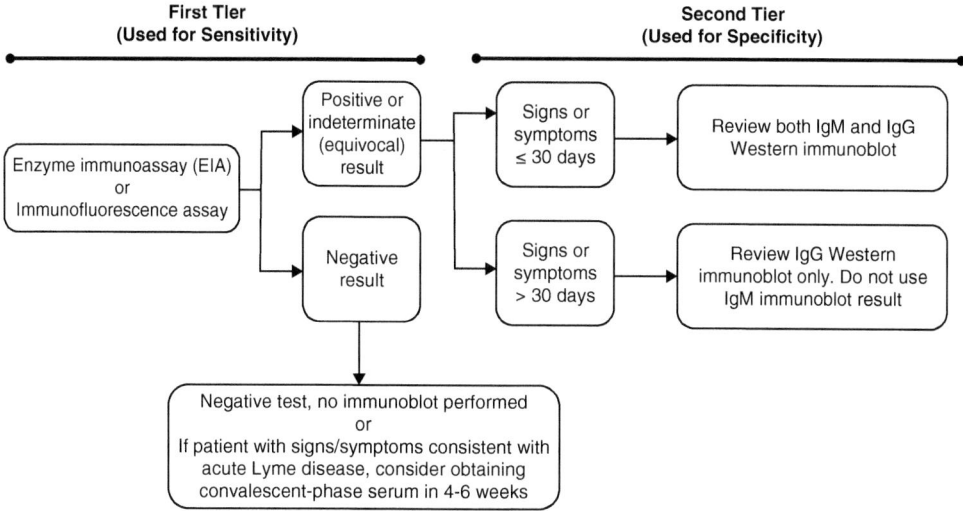

[1]Adapted from MMWR, 1995

Fig. 4.1. Two-tiered serology for Lyme disease, North America. (Adapted from CDC, 1995.)

relative to controls and therefore is a general measure of the amount of potentially specific antibodies present (Aguero-Rosenfeld et al., 2005).

The basis for the EIA used in many US FDA-approved kits is a whole-cell sonicate (WCS) of B. burgdorferi. This approach means that multiple antigens are available, which advances sensitivity. However, it also influences specificity as antibodies to antigens from different pathogens may cross-react (Berardi et al., 1988; Gomes-Solecki et al., 2000; Aguero-Rosenfeld et al., 2005). Over the years, modifications to improve the specificity of the whole-cell lysate approach have included adsorption steps to reduce cross-reacting antibodies, antibody capture techniques, fractionation of the cells and adding synthetically produced antigens such as flagellin, p39 or VlsE (Branda et al., 2010; Marques, 2015).

Performing the second-tier immunoblotting improves specificity, but typically results in delay compared to the more rapid availability of EIA values. A recent report in children suggested that a single high-value EIA reading alone with optical density values ≥3.0 had a positive predictive value of 99.4% (95% confidence intervals (CI), 98.1–99.8%) (Lipsett et al., 2015). This approach, if further validated, would argue against the need to obtain immunoblots that may be otherwise unnecessary or engender delay in diagnosis and treatment with high first-tier values.

Single or few antigen EIA tests for Lyme disease have been FDA-approved and have similar sensitivity to WCS EIAs. Two prominent entries include one based on using the surface lipoprotein, VlsE and the other using the C6 peptide based on the sequence of invariable region 6 of VlsE (Marques et al., 2002; Bacon et al., 2003; Dickeson et al., 2016). These antigens are highly conserved and do not appear to be highly expressed in B. burgdorferi grown in culture systems. Using or adding an antigen such as VlsE or C6 appears to result in earlier detection of specific antibodies than WCS assays in early Lyme disease (EM) including immunoblotting results, but when used alone may be slightly less specific than traditional two-tier testing especially in later disease (Liang et al., 1999; Branda et al., 2011, Wormser et al., 2013b). For example, a study of 403 patients with EM using an FDA-approved single-tier C6 enzyme linked immunosorbent assay (ELISA) kit was 66.5% sensitive while the traditional two-tier testing yield was 35.2%; the tests performed similarly in other populations (early neurologic disease or late Lyme arthritis) while maintaining high specificity of 98.9–99.5% in 2200 controls (Wormser et al., 2013b). Current FDA approval of the single antigen C6 test requires subsequent *B. burgdorferi* immunoblot testing if positive. The C6 antibody EIA appears more sensitive than North American two-tier testing for detecting exposure to Lyme disease acquired in Europe with strains such as *B. afzelii* and *B. garinii* and has been suggested as a standalone test in this scenario (Branda et al., 2013; Wormser et al., 2014).

4.3.2 Second tier

If first-tier testing is judged positive or falls in the equivocal range, testing will proceed to separate IgM and IgG Western blots, also termed immunoblots. This phase of testing also detects antibodies produced against *B. burgdorferi*, though limited to specific standardized antigens (see Fig. 4.2). This process uses proteins derived from *B. burgdorferi* spread across a porous gel by an electrical field. Positions of the proteins are determined by their molecular mass and then transferred to a membrane surface that may be probed by serum that may contain antibodies generated to *B. burgdorferi* bacterial antigens. Such antibody- and antigen-specific binding results in the detection of specific bands on the immunoblot.

The IgM immunoblot is positive if two or three of three bands (21–24, 39 and 41 kDa) stain greater than with control sera, but this finding should only be used if clinical symptoms are 4 weeks or less in duration (CDC, 1995; Engstrom et al., 1995). The IgG immunoblot is considered positive if five or more of 10 predetermined bands (18, 21–24, 28, 30, 39, 41, 45, 58, 66 and 93 kDa) are found. How these blots are scored has been validated for *B. burgdorferi* sensu stricto for Lyme disease in North America but is less reliable for diagnosing other *Borreliella* genospecies in Europe (Wormser et al., 2014).

Numerous retrospective and prospective studies have validated the performance of two-tier serology. For disseminated Lyme disease, the sensitivity ranges from approximately 70–100% with a greater than 95% specificity including more recent studies using contemporary, FDA-approved

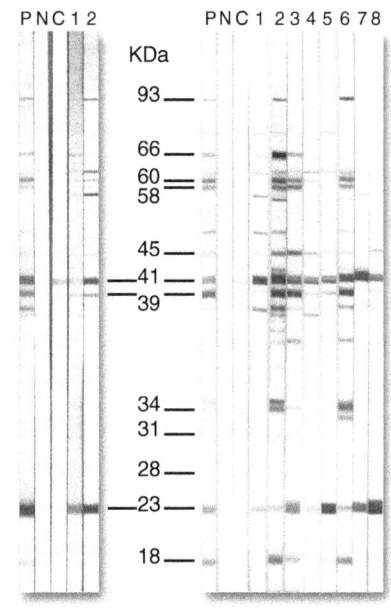

Fig. 4.2. Examples of second-tier, conventional IgM and IgG immunoblots, *Boreliella burgdorferi*. (Left panel) IgM blots. (Right panel) IgG blots. P = positive control serum, N = negative control serum, C = calibration control (weak positive control), patient sample numbers 1–8; kDa, molecular mass, kiloDaltons. Bands shown are part of CDC two-tier criteria (CDC, 1995), additional IgG bands also labeled (outer-surface proteins, OspA and OspB at 31 and 34 kDa, respectively). IgM blots are considered positive if two of the three marked, or five of 10 for IgG blots (excluding OspA and B) with appearance equaling or exceeding the calibration control. IgM blot lane 1 from a patient with acute EM, lane 2 is same patient with convalescent sample demonstrating an increased number and intensity of bands. IgG lanes 1–8 are individual patients with later manifestations of Lyme disease. (Source: CDC, public domain.)

testing kits (Dressler et al., 1993; Johnson et al., 1996; Aguero-Rosenfeld et al., 2005; Branda et al., 2011; Wormser et al., 2013a, b; Molins et al., 2014). Late Lyme arthritis is nearly universally positive according to two-tier criteria as is late neuroborreliosis (Wormser et al., 2013b). Testing for early Lyme disease in the first week of illness may yield rates as low as 14% according to two-tier criteria, not unexpected given the time needed to generate antibodies; seropositivity rises to ~80% by 3–4 weeks after onset of rash in culture-confirmed patients (Wormser et al., 2013b). Moreover, in one study (Wormser et al., 2008) patients with multiple EM rashes were more often initially seropositive on initial testing (~60%) than those with single lesions (~25%).

One of the frequently encountered approaches from alternative testing centers includes non-standard immunoblot criteria to diagnose Lyme disease. Such LDTs are often not well clinically validated, report non-standard combinations of bands and are usually performed without first-tier EIA (CDC, 2005). Relying on such tests may lead to delay, misdiagnosis and overtreatment for conditions that range from chronic fatigue syndrome to neoplasia (Nelson et al., 2015; Patrick et al., 2015).

4.4 Helpful Tips in Two-tier Serological Interpretation (Using FDA-approved Tests)

4.4.1 False negative results

Given the time needed to generate specific antibodies, during the first week or two of infection, two-tier testing sensitivity rates may be as low as 14%; on average less than 50–60% of patients with EM will test positive (Aguero-Rosenfeld et al., 2005; Wormser et al., 2013b). Laboratory testing is unnecessary if a patient presents in a Lyme disease-endemic area with a characteristic rash (Wormser et al., 2006). Testing could falsely lead practitioners to conclude that a rash is not due to B. burgdorferi infection.

There has also been a suggestion that early treatment of Lyme disease may abrogate antibody production so that patients with an EM rash remain seronegative. These studies have used antibody assays no longer in routine use or have methodological issues that have been critiqued (Dattwyler et al., 1988; Schutzer et al., 1990; Bakken et al., 1997; Halperin et al., 2013). Although the aborted generation of antibodies may occur with early treatment, most patients in convalescent phase are seropositive with sensitivity and specificity ranges from 85–99% (Steere et al., 2008).

If clinical suspicion for Lyme disease remains in an individual with suspected early Lyme disease, then follow-up testing after an initial negative result may be considered. For example, a patient without concomitant EM who has a facial palsy but is seronegative on presentation with a lifestyle that places him/her at risk for acquiring B. burgdorferi, convalescent serology 2–4 weeks later would more assuredly rule out infection (CDC, 1995).

While the limitations of serologic testing for early Lyme disease are well-known, typical criticism from Lyme disease advocates off-handedly state the test as being of little value for determining if B. burgdorferi has caused infection as they are more often than not negative despite infection (Furuta et al., 2001; Anonymous, 2017). This information is misleading and often confuses patients who then believe they have Lyme disease when testing is negative, frequently as an explanation for long-standing subjective complaints of fatigue, pain or cognitive disturbances. People evaluated for such problems or who have little likelihood of exposure risk to Lyme disease should not be tested (Tugwell et al., 1997). If serology is performed, negative values should confidently exclude infection. Patients with such chronic, subjective symptoms and positive results are unlikely to benefit from antibiotic treatment (Feder et al., 2007; Klempner et al., 2012; 2013).

4.4.2 False positive results

Although the current testing algorithm is a two-stage procedure, the first EIA tier may be positive due to other infectious or inflammatory processes. WCS ELISAs and especially IgM immunoblots may be scored as positive due to cross-reacting antibodies to other spirochetal diseases including relapsing fever borreliosis, syphilis or leptospirosis as well as viral infections including Epstein–Barr virus, cytomegalovirus and parvovirus B19 (Magnarelli et al., 1987; Magnarelli and Anderson, 1988; Goossens et al., 1999; Tuuminen et al., 2011; Patriquin et al., 2016; Pavletic and Marques, 2017). One study of patients with PCR-confirmed human granulocytic anaplasmosis (then termed ehrlichiosis) found EIA elevations with positive or equivocal Western blots in 60–90% of patients, considered statistically improbable to represent Lyme disease, thereby suggesting the presence of cross-reacting antibodies (Wormser et al., 1997). Auto-immune disorders including systemic lupus erythematosus and rheumatoid arthritis have also caused false positive results (Weiss *et al.*, 1995).

Many laboratories report individual immunoblot bands as present or absent instead of focusing on whether the number of bands present meets diagnostic criteria, which may create confusion for clinicians examining test reports. Patterns with lower numbers of bands may be present due to very early infection or cross-reacting antibodies. For example, many bacteria elaborate heat-shock proteins or have flagellin antigens that elicit strong antibody responses, triggering false readings either in EIA or immunoblot bands (Carreiro *et al.*, 1990). These commonly seen bands include 41 kDa (flagellin) and 58, 60 or 66 kDa. One study found that 43% of healthy people serving as controls had cross-reacting antibodies to bacterial flagellar proteins with little to no risk of Lyme disease exposure (Bacon *et al.*, 2003).

An additional false positive scenario arises when immunoblots are run without first performing an EIA or IFA. If the first tier is negative – indicating the absence of meaningful quantities of anti-borrelial antibodies – immunoblots should not be performed. As immunoblots are not quantitative like first-tier assays, bands may appear with minute amounts of antibody that would not normally trigger a positive first-tier test. First- and second-tier tests are not independent predictors of *B. burgdorferi* infection, yet some believe immunoblots are a more sensitive test than EIA, which is not the case (Wormser *et al.*, 2000). False positive banding patterns occur in other bacterial infections including periodontal inflammation (Johnson *et al.*, 1996; Ledue *et al.*, 1996). Moreover, bypassing the first tier and using immunoblots alone to diagnose Lyme disease has been shown to decrease the specificity from 100% to 92–98.5% in healthy blood donors from non-endemic regions as well as in those with infectious processes other than Lyme disease (Engstrom *et al.*, 1995; Johnson *et al.*, 1996). What this means practically is that more false positives will occur if serotesting for Lyme disease is not performed by the two-tier method.

4.4.3 Background seropositivity and repeated serological testing

In states with high numbers of cases of Lyme disease, rates of positive tests have been noted in epidemiologic studies to be as high as 5% in one New York study (Kugeler *et al.*, 2015). Using ELISA techniques for anti-Borrelia antibodies, a 4.8% rate was described in German children (Dehnert *et al.*, 2012). Among seropositive patients in New York with no symptoms, nearly 60% denied any history consistent with Lyme disease (Hilton *et al.*, 1999). Therefore, indiscriminate use of *B. burgdorferi* antibody testing in such regions in patients without objective symptoms may lead to misdiagnoses and overtreatment, though asymptomatic infection remains possible as well.

An additional factor is that following Lyme disease, antibody responses are long-lived. Using standard two-tier testing, including IgM assays, approximately 40–60% of patients treated for Lyme disease remained seropositive including IgM or IgG Western blots when examined 10–20 years after successful treatment (Kalish *et al.*, 2001). Such antibody persistence with two-tier serology does not connote active infection. IgM positivity sometimes misleads clinicians to believe a new infection has occurred, requiring treatment, or that treatment needs to continue until seronegativity. In contrast, monoantigen C6 peptide antibody levels decline four-fold or become absent in patients with treated single or multiple EM in 89–100% of patients (Philipp *et al.*, 2005).

The scientific basis for such prolonged antibody production is not well understood and is not true for all patients. Remnants of non-viable bacteria or antigenic debris may remain in tissues perhaps due to integrins or other adhesion mechanisms that stimulate antibody production long after sufficient antibiotic courses (Peltomaa *et al.*, 2003; Antonara *et al.*, 2011; Bockenstedt *et al.*, 2012; Wormser *et al.*, 2012). Routine rechecks of serostatus as a test of cure, therefore, have no benefit and may only sow confusion.

4.4.4 IgM immunoblots

Perhaps no other element of serological testing contributes more to confusion regarding whether or not a patient has Lyme disease than IgM immunoblots. Two-tier testing includes both IgM and IgG immunoblots based on the long-known sequence of antibody production following antigen exposure wherein IgM antibodies are produced first, usually within the first 10–14 days after infection, and then IgG antibodies ensue as a primary immune response. IgM immunoblotting is included to assist in the diagnosis of early Lyme disease when characteristic EM is not present, though the two-tier predictive value falls considerably if objective clinical findings are lacking (Sivak et al., 1996; Porwancher, 1999).

While research studies using reference laboratory two-tier approaches have shown specificities of 99% or higher, employing these tests in daily clinical practice has yielded lower rates, mostly due to incorporating faint IgM immunoblot bands or cross-reacting antibodies as positives (Branda et al., 2010; Branda et al., 2011). In a retrospective study of 182 patients evaluated for Lyme disease in Westchester County, New York, 27.5% were judged to be falsely positive based upon the IgM immunoblot with 78% receiving unnecessary antibiotics (Seriburi et al., 2012). A Boston-based pediatric study found 29% had false positives among a total of 167 patients with positive IgM but negative IgG immunoblots (Lantos et al., 2016).

The IgM immunoblot should only be relied upon in patients with less than 30 days of new clinical symptoms, for several reasons. First, problems with specificity as noted earlier mean that the predictive value is low, especially without symptoms and signs typically found with early Lyme disease. Second, by 4 weeks, the IgG immunoblot, which does not suffer from specificity problems, should have positive banding profiles. Some have argued that the IgM range allowance for clinical validity should be extended to 6 weeks if the IgG immunoblot remains negative (Branda et al., 2010). Lastly, IgM antibodies with their pentameric structure bind more non-specifically than monomeric IgG antibodies – hence a single overread or misinterpreted IgM band may result in a positive test as appears to be the case in mainstream commercial laboratories (Seriburi et al., 2012).

4.4.5 Cerebrospinal fluid analytics

Most neuroborreliosis in both North America and Europe occurs early manifesting as cranial neuropathy, lymphocytic meningitis or radiculitis. Much of the diagnostic and treatment literature comes from European studies where neuroborreliosis may be more common, mostly caused by B. garinii compared to B. burgdorferi sensu stricto in North America (Stanek and Strle, 2008; Dessau et al., 2018). Due to strain differences and heterogenous laboratory approaches, synthesizing this literature can be challenging although disease manifestations of North American and European Lyme neuroborreliosis are similar (Koedel et al., 2015).

The result of disseminated B. burgdorferi infection into the central nervous system (CNS), blood serologic testing is usually positive, or positive upon convalescent recheck in the unusual cases wherein neurologic symptoms precede antibody responses (Halperin and Golightly, 1992; Kaiser and Rauer, 1998; Knudtzen et al., 2017). European guidelines for the diagnosis of neuroborreliosis include the presence of cerebrospinal fluid (CSF) pleocytosis and/or intrathecal Borreliella antibody production as a requirement (Mygland et al., 2010), while American-based guidelines require either microbiologic or molecular proof of B. burgdorferi infection or evidence of exposure by immunologic means (Halperin et al., 2007). Despite these recommendations, additional challenges remain when evaluating Borreliella-specific CSF antibodies such that both positive and negative results should be interpreted with caution (see Chapters 8, 9 and 13).

Assessing total B. burgdorferi antibody levels in the CSF in isolation may be misleading due to long-term persistence following earlier antibiotic therapy or merely the result of antibody diffusion passively into the CSF with acute infection without CNS involvement (Martin et al., 1988; Hammers-Berggren et al., 1993; Wang et al., 1993). To avoid a false conclusion, the antibody index (AI) has become the predominant confirmatory method. An AI incorporates normalized CSF and serum protein levels with the generation of a ratio of anti-borrelial antibodies. When measured, an AI CSF:serum ratio >1.2–1.3 is considered confirmatory of bona fide intrathecal antibody production in response to CNS infection, more so if a control antibody index measures <1.0 and an albumin ratio is <0.0078. This approach results in good specificity but more moderate sensitivity, 97% and 75%, respectively, in one study of 40 patients (Blanc et al., 2007). Use of synthetic peptides or recombinant antigen appears to improve both sensitivity and specificity of the AI compared to older studies using WCS-generated antibodies (Henningsson et al., 2014; Stanek et al., 2014). Conversely, assessment early in the case of Lyme neuroborreliosis may produce negative CSF results initially, and even convalescent assessment of CSF antibodies after treatment has been described as also potentially uninformative (Ljostad et al., 2007).

The chemokine CXCL13 has been proposed as an early biomarker for detecting Lyme neuroborreliosis (Yang et al., 2017). This assay is available in some laboratories; CXCL13 concentration has been studied in smaller prospective trials and also appears to decline with antibiotic therapy. However, the role of CSF CXCL13 levels in CNS infections remains unestablished as elevation may occur in other conditions such as HIV infection (Schmidt et al., 2011; Bremell et al., 2013).

4.4.6 Immunoblot testing of fluids other than blood

Two-tier testing for Lyme disease has only been clinically validated for blood. Some commercial testing centers offer to analyze samples other than blood by immunoblot, but these are performed as LDTs without evidence of validity in the literature. For example, one study of patients with identified positive B. burgdorferi immunoblots in synovial fluid found >90% to be without confirmatory evidence to support Lyme arthritis with negative serology in the blood, highly unusual given the nearly 100% seropositive state described in numerous other studies (Barclay et al., 2012). Immunoblot testing of CSF is offered as well by some labs, but they typically acknowledge there are no interpretive criteria for B. burgdorferi Western blots in CSF or other fluids (QuestDiagnostics, 2017).

4.5 PCR and Other Direct Methods

Although PCR technology is offered in many laboratories, it is neither an FDA-approved test nor of established validity in clinical practice. Boreliella burgdorferi DNA detection by PCR is most often used in practice to evaluate Lyme arthritis. While specific, the sensitivity ranges between 46 and 96% assessing late Lyme arthritis synovial fluid (Li et al., 2011). Serology remains the backbone for diagnosis of Lyme arthritis as positive serum anti-B. burgdorferi IgG antibodies are almost universally identified and in the correct clinical context of monoarticular arthritis, usually a swollen knee, this is sufficient to secure the diagnosis (Arvikar and Steere, 2015). Though PCR has been proposed as having a role for assessing antibiotic-resistant Lyme arthritis, its ability to detect residual spirochetal DNA after therapy limits its utility discerning active infection (Nocton et al., 1996; Steere and Angelis, 2006). Therefore, the role of PCR in Lyme arthritis remains adjunctive.

PCR in the CSF for either early or late neuroborreliosis was positive 38% or 25% of the time, respectively, in one North American study (Nocton et al., 1996). In a European cohort with suspected neuroborreliosis, different PCR primer techniques detected borrelial DNA in only 3.2–15.4% of samples (Cerar et al., 2008). In a Scandinavian cohort of hospitalized patients, yield in CSF was 35% (Picha et al., 2005). Given this low range, antibody responses are better relied upon to evaluate abnormal CSF for potential infection, so PCR is not routinely advised for neuroborreliosis evaluation (Auwaerter et al., 2004; Mygland et al., 2010).

PCR has been employed in a number of research studies examining both blood and skin biopsies. Skin biopsies are rarely performed in clinical practice, but PCR positivity ranges from 36–88% (Aguero-Rosenfeld et al., 2005). Analysis of blood in patients with EM or early disseminated Lyme disease in North America or Europe has a much lower yield ranging from 10–18% and is not routinely recommended, given cost and low sensitivity (Aguero-Rosenfeld et al., 2005). In Europe, a recent study examining PCR among eight different clinical laboratories showed good agreement among results but an inability to detect B. spielmanii, B. lusitaniae or B. japonica that infrequently cause human infection (Lager et al., 2017).

4.6 Culture

Boreliella burgdorferi may grow in a number of culture systems, with Barbour–Stoenner–Kelly

(BSK) and Kelly–Pettenkofer media among the most commonly used (Pollack *et al.*, 1993; Ružić-Sabljić *et al.*, 2006). Culture is unavailable in most clinical laboratories, and this method remains impractical in such settings due to high technical demands and slow growth characteristics, often requiring weeks of incubation. Positive growth is confirmed by microscopy using dark field methods or stains such as acridine orange fluorescence detecting characteristic spirochetes, or determined by PCR.

Culture remains a standard method of research studies to assure true infection. However, due to lower organism burden and brief spirochetemia usually seen in early infection, this method is relatively insensitive for detection of *B. burgdorferi* in human disease. In early Lyme disease with EM, the yield of positive blood cultures is approximately 45%, although quantitative PCR techniques using high-volume samples incubated for 2–14 weeks in BSK II media increased rates to 70.8% in one study (Liveris *et al.*, 2011). Positive blood cultures are seen more in patients with multiple EM representing disseminated infection than single EM (Liveris *et al.*, 2011; Liveris *et al.*, 2012). EM lesions biopsied for culture displayed growth in 22–41% of patients judged to have possible or probable Lyme disease in one study, but also have been described in the range of 40–60% (Aguero-Rosenfeld *et al.*, 2005; Coulter *et al.*, 2005).

Clinicians do need to be aware that some alternative laboratories offer culture systems that appear to yield very high rates of positive cultures for *Borreliella* even in patients who have been extensively treated for Lyme disease (Sapi *et al.*, 2013). The credibility of such findings has been severely questioned as laboratory contamination appeared to explain some published results (Johnson *et al.*, 2014; Nelson *et al.*, 2014; Wormser *et al.*, 2017).

4.7 New Testing Algorithms and Other Tests

Due to frequent clinician confusion interpreting two-tier serology reports, as well as the low specificity of IgM immunoblots outside of early Lyme disease, ways to improve the diagnostic accuracy for clinical practice are ongoing. Additionally, immunoblotting is technically cumbersome, prone to faint band interpretation problems and adds costs compared to less expensive methods. A perfect test for Lyme disease would have point-of-care applicability and differentiate between active and treated *B. burgdorferi* infection in all phases of illness – though this aspirational goal is still far from reality.

One approach to avoid immunoblots has been studied by using WCS ELISA and C6 ELISA in either order as a two-test strategy. In a study of non-cutaneous Lyme disease, this algorithm had 96.5% sensitivity and 99.5% specificity, comparing favorably to standard two-tier testing, as well as potentially being more cost-effective (Wormser *et al.*, 2013a; 2013b). Such modified two-tier testing (MTTT) protocols have been examined further against standard two-tier testing (STTT). One study comparing 55 patients with early Lyme disease (EM) to ill patients without Lyme disease and to healthy controls found MTTT – using three different approaches: WCS followed by C6, WCS then VlsE, VlsE then C6 – had sensitivity ranging from 36–54%, compared to 25% STTT and MTTT specificity in all arms at ~99% (Branda *et al.*, 2017). Another study using 471 well-characterized sera from a range of Lyme disease presentations found comparable support for a 2-ELISA-based MTTT algorithm as it performed as well as STTT for later Lyme disease, but outperformed STTT for early Lyme presentations (Molins *et al.*, 2016). Other published reports have reached similar conclusions (Branda *et al.*, 2011; 2013; Lipsett *et al.*, 2016; Molins *et al.*, 2017b). Such encouraging results suggest MTTT approaches may well be an improvement over STTT and obviate the need for immunoblots.

Point-of-care testing with rapid results would help avoid empiric antibiotic treatment as well as a potential delay in diagnosis. Examples include a sufficiently sensitive and specific first-tier only test or the use of a microfluidic platform with current serologic assays (Gomes-Solecki *et al.*, 2001; Nayak *et al.*, 2016). Other technologies under exploration include nanotechnology antigen capture, whole-genome or next-generation sequencing, differential gene expression and comparison of metabolic signatures (Lee *et al.*, 2010; Magni *et al.*, 2015; Molins *et al.*, 2015; Bouquet *et al.*, 2016; Kingry *et al.*, 2016; Molins *et al.*, 2017a).

Xenodiagnosis using the *Ixodes scapularis* tick vector has retrieved borrelial DNA from some patients treated for Lyme disease; the significance of this remains uncertain and it is not likely to become incorporated into clinical practice (Bockenstedt and Radolf, 2014; Marques *et al.*, 2014).

4.8 Summary

Currently available and validated laboratory testing for *B. burgdorferi* cannot be employed in a vacuum, but instead, must be placed into a clinical context of whether a patient has an epidemiological risk for exposure as well as objective clinical findings that make sense and are likely indicative of active infection. Particular care is needed when discussing results with patients who have positive IgM immunoblot testing that may not represent authentic Lyme disease.

Improvements in direct testing methods or new approaches to serologic testing may both eventually assist in the diagnosis of early Lyme disease when EM is not present and reduce difficulties produced with two-tier serology reporting. A Lyme disease serum repository of well-characterized infections has been established by a joint effort between the CDC and the NIH (Molins *et al.*, 2014). Such a resource may be held as a common standard to validate as well as compare testing methodologies.

Lyme disease remains an infection that is both overdiagnosed and underreported. Clinicians and researchers should not be persuaded by thin arguments based on often misleading information concerning currently available FDA-approved serological tests that are based on well-grounded and robustly performed clinical studies. A solid foundation in the laboratory diagnosis of Lyme disease is vital to achieving an accurate diagnosis.

References

Aguero-Rosenfeld, M.E., Nowakowski, J., McKenna, D.F., Carbonaro, C.A. and Wormser, G.P. (1993) Serodiagnosis in early Lyme disease. *Journal of Clinical Microbiology* 31, 3090–3095.

Aguero-Rosenfeld, M.E., Wang, G., Schwartz, I. and Wormser, G.P. (2005) Diagnosis of Lyme borreliosis. *Clinical Microbiology Reviews* 18, 484–509.

Anonymous (2017) *4 Reasons a Lyme Test Will Come Back Negative Even If a Person Truly Has Lyme Disease* [Online]. Available at: www.tiredoflyme.com/4-reasons-a-lyme-test-will-come-back-negative-even-if-a-person-truly-has-lyme-disease.html (accessed 11 March 2017).

Antonara, S., Ristow, L. and Coburn, J. (2011) Adhesion mechanisms of *Borrelia burgdorferi*. *Advances in Experimental Medicine and Biology* 715, 35–49.

Arvikar, S.L. and Steere, A.C. (2015) Diagnosis and treatment of Lyme arthritis. *Infectious Disease Clinics of North America* 29, 269–280.

Aucott, J.N., Crowder, L.A., Yedlin, V. and Kortte, K.B. (2012) Bull's-eye and nontarget skin lesions of Lyme disease: an internet survey of identification of erythema migrans. *Dermatology Research and Practice* 2012, 451727.

Auwaerter, P.G., Aucott, J. and Dumler, J.S. (2004) Lyme borreliosis (Lyme disease): molecular and cellular pathobiology and prospects for prevention, diagnosis and treatment. *Expert Reviews in Molecular Medicine* 6, 1–22.

Auwaerter, P.G., Bakken, J.S., Dattwyler, R.J., Dumler, J.S., Halperin, J.J., McSweegan, E., Nadelman, R.B., O'Connell, S., Shapiro, E.D., Sood, S.K., Steere, A.C., Weinstein, A. and Wormser, G.P. (2011) Antiscience and ethical concerns associated with advocacy of Lyme disease. *Lancet Infectious Diseases* 11, 713–719.

Bacon, R.M., Biggerstaff, B.J., Schriefer, M.E., Gilmore Jr, R.D., Philipp, M.T., Steere, A.C., Wormser, G.P., Marques, A.R. and Johnson, B.J. (2003) Serodiagnosis of Lyme disease by kinetic enzyme-linked immunosorbent assay using recombinant VlsE1 or peptide antigens of *Borrelia burgdorferi* compared with 2-tiered testing using whole-cell lysates. *Journal of Infectious Diseases* 187, 1187–1199.

Bakken, L.L., Case, K.L., Callister, S.M., Bourdeau, N.J. and Schell, R.F. (1992) Performance of 45 laboratories participating in a proficiency testing program for Lyme disease serology. *JAMA* 268, 891–895.

Bakken, L.L., Callister, S.M., Wand, P.J. and Schell, R.F. (1997) Interlaboratory comparison of test results for detection of Lyme disease by 516 participants in the Wisconsin State Laboratory of Hygiene/

College of American Pathologists Proficiency Testing Program. *Journal of Clinical Microbiology* 35, 537–543.

Barclay, S.S., Melia, M.T. and Auwaerter, P.G. (2012) Misdiagnosis of late-onset Lyme arthritis by inappropriate use of *Borrelia burgdorferi* immunoblot testing with synovial fluid. *Clinical and Vaccine Immunology* 19, 1806–1809.

Berardi, V.P., Weeks, K.E. and Steere, A.C. (1988) Serodiagnosis of early Lyme disease: analysis of IgM and IgG antibody responses by using an antibody-capture enzyme immunoassay. *Journal of Infectious Diseases* 158, 754–760.

Blanc, F., Jaulhac, B., Fleury, M., De Seze, J., De Martino, S.J., Remy, V., Blaison, G., Hansmann, Y., Christmann, D. and Tranchant, C. (2007) Relevance of the antibody index to diagnose Lyme neuroborreliosis among seropositive patients. *Neurology* 69, 953–958.

Bockenstedt, L.K. and Radolf, J.D. (2014) Xenodiagnosis for posttreatment Lyme disease syndrome: resolving the conundrum or adding to it? *Clinical Infectious Diseases* 58, 946–948.

Bockenstedt, L.K., Gonzalez, D.G., Haberman, A.M. and Belperron, A.A. (2012) Spirochete antigens persist near cartilage after murine Lyme borreliosis therapy. *Journal of Clinical Investigation* 122, 2652–2660.

Bouquet, J., Soloski, M.J., Swei, A., Cheadle, C., Federman, S., Billaud, J.N., Rebman, A.W., Kabre, B., Halpert, R., Boorgula, M., Aucott, J.N. and Chiu, C.Y. (2016) Longitudinal transcriptome analysis reveals a sustained differential gene expression signature in patients treated for acute lyme disease. *MBio* 7, e00100–e00116.

Branda, J.A., Aguero-Rosenfeld, M.E., Ferraro, M.J., Johnson, B.J., Wormser, G.P. and Steere, A.C. (2010) 2-tiered antibody testing for early and late Lyme disease using only an immunoglobulin G blot with the addition of a VlsE band as the second-tier test. *Clinical Infectious Diseases* 50, 20–26.

Branda, J.A., Linskey, K., Kim, Y.A., Steere, A.C. and Ferraro, M.J. (2011) Two-tiered antibody testing for Lyme disease with use of 2 enzyme immunoassays, a whole-cell sonicate enzyme immunoassay followed by a VlsE C6 peptide enzyme immunoassay. *Clinical Infectious Diseases* 53, 541–547.

Branda, J.A., Strle, F., Strle, K., Sikand, N., Ferraro, M.J. and Steere, A.C. (2013) Performance of United States serologic assays in the diagnosis of Lyme borreliosis acquired in Europe. *Clinical Infectious Diseases* 57, 333–340.

Branda, J.A., Strle, K., Nigrovic, L.E., Lantos, P.M., Lepore, T.J., Damle, N.S., Ferraro, M.J. and Steere, A.C. (2017) Evaluation of modified 2-tiered serodiagnostic testing algorithms for early Lyme disease. *Clinical Infectious Diseases* 64, 1074–1080.

Bremell, D., Mattsson, N., Edsbagge, M., Blennow, K., Andreasson, U., Wikkelso, C., Zetterberg, H. and Hagberg, L. (2013) Cerebrospinal fluid CXCL13 in Lyme neuroborreliosis and asymptomatic HIV infection. *BMC Neurology* 13, 2.

Burgdorfer, W., Barbour, A.G., Hayes, S.F., Benach, J.L., Grunwaldt, E. and Davis, J.P. (1982) Lyme disease - a tick-borne spirochetosis? *Science* 216, 1317–1319.

Burkot, T.R., Schriefer, M.E. and Larsen, S.A. (1997) Cross-reactivity to *Borrelia burgdorferi* proteins in serum samples from residents of a tropical country nonendemic for Lyme disease. *Journal of Infectious Diseases* 175, 466–469.

Carreiro, M.M., Laux, D.C. and Nelson, D.R. (1990) Characterization of the heat shock response and identification of heat shock protein antigens of *Borrelia burgdorferi*. *Infection and Immunity* 58, 2186–2191.

Centers for Disease Control and Prevention (CDC) (1995) Recommendations for test performance and interpretation from the second national conference on serologic diagnosis of Lyme disease. *MMWR Morbidity and Mortality Weekly Report* 44, 590–591.

CDC (2005) Notice to readers: caution regarding testing for Lyme disease. *MMWR Morbidity and Mortality Weekly Report* 54, 125.

Cerar, T., Ogrinc, K., Cimperman, J., Lotric-Furlan, S., Strle, F. and Ružić-Sabljić, E. (2008) Validation of cultivation and PCR methods for diagnosis of Lyme neuroborreliosis. *Journal of Clinical Microbiology* 46, 3375–3379.

Cooper, J.D. and Feder Jr, H.M. (2004) Inaccurate information about Lyme disease on the internet. *Pediatric Infectious Disease Journal* 23, 1105–1108.

Coulter, P., Lema, C., Flayhart, D., Linhardt, A.S., Aucott, J.N., Auwaerter, P.G. and Dumler, J.S. (2005) Two-year evaluation of *Borrelia burgdorferi* culture and supplemental tests for definitive diagnosis of Lyme disease. *Journal of Clinical Microbiology* 43, 5080–5084.

Cutler, S.J. and Wright, D.J. (1989) Comparison of immunofluorescence and enzyme linked immunosorbent assays for diagnosing Lyme disease. *Journal of Clinical Pathology* 42, 869–871.

Dattwyler, R.J., Volkman, D.J., Luft, B.J., Halperin, J.J., Thomas, J. and Golightly, M.G. (1988) Seronegative Lyme disease. Dissociation of specific T- and B-lymphocyte responses to *Borrelia burgdorferi*. *New England Journal of Medicine* 319, 1441–1446.

Dehnert, M., Fingerle, V., Klier, C., Talaska, T., Schlaud, M., Krause, G., Wilking, H. and Poggensee, G. (2012) Seropositivity of Lyme borreliosis and associated risk factors: a population-based study in children and adolescents in Germany (KiGGS). *PLoS One* 7, e41321.

Dessau, R.B., Van Dam, A.P., Fingerle, V. *et al*. (2018) To test or not to test? Laboratory support for the diagnosis of Lyme borreliosis: a position paper of ESGBOR, the ESCMID study group for Lyme borreliosis. *Clinical Microbiology and Infection* 24(2), 118–124.

Dickeson, D.J., Chen, S.C. and Sintchenko, V.G. (2016) Concordance of four commercial enzyme immunoassay and three immunoblot formats for the detection of Lyme borreliosis antibodies in human serum: the two-tier approach remains. *Pathology* 48, 251–256.

Dressler, F., Whalen, J.A., Reinhardt, B.N. and Steere, A.C. (1993) Western blotting in the serodiagnosis of Lyme disease. *Journal of Infectious Diseases* 167, 392–400.

Engstrom, S.M., Shoop, E. and Johnson, R.C. (1995) Immunoblot interpretation criteria for serodiagnosis of early Lyme disease. *Journal of Clinical Microbiology* 33, 419–427.

Fallon, B.A., Pavlicova, M., Coffino, S.W. and Brenner, C. (2014) A comparison of Lyme disease serologic test results from 4 laboratories in patients with persistent symptoms after antibiotic treatment. *Clinical Infectious Diseases* 59, 1705–1710.

Feder Jr, H.M., Johnson, B.J., O'Connell, S. *et al*. (2007) A critical appraisal of 'chronic Lyme disease'. *New England Journal of Medicine* 357, 1422–1430.

Forrester, J.D., Brett, M., Matthias, J., Stanek, D., Springs, C.B., Marsden-Haug, N., Oltean, H., Baker, J.S., Kugeler, K.J., Mead, P.S. and Hinckley, A. (2015) Epidemiology of Lyme disease in low-incidence states. *Ticks and Tick-borne Diseases* 6, 721–723.

Furuta, Y., Kawabata, H., Ohtani, F. and Watanabe, H. (2001) Western blot analysis for diagnosis of Lyme disease in acute facial palsy. *Laryngoscope* 111, 719–723.

Gomes-Solecki, M.J., Dunn, J.J., Luft, B.J., Castillo, J., Dykhuizen, D.E., Yang, X., Glass, J.D. and Dattwyler, R.J. (2000) Recombinant chimeric Borrelia proteins for diagnosis of Lyme disease. *Journal of Clinical Microbiology* 38, 2530–2535.

Gomes-Solecki, M.J., Wormser, G.P., Persing, D.H., Berger, B.W., Glass, J.D., Yang, X. and Dattwyler, R.J. (2001) A first-tier rapid assay for the serodiagnosis of *Borrelia burgdorferi* infection. *Archives of Internal Medicine* 161, 2015–2020.

Goossens, H.A., Nohlmans, M.K. and Van Den Bogaard, A.E. (1999) Epstein-Barr virus and cytomegalovirus infections cause false-positive results in IgM two-test protocol for early Lyme borreliosis. *Infection* 27, 231.

Halperin, J.J. and Golightly, M. (1992) Lyme borreliosis in Bell's palsy. Long Island Neuroborreliosis Collaborative Study Group. *Neurology* 42, 1268–1270.

Halperin, J.J., Shapiro, E.D., Logigian, E., Belman, A.L., Dotevall, L., Wormser, G.P., Krupp, L., Gronseth, G., Bever Jr, C.T., and Quality Standards Subcommittee of the American Academy of Neurology (2007) Practice parameter: treatment of nervous system Lyme disease (an evidence-based review): report of the Quality Standards Subcommittee of the American Academy of Neurology. *Neurology* 69, 91–102.

Halperin, J.J., Baker, P. and Wormser, G.P. (2013) Common misconceptions about Lyme disease. *American Journal of Medicine* 126(264), e1–e7.

Hammers-Berggren, S., Hansen, K., Lebech, A.M. and Karlsson, M. (1993) *Borrelia burgdorferi*-specific intrathecal antibody production in neuroborreliosis: a follow-up study. *Neurology* 43, 169–175.

Hedberg, C.W., Osterholm, M.T., Macdonald, K.L. and White, K.E. (1987) An interlaboratory study of antibody to *Borrelia burgdorferi*. *Journal of Infectious Diseases* 155, 1325–1327.

Henningsson, A.J., Christiansson, M., Tjernberg, I., Lofgren, S. and Matussek, A. (2014) Laboratory diagnosis of Lyme neuroborreliosis: a comparison of three CSF anti-*Borrelia* antibody assays. *European Journal of Clinical Microbiology and Infectious Diseases* 33, 797–803.

Hilton, E., Devoti, J., Benach, J.L., Halluska, M.L., White, D.J., Paxton, H. and Dumler, J.S. (1999) Seroprevalence and seroconversion for tick-borne diseases in a high-risk population in the northeast United States. *American Journal of Medicine* 106, 404–409.

Hinckley, A.F., Connally, N.P., Meek, J.I., Johnson, B.J., Kemperman, M.M., Feldman, K.A., White, J.L. and Mead, P.S. (2014) Lyme disease testing by large commercial laboratories in the United States. *Clinical Infectious Diseases* 59, 676–681.

Johnson, B.J., Robbins, K.E., Bailey, R.E., Cao, B.L., Sviat, S.L., Craven, R.B., Mayer, L.W. and Dennis, D.T. (1996) Serodiagnosis of Lyme disease: accuracy of a two-step approach using a flagella-based ELISA and immunoblotting. *Journal of Infectious Diseases* 174, 346–353.

Johnson, B.J., Pilgard, M.A. and Russell, T.M. (2014) Assessment of new culture method for detection of *Borrelia* species from serum of Lyme disease patients. *Journal of Clinical Microbiology* 52, 721–724.

Kaiser, R. and Rauer, S. (1998) Analysis of the intrathecal immune response in neuroborreliosis to a sonicate antigen and three recombinant antigens of *Borrelia burgdorferi* sensu stricto. *European Journal of Clinical Microbiology and Infectious Diseases* 17, 159–166.

Kalish, R.A., McHugh, G., Granquist, J., Shea, B., Ruthazer, R. and Steere, A.C. (2001) Persistence of immunoglobulin M or immunoglobulin G antibody responses to *Borrelia burgdorferi* 10–20 years after active Lyme disease. *Clinical Infectious Diseases* 33, 780–785.

Kingry, L.C., Batra, D., Replogle, A., Rowe, L.A., Pritt, B.S. and Petersen, J.M. (2016) Whole genome sequence and comparative genomics of the novel Lyme borreliosis causing pathogen, *Borrelia mayonii*. *PLoS One* 11, e0168994.

Klempner, M.S., Halperin, J.J., Baker, P.J., Shapiro, E.D., O'Connell, S., Fingerle, V. and Wormser, G.P. (2012) Lyme borreliosis: the challenge of accuracy. *Netherlands Journal of Medicine* 70, 3–5.

Klempner, M.S., Baker, P.J., Shapiro, E.D., Marques, A., Dattwyler, R.J., Halperin, J.J. and Wormser, G.P. (2013) Treatment trials for post-Lyme disease symptoms revisited. *American Journal of Medicine* 126, 665–669.

Knudtzen, F.C., Andersen, N.S., Jensen, T.G. and Skarphedinsson, S. (2017) Characteristics and clinical outcome of Lyme neuroborreliosis in a high endemic area, 1995–2014: a retrospective cohort study in Denmark. *Clinical Infectious Diseases* 65, 1489–1495.

Koedel, U., Fingerle, V. and Pfister, H.W. (2015) Lyme neuroborreliosis – epidemiology, diagnosis and management. *Nature Reviews Neurology* 11, 446–456.

Kugeler, K.J., Farley, G.M., Forrester, J.D. and Mead, P.S. (2015) Geographic distribution and expansion of human Lyme disease, United States. *Emerging Infectious Diseases* 21, 1455–1457.

Kwit, N.A., Dietrich, E.A., Nelson, C., Taffner, R., Petersen, J., Schriefer, M., Mead, P., Weinstein, S. and Haselow, D. (2017) Notes from the field: high volume of Lyme disease laboratory reporting in a low-incidence state – Arkansas, 2015–2016. *MMWR Morbidity and Mortality Weekly Report* 66, 1156–1157.

Lager, M., Faller, M., Wilhelmsson, P. et al. (2017) Molecular detection of *Borrelia burgdorferi* sensu lato – an analytical comparison of real-time PCR protocols from five different Scandinavian laboratories. *PLoS One* 12, e0185434.

Lantos, P.M., Auwaerter, P.G. and Wormser, G.P. (2014) A systematic review of *Borrelia burgdorferi* morphologic variants does not support a role in chronic Lyme disease. *Clinical Infectious Diseases* 58, 663–671.

Lantos, P.M., Branda, J.A., Boggan, J.C., Chudgar, S.M., Wilson, E.A., Ruffin, F., Fowler, V., Auwaerter, P.G. and Nigrovic, L.E. (2015) Poor positive predictive value of Lyme disease serologic testing in an area of low disease incidence. *Clinical Infectious Diseases* 61, 1374–1380.

Lantos, P.M., Lipsett, S.C. and Nigrovic, L.E. (2016) False positive Lyme disease IgM immunoblots in children. *Journal of Pediatrics* 174, 267–269, e1.

Ledue, T.B., Collins, M.F. and Craig, W.Y. (1996) New laboratory guidelines for serologic diagnosis of Lyme disease: evaluation of the two-test protocol. *Journal of Clinical Microbiology* 34, 2343–2350.

Lee, S.H., Vigliotti, V.S., Vigliotti, J.S., Jones, W., Williams, J. and Walshon, J. (2010) Early Lyme disease with spirochetemia – diagnosed by DNA sequencing. *BMC Research Notes* 3, 273.

Li, X., McHugh, G.A., Damle, N., Sikand, V.K., Glickstein, L. and Steere, A.C. (2011) Burden and viability of *Borrelia burgdorferi* in skin and joints of patients with erythema migrans or Lyme arthritis. *Arthritis and Rheumatism* 63, 2238–2247.

Liang, F.T., Steere, A.C., Marques, A.R., Johnson, B.J., Miller, J.N. and Philipp, M.T. (1999) Sensitive and specific serodiagnosis of Lyme disease by enzyme-linked immunosorbent assay with a peptide based on an immunodominant conserved region of *Borrelia burgdorferi* vlsE. *Journal of Clinical Microbiology* 37, 3990–3996.

Lightfoot Jr, R.W., Luft, B.J., Rahn, D.W., Steere, A.C., Sigal, L.H., Zoschke, D.C., Gardner, P., Britton, M.C. and Kaufman, R.L. (1993) Empiric parenteral antibiotic treatment of patients with fibromyalgia and fatigue and a positive serologic result for Lyme disease. A cost-effectiveness analysis. *Annals of Internal Medicine* 119, 503–509.

Lipsett, S.C., Pollock, N.R., Branda, J.A., Gordon, C.D., Gordon, C.R., Lantos, P.M. and Nigrovic, L.E. (2015) The positive predictive value of Lyme ELISA for the diagnosis of Lyme disease in children. *Pediatric Infectious Disease Journal* 34, 1260–1262.

Lipsett, S.C., Branda, J.A., McAdam, A.J., Vernacchio, L., Gordon, C.D., Gordon, C.R. and Nigrovic, L.E. (2016) Evaluation of the C6 Lyme enzyme immunoassay for the diagnosis of Lyme disease in children and adolescents. *Clinical Infectious Diseases* 63, 922–928.

Liveris, D., Schwartz, I., Bittker, S., Cooper, D., Iyer, R., Cox, M.E. and Wormser, G.P. (2011) Improving the yield of blood cultures from patients with early Lyme disease. *Journal of Clinical Microbiology* 49, 2166–2168.

Liveris, D., Schwartz, I., McKenna, D., Nowakowski, J., Nadelman, R., Demarco, J., Iyer, R., Bittker, S., Cooper, D., Holmgren, D. and Wormser, G.P. (2012) Comparison of five diagnostic modalities for direct detection of *Borrelia burgdorferi* in patients with early Lyme disease. *Diagnostic Microbiology and Infectious Disease* 73, 243–245.

Ljostad, U., Skarpaas, T. and Mygland, A. (2007) Clinical usefulness of intrathecal antibody testing in acute Lyme neuroborreliosis. *European Journal of Neurology* 14, 873–876.

Magnarelli, L.A. and Anderson, J.F. (1988) Enzyme-linked immunosorbent assays for the detection of class-specific immunoglobulins to *Borrelia burgdorferi*. *American Journal of Epidemiology* 127, 818–825.

Magnarelli, L.A., Anderson, J.F. and Johnson, R.C. (1987) Cross-reactivity in serological tests for Lyme disease and other spirochetal infections. *Journal of Infectious Diseases* 156, 183–188.

Magni, R., Espina, B.H., Shah, K. et al. (2015) Application of Nanotrap technology for high sensitivity measurement of urinary outer surface protein A carboxyl-terminus domain in early stage Lyme borreliosis. *Journal of Translational Medicine* 13, 346.

Markowicz, M., Kivaranovic, D. and Stanek, G. (2015) Testing patients with non-specific symptoms for antibodies against *Borrelia burgdorferi* sensu lato does not provide useful clinical information about their aetiology. *Clinical Microbiology and Infection* 21, 1098–1103.

Marques, A.R. (2015) Laboratory diagnosis of Lyme disease: advances and challenges. *Infectious Disease Clinics of North America* 29, 295–307.

Marques, A.R., Martin, D.S. and Philipp, M.T. (2002) Evaluation of the C6 peptide enzyme-linked immunosorbent assay for individuals vaccinated with the recombinant OspA vaccine. *Journal of Clinical Microbiology* 40, 2591–2593.

Marques, A., Telford, S.R. III, Turk, S.P. et al. (2014) Xenodiagnosis to detect *Borrelia burgdorferi* infection: a first-in-human study. *Clinical Infectious Diseases* 58, 937–945.

Martin, R., Martens, U., Sticht-Groh, V., Dorries, R. and Kruger, H. (1988) Persistent intrathecal secretion of oligoclonal, *Borrelia burgdorferi*-specific IgG in chronic meningoradiculomyelitis. *Journal of Neurology* 235, 229–233.

Molins, C.R., Sexton, C., Young, J.W., Ashton, L.V., Pappert, R., Beard, C.B. and Schriefer, M.E. (2014) Collection and characterization of samples for establishment of a serum repository for Lyme disease diagnostic test development and evaluation. *Journal of Clinical Microbiology* 52, 3755–3762.

Molins, C.R., Ashton, L.V., Wormser, G.P., Hess, A.M., Delorey, M.J., Mahapatra, S., Schriefer, M.E. and Belisle, J.T. (2015) Development of a metabolic biosignature for detection of early Lyme disease. *Clinical Infectious Diseases* 60, 1767–1775.

Molins, C.R., Delorey, M.J., Sexton, C. and Schriefer, M.E. (2016) Lyme borreliosis serology: performance of several commonly used laboratory diagnostic tests and a large resource panel of well-characterized patient samples. *Journal of Clinical Microbiology* 54, 2726–2734.

Molins, C.R., Ashton, L.V., Wormser, G.P. et al. (2017a) Metabolic differentiation of early Lyme disease from southern tick-associated rash illness (STARI). *Science Translational Medicine* 9(403), pii: eaal2717. DOI: 10.1126/scitranslmed.aal2717.

Molins, C.R., Delorey, M.J., Replogle, A., Sexton, C. and Schriefer, M.E. (2017b) Evaluation of bioMerieux's dissociated vidas Lyme IgM II and IgG II as a first-tier diagnostic assay for Lyme disease. *Journal of Clinical Microbiology* 55, 1698–1706.

Moore, J.E. and Eagle, H. (1941) The confusing multiplicity of serologic tests for syphilis. *JAMA* 117, 243–247.

Mygland, A., Ljostad, U., Fingerle, V., Rupprecht, T., Schmutzhard, E., Steiner, I. and European Federation of Neurological Science (2010) EFNS guidelines on the diagnosis and management of European Lyme neuroborreliosis. *European Journal of Neurology* 17, 8–16, e1–4.

Nayak, S., Sridhara, A., Melo, R., Richer, L., Chee, N.H., Kim, J., Linder, V., Steinmiller, D., Sia, S.K. and Gomes-Solecki, M. (2016) Microfluidics-based point-of-care test for serodiagnosis of Lyme disease. *Scientific Reports* 6, 35069.

Nelson, C., Hojvat, S., Johnson, B., Petersen, J., Schriefer, M., Beard, C.B., Petersen, L., Mead, P., Centers for Disease Control and Prevention (2014) Concerns regarding a new culture method for *Borrelia burgdorferi* not approved for the diagnosis of Lyme disease. *MMWR Morbidity and Mortality Weekly Report* 63, 333.

Nelson, C., Elmendorf, S. and Mead, P. (2015) Neoplasms misdiagnosed as 'chronic Lyme disease'. *JAMA Internal Medicine* 175, 132–133.

Nocton, J.J., Bloom, B.J., Rutledge, B.J., Persing, D.H., Logigian, E.L., Schmid, C.H. and Steere, A.C. (1996) Detection of *Borrelia burgdorferi* DNA by polymerase chain reaction in cerebrospinal fluid in Lyme neuroborreliosis. *Journal of Infectious Diseases* 174, 623–627.

Nowakowski, J., Schwartz, I., Liveris, D., Wang, G., Aguero-Rosenfeld, M.E., Girao, G., McKenna, D., Nadelman, R.B., Cavaliere, L.F. and Wormser, G.P. (2001) Laboratory diagnostic techniques for patients with early Lyme disease associated with erythema migrans: a comparison of different techniques. *Clinical Infectious Diseases* 33, 2023–2027.

Patrick, D.M., Miller, R.R., Gardy, J.L., Parker, S.M., Morshed, M.G., Steiner, T.S., Singer, J., Shojania, K., Tang, P. and Complex Chronic Disease Study Group (2015) Lyme disease diagnosed by alternative methods: a phenotype similar to that of chronic fatigue syndrome. *Clinical Infectious Diseases* 61, 1084–1091.

Patriquin, G., Leblanc, J., Heinstein, C., Roberts, C., Lindsay, R. and Hatchette, T.F. (2016) Cross-reactivity between Lyme and syphilis screening assays: Lyme disease does not cause false-positive syphilis screens. *Diagnostic Microbiology and Infectious Disease* 84, 184–186.

Pavletic, A.J. and Marques, A.R. (2017) Early disseminated Lyme disease causing false-positive serology for primary Epstein-Barr virus infection: report of 2 cases. *Clinical Infectious Diseases* 65, 336–337.

Peltomaa, M., McHugh, G. and Steere, A.C. (2003) Persistence of the antibody response to the VlsE sixth invariant region (IR6) peptide of *Borrelia burgdorferi* after successful antibiotic treatment of Lyme disease. *Journal of Infectious Diseases* 187, 1178–1186.

Philipp, M.T., Wormser, G.P., Marques, A.R., Bittker, S., Martin, D.S., Nowakowski, J. and Dally, L.G. (2005) A decline in C6 antibody titer occurs in successfully treated patients with culture-confirmed early localized or early disseminated Lyme borreliosis. *Clinical and Vaccine Immunology* 12, 1069–1074.

Picha, D., Moravcova, L., Zdarsky, E., Maresova, V. and Hulinsky, V. (2005) PCR in Lyme neuroborreliosis: a prospective study. *Acta Neurologica Scandinavica* 112, 287–292.

Pollack, R.J., Telford, S.R. III and Spielman, A. (1993) Standardization of medium for culturing Lyme disease spirochetes. *Journal of Clinical Microbiology* 31, 1251–1255.

Porwancher, R. (1999) A reanalysis of IgM Western blot criteria for the diagnosis of early Lyme disease. *Journal of Infectious Diseases* 179, 1021–1024.

Questdiagnostics (2017) Lyme disease antibodies (IgG, IgM), IBL (CSF) [online]. Available at: www.questdiagnostics.com/testcenter/BUOrderInfo.action?tc=70028&labCode=SJC (accessed 11 October 2017).

Radolf, J.D., Caimano, M.J., Stevenson, B. and Hu, L.T. (2012) Of ticks, mice and men: understanding the dual-host lifestyle of Lyme disease spirochaetes. *Nature Reviews Microbiology* 10, 87–99.

Ružić-Sabljić, E., Lotric-Furlan, S., Maraspin, V., Cimperman, J., Logar, M., Jurca, T. and Strle, F. (2006) Comparison of isolation rate of *Borrelia burgdorferi* sensu lato in MKP and BSK-II medium. *International Journal of Medical Microbiology* 296(40), 267–273.

Sanchez, E., Vannier, E., Wormser, G.P. and Hu, L.T. (2016) Diagnosis, treatment, and prevention of Lyme disease, human granulocytic anaplasmosis, and babesiosis: a review. *Jama* 315, 1767–1777.

Sapi, E., Pabbati, N., Datar, A., Davies, E.M., Rattelle, A. and Kuo, B.A. (2013) Improved culture conditions for the growth and detection of *Borrelia* from human serum. *International Journal of Medical Sciences* 10, 362–376.

Schmidt, C., Plate, A., Angele, B., Pfister, H.W., Wick, M., Koedel, U. and Rupprecht, T.A. (2011) A prospective study on the role of CXCL13 in Lyme neuroborreliosis. *Neurology* 76, 1051–1058.

Schutzer, S.E., Coyle, P.K., Belman, A.L., Golightly, M.G. and Drulle, J. (1990) Sequestration of antibody to *Borrelia burgdorferi* in immune complexes in seronegative Lyme disease. *Lancet* 335, 312–315.

Seltzer, E.G. and Shapiro, E.D. (1996) Misdiagnosis of Lyme disease: when not to order serologic tests. *Pediatric Infectious Disease Journal* 15, 762–763.

Seriburi, V., Ndukwe, N., Chang, Z., Cox, M.E. and Wormser, G.P. (2012) High frequency of false positive IgM immunoblots for *Borrelia burgdorferi* in clinical practice. *Clinical Microbiology and Infection* 18, 1236–1240.

Shapiro, E.D. (2014) Clinical practice. Lyme disease. *New England Journal of Medicine* 370, 1724–1731.
Sivak, S.L., Aguero-Rosenfeld, M.E., Nowakowski, J., Nadelman, R.B. and Wormser, G.P. (1996) Accuracy of IgM immunoblotting to confirm the clinical diagnosis of early Lyme disease. *Archives of Internal Medicine* 156, 2105–2109.
Stanek, G. and Strle, F. (2008) Lyme disease: European perspective. *Infectious Disease Clinics of North America* 22, 327–339, vii.
Stanek, G., Wormser, G.P., Gray, J. and Strle, F. (2012) Lyme borreliosis. *Lancet* 379, 461–473.
Stanek, G., Lusa, L., Ogrinc, K., Markowicz, M. and Strle, F. (2014) Intrathecally produced IgG and IgM antibodies to recombinant VlsE, VlsE peptide, recombinant OspC and whole cell extracts in the diagnosis of Lyme neuroborreliosis. *Medical Microbiology and Immunology* 203, 125–132.
Steere, A.C. and Angelis, S.M. (2006) Therapy for Lyme arthritis: strategies for the treatment of antibiotic-refractory arthritis. *Arthritis and Rheumatism* 54, 3079–3086.
Steere, A.C., McHugh, G., Damle, N. and Sikand, V.K. (2008) Prospective study of serologic tests for Lyme disease. *Clinical Infectious Diseases* 47, 188–195.
Tugwell, P., Dennis, D.T., Weinstein, A., Wells, G., Shea, B., Nichol, G., Hayward, R., Lightfoot, R., Baker, P. and Steere, A.C. (1997) Laboratory evaluation in the diagnosis of Lyme disease. *Annals of Internal Medicine* 127, 1109–1123.
Tuuminen, T., Hedman, K., Soderlund-Venermo, M. and Seppala, I. (2011) Acute parvovirus B19 infection causes nonspecificity frequently in *Borrelia* and less often in *Salmonella* and *Campylobacter* serology, posing a problem in diagnosis of infectious arthropathy. *Clinical and Vaccine Immunology* 18, 167–172.
Wang, Z.Y., Hansen, K., Siden, A. and Cruz, M. (1993) Intrathecal synthesis of anti-*Borrelia burgdorferi* antibodies in neuroborreliosis: a study with special emphasis on oligoclonal IgM antibody bands. *Scandinavian Journal of Immunology* 37, 369–376.
Weiss, N.L., Sadock, V.A., Sigal, L.H., Phillips, M., Merryman, P.F. and Abramson, S.B. (1995) False positive seroreactivity to *Borrelia burgdorferi* in systemic lupus erythematosus: the value of immunoblot analysis. *Lupus* 4, 131–137.
Wormser, G.P., Horowitz, H.W., Nowakowski, J., McKenna, D., Dumler, J.S., Varde, S., Schwartz, I., Carbonaro, C. and Aguero-Rosenfeld, M. (1997) Positive Lyme disease serology in patients with clinical and laboratory evidence of human granulocytic ehrlichiosis. *American Journal of Clinical Pathology* 107, 142–147.
Wormser, G.P., Carbonaro, C., Miller, S., Nowakowski, J., Nadelman, R.B., Sivak, S. and Aguero-Rosenfeld, M.E. (2000) A limitation of 2-stage serological testing for Lyme disease: enzyme immunoassay and immunoblot assay are not independent tests. *Clinical Infectious Diseases* 30, 545–548.
Wormser, G.P., Bittker, S., Cooper, D., Nowakowski, J., Nadelman, R.B. and Pavia, C. (2001) Yield of large-volume blood cultures in patients with early Lyme disease. *Journal of Infectious Diseases* 184, 1070–1072.
Wormser, G.P., McKenna, D., Carlin, J., Nadelman, R.B., Cavaliere, L.F., Holmgren, D., Byrne, D.W. and Nowakowski, J. (2005) Brief communication: hematogenous dissemination in early Lyme disease. *Annals of Internal Medicine* 142, 751–755.
Wormser, G.P., Dattwyler, R.J., Shapiro, E.D. *et al.* (2006) The clinical assessment, treatment, and prevention of Lyme disease, human granulocytic anaplasmosis, and babesiosis: clinical practice guidelines by the Infectious Diseases Society of America. *Clinical Infectious Diseases* 43, 1089–1134.
Wormser, G.P., Nowakowski, J., Nadelman, R.B., Visintainer, P., Levin, A. and Aguero-Rosenfeld, M.E. (2008) Impact of clinical variables on *Borrelia burgdorferi*-specific antibody seropositivity in acute-phase sera from patients in North America with culture-confirmed early Lyme disease. *Clinical and Vaccine Immunology* 15, 1519–1522.
Wormser, G.P., Nadelman, R.B. and Schwartz, I. (2012) The amber theory of Lyme arthritis: initial description and clinical implications. *Clinical Rheumatology* 31, 989–994.
Wormser, G.P., Levin, A., Soman, S., Adenikinju, O., Longo, M.V. and Branda, J.A. (2013a) Comparative cost-effectiveness of two-tiered testing strategies for serodiagnosis of Lyme disease with noncutaneous manifestations. *Journal of Clinical Microbiology* 51, 4045–4049.
Wormser, G.P., Schriefer, M., Aguero-Rosenfeld, M.E., Levin, A., Steere, A.C., Nadelman, R.B., Nowakowski, J., Marques, A., Johnson, B.J. and Dumler, J.S. (2013b) Single-tier testing with the C6 peptide ELISA kit compared with two-tier testing for Lyme disease. *Diagnostic Microbiology and Infectious Disease* 75, 9–15.
Wormser, G.P., Tang, A.T., Schimmoeller, N.R., Bittker, S., Cooper, D., Visintainer, P., Aguero-Rosenfeld, M.E., Ogrinc, K., Strle, F. and Stanek, G. (2014) Utility of serodiagnostics designed for use in the United

States for detection of Lyme borreliosis acquired in Europe and vice versa. *Medical Microbiology and Immunology* 203, 65–71.

Wormser, G.P., Shapiro, E.D. and Strle, F. (2017) Studies that report unexpected positive blood cultures for Lyme borrelia – are they valid? *Diagnostic Microbiology and Infectious Disease* 89, 178–181.

Yang, J., Han, X., Liu, A., Bao, F., Peng, Y., Tao, L., Ma, M., Bai, R. and Dai, X. (2017) Chemokine CXC Ligand 13 in cerebrospinal fluid can be used as an early diagnostic biomarker for Lyme neuroborreliosis: a meta-analysis. *Journal of Interferon and Cytokine Research* 37, 433–439.

5 Global Epidemiology of *Borreliella burgdorferi* Infections

Paul S. Mead
Bacterial Diseases Branch, Division of Vector-borne Diseases, National Center for Emerging and Zoonotic Infectious Diseases, Centers for Disease Control and Prevention (CDC), Ft Collins, Colorado, USA

5.1 Introduction

Lyme borreliosis, or Lyme disease, is a multisystem illness caused by certain genospecies of the spirochete *Borreliella burgdorferi* (formerly *Borrelia burgdorferi* sensu lato) (Steere *et al.*, 2016). Although not formally identified until the mid-1970s (Steere *et al.*, 1977; Burgdorfer *et al.*, 1982), the illness is now recognized as the most common vector-borne disease in Europe and North America. The *Borreliella* spirochete is transmitted among animals and to humans by ticks of the *Ixodes ricinus* complex, which are found widely in temperate wooded regions of the northern hemisphere (Piesman and Gern, 2004). Clinical features of human infection include dermatologic, rheumatologic, neurologic and cardiac abnormalities (Steere *et al.*, 2016). An understanding of the disease's epidemiology is vital for clinicians attempting to distinguish infected patients from those with other conditions.

Many factors interact to determine the incidence, distribution and clinical features of Lyme borreliosis. These include the different genospecies of *B. burgdorferi* and their distribution in nature, the abundance and feeding habits of the vector tick species, and the demographic and behavioral traits of the exposed human population. Surveillance practices can alter the perceived features of the disease through underreporting and detection bias. Laboratory-based surveillance, for example, typically detects patients who are seropositive and therefore likely to have later stages of illness (Ertel *et al.*, 2012). Interpretation of surveillance data is further complicated by the existence of clinically similar diseases (Wormser *et al.*, 2005; Mantovani *et al.*, 2007), the vagaries of serologic testing (Hunfeld *et al.*, 2002; Aguero-Rosenfeld, 2003; Ekerfelt *et al.*, 2004) and substantial differences in surveillance practices across jurisdictions. With these limitations in mind, this chapter provides an overview of the epidemiology of *B. burgdorferi* infections in various regions of the world, underscoring similarities and differences across regions.

5.2 Agents, Vectors and Geographic Distribution

At least 20 named genospecies of *B. burgdorferi* sensu lato have been described based on isolates from ticks, rodents and birds (LPSN, 2017). Three of these, *B. afzelii*, *B. garinii* and *B. burgdorferi* sensu stricto (hereafter *B. burgdorferi*), cause the majority of human infections. A fourth genospecies, *B. mayonii*, has been isolated from patients living in the north central United States (Pritt *et al.*, 2016). Other genospecies including *B. bavariensis*, *B. bissetii*, *B. lusitaniae*, *B. spielmanii* and *B. valaisiana* have been detected on rare occasion in humans; however, the clinical features, frequency and overall public health significance of these agents are poorly defined (van Dam, 2002; Diza et al., 2004; da Franca et al., 2005; Maraspin et al., 2006; de Carvalho et al., 2008; Rudenko et al., 2008; 2009; Pritt et al., 2016). The diversity in *Borreliella* genospecies presumably reflects adaptation to different reservoir hosts (van Dam, 2002; Becker et al., 2016), and it seems likely that some genospecies might have greater capacity than others for infecting humans.

Borreliella burgdorferi is transmitted in nature by multiple species of *Ixodes* ticks; however only four of these species commonly bite humans (Fig. 5.1). The most important in North America is *I. scapularis*. This tick is abundant in the mid-Atlantic, northeastern and north central United States and nearby areas of Canada. A less abundant species, *I. pacificus*, occurs in pockets from the central California coast northward into British Columbia. The principal vectors of Lyme borreliosis in Europe and Asia are *I. ricinus* and *I. persulcatus*, respectively. *Ixodes ricinus* is found at elevations below 1300 m throughout western, central and eastern Europe, as well as northern Africa (Piesman and Gern, 2004). *Ixodes persulcatus* is found in western Russia, where its distribution overlaps with *I. ricinus*, and eastward through Mongolia and China to the Pacific Ocean and Japan.

The four tick vectors differ with regard to carriage of *B. burgdorferi* sensu lato genospecies (Fig. 5.1). *Ixodes ricinus* ticks transmit all three major pathogenic genospecies, with some geographic variation. Ticks collected in northern and eastern Europe are more likely to carry *B. afzelii*, while those from western Europe are more often infected with *B. garinii* (Rauter and Hartung, 2005). Carriage of *B. burgdorferi* occurs throughout Europe but is generally less prevalent (Piesman and Gern, 2004). In Asia, *I. persulcatus* transmits *B. afzelii* and Asian and Eurasian variants of *B. garinii*, but it is not known to transmit *B. burgdorferi* (Korenberg, 1994; Korenberg et al., 2002; Masuzawa, 2004). In North America, *I. pacificus* transmits *B. burgdorferi* alone, and *I. scapularis* transmits *B. burgdorferi* and the closely related *B. mayonii* (Steere, 2001; Piesman and Gern, 2004; Dolan et al., 2016).

The geographic distribution of vector tick species generally defines areas of potential risk for Lyme borreliosis in Eurasia and North America. Within these broad areas, however, actual risk of human infection can vary widely due to

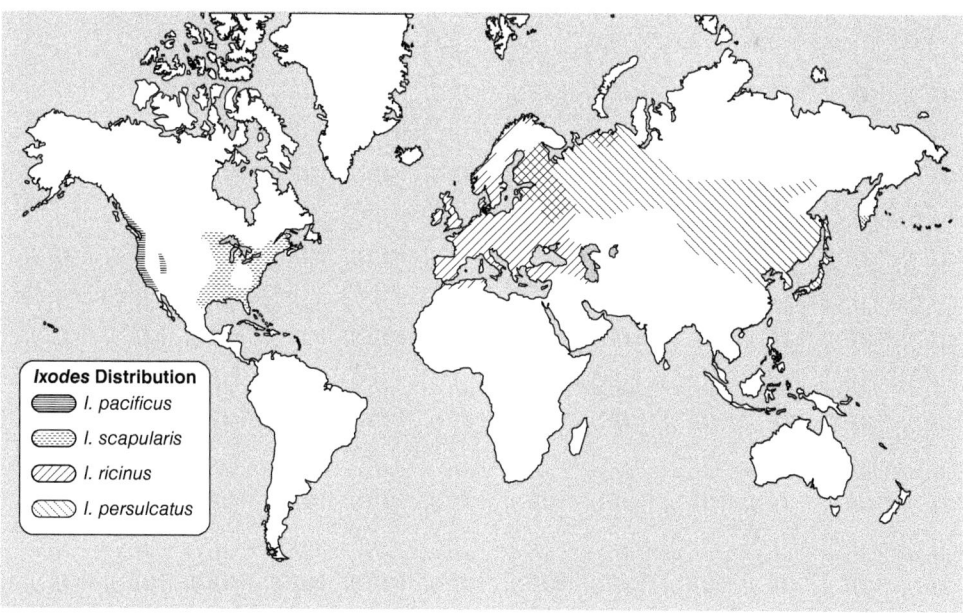

Fig. 5.1. Approximate global distribution of principal *Ixodes* vectors of Lyme borreliosis and associated genospecies of *Borreliella burgdorferi* sensu lato. (Derived from Korenberg, 1994; Masuzawa 2004; Hao et al., 2011; ECDC, 2017.)

differences in tick abundance and infection prevalence. In the northeastern United States, infection prevalence among adult *I. scapularis* can approach 40%, reflecting robust local enzootic cycles. In contrast, *I. scapularis* ticks in the southeastern United States are rarely infected with *B. burgdorferi*, possibly as a result of genetic and local ecologic factors (Piesman and Gern, 2004). It has been hypothesized, for example, that southern *I. scapularis* have been selected to quest below the leaf litter due to a greater risk of desiccation (Ginsberg et al., 2017). In the western United States, *I. pacificus* ticks are also rarely infected with *B. burgdorferi* owing to their preferences for feeding on lizards that are not competent reservoirs for the spirochete (Piesman and Gern, 2004).

5.3 Incidence by Region

Regional comparisons of disease incidence are subject to many limitations and caveats. There is no formal surveillance for Lyme borreliosis in some endemic countries, and even where surveillance is conducted, methods can vary widely. Case ascertainment and reported incidence will be generally greater in areas with active surveillance or those utilizing sentinel sites (e.g. France and Belgium). Because the distribution of disease can be quite focal, the geographic scale at which data are aggregated can further complicate comparisons. For example, while pockets of equally intense transmission may exist in both Russia and Estonia, the overall rate for Russia will be lower due to its vastly greater size. Despite these and other difficulties, several trends are apparent: (i) incidence continues to increase in many countries; (ii) the geographic distribution of disease is expanding in both Europe and North America; and (iii) the absolute risk of infection is substantial in some areas.

5.3.1 North America

The United States currently accounts for the great majority of all Lyme disease cases reported in North America (Table 5.1). The disease was designated a nationally notifiable condition in 1991, and reported cases have increased from ~9000 in 1992 to more than 35,000 in 2015 (Bacon et al., 2008; Schwartz et al., 2017). Because US surveillance data are based on passive surveillance, underreporting is inevitable. Special studies using data from commercial laboratories (Hinckley et al., 2014) and medical claims (Nelson et al., 2015) suggest that the true number of infections is approximately 300,000 annually, roughly eight-fold greater than the number reported.

Within the United States, Lyme disease occurs in two major foci, one in the northeast and mid-Atlantic region, and a second in the upper Midwest (Fig. 5.2; Table 5.2). Fourteen states in these two regions (Connecticut, Delaware, Maine, Massachusetts, Maryland, Minnesota, New Hampshire, New Jersey, New York, Pennsylvania, Rhode Island, Vermont, Virginia and Wisconsin) account for over 95% of all reported cases (Schwartz et al., 2017). Within these states county-level incidence can exceed 200 reported cases per 100,000 population (Bacon et al., 2008). This equates to an annual infection rate of approximately 1–2% after accounting for underreporting. Smaller foci of low-level transmission occur along the west coast in California, Oregon and Washington where *I. pacificus* is an established though rarely infected vector (Piesman and Gern, 2004). Some of the increase in reported cases over time can be attributed to improved surveillance (Connecticut Department of Public Health, 2009); however, there is also evidence that the two major foci of transmission have expanded substantially (Fig. 5.2). In a formal assessment, the number of counties in the northeast meeting criteria for high incidence increased from 43 during 1993–1997 to 182 during 2008–2012, a gain of more than 320%. During the same time period, the number of high incidence counties in the upper Midwest increased ≈250%, from 22 to 78 (Kugeler et al., 2015).

In the United States, cases are reported based on the state in which a patient resides. Consequently, infections acquired during travel or former residence in an endemic area are occasionally reported from states where evidence of local transmission is lacking (Bacon et al., 2008). These reports have sometimes been misinterpreted as evidence that transmission occurs in all states. Strong evidence to the contrary, however, is provided by seroprevalence studies of domestic dogs. Millions of dogs nationwide have been tested for antibodies to the conserved C6

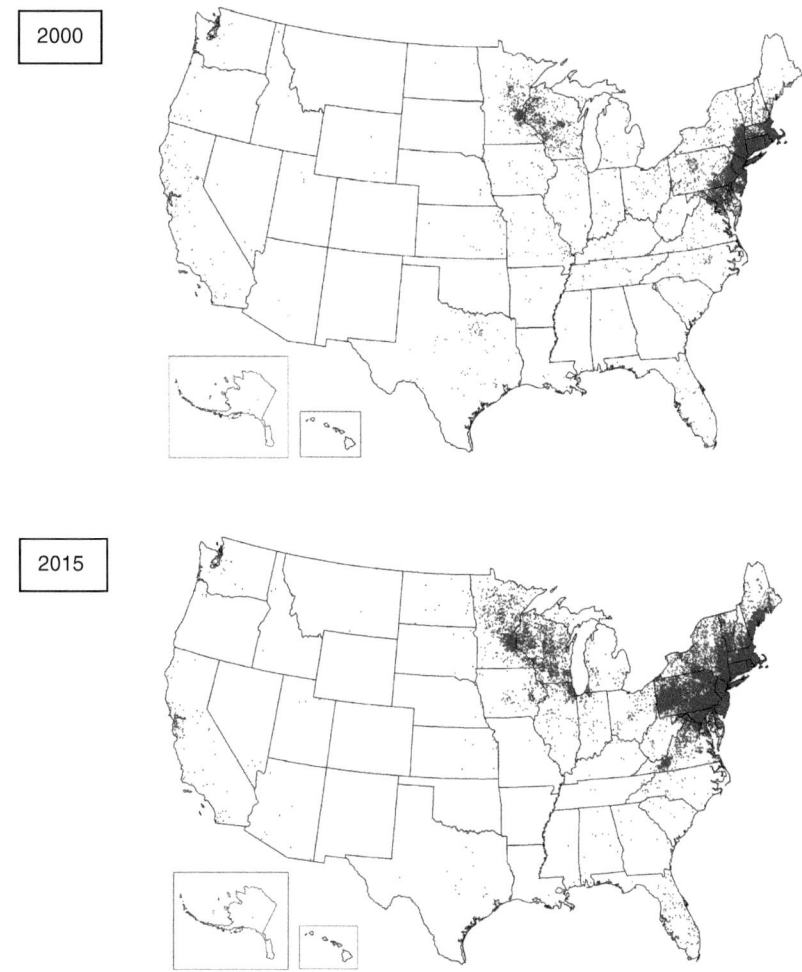

Fig. 5.2. Distribution of US cases of Lyme diseases reported by the Centers for Disease Control and Prevention, 2001 and 2015. Each dot represents one case, placed randomly in the county of patient residence, which is often but not always the county of exposure.

oligopeptide of *B. burgdorferi* (Duncan *et al.*, 2004; Bowman *et al.*, 2009; Little *et al.*, 2014). In Lyme endemic states of the northeast, up to 25% of dogs are seropositive, underscoring the remarkable sensitivity of dogs as sentinels for the presence of *B. burgdorferi* in the environment (Duncan *et al.*, 2004; Mead *et al.*, 2011). In contrast, less than 1% of dogs in the south-east are seropositive (Bowman *et al.*, 2009; Little *et al.*, 2014). This value is wholly explained by the false positive rate of the assay (Duncan *et al.*, 2004; IDEXX, 2010; Stillman *et al.*, 2014) and thus evidence against an appreciable enzootic transmission cycle in these areas.

In Canada, *I. pacificus* ticks are established in coastal areas of southern British Columbia, and populations of *I. scapularis* have been identified along the US border in Manitoba, Ontario, Quebec and Nova Scotia (Ogden *et al.*, 2009). Although less common than in the United States, reports of human Lyme disease have increased substantially in recent years, from 144 in 2009 to 917 in 2015 (Public Health Agency of Canada, 2017). In 2015, three eastern provinces, Ontario, Quebec and Nova Scotia, accounted for over 90% of reported cases. Incidence is greatest in Nova Scotia, at 26 cases per 100,000 population. Consistent with this, a recent serologic study found that 16% of dogs in Nova Scotia had antibodies to *B. burgdorferi*, a far higher prevalence than in other areas (Herrin *et al.*, 2017). There is concern that changing climatic conditions will allow northward expansion of *Ixodes* populations further into Canada, potentially increasing the risk of Lyme disease (Ogden *et al.*, 2006).

Although *I. scapularis* ticks are found in northeastern Mexico and *I. pacificus* are found in Baja (Piesman and Gern, 2004; Gordillo-Perez *et al.*, 2009), evidence for human Lyme borreliosis in Mexico is limited to a few case reports (Gordillo-Perez *et al.*, 2007). Some investigators have reported high rates of *B. burgdorferi* infection among *I. scapularis* ticks collected in Texas and northern Mexico (Feria-Arroyo *et al.*, 2014); however, genetic analysis of these results suggests that they likely represent laboratory contamination (Norris *et al.*, 2015).

5.3.2 Europe

Lyme borreliosis is widespread in Europe, with approximately 65,000 cases occurring annually (Hubalek, 2009; Rizzoli *et al.*, 2011). Endemic foci are found within the range of *I. ricinus*, from Portugal and the British Isles east to Turkey and north into Scandinavia and Russia (Fig. 5.1). Although Lyme borreliosis is not a notifiable condition in many countries, available data suggest that transmission is most intense in central and northeastern Europe (Rizzoli *et al.*, 2011). The Czech Republic, France, Germany, Latvia, Poland and Switzerland report incidence rates ranging from 20–50/100,000 population. Higher rates, some exceeding 100/100,000 population, have been reported from Austria, Belgium, Estonia, Finland, Lithuania, the Netherlands, Slovenia and southern Sweden (Table 5.1). In general, incidence appears to decrease moving northward in Scandinavia, from east to west in central Europe, and southward through France, Spain, Italy and Greece (Lindgren and Jaenson, 2006; Vandenesch *et al.*, 2014). A temporal increase in cases has been reported in several countries over the past two decades, including Poland, east Germany, Slovenia, Bulgaria, Norway, Finland, Belgium, the UK and the Netherlands (Hofhuis *et al.*, 2006; Smith and Takkinen, 2006; Fulop and Poggensee, 2008; Dubrey *et al.*, 2014; Sajanti *et al.*, 2017). As in North America, these increases may reflect a combination of both increased transmission and improved awareness of the disease (Kampen *et al.*, 2004; Hofhuis *et al.*, 2006; Smith and Takkinen, 2006). Stabilization of rates, as seen more recently in Germany, suggests maturation of the surveillance system (Wilking and Stark, 2014).

5.3.3 Asia

Areas at risk for Lyme borreliosis extend across Eurasia, from Japan to the western border of Russia (Fig. 5.1). In Russia, official records on Lyme borreliosis cases have been kept since 1992 (Korenberg, 1994). Reported incidence in endemic areas generally ranges from 5 to 10/100,000 population (Table 5.1). Higher rates have been reported in areas northeast of Moscow in Vologda oblast, in the Sverdlovsk (Urals) region and in western Siberia (World Health Organization, 1995; EpiNorth, 2014). Although infected ticks have been found in Mongolia, information on human cases is scarce in the English literature. At least six genospecies of *B. burgdorferi* sensu lato have been isolated from rodents and ticks in China, and over 2000 human infections have been identified through serologic testing (Ai *et al.*, 1990; Chu *et al.*, 2008; Hao *et al.*, 2011; Zhang *et al.*, 2010; Fang *et al.*, 2015). Based on a small number of clinical isolates, *B. garinii* appears to be the most common cause of human infection, followed by *B. afzelii* and a single isolate of a *B. valasiana*-related genospecies (Fang *et al.*, 2015). Human cases have been reported from most areas but most commonly from the more northern provinces of Xinjiang, Gansu, Inner Mongolia, Jinlin and Heilongjiang (Fang *et al.*, 2015). Although both *B. garinii* and *B. afzelii* have been isolated from patients in Japan, overall incidence is <0.1 per 100,000 population, with most cases occurring on Hokkaido Island in northern Japan and some from exposures in subalpine forested areas in central Japan (Nakama *et al.*, 1994; Hashimoto *et al.*, 2007). Enzootic cycles are established in Korea and Taiwan, and *B. garinii* has been isolated in culture from at least one patient from northern Taiwan (Chao *et al.*, 2010).

Table 5.1. Reported or estimated incidence of Lyme borreliosis for selected countries. Surveillance methods vary widely and values are not directly comparable.

Region/country	Incidence[a]	Year/period	Reference
Albania	0.1	2010	WHO, 2014
Austria[b]	135	2005	Smith and Takkinen, 2006
Belarus	12	2012	EpiNorth, 2014
Belgium	90	2008–2009	Vanthomme et al., 2012
Bulgaria	8	2010	WHO, 2014
Bosnia/Herzegovina	2	2010	WHO, 2014
Canada	<0.1	1995–2006	Ogden et al., 2008
Croatia	11	2010	WHO, 2014
Czech Republic	36	2005	Smith and Takkinen, 2006
Denmark	1	2012	EpiNorth, 2014
Estonia	115	2012	EpiNorth, 2014
Finland[b]	84	2010–2014	Sajanti et al., 2017
France	42	2009–2012	Vandenesch et al., 2014
Georgia	0.4	2010	WHO, 2014
Germany	36.5	2006	Fulop and Poggensee, 2008
Hungary	12.8	2001–2005	Hubalek, 2009
Iceland	0.6	1999–2003	Hubalek, 2009
Italy	<0.1	2001–2005	Hubalek, 2009
Japan	<0.1	2000–2005	Hashimoto et al., 2007
Latvia	35	2012	EpiNorth, 2014
Lithuania	82	2012	EpiNorth, 2014
Moldova	3.0	2010	WHO, 2014
Montenegro	0.3	2010	WHO, 2014
The Netherlands[c]	140	2009–2010	Hofhuis et al., 2015
Norway	5	2012	EpiNorth, 2014
Poland	23	2012	Paradowska-Stankiewicz and Chrzescijanska, 2016
Portugal	0.1	2010	WHO, 2014
Romania	1.2	2010	WHO, 2014
Russia	8	2012	EpiNorth, 2014
Serbia	9.8	2010	WHO, 2014
Slovakia	15	2010	WHO, 2014
Slovenia	273	2011	WHO, 2014
Spain	0.1	2010	WHO, 2014
Switzerland	25.1	1988–1998	Hubalek, 2009
Sweden (southern)	69	1992	Berglund et al., 1996
Turkey	<0.1	1990–2002	Hubalek, 2009
Ukraine	3.6	2012	EpiNorth, 2014
United Kingdom	1.6	2010	Dubrey et al., 2014
United States	8.5	2012–2015	Schwartz et al., 2017

[a]Reported cases per 100,000 population per year.
[b]Estimated.
[c]Combined rates for erythema migrans and disseminated infections.

5.3.4 Tropics and southern hemisphere

A Lyme borreliosis-like illness has been reported on rare occasions in countries of the southern hemisphere, including Australia (Russell, 1995), Brazil (Mantovani et al., 2007) and South Africa (Stanek et al., 1987b). In addition, antibodies reactive to B. burgdorferi sensu lato antigens have been detected in some serosurveys and diagnostic tests on residents in tropical areas (Miranda et al., 2009; Santos et al., 2010). While the possibility of Borreliella-related illness with distinct

Table 5.2. Average annual Lyme Disease incidence, U.S. States, 2012-2015. Data from Schwartz et al., 2017.

State	Incidence[a]
Alabama	0.4
Alaska	0.9
Arizona	0.2
Arkansas	0
California	0.2
Colorado	0
Connecticut	52.9
Delaware	38.3
District of Columbia	7.4
Florida	0.5
Georgia	0.1
Hawaii	0
Idaho	0.5
Illinois	2.2
Indiana	1.5
Iowa	4.2
Kansas	0.5
Kentucky	0.3
Louisiana	0
Maine	82.5
Maryland	16.8
Massachusetts	51.3
Michigan	1.1
Minnesota	21.4
Mississippi	0.1
Missouri	0.1
Montana	0.7
Nebraska	0.3
Nevada	0.2
New Hampshire	59.8
New Jersey	34.7
New Mexico	0
New York	16.2
North Carolina	0.3
North Dakota	1.3
Ohio	0.8
Oklahoma	0
Oregon	0.2
Pennsylvania	49
Rhode Island	49.9
South Carolina	0.5
South Dakota	0.4
Tennessee	0.1
Texas	0.1
Utah	0.2
Vermont	85.5
Virginia	12
Washington	0.2
West Virginia	8.5
Wisconsin	21.7
Wyoming	0.2

[a]Reported cases per 100,000 population per year.

enzootic cycles in these areas cannot be excluded, a great deal more information will be needed to determine the relationship, if any, between these reports and Lyme borreliosis as currently defined. A recent review of data from Australia concluded that there was no credible evidence for the disease in that country (Collignon et al., 2016).

5.4 Seasonality

Like other vector-borne diseases, Lyme borreliosis occurs most often in the warmer months. This temporal pattern is likely the result of both tick questing habits and the recreational tendencies of humans (Ai et al., 1990; Piesman and Gern, 2004; Bacon et al., 2008). Due to their abundance and minute size, nymphal ticks pose a special risk of transmission. Nymphal questing usually peaks in spring or early summer and is followed by an increase in human cases one to several weeks later (Piesman and Gern, 2004). In the United States, human disease onset peaks in early summer, with over half of all cases having onset in June or July (Bacon et al., 2008). In most European countries, acute infections peak slightly later, in July and August, as reported in Estonia (Lindgren and Jaenson, 2006), Finland (Sajanti et al., 2017), France (Vandenesch et al., 2014), Germany (Wilking and Stark, 2014) and Sweden (Berglund et al., 1995). It is unclear whether this temporal difference is due to the more northern latitude of these countries or the recreational patterns of their population. There is evidence that questing behavior responds to meteorological factors (Alekseev and Dubinina, 2000; Eisen et al., 2002), and that the onset of human illness can vary from year to year based on climatic conditions (Bennet et al., 2006; Moore et al., 2014). Due to longer and more variable incubation periods, later stages of disease tend to peak slightly later in the year and show less seasonal fluctuation (Stanek et al., 1987a; Berglund et al., 1995; Strle, 1999; Bacon et al., 2008; Vandenesch et al., 2014; Sajanti et al., 2017).

5.5 Age and Sex

Data on age and sex distribution are often published as case counts rather than incidence rates. Although this hinders comparisons, several trends are generally apparent. With respect to age, the distribution of Lyme borreliosis cases is most often bimodal. Rates peak among children between the ages of 5 and 15 years, decrease among 20- to 25-year-olds, and peak again among adults, typically in those 50 years or older (Fig. 5.3) (Bacon *et al.*, 2008; Fulop and Poggensee, 2008; Hubalek, 2009). The absolute highest rate usually occurs among adults in Europe and among children in North America. These patterns likely reflect behavior-related differences in rates of exposure across populations, although they may also be influenced by age- and sex-specific differences in clinical illness (see clinical features below) and reporting practices. With respect to sex, females account for the majority of cases in most European countries. In series from Austria, Czech Republic, Germany, Italy, Slovenia, Sweden, Switzerland and Poland, 51–60% of identified cases were in females. Where information on incidence is also available, these percentages correspond to higher incidence among females, but often only in adults (Fig. 5.3). Despite the overall preponderance of female cases, incidence is actually higher for boys than girls in both Sweden and Germany (Berglund *et al.*, 1995; Fulop and Poggensee, 2008).

The situation with respect to gender is appreciably different in North America, where incidence is higher among males in nearly all age groups (Fig. 5.3). During 1992–2006, females accounted for only 47% of US cases, yielding an overall incidence of 5.4/100,000 for females, as compared to 6.3/100,000 for males (Bacon *et al.*, 2008). Over time, incidence has increased disproportionately among males, shifting the overall sex ratio for confirmed cases from 51% males in 1992 to 53% in 2006 (Bacon *et al.*, 2008) to 57% males during 2008–2015 (Schwartz *et al.*, 2017). Although unexplained, this gender-specific increase has been most pronounced among children. Age and sex distributions also differ between areas with high and low reported incidence (CDC, 2004). During 2008–2015, the modal age for cases in high incidence states was 8 years with 57% of cases among males, as compared with 44 years with 45% of cases among males in low incidence states (Schwartz *et al.*, 2017). Barring fundamental differences in risk factors for infection, this discrepancy suggests that cases reported in low incidence states are often due to conditions other than Lyme disease. This is consistent with the lower predictive value of clinical and laboratory findings in the setting of low prior probability (Tugwell *et al.*, 1997).

5.6 Clinical Features

As described in detail elsewhere, the clinical manifestations of Lyme borreliosis include erythema migrans (EM), acrodermatitis chronica atrophicans (ACA), lymphocytoma, acute and chronic neuroborreliosis, arthritis, carditis and asymptomatic infection (Feder *et al.*, 1995; Steere, 2001; Stanek and Strle, 2003; Steere and Sikand, 2003; Nau *et al.*, 2009; Steere *et al.*, 2016). EM is universally the most common manifestation, accounting for 60–90% of cases in both North America and Eurasia, and carditis is consistently rare, generally accounting for fewer than 1% of cases in most series (Ai *et al.*, 1988; Steere, 2001; Stanek and Strle, 2003; Schwartz *et al.*, 2017). These overall trends aside, the relative frequency of different clinical features is clearly influenced by the traits of both host and pathogen.

All three major genospecies of *B. burgdorferi* sensu lato can cause dermatologic, neurologic and rheumatologic illness; however, they appear to have differing proclivities. In European studies, isolates from patients with neuroborreliosis are most commonly *B. garinii* (Ružić-Sabljić *et al.*, 2001a), while those from patients with EM – and especially ACA – are predominantly *B. afzelii* (van Dam *et al.*, 1993; Busch *et al.*, 1996; Ornstein *et al.*, 2001; Ružić-Sabljić *et al.*, 2001b). A similar affinity has been suggested for *B. burgdorferi* and arthritic manifestations (Steere, 2001; Steere and Glickstein, 2004). In the United States where human infection is primarily caused by *B. burgdorferi*, 27% of cases reported through national surveillance during 2008–2015 were associated with arthritis, while only 12% had neurological symptoms (usually facial palsy) (Schwartz *et al.*, 2017). In series from Europe, arthritis is generally reported less commonly than neuroborreliosis, sometimes markedly so (Stanek *et al.*, 1987a; Berglund *et al.*, 1995; Letrilliart *et al.*, 2005). Among 1471 Swedish patients, 16% had manifestations of neuroborreliosis, while only 7% had arthritis (Berglund

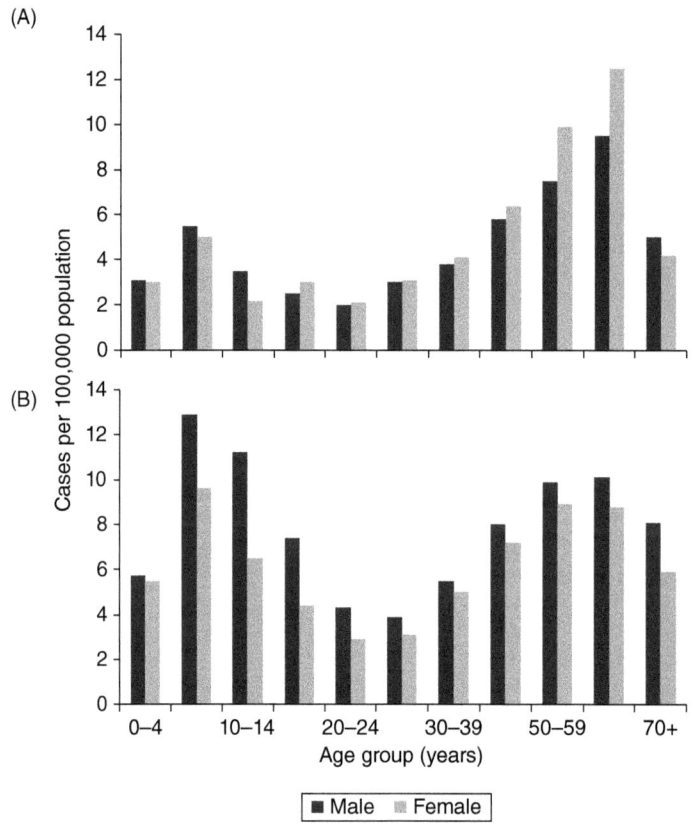

Fig. 5.3. Age- and sex-specific incidence for Lyme borreliosis cases from six German states (A, redrawn from Fulop and Poggensee, 2008) and the United States (B, US Centers for Disease Control and Prevention) for the years 2002–2006.

et al., 1995), and among 873 Austrian patients, 24% had neurologic manifestations, as compared with only 2% with arthritis (Stanek *et al.*, 1987a). The dermatologic manifestations ACA and lymphocytoma are well known in Europe but extremely rare in North America, a reflection of their particular association with *B. afzelii* infection (Busch *et al.*, 1996).

Patient age and sex also appear to influence the clinical features of disease, although unifying patterns are difficult to discern. At least in North America, Lyme arthritis is distinctly more common among children aged 5–15 years (Bacon *et al.*, 2008; Schwartz *et al.*, 2017), suggesting a particular susceptibility during this period of rapid long bone growth. US surveillance data and case series also suggest a disproportionate number of Lyme carditis cases among persons aged 20–40 years, especially men (Forrester and Mead, 2014; Schwartz *et al.*, 2017). In Europe, lymphocytoma and neuroborreliosis are more common in children than adults (Stanek *et al.*, 1987a; Berglund *et al.*, 1995; Huppertz *et al.*, 1999; Hubalek, 2009; Henningsson *et al.*, 2010). In contrast, ACA, with its insidious onset, is a condition of adults, particularly women (Asbrink *et al.*, 1986; Stanek *et al.*, 1987a; World Health Organization, 1995; Hubalek, 2009). Dermatologic features in general appear to be more common among women in Europe, while non-cutaneous manifestations are more common among men (Fulop and Poggensee, 2008; Hubalek, 2009). In a large series of Slovenian patients aged 15 years and older, females accounted for 59% of patients with EM and 69% with ACA, as compared with only 39% of patients with neuroborreliosis and 25% with Lyme arthritis (Strle et al., 2013).

Despite the high frequency of infection, very few deaths due to Lyme borreliosis have been reported in the medical literature (Marcus et al., 1985; Kirsch et al., 1988; Waniek et al., 1995; Tavora et al., 2008). A review of US death certificates for the years 1999–2003 identified 23 records that listed Lyme disease as the underlying cause of death, 11 of which were improperly coded, and only one of which listed a plausible causal sequence (Kugeler et al., 2011). Sudden death due to Lyme carditis may occasionally go undetected, as suggested by a report in which the diagnosis was only recognized during examination of donated organs (CDC, 2013). Nevertheless, a study of over 120,000 patients diagnosed with Lyme disease found that only 0.6% died within a year of diagnosis, a rate less than the expected, all-cause mortality for the population (Forrester et al., 2014).

5.7 Risk Factors and Transmission

In the northeastern United States where homes are located in heavily tick-infested areas, most infections are thought to result from exposures occurring around the home (Falco and Fish, 1988; Maupin et al., 1991; Klein et al., 1996). A series of studies has identified peridomestic risk factors for infection, including the presence of suitable tick habitat, landscaping practices, deer density and outdoor activities such as gardening (Ley et al., 1995; Orloski et al., 1998; Smith et al., 2001; Rand et al., 2003). Lyme borreliosis is also, however, an occupational risk. Increased risk of infection has been noted among forestry workers, farmers, hikers, soldiers, hunters and orienteers in studies from the United States (Schwartz and Goldstein, 1990), Asia (Ai et al., 1994; Nakama et al., 1994), and throughout Europe (Cinco et al., 2004; Kaya et al., 2008; Bilski, 2009; Buczek et al., 2009; Hubalek, 2009; Rizzoli et al., 2011; Richard and Oppliger, 2015). Animal studies and clinical observations indicate that I. scapularis ticks require at least 36 h of attachment in order to transmit B. burgdorferi, supporting a possible preventive role for daily tick checks and showering after exposure (Vazquez et al., 2008; Connally et al., 2009). Unfortunately, similar studies have demonstrated that I. ricinus ticks, especially when infected with B afzelii, can transmit infection efficiently after much shorter periods of attachment (Piesman and Gern, 2004).

Observed patterns of Lyme borreliosis are thoroughly consistent with the well-established mechanism of transmission by Ixodes ticks. Nevertheless, alternate modes of transmission have been investigated. Inoculation of blood with laboratory-adapted strains of B. burgdorferi has demonstrated the organism's ability to survive under blood banking conditions, raising the specter of transfusion-associated infection (Johnson et al., 1990). However, while transfusion-associated infection with less common Ixodes-transmitted pathogens (Babesia, Anaplasma) has been demonstrated repeatedly, no cases of transfusion-associated Lyme borreliosis have ever been documented (McQuiston et al., 2000; CDC, 2008). Similarly, despite a series of studies in animals, there is no credible evidence of transmission through sexual contact, semen, urine or breast milk (Moody and Barthold, 1991; Woodrum and Oliver, 1999). Intrauterine infection has been documented in rare reports of miscarriage and stillbirth in women infected during pregnancy (Schlesinger et al., 1985). A causal relationship to the miscarriage has not been established however, as B. burgdorferi has also been identified in placentas of women with normal pregnancy outcomes (Figueroa et al., 1996), and larger epidemiological studies have identified no definable pattern of teratogenicity (Markowitz et al., 1986; Walsh et al., 2007). Pregnant women who develop Lyme disease have good outcomes if they receive appropriate antimicrobial therapy (Walsh et al., 2007).

5.8 Conclusion

Lyme borreliosis is both a local and a global problem. Areas of risk, though discrete in space and time, are found throughout the northern hemisphere. Etiologic agents, principal vectors and clinical manifestations vary widely by region. A detailed knowledge of Lyme borreliosis epidemiology is both clinically relevant (Makhani *et al.*, 2010) and essential for the development of effective prevention measures. Despite enormous gains in knowledge over the past two decades, a great deal remains to be learned about risk factors for infection, enzootic cycles, the role of other *B. burgdorferi* genospecies, and most importantly, how best to prevent human infection and morbidity.

The findings and conclusions in this article are those of the author and do not necessarily represent the views of the Centers for Disease Control and Prevention.

References

Aguero-Rosenfeld, M.E. (2003) Laboratory aspects of tick-borne diseases: Lyme, human granulocytic ehrlichiosis and babesiosis. *Mount Sinai Journal of Medicine* 70(3), 197–206.

Ai, C.X., Wen, Y.X., Zhang, Y.G., Wang, S.S., Qiu, Q.C., Shi, Z.X., Li, D.Y., Chen, D.Q., Liu, X.D. and Zhao, J.H. (1988) Clinical manifestations and epidemiological characteristics of Lyme disease in Hailin county, Heilongjiang Province, China. *Annals of the New York Academy of Sciences* 539, 302–313.

Ai, C.X., Hu, R.J., Hyland, K.E. *et al.* (1990) Epidemiological and aetiological evidence for transmission of Lyme disease by adult *Ixodes persulcatus* in an endemic area in China. *International Journal of Epidemiology* 19(4), 1061–1065.

Ai, C.X., Zhang, W.F. and Zhao, J.H. (1994) Sero-epidemiology of Lyme disease in an endemic area in China. *Microbiology and Immunology* 38(7), 505–509.

Alekseev, A.N. and Dubinina, H.V. (2000) Abiotic parameters and diel and seasonal activity of *Borrelia*-infected and uninfected *Ixodes persulcatus* (Acarina: Ixodidae). *Journal of Medical Entomology* 37(1), 9–15.

Asbrink, E., Hovmark, A. and Olsson, I. (1986) Clinical manifestations of acrodermatitis chronica atrophicans in 50 Swedish patients. *Zentralblatt fur Bakteriologie Mikrobiologie und Hygiene (A)* 263(1–2), 253–261.

Bacon, R.M., Kugeler, K.J. and Mead, P.S. (2008) Surveillance for Lyme disease – United States, 1992–2006. *MMWR Surveillance Summaries* 57(10), 1–9.

Becker, N.S., Margos, G., Blum, H., Krebs, S., Graf, A., Lane, R.S., Castillo-Ramirez, S., Sing, A. and Fingerle, V. (2016) Recurrent evolution of host and vector association in bacteria of the *Borrelia burgdorferi* sensu lato species complex. *BMC Genomics* 17(1), 734.

Bennet, L., Halling, A. and Berglund, J. (2006) Increased incidence of Lyme borreliosis in southern Sweden following mild winters and during warm, humid summers. *European Journal of Clinical Microbiology and Infectious Diseases* 25(7), 426–432.

Berglund, J., Eitrem, R., Ornstein, K., Lindberg, A., Ringer, A., Elmrud, H., Carlsson, M., Runehagen, A., Svanborg, C. and Norrby, R. (1995) An epidemiologic study of Lyme disease in southern Sweden. *New England Journal of Medicine* 333(20), 1319–1327.

Berglund, J., Eitrem, R. and Norrby, S.R. (1996) Long-term study of Lyme borreliosis in a highly endemic area in Sweden. *Scandinavian Journal of Infectious Diseases* 28(5), 473–478.

Bilski, B. (2009) Occurrence of cases of borreliosis certified as an occupational disease in the province of Wielkopolska (Poland). *Annals of Agricultural and Environmental Medicine* 16(2), 211–217.

Bowman, D., Little, S.E., Lorentzen, L., Shields, J., Sullivan, M.P. and Carlin, E.P. (2009) Prevalence and geographic distribution of *Dirofilaria immitis*, *Borrelia burgdorferi*, *Ehrlichia canis*, and *Anaplasma phagocytophilum* in dogs in the United States: results of a national clinic-based serologic survey. *Veterinary Parasitology* 160(1–2), 138–148.

Buczek, A., Rudek, A., Bartosik, K., Szymanska, J. and Wojcik-Fatla, A. (2009) Seroepidemiological study of Lyme borreliosis among forestry workers in southern Poland. *Annals of Agricultural and Environmental Medicine* 16(2), 257–261.

Burgdorfer, W., Barbour, A.G., Hayes, S.F., Benach, J.L., Grunwaldt, E. and Davis, J.P. (1982) Lyme disease – a tick-borne spirochetosis? *Science* 216(4552), 1317–1319.

Busch, U., Hizo-Teufel, C., Bohmer, R., Fingerle, V., Rossler, D., Wilske, B. and Preac-Mursic, V. (1996) *Borrelia burgdorferi* sensu lato strains isolated from cutaneous Lyme borreliosis biopsies differentiated by pulsed-field gel electrophoresis. *Scandinavian Journal of Infectious Diseases* 28(6), 583–589.

CDC (2008) *Anaplasma phagocytophilum* transmitted through blood transfusion – Minnesota, 2007. *Morbidity and Mortality Weekly Report* 57(42), 1145–1148.

CDC (2013) Three sudden cardiac deaths associated with Lyme carditis – United States, November 2012–July 2013. *Morbidity and Mortality Weekly Report* 62(49), 993–996.

CDC (2004) Lyme disease – United States, 2001–2002. *MMWR Morbidity and Mortality Weekly Report* 53(17), 365–369.

Chao, L.L., Chen, Y.J. and Shih, C.M. (2010) First detection and molecular identification of *Borrelia garinii* isolated from human skin in Taiwan. *Journal of Medical Microbiology* 59(2), 254–257.

Chu, C.Y., Jiang, B.G., Liu, W., Zhao, Q.M., Wu, X.M., Zhang, P.H., Zhan, L., Yang, H. and Cao, W.C. (2008) Presence of pathogenic *Borrelia burgdorferi* sensu lato in ticks and rodents in Zhejiang, south-east China. *Journal of Medical Microbiology* 57(8), 980–985.

Cinco, M., Barbone, F., Grazia Ciufolini, M., Mascioli, M., Anguero Rosenfeld, M., Stefanel, P. and Luzzati, R. (2004) Seroprevalence of tick-borne infections in forestry rangers from northeastern Italy. *Clinical Microbiology and Infection* 10(12), 1056–1061.

Collignon, P.J., Lum, G.D. and Robson, J.M. (2016) Does Lyme disease exist in Australia? *Medical Journal of Australia* 205(9), 413–417.

Connally, N.P., Durante, A.J., Yousey-Hindes, K.M., Meek, J.I., Nelson, R.S. and Heimer, R. (2009) Peridomestic Lyme disease prevention: results of a population-based case-control study. *American Journal of Preventive Medicine* 37(3), 201–206.

Connecticut Department of Public Health (2009) Lyme disease – Connecticut, 2008. *Connecticut Epidemiologist* 29(4), 14–16.

da Franca, I., Santos, L., Mesquita, T., Collares-Pereira, M., Baptista, S., Vieira, L., Viana, I., Vale, E. and Prates, C. (2005) Lyme borreliosis in Portugal caused by *Borrelia lusitaniae*? Clinical report on the first patient with a positive skin isolate. *Wien Klin Wochenschr* 117(11–12), 429–432.

de Carvalho, I.L., Fonseca, J.E., Marques, J.G., Ullmann, A., Hojgaard, A., Zeidner, N. and Nuncio, M.S. (2008) Vasculitis-like syndrome associated with *Borrelia lusitaniae* infection. *Clinical Rheumatology* 27(12), 1587–1591.

Diza, E., Papa, A., Vezyri, E., Tsounis, S., Milonas, I. and Antoniadis, A. (2004) *Borrelia valaisiana* in cerebrospinal fluid. *Emerging Infectious Diseases* 10(9), 1692–1693.

Dolan, M.C., Hojgaard, A., Hoxmeier, J.C., Replogle, A.J., Respicio-Kingry, L.B., Sexton, C., Williams, M.A., Pritt, B.S., Schriefer, M.E. and Eisen, L. (2016) Vector competence of the blacklegged tick, *Ixodes scapularis*, for the recently recognized Lyme borreliosis spirochete *Candidatus Borrelia mayonii*. *Ticks and Tick-borne Diseases* 7(5), 665–669.

Dubrey, S.W., Bhatia, A., Woodham, S. and Rakowicz, W. (2014) Lyme disease in the United Kingdom. *Postgraduate Medical Journal* 90(1059), 33–42.

Duncan, A.W., Correa, M.T., Levine, J.F. and Breitschwerdt, E.B. (2004) The dog as a sentinel for human infection: prevalence of *Borrelia burgdorferi* C6 antibodies in dogs from southeastern and mid-Atlantic states. *Vector-Borne and Zoonotic Diseases* 4(3), 221–229.

ECDC (2017) European Centre for Disease Prevention and Control Tick Species Distribution Maps. Available at: https://ecdc.europa.eu/en/disease-vectors/surveillance-and-disease-data/tick-maps (accessed 12 October 2017).

Eisen, L., Eisen, R.J. and Lane, R.S. (2002) Seasonal activity patterns of *Ixodes pacificus* nymphs in relation to climatic conditions. *Medical and Veterinary Entomology* 16(3), 235–244.

Ekerfelt, C., Ernerudh, J., Forsberg, P., Jonsson, A.L., Vrethem, M., Arlehag, L. and Forsum, U. (2004) Lyme borreliosis in Sweden – diagnostic performance of five commercial *Borrelia* serology kits using sera from well-defined patient groups. *APMIS* 112(1), 74–78.

EpiNorth (2014) A Co-operation Project for Communicable Disease Control in Northern Europe. EpiNorth Data: Lyme borreliosis. Obtained from: https://web.archive.org/web/20130403082748/http://www.epinorth.org/ (accessed 10 July 2014).

Ertel, S.H., Nelson, R.S. and Cartter, M.L. (2012) Effect of surveillance method on reported characteristics of Lyme disease, Connecticut, 1996–2007. *Emerging Infectious Diseases* 18(2), 242–247.

Falco, R.C. and Fish, D. (1988) Prevalence of *Ixodes dammini* near the homes of Lyme disease patients in Westchester County, New York. *American Journal of Epidemiology* 127(4), 826–830.

Fang, L.Q., Liu, K., Li, X.L. *et al*. (2015) Emerging tick-borne infections in mainland China: an increasing public health threat. *Lancet Infectious Diseases* 15(12), 1467–1479.

Feder Jr, H.M., Gerber, M.A., Cartter, M.L., Sikand, V. and Krause, P.J. (1995) Prospective assessment of Lyme disease in a school-aged population in Connecticut. *Journal of Infectious Diseases* 171(5), 1371–1374.

Feria-Arroyo, T.P., Castro-Arellano, I., Gordillo-Perez, G., Cavazos, A.L., Vargas-Sandoval, M., Grover, A., Torres, J., Medina, R.F., de Leon, A.A. and Esteve-Gassent, M.D. (2014) Implications of climate change on the distribution of the tick vector *Ixodes scapularis* and risk for Lyme disease in the Texas-Mexico transboundary region. *Parasites and Vectors* 7, 199.

Figueroa, R., Bracero, L.A., Aguero-Rosenfeld, M., Beneck, D., Coleman, J. and Schwartz, I. (1996) Confirmation of *Borrelia burgdorferi* spirochetes by polymerase chain reaction in placentas of women with reactive serology for Lyme antibodies. *Gynecologic and Obstetric Investigation* 41(4), 240–243.

Forrester, J.D. and Mead, P. (2014) Third-degree heart block associated with Lyme carditis: review of published cases. *Clinical Infectious Diseases* 59(7), 996–1000.

Forrester, J.D., Meiman, J., Mullins, J. *et al.* (2014) Notes from the field: update on Lyme carditis, groups at high risk, and frequency of associated sudden cardiac death – United States. *MMWR Morbidity and Mortality Weekly Report* 63(43), 982–983.

Fulop, B. and Poggensee, G. (2008) Epidemiological situation of Lyme borreliosis in Germany: surveillance data from six Eastern German States, 2002 to 2006. *Parasitology Research* 103(1), S117–120.

Ginsberg, H.S., Albert, M., Acevedo, L., Dyer, M.C., Arsnoe, I.M., Tsao, J.I., Mather, T.N. and LeBrun, R.A. (2017) Environmental factors affecting survival of immature *Ixodes scapularis* and implications for geographical distribution of Lyme disease: the climate/behavior hypothesis. *PLoS One* 12(1), e0168723.

Gordillo-Perez, G., Torres, J., Solorzano-Santos, F., de Martino, S., Lipsker, D., Velazquez, E., Ramon, G., Onofre, M. and Jaulhac, B. (2007) *Borrelia burgdorferi* infection and cutaneous Lyme disease, Mexico. *Emerging Infectious Diseases* 13(10), 1556–1558.

Gordillo-Perez, G., Vargas, M., Solorzano-Santos, F., Rivera, A., Polaco, O.J., Alvarado, L., Munoz, O. and Torres, J. (2009) Demonstration of *Borrelia burgdorferi* sensu stricto infection in ticks from the northeast of Mexico. *Clinical Microbiology and Infection* 15(5), 496–498.

Hao, Q., Hou, X., Geng, Z. and Wan, K. (2011) Distribution of *Borrelia burgdorferi* sensu lato in China. *Journal of Clinical Microbiology* 49, 647–650. DOI: 10.1128/JCM.00725-10.

Hashimoto, S., Kawado, M., Murakami, Y., Izumida, M., Ohta, A., Tada, Y., Shigematsu, M., Yasui, Y., Taniguchi, K. and Nagai, M. (2007) Epidemics of vector-borne diseases observed in infectious disease surveillance in Japan, 2000–2005. *Journal of Epidemiology* 17(Suppl.), S48–55.

Henningsson, A.J., Malmvall, B.E., Ernerudh, J., Matussek, A. and Forsberg, P. (2010) Neuroborreliosis – an epidemiological, clinical and healthcare cost study from an endemic area in the south-east of Sweden. *Clinical Microbiology and Infection* 16(8), 1245–1251.

Herrin, B.H., Peregrine, A.S., Goring, J., Beall, M.J. and Little, S.E. (2017) Canine infection with *Borrelia burgdorferi*, *Dirofilaria immitis*, *Anaplasma* spp. and *Ehrlichia* spp. in Canada, 2013–2014. *Parasites and Vectors* 10(1), 244.

Hinckley, A.F., Connally, N.P., Meek, J.I., Johnson, B.J., Kemperman, M.M., Feldman, K.A., White, J.L. and Mead, P.S. (2014) Lyme disease testing by large commercial laboratories in the United States. *Clinical Infectious Diseases* 59(5), 676–681.

Hofhuis, A., van der Giessen, J.W., Borgsteede, F.H., Wielinga, P.R., Notermans, D.W. and van Pelt, W. (2006) Lyme borreliosis in the Netherlands: strong increase in GP consultations and hospital admissions in past 10 years. *Eurosurveillance* 11(6), E060622–E060622.

Hofhuis, A., Harms, M., Bennema, S., van den Wijngaard, C.C. and van Pelt, W. (2015) Physician reported incidence of early and late Lyme borreliosis. *Parasites and Vectors* 8, 161.

Hubalek, Z. (2009) Epidemiology of Lyme borreliosis. *Current Problems in Dermatology* 37, 31–50.

Hunfeld, K.P., Stanek, G., Straube, E., Hagedorn, H.J., Schorner, C., Muhlschlegel, F. and Brade, V. (2002) Quality of Lyme disease serology. Lessons from the German Proficiency Testing Program 1999–2001. A preliminary report. *Wiener klinische Wochenschrift* 114(13–14), 591–600.

Huppertz, H.I., Bohme, M., Standaert, S.M., Karch, H. and Plotkin, S.A. (1999) Incidence of Lyme borreliosis in the Wurzburg region of Germany. *European Journal of Clinical Microbiology and Infectious Diseases* 18(10), 697–703.

IDEXX (2010) Sensitivity and specificity of the SNAP® 4Dx® Test. Available at: www.idexx.com/view/xhtml/en_us/smallanimal/inhouse/snap/4dx.jsf?selectedTab=Accuracy#tabs (accessed 1 October 2010).

Johnson, S.E., Swaminathan, B., Moore, P., Broome, C.V. and Parvin, M. (1990) *Borrelia burgdorferi*: survival in experimentally infected human blood processed for transfusion. *Journal of Infectious Diseases* 162(2), 557–559.

Kampen, H., Rotzel, D.C., Kurtenbach, K., Maier, W.A. and Seitz, H.M. (2004) Substantial rise in the prevalence of Lyme borreliosis spirochetes in a region of western Germany over a 10-year period. *Applied and Environmental Microbiology* 70(3), 1576–1582.

Kaya, A.D., Parlak, A.H., Ozturk, C.E. and Behcet, M. (2008) Seroprevalence of *Borrelia burgdorferi* infection among forestry workers and farmers in Duzce, north-western Turkey. *New Microbiologica* 31(2), 203–209.

Kirsch, M., Ruben, F.L., Steere, A.C., Duray, P.H., Norden, C.W. and Winkelstein, A. (1988) Fatal adult respiratory distress syndrome in a patient with Lyme disease. *Journal of the American Medical Association* 259(18), 2737–2739.

Klein, J.D., Eppes, S.C. and Hunt, V. (1996) Environmental and life-style risk factors for Lyme disease in children. *Clinical Pediatrics* 35(7), 359–363.

Korenberg, E. (1994) Comparative ecology and epidemiology of Lyme disease and tick-borne encephalitis in the former Soviet Union. *Parasitology Today* 4, 157–160.

Korenberg, E., Gorelova, N. and Kovalevskii, Y. (2002) Ecology of *Borrelia burgdorferi* sensu lato in Russia. In: Gray, J.S., Kahl, O., Lane, R.S. and Stanek, G. (eds) *Lyme Borreliosis: Biology, Epidemiology and Control*. CAB International, Wallingford, UK, pp. 175–200.

Kugeler, K.J., Griffith, K.S., Gould, L.H., Kochanek, K., Delorey, M.J., Biggerstaff, B.J. and Mead, P.S. (2011) A review of death certificates listing Lyme disease as a cause of death in the United States. *Clinical Infectious Diseases* 52(3), 364–367.

Kugeler, K.J., Farley, G.M., Forrester, J.D. and Mead, P.S. (2015) Geographic distribution and expansion of human Lyme disease, United States. *Emerging Infectious Diseases* 21(8), 1455–1457.

Letrilliart, L., Ragon, B., Hanslik, T. and Flahault, A. (2005) Lyme disease in France: a primary care-based prospective study. *Epidemiology and Infection* 133(5), 935–942.

Ley, C., Olshen, E.M. and Reingold, A.L. (1995) Case-control study of risk factors for incident Lyme disease in California. *American Journal of Epidemiology* 142(9), S39–47.

Lindgren, E. and Jaenson, T. (2006) Lyme Borreliosis in Europe: Influences of climate and climate change, epidemiology, ecology and adaptation measures. Available at: www.euro.who.int/__data/assets/pdf_file/0006/96819/E89522.pdf (accessed 1 October 2010).

Little, S.E., Beall, M.J., Bowman, D.D., Chandrashekar, R. and Stamaris, J. (2014) Canine infection with *Dirofilaria immitis*, *Borrelia burgdorferi*, *Anaplasma* spp., and *Ehrlichia* spp. in the United States, 2010–2012. *Parasites and Vectors* 7, 257.

LPSN (2017) List of prokaryotic names with standing in nomenclature: *Borrelia*. Available at: www.bacterio.net/borrelia.html (accessed 1 August 2017).

Makhani, N., Morris, S.K., Page, A.V., Brophy, J., Lindsay, L.R., Banwell, B.L. and Richardson, S.E. (2010) A twist on Lyme: the challenge of diagnosing European Lyme neuroborreliosis. *Journal of Clinical Microbiology* 49, 455–457.

Mantovani, E., Costa, I.P., Gauditano, G., Bonoldi, V.L., Higuchi, M.L. and Yoshinari, N.H. (2007) Description of Lyme disease-like syndrome in Brazil. Is it a new tick borne disease or Lyme disease variation? *Brazilian Journal of Medical and Biological Research* 40(4), 443–456.

Maraspin, V., Ružić-Sabljić, E. and Strle, F. (2006) Lyme borreliosis and *Borrelia spielmanii*. *Emerging Infectious Diseases* 12(7), 1177.

Marcus, L.C., Steere, A.C., Duray, P.H., Anderson, A.E. and Mahoney, E.B. (1985) Fatal pancarditis in a patient with coexistent Lyme disease and babesiosis. Demonstration of spirochetes in the myocardium. *Annals of Internal Medicine* 103(3), 374–376.

Markowitz, L.E., Steere, A.C., Benach, J.L., Slade, J.D. and Broome, C.V. (1986) Lyme disease during pregnancy. *Journal of the American Medical Association* 255(24), 3394–3396.

Masuzawa, T. (2004) Terrestrial distribution of the Lyme borreliosis agent *Borrelia burgdorferi* sensu lato in East Asia. *Japanese Journal of Infectious Diseases* 57(6), 229–235.

Maupin, G.O., Fish, D., Zultowsky, J., Campos, E.G. and Piesman, J. (1991) Landscape ecology of Lyme disease in a residential area of Westchester County, New York. *American Journal of Epidemiology* 133(11), 1105–1113.

McQuiston, J.H., Childs, J.E., Chamberland, M.E. and Tabor, E. (2000) Transmission of tick-borne agents of disease by blood transfusion: a review of known and potential risks in the United States. *Transfusion* 40(3), 274–284.

Mead, P., Goel, R. and Kugeler, K. (2011) Canine serology as adjunct to human Lyme disease surveillance. *Emerging Infectious Diseases* 17(9), 1710–1712.

Miranda, J., Mattar, S., Perdomo, K. and Palencia, L. (2009) [Seroprevalence of Lyme borreliosis in workers from Cordoba, Colombia]. *Revista de Salud Pública (Bogota)* 11(3), 480–489.

Moody, K.D. and Barthold, S.W. (1991) Relative infectivity of *Borrelia burgdorferi* in Lewis rats by various routes of inoculation. *American Journal of Tropical Medicine and Hygiene* 44(2), 135–139.

Moore, S.M., Eisen, R.J., Monaghan, A. and Mead, P. (2014) Meteorological influences on the seasonality of Lyme disease in the United States. *American Journal of Tropical Medicine and Hygiene* 90(3), 486–496.

Nakama, H., Muramatsu, K., Uchikama, K. and Yamagishi, T. (1994) Possibility of Lyme disease as an occupational disease – seroepidemiological study of regional residents and forestry workers. *Asia-Pacific Journal of Public Health* 7(4), 214–217.

Nau, R., Christen, H.J. and Eiffert, H. (2009) Lyme disease – current state of knowledge. *Deutsches Ärzteblatt International* 106(5), 72–81.

Nelson, C.A., Saha, S., Kugeler, K.J., Delorey, M.J., Shankar, M.B., Hinckley, A.F. and Mead, P.S. (2015) Incidence of clinician-diagnosed Lyme disease, United States, 2005–2010. *Emerging Infectious Diseases* 21(9), 1625–1631.

Norris, S.J., Barbour, A.G., Fish, D. and Diuk-Wasser, M.A. (2015) Response to Esteve-Gassent et al.: flaB sequences obtained from Texas PCR products are identical to the positive control strain *Borrelia burgdorferi* B31. *Parasites and Vectors* 8, 310.

Ogden, N.H., Maarouf, A., Barker, I.K., Bigras-Poulin, M., Lindsay, L.R., Morshed, M.G., O'Callaghan, J., Ramay, C.F., Waltner-Toews, D. and Charron, D.F. (2006) Climate change and the potential for range expansion of the Lyme disease vector *Ixodes scapularis* in Canada. *International Journal for Parasitology* 36(1), 63–70.

Ogden, N.H., Lindsay, L.R., Morshed, M., Sockett, P.N. and Artsob, H. (2008) The rising challenge of Lyme borreliosis in Canada. *Canada Communicable Disease Report* 34(1), 1–19.

Ogden, N.H., Lindsay, L.R., Morshed, M., Sockett, P.N. and Artsob, H. (2009) The emergence of Lyme disease in Canada. *Canadian Medical Association Journal* 180(12), 1221–1224.

Orloski, K.A., Campbell, G.L., Genese, C.A., Beckley, J.W., Schriefer, M.E., Spitalny, K.C. and Dennis, D.T. (1998) Emergence of Lyme disease in Hunterdon County, New Jersey, 1993: a case-control study of risk factors and evaluation of reporting patterns. *American Journal of Epidemiology* 147(4), 391–397.

Ornstein, K., Berglund, J., Nilsson, I., Norrby, R. and Bergstrom, S. (2001) Characterization of Lyme borreliosis isolates from patients with erythema migrans and neuroborreliosis in southern Sweden. *Journal of Clinical Microbiology* 39(4), 1294–1298.

Paradowska-Stankiewicz, I. and Chrzescijanska, I. (2016) Lyme disease in Poland in 2014. *Przeglad Epidemiologiczny* 70(3), 395–398.

Piesman, J. and Gern, L. (2004) Lyme borreliosis in Europe and North America. *Parasitology* 129(Suppl), S191–S220.

Pritt, B.S., Mead, P.S., Johnson, D.K. et al. (2016) Identification of a novel pathogenic *Borrelia* species causing Lyme borreliosis with unusually high spirochaetaemia: a descriptive study. *Lancet Infectious Diseases* 16(5), 556–564.

Public Health Agency of Canada (2017) Surveillance of Lyme disease. Available at: https://www.canada.ca/en/public-health/services/diseases/lyme-disease/surveillance-lyme-disease.html (accessed 1 September 2017).

Rand, P.W., Lubelczyk, C., Lavigne, G.R., Elias, S., Holman, M.S., Lacombe, E.H. and Smith Jr, R.P. (2003) Deer density and the abundance of *Ixodes scapularis* (Acari: Ixodidae). *Journal of Medical Entomology* 40(2), 179–184.

Rauter, C. and Hartung, T. (2005) Prevalence of *Borrelia burgdorferi* sensu lato genospecies in *Ixodes ricinus* ticks in Europe: a metaanalysis. *Applied and Environmental Microbiology* 71(11), 7203–7216.

Richard, S. and Oppliger, A. (2015) Zoonotic occupational diseases in forestry workers – Lyme borreliosis, tularemia and leptospirosis in Europe. *Annals of Agricultural and Environmental Medicine* 22(1), 43–50.

Rizzoli, A., Hauffe, H., Carpi, G., Vourc, H.G., Neteler, M. and Rosa, R. (2011) Lyme borreliosis in Europe. *Eurosurveillance* 16(27), pii=19906. https://doi.org/10.2807/ese.16.27.19906-en.

Rudenko, N., Golovchenko, M., Mokracek, A., Piskunova, N., Ruzek, D., Mallatova, N. and Grubhoffer, L. (2008) Detection of *Borrelia bissettii* in cardiac valve tissue of a patient with endocarditis and aortic valve stenosis in the Czech Republic. *Journal of Clinical Microbiology* 46(10), 3540–3543.

Rudenko, N., Golovchenko, M., Ruzek, D., Piskunova, N., Mallatova, N. and Grubhoffer, L. (2009) Molecular detection of *Borrelia bissettii* DNA in serum samples from patients in the Czech Republic with suspected borreliosis. *FEMS Microbiology Letters* 292(2), 274–281.

Russell, R.C. (1995) Lyme disease in Australia-still to be proven! *Emerging Infectious Diseases* 1(1), 29–31.

Ružić-Sabljić, E., Lotric-Furlan, S., Maraspin, V., Cimperman, J., Pleterski-Rigler, D. and Strle, F. (2001a) Analysis of *Borrelia burgdorferi* sensu lato isolated from cerebrospinal fluid. *APMIS* 109(10), 707–713.

Ružić-Sabljić, E., Arnez, M., Lotric-Furlan, S., Maraspin, V., Cimperman, J. and Strle, F. (2001b) Genotypic and phenotypic characterisation of *Borrelia burgdorferi* sensu lato strains isolated from human blood. *Journal of Medical Microbiology* 50(10), 896–901.

Sajanti, E., Virtanen, M., Helve, O., Kuusi, M., Lyytikainen, O., Hytonen, J. and Sane, J. (2017) Lyme borreliosis in Finland, 1995–2014. *Emerging Infectious Diseases* 23(8), 1282–1288.

Santos, M., Ribeiro-Rodrigues, R., Lobo, R. and Talhari, S. (2010) Antibody reactivity to *Borrelia burgdorferi* sensu stricto antigens in patients from the Brazilian Amazon region with skin diseases not related to Lyme disease. *International Journal of Dermatology* 49(5), 552–556.

Schlesinger, P.A., Duray, P.H., Burke, B.A., Steere, A.C. and Stillman, M.T. (1985) Maternal-fetal transmission of the Lyme disease spirochete, *Borrelia burgdorferi*. *Annals of Internal Medicine* 103(1), 67–68.

Schwartz, B.S. and Goldstein, M.D. (1990) Lyme disease in outdoor workers: risk factors, preventive measures, and tick removal methods. *American Journal of Epidemiology* 131(5), 877–885.

Schwartz, A., Hinckley, A., Mead, P., Hook, S. and Kugeler, K. (2017) Surveillance for Lyme disease – United States, 2008–2015. *MMWR Surveillance Summaries* 66, 1–12. DOI: 10.15585/mmwr.ss6622a1.

Smith, R. and Takkinen, J. (2006) Lyme borreliosis: Europe-wide coordinated surveillance and action needed? *Eurosurveillance* 11(6), E060622–E060621.

Smith, G., Wileyto, E.P., Hopkins, R.B., Cherry, B.R. and Maher, J.P. (2001) Risk factors for Lyme disease in Chester County, Pennsylvania. *Public Health Reports* 116(1), 146–156.

Stanek, G. and Strle, F. (2003) Lyme borreliosis. *Lancet* 362(9396), 1639–1647.

Stanek, G., Flamm, H., Groh, V., Hirschl, A., Kristoferitsch, W., Neumann, R., Schmutzhard, E. and Wewalka, G. (1987a) Epidemiology of *Borrelia* infections in Austria. *Zentralblatt fur Bakteriologie, Mikrobiologie, und Hygiene. Series A* 263(3), 442–449.

Stanek, G., Hirschl, A., Stemberger, H., Wewalka, G. and Wiedermann, G. (1987b) Does Lyme borreliosis also occur in tropical and subtropical areas? *Zentralblatt Fur Bakteriologie, Mikrobiologie, Und Hygiene. Series A* 263(3), 491–495.

Steere, A.C. (2001) Lyme disease. *New England Journal of Medicine* 345(2), 115–125.

Steere, A.C. and Glickstein, L. (2004) Elucidation of Lyme arthritis. *Nature Reviews Immunology* 4(2), 143–152.

Steere, A.C. and Sikand, V.K. (2003) The presenting manifestations of Lyme disease and the outcomes of treatment. *New England Journal of Medicine* 348(24), 2472–2474.

Steere, A.C., Malawista, S.E., Snydman, D.R., Shope, R.E., Andiman, W.A., Ross, M.R. and Steele, F.M. (1977) Lyme arthritis: an epidemic of oligoarticular arthritis in children and adults in three Connecticut communities. *Arthritis and Rheumatology* 20(1), 7–17.

Steere, A.C., Strle, F., Wormser, G.P., Hu, L.T., Branda, J.A., Hovius, J.W., Li, X. and Mead, P.S. (2016) Lyme borreliosis. *Nature Reviews Disease Primers* 2, 16090.

Stillman, B.A., Monn, M., Liu, J., Thatcher, B., Foster, P., Andrews, B., Little, S., Eberts, M., Breitschwerdt, E.B., Beall, M.J. and Chandrashekar, R. (2014) Performance of a commercially available in-clinic ELISA for detection of antibodies against *Anaplasma phagocytophilum*, *Anaplasma platys*, *Borrelia burgdorferi*, *Ehrlichia canis*, and *Ehrlichia ewingii* and *Dirofilaria immitis* antigen in dogs. *Journal of the American Veterinary Medical Association* 245(1), 80–86.

Strle, F. (1999) Lyme borreliosis in Slovenia. *Zentralblatt für Bakteriologie* 289(5–7), 643–652.

Strle, F., Wormser, G.P., Mead, P. *et al.* (2013) Gender disparity between cutaneous and non-cutaneous manifestations of Lyme borreliosis. *PLoS One* 8(5), e64110.

Tavora, F., Burke, A., Li, L., Franks, T.J. and Virmani, R. (2008) Postmortem confirmation of Lyme carditis with polymerase chain reaction. *Cardiovascular Pathology* 17(2), 103–107.

Tugwell, P., Dennis, D.T., Weinstein, A., Wells, G., Shea, B., Nichol, G., Hayward, R., Lightfoot, R., Baker, P. and Steere, A.C. (1997) Laboratory evaluation in the diagnosis of Lyme disease. *Annals of Internal Medicine* 127(12), 1109–1123.

van Dam, A.P. (2002) Diversity of *Ixodes*-borne *Borrelia* species – clinical, pathogenetic, and diagnostic implications and impact on vaccine development. *Vector-Borne and Zoonotic Diseases* 2(4), 249–254.

van Dam, A., Kuiper, H., Vos, K., Widjojokusumo, A., De Jongh, B., Spanjaard, L., Ramselaar, A., Kramer, M. and Dankert, J. (1993) Different genospecies of *Borrelia burgdorferi* are associated with distinct clinical manifestations of Lyme borreliosis. *Clinical Infectious Diseases* 17, 708–717.

Vandenesch, A., Turbelin, C., Couturier, E. *et al.* (2014) Incidence and hospitalisation rates of Lyme borreliosis, France, 2004 to 2012. *Eurosurveillance* 19(34), pii=20883. https://doi.org/10.2807/1560-7917.ES2014.19.34.20883.

Vanthomme, K., Bossuyt, N., Boffin, N. and Van Casteren, V. (2012) Incidence and management of presumption of Lyme borreliosis in Belgium: recent data from the sentinel network of general practitioners. *European Journal of Clinical Microbiology and Infectious Diseases* 31(9), 2385–2390.

Vazquez, M., Muehlenbein, C., Cartter, M., Hayes, E.B., Ertel, S. and Shapiro, E.D. (2008) Effectiveness of personal protective measures to prevent Lyme disease. *Emerging Infectious Diseases* 14(2), 210–216.

Walsh, C.A., Mayer, E.W. and Baxi, L.V. (2007) Lyme disease in pregnancy: case report and review of the literature. *Obstetrical and Gynecological Survey* 62(1), 41–50.

Waniek, C., Prohovnik, I., Kaufman, M.A. and Dwork, A.J. (1995). Rapidly progressive frontal-type dementia associated with Lyme disease. *Journal of Neuropsychiatry and Clinical Neurosciences* 7(3), 345–347.

Wilking, H. and Stark, K. (2014) Trends in surveillance data of human Lyme borreliosis from six federal states in eastern Germany, 2009–2012. *Ticks and Tick Borne Diseases* 5(3), 219–224.

Woodrum, J.E. and Oliver Jr, J.H. (1999) Investigation of venereal, transplacental, and contact transmission of the Lyme disease spirochete, *Borrelia burgdorferi*, in Syrian hamsters. *Journal of Parasitology* 85(3), 426–430.

World Health Organization (1995) *Report of WHO workshop on Lyme Borreliosis Diagnosis and Surveillance (who/cds/vph/95141-1)*. World Health Organization, Geneva.

World Health Organization/Europe (2014) Centralized information system for infectious diseases (CISID) *Lyme disease – Incidence (Table)*. Available at http://data.euro.who.int/cisid/?TabID=67 (accessed 15 February 2018).

Wormser, G.P., Masters, E., Nowakowski, J., McKenna, D., Holmgren, D., Ma, K., Ihde, L., Cavaliere, L.F. and Nadelman, R.B. (2005) Prospective clinical evaluation of patients from Missouri and New York with erythema migrans-like skin lesions. *Clinical Infectious Diseases* 41(7), 958–965.

Zhang, F., Gong, Z., Zhang, J. and Liu, Z. (2010) Prevalence of *Borrelia burgdorferi* sensu lato in rodents from Gansu, northwestern China. *BMC Microbiology* 10, 157.

6 Antibiotic Therapy for Infection Caused by *Borrelia Burgdorferi* Sensu Lato

Gary P. Wormser
New York Medical College, Valhalla, New York, USA

6.1 Introduction

Lyme disease, or Lyme borreliosis, is the term usually applied to infection with *Borrelia burgdorferi* sensu lato (Bbsl). Because this term is now often used inaccurately to describe patients with a wide range of conditions but who have no evidence of Bbsl infection (Steere *et al.*, 1993; Feder *et al.*, 2007; Hassett *et al.*, 2008; Hassett *et al.*, 2009), in this chapter the term Bbsl infection will be used instead. Human disease is principally caused by three genospecies of Bbsl – primarily *B. burgdorferi* sensu stricto (Bbss) in North America, and *B. afzelii* and *B. garinii* in Europe (Stanek *et al.*, 2012). Although each of the three major Bbsl species can cause erythema migrans (EM) and/or neurologic manifestations, *B. afzelii* is most closely associated with skin manifestations, *B. garinii* appears to be the most neurotropic and Bbss is the most likely to cause arthritis (Stanek *et al.*, 2012; Wormser, 2016).

The objective clinical manifestations of Bbsl infection are thought to be due to an inflammatory reaction, presumably to live spirochetes or their undegraded antigens (Malawista and Bockenstedt, 2007; Steere, 2010; Steere *et al.*, 2016). Localized infection is typically manifested by a single focus of infection in the skin, EM. Systemic symptoms such as fatigue or arthralgia accompany EM in approximately 65% of United States patients compared with about 35% of European patients (Tibbles and Edlow, 2007).

Disseminated disease is usually characterized by multiple EM skin lesions or by an objective neurologic, cardiac or musculoskeletal manifestation of Bbsl infection (Wormser *et al.*, 2006; Sanchez *et al.*, 2016). Clinical evidence of dissemination may appear within days of the appearance of the EM skin lesion, but arthritis, the skin condition known as acrodermatitis chronica atrophicans or certain rare late neurologic manifestations typically only become apparent after months to years.

6.2 Antibiotic Susceptibility

The preferred antibiotic for a bacterial infection is usually based on the organism's sensitivity to it *in vitro*, taking into consideration the drug's pharmacokinetics, pharmacodynamics, safety, ease of administration and cost. Unfortunately, *in vitro* studies of Bbsl's sensitivity to antibiotics have lacked standardized methodologies and used a variety of end points (Nowakowski and Wormser, 1993; Terekhova *et al.*, 2002), making interpretation challenging.

Variations in minimum bactericidal concentration (MBC) values have generally been greater than those for minimum inhibitory concentrations (MICs). Therefore, inconsistencies among published studies in the reported MICs and MBCs for various antibiotics against Bbsl may be related more to differences in assay techniques than to true strain variations. In five different studies MBC values of the B31 strain of Bbss to doxycycline have been reported to be 0.80 (Baradaran-Dilmaghani and Stanek, 1996), ≤4.0 (Levin et al., 1993), 8.0 (Sicklinger et al., 2003), 16 (Morgenstern et al., 2009) and 25 (Barthold et al., 2010), representing a more than 30-fold range of reported values. Alternatively, it may be that the studied strains were not actually all B31, since it is unclear that the isolates were cloned before testing.

Strains of Bbsl are susceptible to tetracyclines, most penicillins, and many second and third generation cephalosporins, but first generation cephalosporins are not active in vitro nor are they effective clinically (Nowakowski et al., 2000). Bbsl strains are also resistant to certain fluoroquinolones and rifampin in vitro (Wormser et al., 2006). Treatment of patients or laboratory animals with certain macrolide antibiotics has been less successful than in vitro testing might have predicted (Wormser et al., 2006; Wormser and O'Connell, 2011).

Multidrug efflux pumps exist in Bbsl (Bunikis et al., 2008), as they do in virtually all gram-negative bacteria. These pumps are believed to be biologically important and potentially involved in the processes of detoxification of intracellular metabolites, bacterial virulence, cell homeostasis and intercellular signal trafficking (Martinez et al., 2009). Tetracycline-specific efflux pumps, which confer resistance to this class of drugs, however, would not be expected and have not been demonstrated in Bbsl.

6.3 Prevention

As with any infection, the best strategy is to avoid Bbsl infection – specifically by avoiding tick-infested environments, and, when in such environments, covering bare skin and using tick repellents. Bathing within 2 h of tick exposure has been shown to decrease the risk of Bbsl infection (Connally et al., 2009).

Transmission of Bbsl requires >36 h of attachment (≤24 h for some European Bbsl species) (des Vignes et al., 2001; Hojgaard et al., 2008). A daily tick check, encompassing the entire skin surface (including scalp) with removal of any attached ticks may help to prevent infection. In highly endemic regions of the United States, fewer than 4% of individuals who find and remove an attached I. scapularis tick will become infected with Bbsl (Wormser, 2006; Warshafsky et al., 2010a). If the tick is not removed in a timely fashion or not found at all, the probability of infection appears to approach the infection rate in the regional tick population (typically 25% of nymphal stage I. scapularis ticks in highly endemic areas of the northeast and Midwest United States) (Nadelman et al., 2001; Tokarz et al., 2010). No vaccine is currently available to prevent Bbsl infection in humans.

6.4 Treatment of Incubating Bbsl Infection (Chemoprophylaxis)

The relatively small number of spirochetes present very early in Bbsl or other spirochetal infections provides an opportunity to eradicate them with a much shorter course of treatment than otherwise needed, as demonstrated in rabbits experimentally infected with Treponema pallidum (Magnuson and Eagle, 1945; Eagle et al., 1950; Hollander et al., 1952). Successful short-course early post-exposure antibiotic treatment of spirochetal diseases is well-documented including single-dose procaine penicillin G for syphilis (Schroeter et al., 1971), a 4-day course of doxycycline for relapsing fever (Hasin et al., 2006) and a once-weekly 200-mg dose of doxycycline for leptospirosis in United States military personnel (Takafuji et al., 1984). Similarly, the likelihood of developing Bbsl infection can be reduced by a single 200-mg dose of doxycycline given within 72 h of I. scapularis tick removal (Nadelman et al., 2001) – a strategy found to be 87% effective in preventing EM at the tick bite site. Studies have not been conducted on the efficacy of antibiotic prophylaxis for I. ricinus tick bites.

The pharmacodynamics and pharmacokinetics of the specific antibiotic administered affect its efficacy in preventing Bbsl infection following a tick bite (Lee and Wormser, 2008). A single parenteral dose of a long-acting doxycycline preparation was 100% effective in eliminating Bbss from mice in two different studies (Zeidner et al., 2004; 2008), whereas a single oral dose of doxycycline was 43% effective in the original murine study (Zeidner et al., 2004). Although the 43% efficacy rate is less than the

87% efficacy rate observed in the human trial of single-dose doxycycline (Nadelman *et al.*, 2001), a single dose of doxycycline given orally to mice was nevertheless significantly more effective than no antibiotic treatment ($P = 0.02$) (Zeidner *et al.*, 2004), thus providing proof of concept (Warshafsky *et al.*, 2010b).

The lower observed efficacy of a single dose of oral doxycycline in mice compared to humans is probably explained by the fact that the antibiotic exposure in the mouse species studied differed substantively from that in humans. Following a single 200-mg dose of doxycycline the area under the curve of unbound doxycycline (fAUC0–∞) in humans was 2.25 times greater than that provided by the doxycycline dose used in the mouse study (Lee and Wormser, 2008).

Interestingly, feeding mice doxycycline *at the time of tick feeding* was even more effective. Allowing five ticks infected with Bbss to feed to repletion (≤96 h) (Dolan *et al.*, 2008) on mice consuming bait containing doxycycline resulted in none of the mice becoming infected. Remarkably Bbss could no longer be cultured from the ticks that had fed on mice that received the higher of the two concentrations of doxycycline in the bait. Eradication of Bbss in the tick itself suggests how potent doxycycline is against this spirochete (Wormser and O'Connell, 2011).

Importantly, failure of antibiotic prophylaxis for spirochetal infections has not been found to change the presentation of the disease or cause seronegative persistent infection (Magnuson and Eagle, 1945; Hollander *et al.*, 1952; Korenberg *et al.*, 1996; Nadelman *et al.*, 2001). In one study (Hollander *et al.*, 1952), rabbits that received penicillin for incubating syphilis were 'either cured or subsequently developed clinically recognizable lesions'. Single subcurative doses of penicillin only prolonged the 'incubation period of experimental syphilis ... up to a limit of 30–40 days'. After lesions developed, all animals become seropositive.

6.5 Treatment of Localized Infection

Although clinical manifestations of Bbsl infection (Steere *et al.*, 1987) usually eventually resolve without treatment, antibiotic therapy accelerates the rate of resolution and prevents later sequelae (Kalish *et al.*, 2001; Wormser *et al.*, 2006). In the United States and Europe oral doxycycline, amoxicillin and cefuroxime axetil are recommended for EM (Table 6.1) (Wormser *et al.*, 2006; Sanchez *et al.*, 2016). Phenoxymethylpenicillin is also used for this indication in Europe (Stanek and Strle, 2003; Wormser and O'Connell, 2011; Steere *et al.*, 2016). Macrolides are somewhat less effective than other oral antibiotics (Luft *et al.*, 1996); hence these agents are usually second line therapy (Wormser *et al.*, 2006; Sanchez *et al.*, 2016). Azithromycin is the preferred agent in this class.

Up to 15% of United States patients with EM may experience an increase in the size or intensity of the erythema, with more intense systemic symptoms within 24 h of starting antimicrobial therapy, which has been interpreted to represent a Jarisch–Herxheimer-like reaction. Contrary to the opinion of some (Oksi *et al.*, 2007), however, such reactions do not occur at later times during treatment. Fever, if present, should resolve within 48 h and the skin lesion itself usually within 7–14 days (Wormser *et al.*, 2006). Subjective symptoms, such as fatigue or arthralgia, tend to improve but do not invariably resolve within this time frame, lasting for more than 3 months in approximately one-quarter of United States patients (Wormser *et al.*, 2003). Extending the initial course of treatment does not result in faster or more complete relief of symptoms (Wormser *et al.*, 2003).

6.6 Oral Doxycycline for Nervous System Bbsl Infection

Doxycycline is highly lipophilic, allowing ready entry into many tissues including the nervous system, and has very high oral bioavailability (>90%), such that blood concentrations are generally similar whether the drug is given intravenously or orally (Wormser and Halperin, 2008). Not surprisingly then, this agent demonstrated efficacy comparable to ceftriaxone in a double-blind, multicenter treatment trial in which 118 Norwegian patients were randomized to receive 14 days of oral doxycycline or intravenous ceftriaxone for presumed neurologic Bbsl infection (Ljostad *et al.*, 2008). Similar efficacy was shown at 4 and 12 months follow-up (Ljostad and

Table 6.1. Recommended therapy for adult patients with Bbsl infection.[a] (Modified from Wormser et al. 2006; Sanchez et al., 2016.)

Manifestation	Duration	Therapy
Erythema migrans	10–14 days[b]	Doxycycline 100 mg PO BID or
Borrelial lymphocytoma	14 days	Amoxicillin 500 mg PO TID or
Acrodermatitis chronica atrophicans	21–28 days	Cefuroxime axetil 500 mg PO BID
Lyme arthritis	28 days	
Lyme carditis – mild	14–21 days	
Cranial neuropathy	14 days[c]	
Lyme meningitis, cranial neuropathy or radiculoneuropathy	14 days	Doxycycline 200 mg PO per day or 100 mg PO BID
Lyme arthritis that failed oral therapy	14–28 days	Ceftriaxone 2 g IV daily
Late or severe neurologic Lyme disease	14–28 days	
Hospitalized patient with Lyme carditis	14–21 days[d]	
Hospitalized patient with Lyme meningitis	14 days	
Erythema migrans in a patient intolerant of doxycycline and beta-lactam antibiotics	7–10 days	Azithromycin 500 mg PO daily

[a]Regardless of the clinical manifestations of Lyme disease, complete response to treatment may be delayed beyond the treatment duration. Relapse may occur with any of these regimens; patients with objective signs of relapse may need another course of treatment.
[b]A 10-day course of doxycycline is sufficient for erythema migrans.
[c]Although any one of the first line oral antibiotics appears to be effective in patients with cranial neuropathy, there is only limited experience in patients with a cranial neuropathy other than seventh nerve palsy or with agents other than doxycycline.
[d]On hospital discharge, may complete the course of treatment with any of the first line oral antimicrobials used to treat erythema migrans.

Mygland, 2010). None of the patients required additional antibiotic treatment. These results are consistent with a previous meta-analysis of prior reports of European patients with early neurologic Bbsl infection, which found the response rate to doxycycline to be comparable to that of parenteral penicillin or ceftriaxone (95% CI 94.8–102.5%) (Halperin et al., 2007).

In sum, there is compelling evidence that European patients with early neurologic Bbsl infection will respond as well, overall, to a 2-week course of oral doxycycline as to a 2-week course of ceftriaxone. Whether similar results could be attained with an oral β-lactam agent, such as amoxicillin, with its less favorable pharmacokinetic profile, is unclear, but seems less likely (Wormser and O'Connell, 2011). Also unclear is whether the efficacy of oral doxycycline and parenteral beta lactams would be comparable in North American neuroborreliosis, but a priori there would be no reason to expect a difference (Wormser and Halperin, 2008; Sanchez et al., 2016). Finally, since the effectiveness of oral doxycycline has not been unequivocally established for patients with severe neurological manifestations (Bremell and Dotevall, 2014), including parenchymal brain involvement, a parenteral antibiotic, such as ceftriaxone, remains the recommended agent in such exceptional cases (Wormser and Halperin, 2008).

6.7 Role of Parenteral Antimicrobial Therapy

Oral antibiotics are recommended as first line treatment for the other cutaneous manifestations of Bbsl infection (Wormser et al., 2006; Sanchez et al., 2016). However, parenteral antibiotics are recommended for patients with certain neurologic manifestations and initially for those with cardiac Bbsl infection during the time they are hospitalized (Wormser et al., 2006; Sanchez et al., 2016). Parenteral antibiotics are often given to patients with Bbsl arthritis who have failed to respond to one or more courses of oral antibiotic treatment, although the risks and benefits of this treatment strategy have never been systematically studied (Wormser et al., 2006; Wormser and O'Connell, 2011; Steere et al., 2016).

Ceftriaxone is the preferred parenteral agent because of its *in vitro* activity against Bbsl, its ability to readily cross the blood–brain barrier and its long serum half-life allowing for the convenience of once daily administration (Wormser *et al.*, 2006; Sanchez *et al.*, 2016). Cefotaxime is similarly effective and does not cause biliary concretions or cholecystitis, recognized adverse effects of ceftriaxone, but this drug may cause leukopenia. High-dose IV penicillin is a third alternative.

6.8 Treatment Duration

Clinical experience with most infections indicates that treating until all symptoms resolve, until a cerebrospinal fluid (CSF) pleocytosis disappears or until serologic tests revert to negative is neither necessary nor rational. Prolonged courses of antibiotics substantially increase the risk of serious adverse events, increase costs and promote antibiotic resistance. Both a prospective, randomized, double-blind treatment trial of 180 United States patients (Wormser *et al.*, 2003) and a large retrospective cohort study of 607 United States patients (Kowalski *et al.*, 2010) have demonstrated that a 10-day course of doxycycline is just as effective as longer courses of treatment with this antibiotic for patients with EM. Fourteen days of an appropriate oral beta-lactam antibiotic also seems to be as effective as longer courses of treatment with these agents, but systematic comparisons are lacking (Wormser *et al.*, 2006; Sanchez *et al.*, 2016). Even shorter durations of treatment may well be effective for early Bbsl infection. In one German study of 73 patients with EM, 5 days of ceftriaxone was just as effective as 12 days of oral penicillin (Weber *et al.*, 1990). Moreover, prolonged courses of antibiotics have never been needed in other spirochetal infections (Wormser, 1995).

At least nine studies – including patients with early localized infection (e.g. single EM skin lesion), early disseminated infection (e.g. multiple EM skin lesions) and late infection – have compared different durations of treatment for Bbsl infection. None has shown a beneficial effect for courses of therapy longer than what is recommended in Table 6.1 (Weber *et al.*, 1990; Wormser *et al.*, 2002; 2003; 2006; Dattwyler *et al.*, 2005; Oksi *et al.*, 2007; Kowalski *et al.*, 2010; Stupica *et al.*, 2012).

6.9 Bbsl Arthritis

Relatively long courses of oral antibiotics are recommended as first line treatment for Bbsl arthritis (Wormser *et al.*, 2006; Arvikar and Steere, 2015; Sanchez *et al.*, 2016). Patients with Bbsl arthritis with persistent joint swelling following completion of 28 days of oral antibiotics are often retreated with either another 28-day course of oral antibiotics or with 14–28 days of ceftriaxone – a recommendation based on expert opinion rather than randomized trials. Although patients treated following this protocol have been shown to have excellent outcomes (Tory *et al.*, 2010), additional studies are warranted to determine the optimal treatment approach for such individuals.

Although Bbsl arthritis typically responds to antibiotic treatment (often combined with non-steroidal anti-inflammatory agents (NSAIDs)) (Wormser *et al.*, 2006; Sanchez *et al.*, 2016), approximately 10% of United States patients do not respond clinically and are said to have antibiotic-refractory arthritis. This condition has been defined as synovitis persisting for at least 2 months after completion of IV ceftriaxone (or 1 month after completion of two 4-week courses of oral antibiotics), in conjunction with negative polymerase chain reaction (PCR) testing on synovial fluid and on synovial tissue if available (Steere and Angelis, 2006). These patients are not believed to be actively infected and are treated with NSAIDs, intra-articular injections of corticosteroids or disease modifying anti-rheumatic drugs (DMARDs) (typically 6–12-month courses of DMARDs are curative (Arvikar and Steere, 2015; Steere *et al.*, 2016)), rather than with additional courses of antimicrobial therapy (Wormser *et al.*, 2006). If these modalities are ineffective, arthroscopic synovectomy may be successful.

6.10 Co-infection

Ixodes ticks potentially carry additional pathogens such as *Anaplasma phagocytophilum*, the cause of human granulocytic anaplasmosis (HGA), *Babesia* spp., including *B. microti*, the primary cause of babesiosis in the United States, and certain viruses that may cause encephalitis (tick-borne encephalitis virus in Europe and the deer tick virus subtype of Powassan virus in the United States) (Swanson et al., 2006; Sanchez et al., 2016). Co-infection is generally uncommon, but depends on the particular species of *Ixodes* tick and on the geographic area. Co-infection should be considered in patients who have high-grade fever for more than 48 h or develop recurrent fever during treatment of Bbsl infection, and in those who have unexplained leukopenia, thrombocytopenia or anemia. *Anaplasma phagocytophilum*-Bbsl co-infection is treated with doxycycline, since HGA does not respond to beta-lactam antibiotics (Biggs et al., 2016). Patients co-infected with babesiosis require additional treatment with azithromycin plus atovaquone or clindamycin plus quinine (Wormser et al., 2006; Sanchez et al., 2016).

6.11 Post-treatment Persistent Subjective Symptoms

As discussed elsewhere in this volume, there has been considerable concern about individuals in whom subjective symptoms persist following treatment that is usually microbiologically curative. Such subjective symptoms must be distinguished from those due to significant tissue damage occurring prior to treatment, with residual objective problems due to as yet incomplete healing following resolution of the infective process (Wormser and O'Connell, 2011). Active co-infection with a second *Ixodes*-transmitted pathogen (*A. phagocytophilum* or *B. microti*) has been investigated and generally excluded as the explanation for such persistent symptoms (Klempner et al., 2001).

Estimates of the frequency and severity of these purely subjective symptoms following treated Bbsl infection are inconsistent, with symptoms persisting for ≥6 months after antibiotic treatment in from none to 40.8% (median 11.5%) in eight randomized treatment trials of United States patients with EM, and from none to 23.4% in five European studies (median 15.4%) (summarized in Cerar et al., 2010). Patients with symptoms that are *disabling* and *persistent for at least 6 months* following treatment for Bbsl infection are sometimes referred to as having post-treatment Lyme disease syndrome (PTLDS) (Wormser et al., 2006) (see Chapters 16 and 17). Since similar symptoms occur not infrequently in the general population (Hassett et al., 2008; 2009), it is difficult to know if the incidence of PTLDS exceeds that of a chance association; few hard data are available. Of interest, two recent prospective European treatment studies incorporated a control group without Bbsl infection (Skogman et al., 2008; Cerar et al., 2010) – one evaluated children with neurologic Bbsl infection (Skogman et al., 2008), the other adults with a single EM (Cerar et al., 2010). In neither did the frequency of subjective symptoms present at >6 months differ between treated patients and uninfected controls. Although it has been suggested that symptoms might be due to spirochetes persisting despite antibiotic treatment (Cameron et al., 2004), carefully performed microbiologic evaluations have failed to find any credible evidence supporting this hypothesis, including studies focusing on possible occult CNS infection (Klempner et al., 2001; Kaplan et al., 2003; Krupp et al., 2003; Fallon et al., 2008; Dersch et al., 2016).

Four NIH-sponsored, randomized, placebo-controlled trials of intensive antibiotic retreatment of United States patients with persisting symptoms following treatment for Bbsl infection (Klempner et al., 2001; 2013; Krupp et al., 2003; Fallon et al., 2008) have failed to provide any evidence of a measurable benefit that outweighed treatment-associated risks. The investigators in these trials concluded that prolonged use of antibiotics is not in the best interest of these patients (Klempner et al., 2001; Kaplan et al., 2003; Krupp et al., 2003; Fallon et al., 2008). These results are therefore consistent with the negative microbiologic findings. A fifth retreatment study done in the Netherlands also failed to find any benefit (Berende et al., 2016). A sixth study by a single physician (Cameron, 2008) was too flawed to interpret, as described elsewhere (Wormser et al., 2009). Therefore, symptomatic treatment is the recommended approach for such patients (Wormser et al., 2006).

6.12 Guidelines

In 2006, the Infectious Diseases Society of America (IDSA) published updated guidelines for the diagnosis, treatment and prevention of Bbsl infection (Wormser et al., 2006). Following an unprecedented degree of external politicization after the guidelines' publication, the IDSA convened an independent panel, vetted by an ombudsman for potential conflicts of interest, to review these guidelines. The eight-member panel reviewed the 2006 guidelines and the supporting evidence in their entirety and concluded that the recommendations were medically and scientifically sound and that no changes were necessary (Lantos et al., 2010).

Although the IDSA guidelines were intended for use in North America, they are remarkably similar to diagnostic and treatment guidelines prepared independently by specialist societies and expert groups in various European countries (Wormser and O'Connell, 2011). No evidence-based European guideline recommends prolonged or multiple courses of antibiotics for persistent symptoms following previously treated Bbsl infection. Comprehensive review articles have recently been published that provide guidance on the management of Bbsl infection (Sanchez et al., 2016).

6.13 What Constitutes Cure of an Infection?

Fundamental to much of this 'debate' is an understanding of the appropriate standard by which to judge successful treatment of an infectious disease. Patients treated for pneumonia usually do not feel back to normal at the end of their course of antibiotic therapy and do not yet have clear chest x-rays. Patients treated for meningitis often still have cerebrospinal fluid abnormalities at the end of successful antibiotic treatment, with persisting headaches and malaise for quite some time. In most infections treatment is judged successful based on the historic observation that patients receiving that course no longer worsen or relapse, and in fact improve with time – a reasonable standard for therapeutic success (Wormser and O'Connell, 2011).

From a microbiologic perspective, similarly, it is probably unrealistic to expect that antimicrobial therapy will eradicate every last microorganism from an infected host; moreover, such an action is rarely if ever required for a successful outcome (Baker and Wormser, 2017). Antimicrobial therapy can be thought to 'tip the balance' in favor of the host's own defenses in their fight against a pathogen (Wormser and Schwartz, 2009). For many infectious diseases antibiotic treatment that only inhibits rather than kills a microorganism is highly effective (Pankey and Sabath, 2004; Wormser and Schwartz, 2009; Baker and Wormser, 2017). The host's immunologic response against spirochetal infections plays a crucial role – as evidenced by the observation that most of the objective clinical manifestations of Bbsl infection will eventually resolve even in the absence of antibiotic treatment (Steere et al., 1987).

It has been suggested that the observation, exclusively in animal systems, of post-antibiotic-treatment PCR positivity for Bbsl DNA – in the absence of culture positivity – could provide an explanation for PTLDS (Hodzic et al., 2008). Bbsl cells remaining after treatment in these animal systems do not elicit a local inflammatory response (Wormser and Schwartz, 2009; Barthold et al., 2010; Baker and Wormser, 2017). Antibody responses to Bbsl decline, suggesting a reduction in the overall immunologic response to the spirochete (Philipp et al., 2001). Since Bbsl does not appear to elaborate a systemic toxin (Fraser et al., 1997), it is difficult to imagine how residual spirochetes – in the absence of a detectable local or generalized immunologic or inflammatory response by the host – could cause chronic subjective symptoms (Wormser and Schwartz, 2009; Baker and Wormser, 2017). Certainly, latent infections with other microorganisms are generally clinically silent.

Whether a few spirochetes might persist is irrelevant in judging the outcome of treatment, unless these residual organisms can be shown to cause objectively demonstrable disease. Recent interest in a 'test of cure' beyond that of clinical resolution of EM, carditis, meningitis or other neurologic manifestations, or arthritis is arguably misdirected, and inconsistent with the way treatment success is judged for almost every other infectious disease (Wormser and O'Connell, 2011; Baker and Wormser, 2017).

6.14 Conclusions

Treatment of Bbsl infection is usually successfully accomplished with 10–28 days of an appropriate oral or parenteral antibiotic. A course of therapy as brief as a single dose of doxycycline is often effective if given during the incubation period within 72 h of inoculation of Bbss by a tick bite (Nadelman et al., 2001; Wormser et al., 2006).

The objective clinical manifestations of Bbsl infection are thought to be due to an inflammatory reaction to live spirochetes or to their undegraded antigens (Malawista and Bockenstedt, 2007; Steere 2010; Steere et al., 2016). Post-treatment subjective symptoms, presumably related to residual inflammation, may last for 3 or more months after initiation of antibiotic therapy and are unaffected by prolonging the initial course of treatment (Wormser et al., 2003; 2006).

It remains unclear whether the frequency of subjective symptoms at 6 months after treatment exceeds the background rates of these symptoms in the general population (Cerar et al., 2010). Clarification of this issue should be a research priority. Microbiologic studies have failed to find evidence of Bbsl infection or of a co-infection in such patients, and patients with post-treatment symptoms clearly are not benefited by additional courses of antibiotic treatment. Future research should address other potential explanations of post-treatment symptoms and alternative therapeutic approaches for their management (Melia and Auwaerter, 2016).

Acknowledgments

The authors thank Lisa Giarratano and Julia Singer for assistance.

References

Arvikar, S.L. and Steere, A.C. (2015) Diagnosis and treatment of Lyme arthritis. *Infectious Diseases Clinics of North America* 29, 269–280.

Baker, P.J. and Wormser, G.P. (2017) The clinical relevance of studies on *Borrelia burgdorferi* persisters. *American Journal of Medicine* 130, 1009–1010.

Baradaran-Dilmaghani, R. and Stanek, G. (1996) In vitro susceptibility of thirty *Borrelia* strains from various sources against eight antimicrobial chemotherapies. *Infection* 24, 60–63.

Barthold, S.W., Hodzic, E., Imai, D.M., Feng, S., Yang, X. and Luft, B.J. (2010) Ineffectiveness of tigecycline against persistent *Borrelia burgdorferi*. *Antimicrobial Agents and Chemotherapy* 54, 643–651.

Berende, A., ter Hofstede, H.J., Vos, F.J., van Middendorp, H., Vogelaar, M.L., Tromp, M., van den Hoogen, F.H., Donders, A.R.T., Evers, A.W. and Kullberg, B.J. (2016) Randomized trial of longer-term therapy for symptoms attributed to Lyme disease. *New England Journal of Medicine* 374, 1209–1220.

Biggs, H.M., Behravesh, C.B., Bradley, K.K. et al. (2016) Diagnosis and management of tickborne rickettsial diseases: rocky mountain spotted fever and other spotted fever group rickettsioses, ehrlichioses, and anaplasmosis – United States. *MMWR Recommendations and Reports* 65, 1–44.

Bremell, D. and Dotevall, L. (2014) Oral doxycycline for Lyme neuroborreliosis with symptoms of encephalitis, myelitis, vasculitis, or intracranial hypertension. *European Journal of Neurology* 21, 1162–1167.

Bunikis, I., Denker, K., Ostberg, Y., Andersen, C., Benz, R. and Bergström, S. (2008) An RND-type efflux system in *Borrelia burgdorferi* is involved in virulence and resistance to antimicrobial compounds. *Public Library of Science Pathogens* 4(2), e1000009.

Cameron, D. (2008) Severity of Lyme disease with persistent symptoms. Insights from a double-blind placebo-controlled clinical trial. *Minerva Medica* 99, 489–496.

Cameron, D., Gaito, A., Harris, N. et al. (2004) Evidence-based guidelines for the management of Lyme disease. *Expert Review of Anti-Infective Therapy* 2 (1 supplement), S1–S13.

Cerar, D., Cerar, T., Ružić-Sabljić, E., Wormser, G.P. and Strle, F. (2010) Subjective symptoms after treatment of early Lyme disease. *American Journal of Medicine* 123, 79–86.

Connally, N.P., Durante, A.J., Yousey-Hindes, K.M., Meek, J.I., Nelson, R.S. and Heimer, R. (2009) Peridomestic Lyme disease prevention: results of a population-based case-control study. *American Journal of Preventative Medicine* 37, 201–206.

Dattwyler, R.J., Wormser, G.P., Rush, T.J., Finkel, M.F., Schoen, R.T., Grunwaldt, E., Franklin, M., Hilton, E., Bryant, G.L., Agger, W.A. and Maladorno, D. (2005) A comparison of two treatment regimens of ceftriaxone in late Lyme disease. *Wiener Klinische Wochenschrift* 117, 393–397.

Dersch, R., Sommer, S., Rauer, S. and Meerpohl, J.J. (2016) Prevalence and spectrum of residual symptoms in Lyme neuroborreliosis after pharmacological treatment: a systematic review. *Journal of Neurology* 263, 17–24.

des Vignes, F., Piesman, J., Heffernan, R., Schulze, T.L., Stafford III, K.C. and Fish, D. (2001) Effect of tick removal on transmission of *Borrelia burgdorferi* and *Ehrlichia phagocytophila* by *Ixodes scapularis* nymphs. *Journal of Infectious Diseases* 183, 773–778.

Dolan, M.C., Zeidner, N.S., Gabitzsch, E., Dietrich, G., Borchert, J.N., Poché, R.M. and Piesman, J. (2008) Short report: a doxycycline hyclate rodent bait formulation for prophylaxis and treatment of tick-transmitted *Borrelia burgdorferi*. *American Journal of Tropical Medicine and Hygiene* 78, 803–805.

Eagle, H., Fleischman, R. and Musselman, A.D. (1950) Effect of schedule of administration on the therapeutic efficacy of penicillin. Importance of aggregate time penicillin remains at effectively bactericidal levels. *American Journal of Medicine* 9, 280–299.

Fallon, B.A., Keilp, J.G., Corbera, K.M., Petkova, E., Britton, C.B., Dwyer, E., Slavov, I., Cheng, J., Dobkin, J., Nelson, D.R. and Sackeim, H.A. (2008) A randomized, placebo-controlled trial of repeated IV antibiotic therapy for Lyme encephalopathy. *Neurology* 70, 992–1003.

Feder, H.M., Johnson, B.J., O'Connell, S. *et al.* (2007) A critical appraisal of 'chronic Lyme disease'. *New England Journal of Medicine* 357, 1422–1430.

Fraser, C.M., Casjens, S., Huang, W.M. *et al.* (1997) Genomic sequence of a Lyme disease spirochete, *Borrelia burgdorferi*. *Nature* 390, 580–586.

Halperin, J.J., Shapiro, E.D., Logigian, E., Belman, A.L., Dotevall, L., Wormser, G.P., Krupp, L., Gronseth, G. and Bever, C.T. (2007) Practice parameter: treatment of nervous system Lyme disease (an evidence-based review): report of the quality standards subcommittee of the American Academy of Neurology. *Neurology* 69, 91–102.

Hasin, T., Davidovitch, N., Cohen, R. *et al.* (2006) Postexposure treatment with doxycycline for the prevention of tick-borne relapsing fever. *New England Journal of Medicine* 355, 148–155.

Hassett, A.L., Radvanski, D.C., Buyske, S., Savage, S.V., Gara, M., Escobar, J.I. and Sigal, L.H. (2008) Role of psychiatric comorbidity in chronic Lyme disease. *Arthritis and Rheumatism* 59, 1742–1749.

Hassett, A.L., Radvanski, D.C., Buyske, S., Savage, S.V. and Sigal, L.H. (2009) Psychiatric comorbidity and other psychological factors in patients with 'chronic Lyme disease'. *American Journal of Medicine* 122, 843–850.

Hodzic, E., Feng, S., Holden, K., Freet, J. and Barthold, S.W. (2008) Persistence of *Borrelia burgdorferi* following antibiotic treatment in mice. *Antimicrobial Agents and Chemotherapy* 52, 1728–1736.

Hollander, D.H., Turner, T.B. and Nell, E.E. (1952) The effect of long continued subcurative doses of penicillin during the incubation period of experimental syphilis. *Bulletin of the Johns Hopkins Hospital* 90, 105–120.

Hojgaard, A., Eisen, R.J. and Piesman, J. (2008) Transmission dynamics of *Borrelia burgdorferi* s.s. during the key third day of feeding by nymphal *Ixodes scapularis* (Acari:Ixodidae). *Journal of Medical Entomology* 45, 732–736.

Kalish R.A., Kaplan, R.F., Taylor, E., Jones-Woodward, L., Workman, K. and Steere, A.C. (2001) Evaluation of study patients with Lyme disease, 10–20 year follow-up. *Journal of Infectious Diseases* 183, 453–460.

Kaplan, R.F., Trevino, R.P., Johnson, G.M., Levy, L., Dornbush, R., Hu, L.T., Evans, J., Weinstein, A., Schmid, C.H. and Klempner, M.S. (2003) Cognitive function in post-treatment Lyme disease. *Neurology* 60, 1916–1922.

Klempner, M.S., Hu, L.T., Evans, J., Schmid, C.H., Johnson, G.M., Trevino, R.P., Norton, D., Levy, L., Wall, D., McCall, J., Kosinski, M. and Weinstein, A. (2001) Two controlled trials of antibiotic treatment in patients with persistent symptoms and a history of Lyme disease. *New England Journal of Medicine* 345, 85–92.

Klempner, M.S., Baker, P.J., Shapiro, E.D., Marques, A., Dattwyler, R.J., Halperin, J.J. and Wormser, G.P. (2013) Treatment trials for post-Lyme disease symptoms revisted. *American Journal of Medicine* 126, 665–669.

Korenberg, E.I., Vorobyeva, N.N., Moskvitina, H.G. and Gorbań, L.Y. (1996) Prevention of borreliosis in persons bitten by infected ticks. *Infection* 24, 187–189.

Kowalski, T.J., Tata, S., Berth, W., Mathiason, M.A. and Agger, W.A. (2010) Antibiotic treatment duration and long-term outcomes of patients with early Lyme disease from a Lyme disease-hyperendemic area. *Clinical Infectious Diseases* 50, 512–520.

Krupp, L.B., Hyman, L.G., Grimson, R., Coyle, P.K., Melville, P., Ahnn, S., Dattwyler, R. and Chandler, B. (2003) Study and treatment of post Lyme disease (Stop-LD). A randomized double-masked clinical trial. *Neurology* 60, 1923–1930.

Lantos, P.M., Charini, W.A., Medoff, G., Moro, M.H., Mushatt, D.M., Parsonnet, J., Sanders, J.W. and Baker, C.J. (2010) Final report of the Lyme disease review panel of the Infectious Diseases Society of America. *Clinical Infectious Diseases* 51, 1–5.

Lee, J. and Wormser, G.P. (2008) Pharmacodynamics of doxycycline for chemoprophylaxis of Lyme disease: preliminary findings and possible implications for other antimicrobials. *International Journal of Antimicrobial Agents* 31, 235–239.

Levin, J.M., Nelson, J.A., Segreti, J., Harrison, B., Benson, C.A. and Strle, F. (1993) In vitro susceptibility of *Borrelia burgdorferi* to 11 antimicrobial agents. *Antimicrobial Agents and Chemotherapy* 37, 1444–1446.

Ljostad, U. and Mygland, A. (2010) Remaining complaints one year after treatment for acute Lyme neuroborreliosis; frequency, pattern and risk factors. *European Journal of Neurology* 17, 118–123.

Ljostad, U., Skogvoll, E., Eikeland, R., Midgard, R., Skarpaas, T., Berg, A. and Mygland, A. (2008) Oral doxycycline versus intravenous ceftriaxone for European Lyme neuroborreliosis: a multicentre, non-inferiority, double-blind, randomised trial. *Lancet Neurology* 7, 690–695.

Luft, B.J., Dattwyler, R.J., Johnson, R.C., Luger, S.W., Bosler, E.M., Rahn, D.W., Masters, E.J., Grunwaldt, E. and Gadgil, S.D. (1996) Azithromycin compared with amoxicillin in the treatment of erythema migrans. A double-blind, randomized, controlled trial. *Annals of Internal Medicine* 124, 785–791.

Magnuson, H.J. and Eagle, H. (1945) The retardation and suppression of experimental early syphilis by small doses of penicillin comparable to those used in the treatment of gonorrhea. *American Journal of Syphilis, Gonorrhea, and Venereal Diseases* 29, 587–596.

Malawista, S.E. and Bockenstedt, L.K. (2007) Lyme disease, 23rd edn. In: Goldman, L. and Ausiello, D.A. (eds) *Cecil Textbook of Medicine*. Saunders Elsevier, Philadelphia, Pennsylvania, pp. 2289–2294.

Martinez, J.L., Sánchez, M.B., Martínez-Solano, L., Hernandez, A., Garmendia, L., Fajardo, A. and Alvarez-Ortega, C. (2009) Functional role of bacterial multidrug efflux pumps in microbial natural ecosystems. *Federation of European Microbiological Societies Microbiology Reviews* 33, 430–449.

Melia, M.T. and Auwaerter, P.G. (2016) Time for a different approach to Lyme disease and long-term symptoms. *New England Journal of Medicine* 374, 1277–1278.

Morgenstern, K., Baljer, G., Norris, D.E., Kraiczy, P., Hanssen-Hubner, C. and Hunfield, K.-P. (2009) In vitro susceptibility of *Borrelia spielmanii* to antimicrobial agents commonly used for treatment of Lyme disease. *Antimicrobial Agents and Chemotherapy* 53, 1281–1284.

Nadelman, R.B., Nowakowski, J., Fish, D., Falco, R.C., Freeman, K., McKenna, D., Welch, P., Marcus, R., Agüero-Rosenfeld, M.E., Dennis, D.T. and Wormser, G.P. (2001) Prophylaxis with single-dose doxycycline for the prevention of Lyme disease after an *Ixodes scapularis* tick bite. *New England Journal of Medicine* 345, 79–84.

Nowakowski, J. and Wormser, G.P. (1993) Treatment of early Lyme disease: infection associated with erythema migrans. In: Coyle, P.K. (ed.) *Lyme Disease*. Mosby Year Book, St. Louis, Missouri, pp. 149–162.

Nowakowski, J., McKenna, D., Nadelman, R.B., Cooper, D., Bittker, S., Holmgren, D., Pavia, C., Johnson, R.C. and Wormser, G.P. (2000) Failure of treatment with cephalexin for Lyme disease. *Archives of Family Medicine* 9, 563–567.

Oksi, J., Nikoskelainen, J., Hiekkanen, H., Lauhio, A., Peltomaa, M., Pitkäranta, A., Nyman, D., Granlund, H., Carlsson, S.A., Seppälä, I., Valtonen, V. and Viljanen, M. (2007) Duration of antibiotic treatment in disseminated Lyme borreliosis: a double-blind, randomized, placebo-controlled, multicenter clinical study. *European Journal of Clinical Microbiology and Infectious Diseases* 26, 571–581.

Pankey, G.A. and Sabath, L.D. (2004) Clinical relevance of bacteriostatic versus bactericidal mechanisms of action in the treatment of gram-positive bacterial infections. *Clinical Infectious Diseases* 38, 864–870.

Philipp, M.T., Bowers, L.C., Fawcett, P.T., Jacobs, M.B., Liang, F.T., Marques, A.R., Mitchell, P.D., Purcell, J.E., Ratterree, M.S. and Straubinger, R.K. (2001) Antibody response to IR6, a conserved mmunodominant region of the VlsE lipoprotein, wanes rapidly after antibiotic treatment of *Borrelia burgdorferi* infection in experimental animals and in humans. *Journal of Infectious Diseases* 184, 870–878.

Sanchez, E., Vannier, E., Wormser, G.P. and Hu, L.T. (2016) Diagnosis, treatment and prevention of Lyme disease, human granulocytic anaplasmosis, and babesiosis. *Journal of the American Medical Association* 315, 1767–1777.

Schroeter, A.L., Turner, R.H., Lucas, J.B. and Brown, W.J. (1971) Therapy for incubating syphilis: effectiveness of gonorrhea treatment. *Journal of the American Medical Association* 218, 711–713.

Sicklinger, M., Wieneche, R. and Neubert, U. (2003) In vitro susceptibility testing of four antibiotics against *Borrelia burgdorferi*: a comparison of results of the three genospecies *Borrelia afzelii*, *Borrelia garinii*, and *Borrelia burgdorferi* sensu stricto. *Journal of Clinical Microbiology* 41, 1791–1793.

Skogman, B.H., Croner, S., Nordwall, M., Eknefelt, M., Ernerudh, J. and Forsberg, P. (2008) Lyme neuroborreliosis in children: a prospective study of clinical features, prognosis and outcome. *Pediatric Infectious Disease Journal* 27, 1089–1094.

Stanek, G. and Strle, F. (2003) Lyme borreliosis. *Lancet* 362, 1639–1647.

Stanek, G., Wormser, G.P., Gray, J. and Strle, F. (2012) Lyme borreliosis. *Lancet* 379, 461–473.

Steere, A.C. (2010) *Borrelia burgdorferi* (Lyme disease, Lyme borreliosis), 7th edn. In: Mandell, G.L., Bennett, J.E. and Dolin, R. (eds) *Mandell, Douglas, and Bennett's Principles and Practice of Infectious Diseases.* Churchill, Livingstone, Elsevier, Philadelphia, Pennsylvania, pp. 3071–3081.

Steere, A.C. and Angelis, S. (2006) Therapy for Lyme arthritis: strategies for the treatment of antibiotic-refractory arthritis. *Arthritis and Rheumatism* 54, 3079–3085.

Steere, A.C., Schoen, R.T. and Taylor, E. (1987) The clinical evolution of Lyme arthritis. *Annals of Internal Medicine* 107, 725–731.

Steere, A.C., Taylor, E., McHugh, G.L. and Logigian, E.L. (1993) The over-diagnosis of Lyme disease. *Journal of the American Medical Association* 269, 1812–1816.

Steere, A.C., Strle, F., Wormser, G.P., Hu, L.T., Brande, J.A., Hovius, J.W.R., Li, X. and Mead, P.S. (2016) Lyme borreliosis. *Nature Reviews Disease Primers* 2, 16090. DOI: 10.1038/nrdp.2016.90.

Stupica, D., Lusa, L., Ružić-Sabljić, E., Cerar, T. and Strle, F. (2012) Treatment of erythema migrans with doxycycline for 10 days versus 15 days. *Clinical Infectious Diseases* 55, 343–350.

Swanson, J.S., Neitzel, D., Reed, K.D. and Belongia, E.A. (2006) Coinfections acquired from *Ixodes* ticks. *Clinical Microbiology Reviews* 19, 708–727.

Takafuji, E.T., Kirkpatrick, J.W., Miller, R.N., Karwacki, J.J., Kelley, P.W., Gray, M.R., McNeil, K.M., Timboe, H.L., Kane, R.E. and Sanchez, J.L. (1984) An efficacy trial of doxycycline prophylaxis against leptospirosis. *New England Journal of Medicine* 310, 497–500.

Terekhova, D., Sartakova, M.L., Wormser, G.P., Schwartz, I. and Cabello, F.C. (2002) Erythromycin resistance in *Borrelia burgdorferi*. *Antimicrobial Agents and Chemotherapy* 46, 3637–3640.

Tokarz, R., Jain, K., Bennett, A., Briese, T. and Lipkin, W.I. (2010) Assessment of polymicrobial infections in ticks in New York State. *Vector-Borne and Zoonotic Diseases* 10, 217–221.

Tory, H.O., Zurakowski, D. and Sundel, R.P. (2010) Outcomes of children treated for Lyme arthritis: results of a large pediatric cohort. *Journal of Rheumatology* 37, 1049–1055.

Tibbles, C.D. and Edlow, J.A. (2007) Does this patient have erythema migrans? *Journal of the American Medical Association* 297, 2617–2627.

Warshafsky, S., Lee, D.H., Francois, L.K., Nowakowski, J., Nadelman, R.B. and Wormser, G.P. (2010a) Efficacy of antibiotic prophylaxis for the prevention of Lyme disease: an updated systematic review and meta-analysis. *Journal of Antimicrobial Chemotherapy* 65, 1137–1144.

Warshafsky, S., Lee, D.H., Nadelman, R.B. and Wormser, G.P. (2010b) Efficacy of antibiotic prophylaxis for the prevention of Lyme disease: an updated systematic review and metanalysis – authors' response. *Journal of Antimicrobial Chemotherapy* 65, 2271–2273.

Weber, K., Preac-Mursic, V., Wilske, B., Thurmays, R., Neubert, U. and Scherwitz, C. (1990) A randomized trial of ceftriaxone versus oral penicillin for the treatment of early European Lyme borreliosis. *Infection* 18, 91–96.

Wormser, G.P. (1995) Lyme disease. Insights into the use of antimicrobials for prevention and treatment in the context of experience with other spirochetal infections. *Mount Sinai Journal of Medicine* 62, 188–195.

Wormser, G.P. (2006) Clinical practice. Early Lyme disease. *New England Journal of Medicine* 354, 2794–2801.

Wormser, G.P. (2016) Lyme Disease, 25th edn. In Goldman, L. and Schafer, A.I. (eds) *Goldman-Cecil Medicine* (Chapter 321). Elsevier, Philadelphia, Pennsylvania, pp. 2021–2027.

Wormser, G.P. and Halperin, J.J. (2008) Oral doxycycline for neuroborreliosis. *Lancet Neurology* 7, 665–666.

Wormser, G.P. and O'Connell, S. (2011) Treatment of infection caused by *Borrelia burgdorferi* sensu lato. *Expert Review of Anti-Infective Therapy* 9, 245–260.

Wormser, G.P. and Schwartz, I. (2009) Antibiotic treatment of animals infected with *Borrelia burgdorferi*. *Clinical Microbiology Reviews* 22, 387–395.

Wormser, G.P., Nowakowski, J. and Nadelman, R.B. (2002) Duration of treatment for Lyme borreliosis: time for a critical reappraisal. *Wiener Klinische Wochenschrift* 114, 613–615.

Wormser, G.P., Ramanathan, R., Nowakowski, J., McKenna, D., Holmgren, D., Visintainer, P., Dornbush, R., Singh, B. and Nadelman, R.B. (2003) Duration of antibiotic therapy for early Lyme disease. A randomized, double-blind, placebo-controlled trial. *Annals of Internal Medicine* 138, 697–704.

Wormser, G.P., Dattwyler, R.J., Shapiro, E.D. *et al.* (2006) The clinical assessment, treatment, and prevention of Lyme disease, human granulocytic anaplasmosis, and babesiosis: clinical practice guidelines by the Infectious Diseases Society of America. *Clinical Infectious Diseases* 43, 1089–1134.

Wormser, G.P., Shapiro, E.D., Halperin, J.J. *et al.* (2009) Analysis of a flawed double-blind, placebo-controlled, clinical trial of patients claimed to have persistent Lyme disease following treatment. *Minerva Medica* 100, 171–172.

Zeidner, N.S., Brandt, K.S., Dadey, E., Dolan, M.C., Happ, C. and Piesman, J. (2004) Sustained-release formulation of doxycycline hyclate for prophylaxis of tick bite infection in a murine model of Lyme borreliosis. *Antimicrobial Agents and Chemotherapy* 48, 2697–2699.

Zeidner, N.S., Massung, R.F., Dolan, M.C., Dadey, E., Gabitzsch, E., Dietrich, G. and Levin, M.L. (2008) A sustained-release formulation of doxycycline hyclate (Atridox) prevents simultaneous infection of *Anaplasma phagocytophilum* and *Borrelia burgdorferi* transmitted by tick bite. *Journal of Medical Microbiology* 57, 463–468.

7 Lyme Borreliosis: The European Perspective

Franc Strle,[1] Gerold Stanek[2] and Klemen Strle[3]

[1]*Department of Infectious Diseases, University Medical Center Ljubljana, Ljubljana, Slovenia;* [2]*Medical University of Vienna, Institute for Hygiene and Applied Immunology, Vienna, Austria;* [3]*Division of Rheumatology, Allergy and Immunology, Center for Immunology and Inflammatory Diseases, Massachusetts General Hospital, Boston, Massachusetts, USA*

7.1 History of Lyme Borreliosis

Lyme borreliosis (LB) encompasses several clinical manifestations that may affect multiple organ systems, most commonly the skin, heart, nervous system or joints. Although this constellation of rather diverse manifestations now falls under a common term (Lyme borreliosis/Lyme disease), most individual manifestations were described in Europe several decades before the discovery of the etiological agent, *Borrelia burgdorferi* (as discussed in Chapter 2, the genus has now been renamed *Borrelia*) (Adeolu and Gupta, 2014; Barbour *et al.*, 2017). Because of the many references that used the genus name Borrelia in this chapter we use this term. The history of LB can be divided rather scholastically into three periods.

7.1.1 First (pre-antibiotic) phase

Initially, the clinical manifestations of LB were described independently. In 1883, Alfred Buchwald from Breslau described a diffuse idiopathic skin atrophy (Buchwald, 1883) which was subsequently named acrodermatitis chronica atrophicans (ACA) by Karl Herxheimer and Kuno Hartmann in 1902 (Herxheimer and Hartmann, 1902). These studies described most symptoms associated with ACA, including macular atrophy, focal loss of dermal elastic tissue, sclerodermal changes, ulnar bands, fibrous peri-articular nodules, livid discoloration of the skin, preferred involvement of the dorsal sides of the extremities, atrophy of the skin akin to shriveled cigarette paper, and finally involvement of bones and joints. However, a connection with tick bite was not made at the time. A moulage of an ACA on one entire leg and gluteal region of a patient, entitled '*atrophia cutis idiopathica diffusa*' from 1905, is on display at the pathologic-anatomical collection in Vienna. ACA with such extensive expansion likely developed over at least two decades.

A distinct skin disease, erythema chronicum migrans, was recognized in the beginning of the 20th century. Benjamin Lipschütz (1878–1931), a dermatologist in Vienna, described an erythema that began as a red spot on the left hip and expanded over many months (Lipschütz, 1913). He stated that this skin lesion is rare, always solitary, mainly located on the lower extremities, and continues to expand for weeks to months and can reach vast diameters. Lipschütz stated that the edges of the erythema are usually accented, the central area usually only slightly colored and the clinical course is fever-free, accompanied only occasionally by mild subjective symptoms; the distinguishing feature of erythema chronicum migrans is 'expanding'. In a later publication Lipschütz (1923) stated that '...attention should be directed toward microscopic/bacteriologic investigations of the intestinal and salivary gland secretions of the tick'. The statement was presumably based on an earlier publication by Arvid Afzelius (1857–1923), who was a student in Vienna at the time of dermatologist Moriz Kaposi (1837–1902), and who at a meeting in Stockholm in 1909 reported a patient who developed an erythema migrans (EM) after the bite of the common castor bean tick (Afzelius, 1910). It remains enigmatic why no one in Europe followed this proposal at that time.

Another key report came from the French physicians Garin and Bujadoux in 1922 of a sheep farmer who was always healthy until he was bitten by an ixodid tick (Garin and Bujadoux, 1922). Three weeks later he developed radicular pain concomitantly with a red spot on the left buttock, which extended rapidly and covered the right buttock and right thigh down to the knee, followed by palsies. Cerebrospinal fluid, taken 4 months later, showed elevated white cell count and increased protein level. The patient was subsequently treated with substances that were at that time used for treating syphilis and recovered with occasional sequelae. This case is considered the first report of typical borrelia meningoradiculoneuritis; although it was questioned recently that it was caused by *Borrelia* infection (Wormser and Wormser, 2016). In 1930 Sven Hellerström from Sweden reported on a patient who developed meningoencephalitis 3 months after the onset of an EM; he reinforced the relationship between tick bite, EM and nervous system disorders (Hellerström, 1930). In 1941, Bannwarth from Munich carefully studied several patients with chronic lymphocytic meningitis and identified three groups, one with intensive radicular pain, one with facial palsy and one with chronic lymphocytic meningitis and cerebral symptoms (Bannwarth, 1941). Although Bannwarth missed the connection with tick bites and erroneously concluded that these symptoms are due to a rheumatic-allergic cause, his name is now synonymous with the full clinical picture of the most typical manifestations of early European Lyme neuroborreliosis (LNB): meningo-poly-radiculo-neuritis (Bannwarth's syndrome).

Finally, Bäfverstedt from Stockholm studied the benign course of pseudolymphomas of the skin and showed a relation with EM in some cases. He defined the predilection sites ear lobe, nipple and scrotum for these manifestations (Bäfverstedt, 1943), later named borrelial lymphocytoma (BL).

7.1.2 Second (penicillin) phase

In the second phase the beneficial effects of penicillin suggested a bacterial etiology of the various clinical manifestations.

Penicillin came into general usage after the Second World War. It was very effective in treatment of ACA (Thyresson, 1949; Brunner, 1951; Götz and Ludwig, 1951; Hopf, 1966), but also of EM (Hollström, 1951) and of BL (Bianchi, 1950). In a publication in 1974 (Weber, 1974) Klaus Weber from Munich posed the question of whether 'erythema migrans meningitis' is a bacterial infectious disease. Serological testing excluded all possible viral and bacteriological causes except *Borrelia*. However, *Borrelia* was excluded because of the acarologist's opinion that hard ticks do not carry borrelia, and thus Weber abandoned this hypothesis.

Clinical courses of 'chronic aseptic meningitis' and meningo-radiculoneuritis, and the cytology of the cerebrospinal fluid were most carefully studied in the 1960s and 1970s (Schaltenbrand, 1962; Bammer and Schenk, 1965; Hörstrup and Ackermann, 1973). In 1983 Kristoferitsch et al. described in detail the spontaneous course of meningopolyneuritis (Kristoferitsch et al., 1983). The same year Sköldenberg et al. reported the beneficial effect of penicillin G in 21 patients who suffered from 'chronic meningitis' (Sköldenberg et al., 1983); noting that 'the patients improved or recovered, sometimes dramatically, during a 2-week course of intravenous penicillin G'. LNB was later confirmed in both studies.

In 1977 Allen C Steere and co-authors described a new type of arthritis, termed Lyme arthritis, which was defined as a separate entity because of the geographical clustering of children with arthritis in the towns of Lyme, Old Lyme and East Haddam, Connecticut (Steere et al., 1977). When the connection with tick bites was made, Lyme arthritis, along with EM, heart and neurological abnormalities were collectively defined as Lyme disease (Steere et al., 1977).

7.1.3 Third phase – Lyme disease/Lyme borreliosis, a borrelial infectious disease

The third phase started with the discovery of spirochetes in the hard tick *Ixodes scapularis* (then called *Ixodes dammini*) by Willy Burgdorfer and colleagues (Burgdorfer *et al.*, 1982). Alan G. Barbour was able to cultivate these spirochetes and characterized their antigenic structure (Barbour, 1984). Culture and serology confirmed that spirochetes were the causative agent of Lyme disease (Benach *et al.*, 1983; Steere *et al.*, 1983) and the related disease in Europe (Preac-Mursic *et al.*, 1984; Asbrink and Hovmark, 1985; Stanek *et al.*, 1985a). A new nosologic entity of a worldwide tick-borne disease has emerged. In 1984, the spirochetes were defined as a new species, now referred to as *Borrelia burgdorferi*, within the genus *Borrelia* (Johnson *et al.*, 1984).

Barbour raised a monoclonal antibody (H5332) against the isolate B31 from *I. scapularis* ticks, which reacted with an outer surface protein (Osp) of a molecular weight of 31 kD – later named OspA. This monoclonal antibody reacted with spirochetes isolated from mammals and patients with Lyme disease in the United States (Barbour *et al.*, 1983); however, the antibody failed to react with most European patients' isolates (Stanek *et al.*, 1985b; Wilske *et al.*, 1985). In retrospect, this was the prelude to the OspA typing scheme of hard tick-borne borrelia. By delineation of three genospecies (*B. burgdorferi*, *Borrelia garinii* and a genospecies later called *Borrelia afzelii*), Guy Baranton established the naming of the 'Lyme disease spirochetes' (Baranton *et al.*, 1992). These genospecies compared quite well with OspA serotypes (Wilske *et al.*, 1993). Bettina Wilske *et al.* isolated *Borrelia* strains from ticks, human skin and cerebrospinal fluid from various geographical regions and interrogated them by Western blotting using eight monoclonal antibodies against different epitopes of OspA. These studies identified seven OspA serotypes, which correlated directly with the delineated genospecies (Baranton *et al.*, 1992). The most prevalent genospecies among European skin isolates was Serotype 2 (group VS461), now known as *B. afzelii*.

Collectively, these data demonstrated that LB is caused by different *Borrelia* genospecies, which appear to vary in geographic distribution, pathogenic potential, and organotropism. In the United States, *B. burgdorferi* was the only causative agent of LB, whereas three genospecies caused the disease in Europe, namely *B. afzelii*, *B. garinii* and *B. burgdorferi*. New genospecies that cause disease in humans have since been identified: *B. bavariensis* (former *B. garinii* OspA-type 4) in Europe, and *B. mayonii* in North America. Currently more than 20 *Borrelia* genospecies have been named (Casjens *et al.*, 2011; Stanek and Reiter, 2011; Wei-Gang and Martin, 2014).

7.2 Epidemiology

The main vector of Lyme borreliae in Europe is *Ixodes ricinus*. *Ixodes persulcatus* is a vector in the northeastern parts of Europe. The principal vertebrate reservoirs for Lyme borreliae are small mammals, such as mice and voles, and certain species of birds. Feeding activity of *I. ricinus* nymphs is highest in late spring to early summer; however, depending on weather conditions, questing ticks may be found throughout the year, even in wintertime. A web resource run by 'tick-radar Ltd', established by German acarologists, provides information regarding the activity of *I. ricinus* ticks in Germany (www.zeckenwetter.de) as well as valuable information about management of tick bites.

Humans are most frequently exposed to tick bites during the height of tick activity season between April and October, usually peaking in the summer, when people are most frequently outdoors and in direct contact with vegetation and tick habitats. Comparison of children and adults revealed that tick bites in children are more frequently localized on the head, while in adults they are on the lower limbs and on the abdominal and gluteal region (Berglund *et al.*, 1995), reflecting the common location of questing ticks on grasses and shrubs.

A recent meta-analysis of studies from 23 European countries, encompassing the period from 2010 to 2016, investigated the prevalence of *Borrelia* strains in 115,028 questing *I. ricinus* ticks. This analysis revealed significantly higher infection rates in adult ticks compared to nymph ticks (17.8% versus 14.2%) and in female compared to male ticks (18.4% versus 15.7%). In addition, the data demonstrated significant differences between various European regions, with the highest infection rates in Central Europe (19.3% of ticks) and the lowest in the British Isles (3.6%). The most common genospecies found in ticks were *B. afzelii*, *B. garinii* and *B. valaisiana*. No statistically significant differences were found among the prevalence rates of the three *Borrelia* species determined by conventional polymerase chain reaction (PCR), nested PCR and real-time PCR (Strnad et al., 2017). Additional information about the eco-epidemiology of *Borrelia* strains in Europe can be obtained from articles in the book *Lyme Borreliosis: Biology, Epidemiology and Control* (Gray et al., 2002).

LB is the most common tick-borne infection in humans throughout Europe and North America, but little is known about the actual incidence of the disease in Europe (Rizzoli et al., 2011; Stanek et al., 2012; Vandenesch et al., 2014; Wilking and Stark, 2014; Hofhuis et al., 2015). Hubalek estimated that 65,500 cases of LB occur each year (Hubalek, 2009). Similarly, the World Health Organization (Lindgren and Jaenson, 2006) estimated that the annual number of LB cases in Europe exceeds 85,000, with several regions of high incidence (Stanek et al., 2012; Vandenesch et al., 2014; Wilking and Stark, 2014; Hofhuis et al., 2015; Kraigher et al., 2016; Eliassen et al., 2017). In contrast, a recently published article, estimated the burden of LB in western Europe to be ~56.3 new cases per 100,000 inhabitants each year, equating to more than 232,000 new cases annually in western Europe (based on a total population of 412.2 million in 2011), with a population-weighted average incidence rate of 22.05 cases per 100,000 person-years (Sykes and Makiello, 2017).

However, only a few countries have required the reporting of LB cases; the true incidence in these countries likely exceeds the number of reported cases. Moreover, the incidence of LB has increased markedly (Wilking and Stark, 2014; Kraigher et al., 2016; van den Wijngaard et al., 2017), partly due to expansion of the geographic distribution as observed in Finland (Sajanti et al., 2017).

Reports from several European countries demonstrate a bimodal age distribution of LB. The incidence peaks in children aged 5 to 9 years and in adults aged 45 to 75 years, with female patients more frequently affected than males (Fülöp and Poggensee, 2008; Kraigher et al., 2016; Sajanti et al., 2017). About 70% of all cases of LB occur between June and September, with EM being the most frequently diagnosed clinical manifestation, accounting for about 90% of all cases in Slovenia (Kraigher et al., 2016).

Analysis of 1114 isolates obtained in prospective studies from Slovenian patients with various manifestations of LB indicated that three genospecies of Lyme borreliae, namely *B. afzelii*, *B. garinii* and *B. burgdorferi*, are important human pathogens in Europe (Ružić-Sabljić et al., 2002; Strle et al., 2006; Stupica et al., 2011; Stupica et al., 2012; O'Rourke et al., 2013; Ogrinc et al., 2013; 2016; Maraspin et al., 2016). The proportion of each genospecies across different clinical manifestations is depicted in Table 7.1. Of the 780 *Borrelia* strains isolated from skin of patients with solitary EM, 698 (89.5%) were *B. afzelii*, 73 (9.4%) *B. garinii* and only 9 (1.1%) *B. burgdorferi*. Similar predominance of *B. afzelii* was shown for isolates from skin and blood of patients with multiple EM. Similarly, the

Table 7.1. The proportion of main *Borrelia* species isolated from Slovenian patients with different clinical manifestations of Lyme borreliosis. (Ružić-Sabljić et al., 2002; Strle et al., 2006; Stupica et al., 2011; Stupica et al., 2012; O'Rourke et al., 2013; Ogrinc et al., 2013; 2016; Maraspin et al., 2017.)

Manifestation	Source	Number of specimens	B. afzelii	B. garinii	B. burgdorferi
Solitary EM	Skin	780	698 (89.5%)	73 (9.4%)	9 (1.1%)
Solitary EM	Blood	55	47 (85.5%)	8 (14.5%)	0
MEM	Skin	46	44 (95.7%)	2 (4.3%)	0
MEM	Blood	10	9 (90%)	1 (10%)	0
BL	Skin	19	17 (89.5%)	1 (5.3%)	1 (5.3%)
ACA	Skin	104	7 (6.1%)	3 (2.6%)	0
LNB	CSF	75	14 (18.7%)	59 (78.7%)	2 (2.7%)
LNB	Skin	25	3 (12%)	22 (88%)	0

EM, erythema migrans; MEM, multiple erythema migrans; BL, borrelial lymphocytoma; ACA, acrodermatitis chronica atrophicans; LNB, Lyme neuroborreliosis; CSF, cerebrospinal fluid.

large majority of isolates from BL were *B. afzelii*, however there was also a single isolate of *B. garinii*, *B. burgdorferi* and *B. bisettii*, suggesting that several species may cause EM or BL. Out of 114 ACA skin lesion isolates, 104 (91.2%) were typed as *B. afzelii*, 7 (6.1%) as *B. garinii* and 3 (2.6%) as *B. burgdorferi*. In contrast, >75% of isolates from cerebrospinal fluid of patients with LNB were *B. garinii* (Ružić-Sabljić *et al.*, 2002; Strle *et al.*, 2006; Ogrinc *et al.*, 2013; 2016). Interestingly, the frequency distribution of isolates from patients does not match that found in ticks (Picken *et al.*, 1996).

Thus, of the more than 20 *Borrelia* genospecies found in ticks, three genospecies, *B. afzelii*, *B. garinii* and *B. burgdorferi* most commonly cause the disease in humans in Europe. *B. afzelii* is associated with skin manifestations, and *B. garinii* particularly with neurologic involvement. Several *B. garinii* strains probably belong to *B. bavariensis* species.

7.3 Clinical Manifestations

LB is a complex disease with diverse clinical presentations. Thorough understanding of the signs and symptoms of each manifestation is critically important in diagnosing LB. It is obvious – albeit too often neglected – that there can be no diagnosis of LB in the absence of clinical manifestations. Good clinical knowledge requires clinical training and experience. In addition, case definitions, guidelines, reviews and seminar articles in peer-reviewed publications serve as good resources to learn about evidence-based knowledge of LB (Wormser *et al.*, 2006; Strle and Stanek, 2009; Mygland *et al.*, 2010; Stanek *et al.*, 2011; 2012; Sanchez *et al.*, 2016; Steere *et al.*, 2016). It is important to note that the web contains hundreds of sites (Sood, 2002) with misinformation on the disease complex, which should be avoided.

Differences in the clinical presentation of LB have been noted between Europe and North America, particularly the northeastern United States. Although EM is the most common early manifestation of the disease on both continents, patients with EM in the US have greater numbers and severity of constitutional symptoms compared to EM patients in Europe. Even greater distinctions between the two continents are observed with later manifestations of disease. Patients in Europe may present with skin manifestations, namely ACA and BL, which are rarely if ever observed in North America. Moreover, European patients more often develop meningoradiculitis (a rather specific form of early LNB named Bannwarth's syndrome), but have lower incidence of Lyme arthritis, which is the most common late manifestation of the disease in the northeastern US (Stanek *et al.*, 2012).

The differences in clinical presentation are probably the consequence of the different pathogenic species of Lyme borreliae on the two sides of Atlantic. Among over 20 genomic species of Lyme borreliae, eight have been found to cause disease in Europe; namely, *B. afzelii*, *B. garinii*, *B. bavariensis*, *B. burgdorferi*, *B. spielmanii*, *B. lusitaniae*, *B. bissettii* and *B. valaisiana*. *B. afzelii* is most frequently isolated from skin biopsies of patients with EM, BL and ACA, while *B. garinii* is predominantly isolated from patients suffering from LNB. *Borrelia burgdorferi* is only rarely cultivated from such specimens, and the remaining genomic species were detected only in single cases. In contrast, the infection in the US is almost exclusively caused by *B. burgdorferi*, although other new species have recently been identified in a cluster of patients in midwestern US (Pritt *et al.*, 2016).

Since borrelia does not produce its own toxins or extracellular matrix, clinical presentation of disease depends upon host immune response to the spirochetal infection (Steere *et al.*, 2016). Several studies have shown that different *Borrelia* species (and subspecies within individual species) elicit distinct host immune responses (Strle *et al.*, 2009; Strle *et al.*, 2011). Moreover, the immune responses to different *Borrelia* strains are likely further shaped by host genetics, such as single nucleotide polymorphisms in the host TLR1 gene, the major pathogen-sensing receptor for borrelia (Strle *et al.*, 2012). Knowledge of specific spirochetal virulence factors and host genetic variants, and their contribution to shaping the range of clinical manifestations and severity of disease remain to be elucidated.

7.3.1 Skin manifestations

Skin is the most frequently involved tissue in LB, and usually clinically the most distinctive, and thus provides clues for the diagnosis and treatment (Strle and Stanek, 2009). Manifestations of LB that involve skin include EM, BL and ACA. All these manifestations were well known as distinct skin disorders long before the discovery of the causative agent. It has been suggested that Lyme borreliae might also be associated with a subset of patients with scleroderma circumscripta, lichen sclerosus et atrophicus and cutaneous B-cell lymphoma.

7.3.1.1 Erythema migrans

EM is by far the most frequent manifestation of LB in Europe. In epidemiological studies in Sweden and Germany, EM represented 77% to 89% of all presentations (Berglund et al., 1995; Huppertz et al., 1999). In Slovenia, where notification of LB has been mandatory for 30 years, EM occurs in about 90% of registered cases (Kraigher et al., 2016).

EM is defined as an erythematous skin lesion that develops within days to weeks after a tick bite and infection with borrelia. The lesion develops at the site of the tick bite, typically as a red macula or papule and expands over days to weeks with or without central clearing. The advancing edge is typically distinct and often intensely colored but not markedly elevated. For a reliable diagnosis a lesion must reach ≥5 cm in diameter. A lesion <5 cm qualifies for the diagnosis of EM only if it develops at the site of a tick bite, if its onset has a time interval from a tick bite of at least 2 days and if the lesion is enlarging (Stanek et al., 2012). Multiple EM is defined as the presence of two or more skin lesions, at least one of which must fulfill the size criteria for solitary EM.

In cases with typical EM, the clinical diagnosis is made without laboratory support. In uncertain cases, detection of borrelia by culture and/or PCR from a skin biopsy may be supportive (Stanek et al., 2011). Isolation rate of Borrelia strains from EM skin lesions in Europe is ~40–65% (Ružić-Sabljić et al., 2002; Stupica et al., 2011; 2012; O'Rourke et al., 2013; Ogrinc et al., 2013) while the proportion of patients with positive skin PCR results may be even higher (Picken et al., 1997a; Zore et al., 2002; O'Rourke et al., 2013). However, borrelia culture and PCR are only available from specialized laboratories. As the most frequently observed manifestation in LB, EM can provide clues in the diagnosis of other manifestations of the disease.

According to borrelia skin culture results, EM in western, central and probably also eastern Europe is caused predominantly by B. afzelii (70–90%), less frequently by B. garinii (10–20%), rarely by B. burgdorferi, and only exceptionally by other species such as B. bissettii or B. spielmanii (Strle et al., 1997; Ornstein et al., 2001; Ružić-Sabljić et al., 2002; Foldvari et al., 2005; Maraspin et al., 2006). However, in northeastern Europe, EM is most commonly caused by B. garinii (Oksi et al., 2001; Stanek et al., 2012). Co-infection with two or more genospecies of Lyme borreliae may occur, as indicated by PCR and culture (Ciceroni et al., 2001; Ružić-Sabljić et al., 2001a; 2005; Cerar et al., 2008); however, this is typically rare.

EM may be accompanied by local symptoms such as mild itching, burning or pain in approximately half of European patients. Constitutional symptoms such as fatigue and malaise, headache, myalgia and arthralgia may occur in a smaller proportion of patients. However, fever is rare in European patients with EM and the skin lesion is generally the only abnormality found on physical examination (Asbrink et al., 1986a; Strle et al., 1996a; 1999; 2002; Stupica et al., 2011; 2012; O'Rourke et al., 2013; Ogrinc et al., 2013). European patients with EM less often report systemic symptoms than patients in the US (Strle et al., 1999; 2011; Tibbles and Edlow, 2007; Jones et al., 2008; Cerar et al., 2016).

7.3.1.2 Borrelial lymphocytoma

BL is a rare skin manifestation of European LB. It appears as a small skin induration that slowly enlarges to a solitary bluish-red nodule or plaque with a diameter up to a few centimeters. Histologically, there is an intense polyclonal lymphocytic infiltration of the cutis and subcutis with a predominance of B lymphocytes and sometimes the presence of germinal centers (Asbrink and Hovmark, 1987; 1988; Hovmark et al., 1993; Strle et al., 1992; Maraspin et al., 2016); CD20(+) B cells and high levels of the B-cell-active chemokine CXCL13 have been reported (Müllegger et al., 2007). It is more frequent in children, in whom it is typically located on the ear lobe. A long-term study revealed that BL was localized on the ear lobe in 47% of patients, on the breast in 42%, and on the nose, arm, shoulder or scrotum in 11%. Patients with BL on the earlobe were younger than those with the lesion on the breast, with a median age of 12 years versus 42 years (Strle et al., 1992). Although systemic symptoms are rare and mild in patients with earlobe BL, about 80% of patients with breast BL complain of mostly mild constitutional symptoms and localized discomfort in the region of the areola mammae. Because of the differential diagnosis, histologic examination is usually required in lymphocytoma on the breast or in other locations with the exception of the earlobe (Strle et al., 1992; Strle and Stanek, 2009; Maraspin et al., 2016). A recent or concomitant EM may facilitate the diagnosis. In a recent study of 144 patients with BL, 81 (56%) patients recalled a tick bite and 104 (72%) had a concomitant EM skin lesion. In all but a few patients, the tick bites were in close proximity to BL, and EM lesions were in the area surrounding BL. This suggested that, like EM, BL also develops at the site of inoculation of borrelia into skin (Maraspin et al., 2016). Although BL may appear before or simultaneously with EM (Maraspin et al., 2002a; 2016; Glatz et al., 2015), the median time interval from the tick bite to development of BL is 21 days. Thus, the incubation period for BL is generally somewhat longer than the ~14–17 days reported for EM in Europe (Strle et al., 1999; Stupica et al., 2012).

Approximately 50% of BL patients are positive by serology and *Borrelia* isolation from BL tissue is possible in about 33% of patients. Of the 13 isolates recovered from BL tissue, 11 were *B. afzelii*, one was *B. garinii* and one *B. bissettii* (Maraspin et al., 2016). Until now, four *Borrelia* species have been identified as causing BL: *B. afzelii* (Busch et al., 1995; Picken et al., 1997b; Ružić-Sabljić et al., 2002; Müllegger et al., 2007; Lenormand et al., 2009; Maraspin et al., 2016), *B. garinii* (Busch et al., 1995; Lenormand et al., 2009; Maraspin et al., 2016), *B. burgdorferi* (Müllegger et al., 2007; Lenormand et al., 2009; Cerar et al., 2016) and *B. bissettii* (Picken et al., 1997b; Ružić-Sabljić et al., 2002; Maraspin et al., 2016). Thus, although several *Borrelia* species can cause BL, *B. afzelii* is the causative agent of BL in the majority of patients.

7.3.1.3 Acrodermatitis chronica atrophicans

ACA is a chronic skin manifestation of European LB. It is more often diagnosed in women than in men and occurs only exceptionally in children. Patients are generally over 40 years old. The reasons for the association with older age and female predominance are unclear (Strle et al., 2013). Recently published data suggest that ACA occurs more commonly in older individuals because these patients have greater likelihood of having age-related anatomic or physiologic changes in the extremities that may predispose them to this particular skin lesion. The older age of ACA patients does not appear to be primarily related to a markedly long latency period, but the exact pathogenetic explanation is not yet known (Ogrinc et al., 2017).

ACA is defined as a long-standing red or bluish-red lesion, usually located on the extensor surfaces of the extremities. The initial lesion is typically unilateral; later, it may become bilateral and symmetrical. It starts with reddish-blue discoloration and doughy swelling of the skin (an inflammatory phase). Over months to several years the affected skin may become atrophic and skin induration and fibroid nodules may develop over bony prominences. If left untreated, peripheral neuropathy and/or arthropathy may occur, primarily in the area of impaired skin but may happen also outside ACA skin lesions (Hopf, 1966; 1975; Kristoferitsch et al., 1988; Kindstrand et al., 1997). In about 20% of patients ACA might be preceded by an earlier manifestation of LB, such as EM, or very rarely by other manifestations, however in most patients ACA is generally the first and only clinical sign of LB. Unlike EM and BL, ACA does not disappear spontaneously (Asbrink and Hovmark, 1988).

Serum IgG antibodies to Lyme borreliae are present in high concentrations in most ACA patients, presumably due to longer duration and the maturation of the immune response. Lyme borreliae may also be demonstrated in biopsies of lesional skin by culture and/or PCR. Genotyping of these isolates demonstrated that ACA is predominantly caused by *B. afzelii* (Rijpkema et al., 1997; Maraspin et al., 2002b), however in a few instances *B. garinii* and *B. burgdorferi* have also been isolated from ACA, indicating that *B. afzelii* is the predominant, but not exclusive, etiologic agent of ACA (Picken et al., 1998; Ružić-Sabljić et al., 2002). The most characteristic and constant histologic findings are lymphocytic infiltrate with plasma cells and telangiectasias. The histopathologic pattern is not diagnostic in itself, but characteristic enough to alert an experienced pathologist.

Sclerotic lesions may develop in about 10% of patients with typical ACA (Asbrink and Hovmark, 1987). Some such lesions are clinically and histologically indistinguishable from localized scleroderma (morphea) or lichen sclerosus et atrophicus, suggesting a possible relationship between these two skin conditions. Peripheral neuropathy is associated with long-standing ACA (Hopf, 1966; 1975; Kristoferitsch et al., 1988). Joints and bones may also become affected in the area of the skin lesion (Asbrink et al., 1986b; 1986c). When present on lower extremities, ACA is often misinterpreted as vascular insufficiency (Müllegger, 2004; Strle and Stanek, 2009).

7.3.1.4 Other skin manifestations of potential borrelial etiology

Isolation of Lyme borrelia from lesional skin of patients suffering from scleroderma circumscripta (morphea) and lichen sclerosus et atrophicus has been reported (Breier et al., 1999; Müllegger, 2004). These observations might indicate either that a subset of these disorders could be of borrelial origin or that these patients in fact have ACA with sclerotic lesions, clinically and histologically indistinguishable from morphea or lichen sclerosus et atrophicus (Asbrink et al., 1986c). A well designed, multicenter, prospective clinical study is needed to help elucidate this question.

7.3.1.5 Cutaneous lymphoma

Similarly, controversial observations have raised the possibility of an association between primary cutaneous B-cell lymphomas and infection with Lyme borreliae (Müllegger, 2004; Schöllkopf et al., 2008). In response to these findings, the European Organization for Research and Treatment of Cancer and the International Society for Cutaneous Lymphoma in 2008 published consensus recommendations on management of cutaneous B-cell lymphomas. In this article, treatment with antibiotics is proposed for patients with primary cutaneous marginal zone lymphoma and evidence of borrelia infection (Senff et al., 2008). It is important to note that European results differ from findings in the USA and Asia, where neither molecular nor epidemiologic studies have demonstrated an etiopathogenetic role for Lyme borreliae in cutaneous B-cell lymphoma. A multicenter scientific effort is required to obtain conclusive information regarding the possible association of Borrelia infection and cutaneous B-cell lymphoma.

7.3.2 Lyme neuroborreliosis

LNB is defined as involvement of central and/or peripheral nervous system due to infection with Lyme borreliae. Diagnosis of LNB in Europe requires the fulfillment of the European Federation of Neurological Societies (EFNS) criteria (Mygland et al., 2010). With the exception of peripheral neuropathy in patients with ACA, peripheral nervous system involvement is most often associated with involvement of the central nervous system. In Europe, LNB is caused predominantly by B. garinii, and in a small proportion of patients by B. afzelii (Busch et al., 1995; Peter et al., 1997; Ružić-Sabljić et al., 2001b; 2002; Ornstein et al., 2002; Strle et al., 2006; Ogrinc et al., 2013; 2016). Borrelia burgdorferi is rarely a cause of LNB in Europe, however, the proportion of patients infected with B. burgdorferi who develop LNB might be relatively high (Jungnick et al., 2015). Other Borrelia species such as B. valaisiana (Peter et al., 1997; Ryffel et al., 1999), B. bissettii (Strle et al., 1997; Fingerle et al., 2008) or species reported as not yet identified, were only found in single cases (Lebech et al., 1998; Ružić-Sabljić et al., 2001b; 2002; Ornstein et al., 2002).

Early European LNB typically appears during the first few weeks or months after the onset of infection and usually presents with lymphocytic meningitis and involvement of cranial and/or peripheral nerves (Kristoferitsch, 1991). The most prominent feature, considered the hallmark of European LNB, is meningoradiculitis, an entity named Bannwarth's syndrome long before the etiology of LNB was established (Bannwarth, 1941). The most pronounced clinical symptom of European LNB in adults is pain due to radiculoneuritis. The pain is usually severe with increasing intensity during the night, and is thus often associated with severe sleep disorders. Involvement of motor nerves may lead to pareses, which are usually asymmetric and not always clinically prominent. If untreated, the neurologic signs and symptoms can persist for many weeks (Kristoferitsch et al., 1987; Kristoferitsch, 1991; Hansen, 1994).

The diagnosis of borrelia meningoadiculoneuritis has been a challenge. In a recent report (Ogrinc et al., 2016) on 77 consecutive patients with borrelia meningoradiculitis (Bannwarth's syndrome), the median duration of illness before diagnosis was 30 (IQR 14−60) days and in 12 (16%) patients it was >2 months. Approximately 60% of patients had EM during the course of the disease and in about 50% the lesion was still visible at enrolment. The large diameter of EM (median 35 cm) is consistent with infection with the etiologic agent of LNB, B. garinii, which has been associated with faster spread of EM than when caused by other species of Borreliae (Strle et al., 2011; Ogrinc et al., 2013). At the time of presentation no patients were febrile; only 15 of 77 (20%) had meningeal signs, 6 (8%) had motor weakness and 28 (36%) had facial nerve palsy (bilateral in 3) and in none did the palsy precede radicular symptoms (Halperin, 2016; Ogrinc et al., 2016). One patient had complete heart block that resolved after treatment.

Patients with borrelia meningitis usually suffer from mild intermittent headache, but in some cases headache may be severe. Adult patients usually do not present with fever, nausea and vomiting, and meningeal signs are typically absent (Kristoferitsch, 1991; Hansen, 1994). The abnormal cerebrospinal fluid findings consist of a lymphocytic pleocytosis of up to several hundred million cells per liter, normal or slightly to moderately elevated protein concentration, and normal or mildly decreased glucose concentration. The course of borrelia meningitis resembles a relatively mild, but unusually protracted viral meningitis with intermittent improvement and deterioration (Stanek and Strle, 2003).

Early LNB is characterized by frequent involvement of the facial nerve although any cranial nerve may be affected. Bilateral peripheral facial palsy is uncommon but more indicative of early LNB than is unilateral involvement (Lotric-Furlan et al., 1999; Halperin, 2008; Ogrinc et al., 2016). Lymphocytic pleocytosis is often present in patients with borrelia peripheral facial palsy, even if patients do not show any sign or symptom of meningitis (Halperin, 2008). However, shortly after the onset of symptoms, cerebrospinal fluid pleocytosis may be absent (mainly in children with facial palsy), and intrathecal production of borrelial antibodies may not be detectable. In children, painful radiculoneuritis is rare, but isolated meningitis and peripheral facial palsy are more common than in adults (Stanek and Strle, 2003; Strle and Stanek, 2009). Although the outcome of borrelia facial palsy is said to be excellent (Halperin and Golightly, 1992; Halperin, 2008), some studies report a relatively high proportion of sequelae. In a Swedish study clinical and neurophysiologic examination 3–5 years after peripheral facial palsy associated with LNB showed mild sequelae in half of evaluated children (Bagger-Sjoback et al., 2005). Another study from Sweden revealed that one-fifth of children with acute facial palsy have permanent mild-to-moderate dysfunction of the facial nerve, without other neurologic symptoms or health problems (Skogman et al., 2003). Treatment of LNB did not seem to affect the clinical outcome of peripheral facial palsy (Skogman et al., 2003).

It is worth mentioning that the clinical presentation of early LNB, as described above, is associated with B. garinii, but not B. afzelii, infection. The majority of patients with suspected LNB in whom B. afzelii was isolated from CSF, did not fulfill the diagnostic criteria for LNB in Europe (Strle et al., 2006).

Late LNB appears to be very rare in Europe, as it is in the US. An exception is peripheral neuritis which is associated with long-lasting ACA that occurs in about half of these patients (Kristoferitsch et al., 1988).

7.3.3 Lyme carditis

Acute cardiac involvement, typically presenting with varying degrees of intermittent atrioventricular (A-V) heart block and sometimes with clinical evidence of myopericarditis, is rarely observed in Europe (Berglund et al., 1995). Among 77 patients treated for Bannwarth's syndrome at LB Outpatients Clinic in Ljubljana, only one had complete heart block (Ogrinc et al., 2016). European Lyme carditis appears similar to Lyme carditis in North America: it most often occurs either in the course of EM or within a few weeks after onset of infection and seems to be transient and self-limiting. The diagnosis of Lyme carditis requires objective evidence of heart involvement, demonstration of borrelia infection and exclusion of other explanations for cardiac abnormalities. Presence of other manifestations of LB, such as EM or LNB (lymphocytic pleocytosis) is helpful in making the diagnosis as the differential diagnosis in Lyme carditis is very broad (Strle and Stanek, 2009).

7.3.4 Joint involvement

Lyme arthritis is considered a rare manifestation in Europe. However, a nationwide survey in Germany, based on responses to a questionnaire, suggests that borrelia arthritis may be more frequent in Europe than once thought (Priem *et al.*, 2003). Arthritis occurs within several months of the initial borrelial infection and most often affects individuals in the fourth decade of life. It may be preceded by other manifestations such as EM, or may represent the initial manifestation of LB. The arthritis most frequently involves the large joints particularly the knee (about 50% of all cases), followed by the ankle, wrist and elbow, and rarely smaller joints (Herzer, 1991). The isolation rate of borrelia from joint fluid and synovia is very low (Markowicz *et al.*, 2015). Information on the etiology in Europe is limited. *Borrelia burgdorferi* is the principal but not the only *Borrelia* species involved in Lyme arthritis in Europe, however, other genospecies have been detected in patients' synovial specimens by PCR (Eiffert *et al.*, 1998; Vasiliu *et al.*, 1998; Jaulhac *et al.*, 2000; Marlovits *et al.*, 2004).

7.3.5 Eye involvement

Eye involvement in the course of LB appears to occur very rarely and may often be associated with other signs of the illness (Mikkila *et al.*, 2000; Strle and Stanek, 2009) such as EM, LNB (Mahne *et al.*, 2015) or Lyme arthritis, but can be the sole manifestation of the disease. The diagnosis of borrelial ocular involvement is difficult and with the absence of other manifestations of LB is more often presumed than confirmed.

7.3.6 Other potential rare manifestations of Lyme borreliosis

Lyme borreliae have been suggested as a possible cause of scleroderma circumscripta, progressive facial hemiatrophia, eosinophilic fasciitis (Shulman syndrome) (Stanek *et al.*, 1987; Granter *et al.*, 1994; Hashimoto *et al.*, 1996; Müllegger, 2004), myositis (Müller-Felber *et al.*, 1993), dermatomyositis (Waton *et al.*, 2007), nodular fasciitis (Schnarr *et al.*, 2002), panniculitis (Hassler *et al.*, 1992; Viljanen *et al.*, 1992) and osteomyelitis (Oksi *et al.*, 1994). There are also reports of effects on individual organs or organ systems such as liver, lymphatic system, respiratory tract, urinary tract and genitalia. Proof of the existence of such involvement in humans is lacking.

7.4 Laboratory Diagnosis

Laboratory testing should only be performed if there are signs and/or symptoms of disease. Specifically, there cannot be a diagnosis of LB in the absence of any clinical manifestation. The only sign that enables a reliable clinical diagnosis of LB in Europe is a typical EM. Ear lobe BL, meningo-radiculoneuritis (Bannwarth's syndrome) and ACA are also highly suggestive of the diagnosis. The clinical case definitions for diagnosis and management of LB in Europe were developed to support this approach (Stanek *et al.*, 2011). Laboratory evidence is essential in most clinical manifestations and consists predominantly of serology. Other approaches, particularly the currently available methods for direct detection of *Borrelia* are both more demanding and time consuming, and often have lower sensitivity in manifestations other than EM (Wilske *et al.*, 2000; Stanek *et al.*, 2011; 2012).

In brief, in typical EM the diagnosis is clinical; serology is not essential. Early treatment can result in a cure and the absence of a detectable specific antibody response. Serological findings are important for the reliable diagnosis of BL. For the diagnosis of early LNB, the demonstration of a CSF pleocytosis is essential. Intrathecal anti-borrelia IgG antibody production is typically demonstrable, a determination that requires simultaneously drawn blood and CSF samples. However, the absence of intrathecal specific antibody synthesis does not exclude LNB in those with short duration of symptoms.

For the diagnosis of Lyme carditis, it is essential to demonstrate specific antibodies or a significant change in the concentration of specific IgG antibody to Lyme borreliae in paired serum samples. For the diagnosis of ACA or Lyme arthritis, it is essential to demonstrate the presence of specific IgG antibodies, usually in high levels.

Assessment of the performance and utility of serodiagnostics designed for use in the US for detection of LB acquired in Europe and vice versa revealed that two-tier serologic testing with the US test kits may be unsatisfactory for detection of LB acquired in Europe. First-tier testing with an assay such as the C6 enzyme linked immunosorbent assay (ELISA) should be considered as a stand-alone diagnostic strategy in such cases (Branda et al., 2013; Stanek et al., 2014; Wormser et al., 2014).

An important observation in LB is that peripheral blood clinical laboratory parameters indicative of an infectious disease are usually absent. Almost all patients have normal or only slightly elevated C-reactive protein (CRP) values and white blood cell counts are usually normal (Strle, 1999; Steere, 2001; Strle and Stanek, 2009; Steere et al., 2016).

7.5 Treatment and Prophylaxis

Treatment with antibiotics is effective for all clinical manifestations; however, it has been most effective early in the course of the illness (Strle, 1999; Stanek and Strle, 2003; Stanek et al., 2012; Steere et al., 2016). In Europe, various antibiotics are used for treatment of LB, depending on the type of manifestations of disease. Patients with solitary EM and BL are treated with doxycycline, amoxicillin, phenoxymethylpenicillin (penicillin V), cefuroxime axetil or azithromycin. The last is used predominantly for young children allergic to ß-lactam antibiotics. The usual duration of treatment is 14 days. However, 10-day treatment with doxycycline 100 mg bid was found to be non-inferior to 15-day treatment (Stupica et al., 2012). Limited data indicate that the same antibiotics, using the same dose and duration as for EM, are also effective for treating BL (Strle et al., 1996b; Maraspin et al., 2016). Nervous system involvement and Lyme carditis are treated with intravenous ceftriaxone or penicillin G, usually for 2 weeks, or oral doxycycline. Oral doxycycline or amoxicillin, or intravenous ceftriaxone are used for the treatment of ACA and arthritis. Duration of treatment is usually 3–4 weeks for ACA and 4 weeks in the case of oral therapy for arthritis (Stanek and Strle, 2018).

In terms of prophylaxis, antibiotic treatment of a tick bite is not recommended in Europe (Stanek and Kahl, 1999; Stanek and Strle, 2003). The principle of 'watch and wait' is advocated for *I. ricinus* tick bites, because studies on the efficacy of antibiotic prophylaxis are limited (Schwameis et al., 2017), because overuse of antibiotics should be avoided, and because the efficacy of antibiotic treatment of manifestations of LB has been established (Stanek and Kahl, 1999; Stanek et al., 2012). Immunoprophylaxis of LB for humans is currently unavailable in Europe or the US.

Removal of an attached tick as soon as possible – on the same day – will largely avoid transmission of Lyme borreliae. It seems that transmission of Lyme borreliae from the tick vector to host is faster in Europe than in North America. According to the results of experimental studies with gerbils performed in Europe, *Borrelia* infection was demonstrable in up to 50%, 17 h after attachment. This study also demonstrated that the method by which ticks were removed (pulling out with forceps, or after 3 min of intensive squeezing, or after applying nail polish to ticks about 1 h before removal) did not significantly influence the risk of becoming infected with Lyme borreliae (Kahl et al., 1998).

References

Adeolu, M. and Gupta, R.S. (2014) A phylogenomic and molecular marker based proposal for the division of the genus *Borrelia* into two genera: the emended genus *Borrelia* containing only the members of the relapsing fever Borrelia, and the genus *Borreliella* gen. nov. containing the members of the Lyme disease Borrelia (*Borrelia burgdorferi* sensu lato complex). *Antonie Van Leeuwenhoek* 105, 1049–1072.

Afzelius, A. (1910) Verhandlungen der Dermatologischen Gesellschaft zu Stockholm, 28 Oct 1909. *Archives of Dermatology and Syphilis* 101, 404.
Asbrink, E. and Hovmark, A. (1985) Successful cultivation of spirochetes from skin lesions of patients with erythema chronicum migrans Afzelius and acrodermatitis chronic atrophicans. *Acta Pathologica, Microbiologica, et Immunologica Scandinavica B* 93, 161–163.
Asbrink, E. and Hovmark, A. (1987) Cutaneous manifestations in *Ixodes*-borne borrelial spirochetosis. *International Journal of Dermatology* 26, 215–223.
Asbrink, E. and Hovmark, A. (1988) Early and late cutaneous manifestations in *Ixodes*-borne borreliosis (erythema migrans borreliosis, Lyme borreliosis). *Annals of the New York Academy of Sciences* 539, 4–15.
Asbrink, E., Olsson, I. and Hovmark, A. (1986a) Erythema chronicum migrans Afzelius in Sweden. A study on 231 patients. *Zentralblatt für Bakteriologie, Mikrobiologie und Hygiene A* 263, 229–236.
Asbrink, E., Hovmark, A. and Olsson, I. (1986b) Clinical manifestations of acrodermatitis chronica atrophicans in 50 Swedish patients. *Zentralblatt für Bakteriologie, Mikrobiologie und Hygiene A* 263, 253–261.
Asbrink, E., Brehmer-Andersson, E. and Hovmark, A. (1986c) Acrodermatitis chronica atrophicans – a spirochetosis. Clinical and histopathological picture based on 32 patients. *American Journal of Dermatopathology* 8, 209–219.
Bäfverstedt, B. (1943) Über Lymphadenitis benigna cutis. *Archiv für Dermatologie und Venereologie (Stockholm)* 24, 1–202.
Bagger-Sjoback, D., Remahl, S. and Ericsson, M. (2005) Long-term outcome of facial palsy in neuroborreliosis. *Otology and Neurotology* 26, 790–795.
Bammer H. and Schenk, K. (1965) Meningo-Myelo-Radikulitis nach Zeckenbiß mit Erythem. *Dtsch Z Nervenheilkd* 187, 25–34.
Bannwarth, A. (1941) Chronische lymphozytäre Meningitis, entzündliche Polyneuritis und 'Rheumatismus'. *Archiv psychiatrischer Nervenkrankheiten* 113, 284–376.
Baranton, G., Postic, D., Saint Girons, I., Boerlin, P., Piffaretti, J.C., Assous, M. and Grimont, P.A. (1992) Delineation of *Borrelia burgdorferi* sensu stricto, *Borrelia garinii* sp. nov., and group VS461 associated with Lyme borreliosis. *International Journal of Systematic and Evolutionary Microbiology* 42, 378–383.
Barbour, A.G. (1984) Isolation and cultivation of Lyme disease spirochetes. *Yale Journal of Biology and Medicine* 57, 521–525.
Barbour, A.G., Tessier, S.L. and Todd, W.J. (1983) Lyme disease spirochetes and ixodid tick spirochetes share a common surface antigenic determinant defined by a monoclonal antibody. *Infection and Immunity* 41, 795–804.
Barbour, A.G., Adeolu, M. and Gupta, R.S. (2017) Division of the genus *Borrelia* into two genera (corresponding to Lyme disease and relapsing fever groups) reflects their genetic and phenotypic distinctiveness and will lead to a better understanding of these two groups of microbes (Margos *et al*. (2016) There is inadequate evidence to support the division of the genus *Borrelia*. *International Journal of Systematic and Evolutionary Microbiology*. DOI: 10.1099/ijsem.0.001717). *International Journal of Systematic and Evolutionary Microbiology* 67, 2058–2067.
Benach, J.L., Bosler, E.M., Hanrahan, J.P., Coleman, J.L., Habicht, G.S., Bast, T.F., Cameron, D.J., Ziegler, J.L., Barbour, A.G., Burgdorfer, W., Edelman, R. and Kaslow, R.A. (1983) Spirochetes isolated from the blood of two patients with Lyme disease. *New England Journal of Medicine* 308, 740–742.
Berglund, J., Eitrem, R., Ornstein, K., Lindberg, A., Ringer, A., Elmrud, H., Carlsson, M., Runehagen, A., Svanborg, C. and Norrby, R. (1995) An epidemiologic study of Lyme disease in southern Sweden. *New England Journal of Medicine* 333, 1319–1327.
Bianchi, G.E. (1950) Die Penicillinbehandlung der Lymphocytome. *Dermatologica* 100, 270–273.
Branda, J.A., Strle, F., Strle, K., Sikand, N., Ferraro, M.J. and Steere, A.C. (2013) Performance of United States serologic assays in the diagnosis of Lyme borreliosis acquired in Europe. *Clinical Infectious Diseases* 57, 333–340.
Breier, F.H., Aberer, E., Stanek, G., Khanakaha, G., Schlick, A. and Tappeiner, G. (1999) Isolation of *Borrelia afzelii* from circumscribed scleroderma. *British Journal of Dermatology* 140, 925–930.
Brunner, N. (1951) Zur Penicillinbehandlung bei Sklerodermie und Akrodermatitis atrophicans Herxheimer. *Hautarzt* 2, 545–547.
Buchwald, A. (1883) Ein Fall von diffuser idiopathischer Haut-Atrophie. *Archiv Fur Dermatologie Und Syphilis* 10, 553–556.

Burgdorfer, W., Barbour, A.G., Hayes, S.F., Benach, J.L., Grunwaldt, E. and Davis, J.P. (1982) Lyme disease – a tick-borne spirochetosis? *Science* 216, 1317–1319.

Busch, U., Hizo-Teufel, C., Boehmer, R., Wilske, B. and Preac-Mursic, V. (1995) Molecular characterisation of *Borrelia burgdorferi* sensu lato strains by pulsed-field gel electrophoresis. *Electrophoresis* 16, 744–747.

Casjens, S.R., Fraser-Liggett, C.M., Mongodin, E.F., Qiu, W.G., Dunn, J.J., Luft, B.J. and Schutzer, S.E. (2011) Whole genome sequence of an unusual *Borrelia burgdorferi* sensu lato isolate. *Journal of Bacteriology* 193, 1489–1490.

Cerar, T., Ružić-Sabljić, E., Glinsek, U., Zore, A. and Strle, F. (2008) Comparison of PCR methods and culture for the detection of *Borrelia* spp. in patients with erythema migrans. *Clinical Microbiology and Infection* 14, 653–658.

Cerar, T., Strle, F., Stupica, D., Ružić-Sabljić, E., McHugh, G., Steere, A.C. and Strle, K. (2016) Differences in genotype, clinical features, and inflammatory potential of *Borrelia burgdorferi* sensu stricto strains from Europe and the United States. *Emerging Infectious Diseases* 22, 818–827.

Ciceroni, L., Ciarrochi, S., Ciervo, A., Mondarini, V., Guzzo, F., Caruso, G., Murgia, R. and Cinco, M. (2001) Isolation and characterization of *Borrelia burgdorferi* sensu lato strains in an area of Italy where Lyme borreliosis is endemic. *Journal of Clinical Microbiology* 39, 2254–2260.

Eiffert, H., Karsten, A., Thomssen, R. and Christen, H.J. (1998) Characterization of *Borrelia burgdorferi* strains in Lyme arthritis. *Scandinavian Journal of Infectious Diseases* 30, 265–268.

Eliassen, K.E., Berild, D., Reiso, H., Grude, N., Christophersen, K.S., Finckenhagen, C. and Lindbæk, M. (2017) Incidence and antibiotic treatment of erythema migrans in Norway 2005–2009. *Ticks and Tick Borne Diseases* 8, 1–8.

Fingerle, V., Schulte-Spechtel, U.C., Ružić-Sabljić, E., Leonhard, S., Hofmann, H., Weber, K., Pfister, K., Strle, F. and Wilske, B. (2008) Epidemiological aspects and molecular characterization of *Borrelia burgdorferi* s.l. from southern Germany with special respect to the new species *Borrelia spielmanii* sp. nov. *International Journal of Medical Microbiology* 298, 279–290.

Foldvari, G., Farkas, R. and Lakos, A. (2005) *Borrelia spielmanii* erythema migrans, Hungary. *Emerging Infectious Diseases* 11, 1794–1795.

Fülöp, B. and Poggensee, G. (2008) Epidemiological situation of Lyme borreliosis in Germany: surveillance data from six Eastern German States, 2002 to 2006. *Parasitology Research* 103, S117–S120.

Garin, C. and Bujadoux, A. (1922) Paralysie par les tiques. *Journal De Medecine De Lyon* 71, 765–767.

Glatz, M., Resinger, A., Semmelweis, K., Ambros-Rudolph, C.M. and Müllegger, R.R. (2015) Clinical spectrum of skin manifestations of Lyme borreliosis in 204 children in Austria. *Acta Dermato Venereologica* 95, 565–571.

Götz, H. and Ludwig, E. (1951) Die Behandlung der Akrodermatitis chronica atrophicans Herxheimer mit Penicillin. *Hautarzt* 2, 6–14.

Granter, S.R., Barnhill, R.L., Hewins, M.E. and Duray, P.H. (1994) Identification of *Borrelia burgdorferi* in diffuse fasciitis with peripheral eosinophilia: borrelial fasciitis. *Journal of the American Medical Association* 272, 1283–1285.

Gray, J.S., Kahl, O., Lane, R.S. and Stanek, G. (eds) (2002) *Lyme Borreliosis: Biology, Epidemiology and Control*. CAB International, Wallingford, UK.

Halperin, J.J. (2008) Nervous system Lyme disease. *Infectious Disease Clinics of North America* 22, 261–274.

Halperin, J. (2016) Neuroborreliosis: what is it, what isn't it? *Clinical Infectious Diseases* 63, 354–555.

Halperin, J.J. and Golightly, M. (1992) Lyme borreliosis in Bell's palsy. Long Island Neuroborreliosis Collaborative Study Group. *Neurology* 42, 1268–1270.

Hansen, K. (1994) Lyme neuroborreliosis: improvements of the laboratory diagnosis and a survey of epidemiological and clinical features in Denmark 1985–1990. *Acta Neurologica Scandinavica* 89 (Suppl. 151), 7–44.

Hashimoto, Y., Takahashi, H., Matsuo, S., Hirai, K., Takemori, N., Nakao, M., Miyamoto, K. and Iizuka, H. (1996) Polymerase chain reaction of *Borrelia burgdorferi* flagellin gene in Shulman syndrome. *Dermatology* 192, 136–139.

Hassler, D., Zorn, J., Zoller, L., Neuss, M., Weyand, C., Goronzy, J., Born, I.A. and Preac-Mursic, V. (1992) Nodular panniculitis: a manifestation of Lyme borreliosis? *Hautarzt* 43, 134–138.

Hellerström, S. (1930) Erythema chronicum migrans Afzelii. *Acta Dermato Venereologica (Stockh)* 11, 315–312.

Herxheimer, K. and Hartmann, K. (1902) Über Acrodermatitis chronica atrophicans. *Archiv Fur Dermatologie Und Syphilis* 61, 57–67.

Herzer, P. (1991) Joint manifestations of Lyme borreliosis in Europe. *Scandinavian Journal of Infectious Diseases* 77, 55–63.

Hofhuis, A., Harms, M., van den Wijngaard, C., Sprong, H. and van Pelt, W. (2015) Continuing increase of tick bites and Lyme disease between 1994 and 2009. *Ticks and Tick Borne Diseases* 6, 69–74.

Hollström, E. (1951) Successful treatment of erythema migrans Afzelius. *Acta Dermato Venereologica (Stockh)* 31, 235–289.

Hopf, H.C. (1966) Acrodermatitis chronica atrophicans (Herxheimer) und Nervensystem. (Monographien aus dem Gesamtgebiet der Neurologie und Psychiatrie, vol 114) Springer, Berlin, Heidelberg, New York.

Hopf, H.C. (1975) Peripheral neuropathy in acrodermatitis chronica atrophicans (Herxheimer). *Journal of Neurology, Neurosurgery, and Psychiatry* 38, 452–458.

Hörstrup, P. and Ackermann, R. (1973) Durch Zecken übertragene Meningopolyneuritis (Garin-Bujadoux-Bannwarth). *Fortschritte der Neurologie und Psychiatrie* 41, 583–606.

Hovmark, A., Asbrink, E., Weber, K. and Kaudevitz, P. (1993) Borrelial lymphocytoma. In: Weber, K., Burgdorfer, W., Schierz, G. (eds) *Aspects of Lyme Borreliosis*. Springer, Berlin, pp. 122–130.

Hubálek, Z. (2009) Epidemiology of Lyme borreliosis. *Current Problems in Dermatology* 37, 31–50.

Huppertz, H.I., Böhme, M., Standaert, S.M., Karch, H. and Plotkin, S.A. (1999) Incidence of Lyme borreliosis in the Würzburg region of Germany. *European Journal of Clinical Microbiology and Infectious Diseases* 18, 697–703.

Jaulhac, B., Heller, R., Limbach, F.X., Hansmann, Y., Lipsker, D., Monteil, H., Sibilia, J. and Piemont, Y. (2000) Direct molecular typing of *Borrelia burgdorferi* sensu lato species in synovial samples from patients with Lyme arthritis. *Journal of Clinical Microbiology* 38, 1895–1900.

Johnson, R.C., Schmid, G.P., Hyde, F.W., Steigerwalt, A.G. and Brenner D.J. (1984) *Borrelia burgdorferi* sp. nov.: etiologic agent of Lyme disease. *International Journal of Systematic and Evolutionary Microbiology* 34, 496–497.

Jones, K.L., Muellegger, R.R., Means, T.K., Lee, M., Glickstein, L.J., Damle, N., Sikand, V.K., Luster, A.D. and Steere A.C. (2008) Higher mRNA levels of chemokines and cytokines associated with macrophage activation in erythema migrans skin lesions in patients from the United States than in patients from Austria with Lyme borreliosis. *Clinical Infectious Diseases* 46, 85–92.

Jungnick, S., Margos, G., Rieger, M., Dzaferovic, E., Bent, S.J., Overzier, E., Silaghi, C., Walder, G., Wex, F., Koloczek, J., Sing, A. and Fingerle, V. (2015) *Borrelia burgdorferi* sensu stricto and *Borrelia afzelii*: population structure and differential pathogenicity. *International Journal of Medical Microbiology* 305, 673–681.

Kahl, O., Janetzki-Mittmann, C., Gray, J.S., Jonas, R., Stein, J. and de Boer, R. (1998) Risk of infection with *Borrelia burgdorferi* sensu lato for a host in relation to the duration of nymphal *Ixodes ricinus* feeding and the method of tick removal. *Zentralblatt Bakteriol* 287, 41–52.

Kindstrand, E., Nilsson, B.Y., Hovmark, A., Pirskanen, R. and Asbrink, E. (1997) Peripheral neuropathy in acrodermatitis chronica atrophicans – effect of treatment. *Acta Neurologica Scandinavica* 106, 253–257.

Kraigher, A., Socan, M., Klavs, I., Frelih, T., Grilc, E., Grgič Vitek, M., Učakar, V. and Kolman, J. (2016) Surveillance of communicable diseases, Slovenia, 2015. National Institute of Public Health, Ljubljana, 2016. Available at: www.nijz.si/sites/www.nijz.si/files/datoteke/epidemiolosko_spremljanje_nb_v_letu_2015.pdf (in Slovenian) (accessed 14 June 2018).

Kristoferitsch, W. (1991) Neurological manifestations of Lyme borreliosis: clinical definition and differential diagnosis. *Scandinavian Journal of Infectious Diseases* 77, 64–73.

Kristoferitsch, W., Spiel, G. and Wessely, P. (1983) Zur Meningopolyneuritis (Garin-Bujadoux-Bannwarth). *Nervenarzt* 54, 640–646.

Kristoferitsch, W., Baumhackl, U., Sluga, E., Stanek, G. and Zeiler, K. (1987) High-dose penicillin therapy in meningopolyneuritis Garin-Bujadoux-Bannwarth. Clinical and cerebrospinal fluid data. *Zentralblatt für Bakteriologie, Mikrobiologie und Hygiene A* 263, 357–364.

Kristoferitsch, W., Sluga, E., Graf, M., Partsch, H., Neumann, R., Stanek, G. and Budka, H. (1988) Neuropathy associated with acrodermatitis chronica atrophicans: clinical and morphological features. *Annals of the New York Academy of Sciences* 539, 35–45.

Lebech, A.M., Hansen, K., Rutledge, B.J., Kolbert, C.P., Rys, P.N. and Pershing, D.H. (1998) Diagnostic detection and direct genotyping of *Borrelia burgdorferi* by polymerase chain reaction in cerebrospinal fluid in Lyme neuroborreliosis. *Journal of Molecular Diagnostics* 3, 131–141.

Lenormand, C., Jaulhac, B., De Martino, S., Barthel, C. and Lipsker, D. (2009) Species of *Borrelia burgdorferi* complex that cause borrelial lymphocytoma in France. *British Journal of Dermatology* 161, 174–176.

Lindgren, E. and Jaenson, T.G. (2006) *Lyme Borreliosis in Europe: Influences of Climate and Climate Change, Epidemiology, Ecology and Adaptation Measures*. World Health Organization Europe, Copenhagen, 1–34.

Lipschütz, B. (1913) Über eine seltene Erythemform (Erythema chronicum migrans). *Archives of Dermatology and Syphilis* 118, 349–356.

Lipschütz, B. (1923) Weiterer Beitrag zur Kenntnis der 'Erythema chronicum migrans'. *Archives of Dermatology and Syphilis* 143, 365–374.

Lotric-Furlan, S., Cimperman, J., Maraspin, V., Ružić-Sabljić, E., Logar, M., Jurca, T. and Strle, F. (1999) Lyme borreliosis and peripheral facial palsy. *Wiener klinische Wochenschrift* 111, 970–975.

Mahne, J., Kranjc, B.S., Strle, F., Ružić-Sabljić, E. and Arnež, M. (2015) Panuveitis caused by *Borrelia burgdorferi* sensu lato infection. *Pediatric Infectious Disease Journal* 34, 102–104.

Maraspin, V., Cimperman, J., Lotrič-Furlan, S., Ruzić-Sabljić, E., Jurca, T., Picken, R.N. and Strle, F. (2002a) Solitary borrelial lymphocytoma in adult patients. *Wiener klinische Wochenschrift* 114, 515–523.

Maraspin, V., Ružić-Sabljić, E. and Strle, F. (2002b) Isolation of *Borrelia burgdorferi* sensu lato from a fibrous nodule in a patient with acrodermatitis chronica atrophicans. *Wiener klinische Wochenschrift* 114, 533–534.

Maraspin, V., Ružić-Sabljić, E. and Strle, F. (2006) Lyme borreliosis and *Borrelia spielmanii*. *Emerging Infectious Diseases* 12, 1177.

Maraspin, V., Nahtigal Klevišar, M., Ružić-Sabljić, E., Lusa, L. and Strle, F. (2016) Borrelial lymphocytoma in adult patients. *Clinical Infectious Diseases* 63, 914–921.

Markowicz, M., Ladstatter, S., Schotta, A.M., Reiter, M., Pomberger, G. and Stanek, G. (2015) Oligoarthritis caused by *Borrelia bavariensis*, Austria, 2014. *Emerging Infectious Diseases* 21, 1052–1054.

Marlovits, S., Khanakah, G., Striessnig, G., Vécsei, V. and Stanek, G. (2004) Emergence of Lyme arthritis after autologous chondrocyte transplantation. *Arthritis Rheumatism* 50, 259–264.

Mikkila, H.O., Seppala, I.J., Viljanen, M.K., Peltomaa, M.P. and Karma, A. (2000) The expanding clinical spectrum of ocular Lyme borreliosis. *Ophthalmology* 107, 581–587.

Müllegger, R.R. (2004) Dermatological manifestations of Lyme borreliosis. *Journal of the European Academy of Dermatology and Venereology* 14, 296–309.

Müllegger, R.R., Means, T.K., Shin, J.J., Lee, M., Jones, K.L., Glickstein, L.J., Luster, A.D. and Steere, A.C. (2007) Chemokine signatures in the skin disorders of Lyme borreliosis in Europe: predominance of CXCL9 and CXCL10 in erythema migrans and acrodermatitis and CXCL13 in lymphocytoma. *Infection and Immunity* 75, 4621–4628.

Müller-Felber, W., Reimers, C.D., de Koning, J., Fischer, P., Pilz, A. and Pongratz, D.E. (1993) Myositis in Lyme borreliosis: an immunohistochemical study of seven patients. *Journal of the Neurological Sciences* 118, 207–212.

Mygland, A., Ljøstad, U., Fingerle, V., Rupprecht, T., Schmutzhard, E., Steiner, I. and European Federation of Neurological Societies (2010) EFNS guidelines on the diagnosis and management of European Lyme neuroborreliosis. *European Journal of Neurology* 17, 8–16.

Ogrinc, K., Lotrič-Furlan, S., Maraspin, V., Lusa, L., Cerar, T., Ružić-Sabljić, E. and Strle, F. (2013) Suspected early Lyme neuroborreliosis in patients with erythema migrans. *Clinical Infectious Diseases* 57, 501–509.

Ogrinc, K., Lusa, L., Lotrič-Furlan, S., Bogovič, P., Stupica, D., Cerar, T., Ružić-Sabljić, E. and Strle, F. (2016) Course and outcome of early European Lyme neuroborreliosis (Bannwarth syndrome): clinical and laboratory findings. *Clinical Infectious Diseases* 63, 346–353.

Ogrinc, K., Wormser, G.P., Visintainer, P., Maraspin, V., Lotrič-Furlan, S., Cimperman, J., Ružić-Sabljić, E., Bogovič, P., Rojko, T., Stupica, D. and Strle, F. (2017) Pathogenetic implications of the age at time of diagnosis and skin location for acrodermatitis chronica atrophicans. *Ticks and Tick Borne Diseases* 8, 266–269.

Oksi, J., Mertsola, J., Reunanen, M., Marjamaki, M. and Viljanen, M.K. (1994) Subacute multiple-site osteomyelitis caused by *Borrelia burgdorferi*. *Clinical Infectious Diseases* 19, 891–896.

Oksi, J., Marttila, H., Soini, H., Aho, H., Uksila, J. and Viljanen, M.K. (2001) Early dissemination of *Borrelia burgdorferi* without generalized symptoms in patients with erythema migrans. *APMIS* 109, 581–588.

Ornstein, K., Berglund, J., Nilsson, I., Norrby, R. and Bergstrom, S. (2001) Characterization of Lyme borreliosis isolates from patients with erythema migrans and neuroborreliosis in southern Sweden. *Journal of Clinical Microbiology* 39, 1294–1298.

Ornstein, K., Berglund, J., Bergstrom, S., Norrby, R. and Barbour, A.G. (2002) Three major Lyme *Borrelia* genospecies (*Borrelia burgdorferi* sensu stricto, *B. afzelii* and *B. garinii*) identified by PCR in cerebrospinal fluid from patients with neuroborreliosis in Sweden. *Scandinavian Journal of Infectious Diseases* 34, 341–346.

O'Rourke, M., Traweger, A., Lusa, L., Stupica, D., Maraspin, V., Barrett, P.N., Strle, F. and Livey, I. (2013) Quantitative detection of *Borrelia burgdorferi* sensu lato in erythema migrans skin lesions using internally controlled duplex real time PCR. *PLoS One* 8(5), e63968. DOI: 10.1371/journal.pone.0063968.

Peter, O., Bretz, A.G., Postic, D. and Dayer, E. (1997) Association of distinct species of *Borrelia burgdorferi* sensu lato with neuroborreliosis in Switzerland. *Clinical Microbiology and Infection* 3, 423–431.

Picken, R.N., Cheng, Y., Strle, F., Cimperman, J., Maraspin, V., Lotric-Furlan, S., Ružić-Sabljić, E., Han, D., Nelson, J.A., Picken, M.M. and Trenholme, G.M. (1996) Molecular characterization of *Borrelia burgdorferi* sensu lato from Slovenia revealing significant differences between tick and human isolates. *European Journal of Clinical Microbiology and Infectious Diseases* 15, 313–323.

Picken, M.M., Picken, R.N., Han, D., Cheng, Y., Ružić-Sabljić, E., Cimperman, J., Maraspin, V., Lotric-Furlan, S. and Strle, F. (1997a) A two year prospective study to compare culture and polymerase chain reaction amplification for the detection and diagnosis of Lyme borreliosis. *Molecular Pathology* 50, 186–193.

Picken, R.N., Strle, F., Ružić-Sabljić, E., Maraspin, V., Lotric-Furlan, S., Cimperman, J., Cheng, Y. and Picken, M.M. (1997b) Molecular subtyping of *Borrelia burgdorferi* sensu lato isolates from five patients with solitary lymphocytoma. *Journal of Investigative Dermatology* 108, 92–97.

Picken, R.N., Strle, F., Picken, M.M., Ružić-Sabljić, E., Maraspin, V., Lotrič-Furlan, S. and Cimperman, J. (1998) Identification of three species of *Borrelia burgdorferi* sensu lato (*B. burgdorferi* sensu stricto, *B. garinii*, *B. afzelii*) among isolates from acrodermatitis chronica atrophicans lesions. *Journal of Investigative Dermatology* 110, 211–214.

Preac-Mursic, V., Schierz, G., Pfister, H.W., Pfister, H.W. and Einhäupl, K. (1984) Isolation of a spirochete from cerebrospinal fluid of a patient with meningoradiculitis Bannwarth. *Munchener Medizinische Wochenschrift* 126, 275–276.

Priem, S., Munkelt, K., Franz, J.K., Schneider, U., Werner, T., Burmester, G.R. and Krause, A. (2003) Epidemiology and therapy of Lyme arthritis and other manifestations of Lyme borreliosis in Germany: results of a nationwide survey. *Zeitschrift für Rheumatologie* 62, 450–458.

Pritt, B.S., Mead, P.S., Johnson, D.K.H., Neitzel, D.F., Respicio-Kingry, L.B. et al. (2016) Identification of a novel pathogenic Borrelia species causing Lyme borreliosis with unusually high spirochaetaemia: a descriptive study. *Lancet Infectious Diseases* 16, 556–564.

Rijpkema, S.G.T., Tazelaar, D.J., Molkenboer, M.J.C.H., Noordhoek, G.T., Plantinga, G., Schouls, L. and Schellekens, J.F.P. (1997) Detection of *Borrelia afzelii*, *Borrelia burgdorferi* sensu stricto, *Borrelia garinii* and group VS116 by PCR in skin biopsies of patients with erythema migrans and acrodermatitis chronica atrophicans. *Clinical Microbiology and Infection* 3, 109–116.

Rizzoli, A., Hauffe, H.C., Carpi, G., Vourc, H.G., Neteler, M. and Rosa, R. (2011) Lyme borreliosis in Europe. *Eurosurveillance* 16, 1–8.

Ružić-Sabljić, E., Arnez, M., Lotric-Furlan, S., Maraspin, V., Cimperman, J. and Strle, F. (2001a) Genotypic and phenotypic characterisation of *Borrelia burgdorferi* sensu lato strains isolated from human blood. *Journal of Medical Microbiology* 50, 896–901.

Ružić-Sabljić, E., Lotrič-Furlan, S., Maraspin, V., Cimperman, J., Pleterski-Rigler, D. and Strle, F. (2001b) Analysis of *Borrelia burgdorferi* sensu lato isolated from cerebrospinal fluid. *APMIS* 109, 707–713.

Ružić-Sabljić, E., Maraspin, V., Lotrič-Furlan, S., Jurca, T., Logar, M., Pikelj-Pečnik, A. and Strle, F. (2002) Characterization of *Borrelia burgdorferi* sensu lato strains isolated from human material in Slovenia. *Wiener klinische Wochenschrift* 114, 544–550.

Ružić-Sabljić, E., Arnez, M., Logar, M., Maraspin, V., Lotric-Furlan, S., Cimperman, J. and Strle, F. (2005) Comparison of *Borrelia burgdorferi* sensu lato strains isolated from specimens obtained simultaneously from two different sites of infection in individual patients. *Journal of Clinical Microbiology* 43, 2194–2200.

Ryffel, K., Peter, O., Rutti, B., Suard, A. and Dayer, E. (1999) Scored antibody reactivity determined by immunoblotting shows an association between clinical manifestations and presence of *Borrelia burgdorferi* sensu stricto, *B. garinii*, *B. afzelii*, and *B. valaisiana* in humans. *Journal of Clinical Microbiology* 37, 4086–4092.

Sajanti, E., Virtanen, M., Helve, O., Kuusi, M., Lyytikäinen, O., Hytönen, J. and Sane, J. (2017) Lyme borreliosis in Finland, 1995–2014. *Emerging Infectious Diseases* 23, 1282–1288.

Sanchez, E., Vannier, E., Wormser, G.P. and Hu, L.T. (2016) Diagnosis, treatment, and prevention of Lyme disease, human granulocytic anaplasmosis, and babesiosis. A review. *JAMA* 315, 1767–1777.

Schaltenbrand, G. (1962) Radikulomyelomeninigitis nach Zeckenbiß. *Munchener Medizinische Wochenschrift* 104, 820–834.

Schnarr, S., Wahl, A., Jurgens-Saathoff, B., Mengel, M., Kreipe, H.H. and Zeidler, H. (2002) Nodular fasciitis, erythema migrans, and oligoarthritis: manifestations of Lyme borreliosis caused by *Borrelia afzelii*. *Scandinavian Journal of Rheumatology* 31, 184–186.

Schöllkopf, C., Melbye, M., Munksgaard, L., Ekström-Smedby, K., Rostgaard, K., Glimelius, B., Chang, E.T., Roos, G., Hansen, M., Adami, H.O. and Hjalgrim, H. (2008) Borrelia infection and risk of non-Hodgkin lymphoma. *Blood* 111, 5524–5529.

Schwameis, M., Kündig, T., Huber, G. *et al*. (2017) Topical azithromycin for the prevention of Lyme borreliosis: a randomised, placebo-controlled, phase 3 efficacy trial. *Lancet Infectious Diseases* 17, 322–329.

Senff, N.J., Noordijk, E.M., Youn, H. *et al*. (2008) European organization for research and treatment of cancer and international society for cutaneous Lymphoma consensus recommendations for the management of cutaneous B-cell lymphomas. *Blood* 112, 1600–1609.

Skogman, B.H., Croner, S. and Odkvist, L. (2003) Acute facial palsy in children – a 2-year follow-up study with focus on Lyme neuroborreliosis. *International Journal of Pediatric Otorhinolaryngology* 67, 597–602.

Sköldenberg, B., Stiernstedt, G., Gårde, A., Kolmodin, G., Carlström, A. and Nord, C.E. (1983) Chronic meningitis caused by a penicillin-sensitive microorganism? *Lancet* 2(8341), 75–78.

Sood, S.K. (2002) Effective retrieval of Lyme disease information on the web. *Clinical Infectious Diseases* 35, 451–464.

Stanek, G. and Kahl, O. (1999) Chemoprophylaxis for Lyme borreliosis? *Zentralblatt für Bakteriologie* 289, 655–665.

Stanek, G. and Reiter, M. (2011) The expanding Lyme Borrelia complex – clinical significance of genomic species? *Clinical Microbiology and Infection* 17, 487–493.

Stanek, G. and Strle, F. (2003) Lyme borreliosis. *Lancet* 362, 1639–1647.

Stanek, G. and Strle, F. (2018) Lyme borreliosis – from tick bite to diagnosis and treatment. *FEMS Microbiological Review*, doi.org/10.1093/femsre/fux047.

Stanek, G., Wewalka, G., Groh, V. and Neumann, R. (1985a) Isolations of spirochetes from the skin of patients with erythema chronicum migrans in Austria. *Zentralblatt für Bakteriologie, Mikrobiologie und Hygiene A* 260, 88–90.

Stanek, G., Wewalka, G., Groh, V., Neumann, R. and Kristoferitsch, W. (1985b) Differences between Lyme disease and European arthropod-borne Borrelia infections. *Lancet* 1(8425), 401.

Stanek, G., Konrad, K., Jung, M. and Ehringer, H. (1987) Shulman syndrome, a scleroderma subtype caused by *Borrelia burgdorferi*? *Lancet* 1(8548), 1490.

Stanek, G., Fingerle, V., Hunfeld, K.P., Jaulhac, B., Kaiser, R., Krause, A., Kristoferitsch, W., O'Connell, S., Ornstein, K., Strle, F. and Gray, J. (2011) Lyme borreliosis: clinical case definitions for diagnosis and management in Europe. *Clinical Microbiology and Infection* 2011, 69–79.

Stanek, G., Wormser, G.P., Gray, J. and Strle, F. (2012) Lyme borreliosis. *Lancet* 379, 461–473.

Stanek, G., Lusa, L., Ogrinc, K., Markowicz, M. and Strle, F. (2014) Intrathecally produced IgG and IgM antibodies to recombinant VlsE, VlsE peptide, recombinant OspC and whole cell extracts in the diagnosis of Lyme neuroborreliosis. *Medical Microbiology and Immunology* 203, 125–132.

Steere, A.C. (2001) Lyme disease. *New England Journal of Medicine* 345, 115–125.

Steere, A.C., Malawista, S.E., Snydman, D.R., Shope, R.E., Andiman, W.A., Ross, M.R. and Steele, F.M. (1977) Lyme arthritis. An epidemic of oligoarticular arthritis in children and adults in three Connecticut communities. *Arthritis and Rheumatology* 20, 7–17.

Steere, A.C., Grodzicki, R.L., Kornblatt, A.N., Craft, J.E., Barbour, A.G., Burgdorfer, W., Schmid, G.P., Johnson, E. and Malawista, S.E. (1983) The spirochetal etiology of Lyme disease. *New England Journal of Medicine* 308, 733–740.

Steere, A.C., Strle, F., Wormser, G.P., Hu, L.T., Branda, J.A., Hovius, J.W., Li, X. and Mead, P.S. (2016) Lyme borreliosis. *Nature Reviews Disease Primers* 2, 16090. DOI: 10.1038/nrdp.2016.90.

Strle, F. (1999) Principles of the diagnosis and antibiotic treatment of Lyme borreliosis. *Wiener klinische Wochenschrift* 111, 911–915.

Strle, F. and Stanek, G. (2009) Clinical manifestations and diagnosis of Lyme borreliosis. *Current Problems in Dermatology* 37, 51–110.

Strle, F., Pleterski-Rigler, D., Stanek, G., Pejovnik-Pustinek, A., Ruzic, E. and Cimperman, J. (1992) Solitary borrelial lymphocytoma: report of 36 cases. *Infection* 20, 201–206.

Strle, F., Nelson, J.A., Ružić-Sabljić, E., Cimperman, J., Maraspin, V., Lotrič-Furlan, S., Cheng, Y., Picken, M.M., Trenholme, G. and Picken, R.N. (1996a) European Lyme borreliosis: 231 culture-confirmed cases involving patients with erythema migrans. *Clinical Infectious Diseases* 23, 61–65.

Strle, F., Maraspin, V., Pleterski-Rigler, D., Lotric-Furlan, S., Ružić-Sabljić, E., Jurca, T. and Cimperman, J. (1996b) Treatment of borrelial lymphocytoma. *Infection* 24, 80–84.

Strle, F., Picken, R.N., Cheng, Y., Cimperman, J., Maraspin, V., Lotric-Furlan, S., Ružić-Sabljić, E. and Picken, M.M. (1997) Clinical findings for patients with Lyme borreliosis caused by *Borrelia burgdorferi* sensu lato with genotypic and phenotypic similarities to strain 25015. *Clinical Infectious Diseases* 25, 273–280.

Strle, F., Nadelman, R.B., Cimperman, J., Nowakowski, J., Picken, R.N., Schwartz, I., Maraspin, V., Aguero-Rosenfeld, M.E., Varde, S., Lotric-Furlan, S. and Wormser, G.P. (1999) Comparison of culture-confirmed erythema migrans caused by *Borrelia burgdorferi* sensu stricto in New York State and *Borrelia afzelii* in Slovenia. *Annals of Internal Medicine* 130, 32–36.

Strle, F., Videcnik, J., Zorman, P., Cimperman, J., Lotric-Furlan, S. and Maraspin, V. (2002) Clinical and epidemiological findings for patients with erythema migrans. Comparison of cohorts from the years 1993 and 2000. *Wiener klinische Wochenschrift* 114, 493–497.

Strle, F., Ružić-Sabljić, E., Cimperman, J., Lotrič-Furlan, S. and Maraspin, V. (2006) Comparison of findings for patients with *Borrelia garinii* and *Borrelia afzelii* isolated from cerebrospinal fluid. *Clinical Infectious Diseases* 43, 704–710.

Strle, F., Ružić-Sabljić, E., Logar, M., Maraspin, V., Lotrič-Furlan, S., Cimperman, J., Ogrinc, K., Stupica, D., Nadelman, R.B., Nowakowski, J. and Wormser, G.P. (2011) Comparison of erythema migrans caused by *Borrelia burgdorferi* and *Borrelia garinii*. *Vector-Borne and Zoonotic Diseases* 11, 1252–1258.

Strle, F., Wormser, G.P., Mead, P. et al. (2013) Gender disparity between cutaneous and non-cutaneous manifestations of Lyme borreliosis. *PLoS ONE*. DOI: 10.1371/journal.pone.0064110.

Strle, K., Drouin, E.E., Shen, S., El Khoury, J., McHugh, G., Ružić-Sabljic, E., Strle, F. and Steere, A.C. (2009) Borrelia burgdorferi stimulates macrophages to secrete higher levels of cytokines and chemokines than Borrelia afzelii or Borrelia garinii. *Journal of Infectious Diseases* 200, 1936–1943.

Strle, K., Jones, K.L., Drouin, E.E., Li, X. and Steere, A.C. (2011) *Borrelia burgdorferi* RST1 (OspC type A) genotype is associated with greater inflammation and more severe Lyme disease. *American Journal of Pathology* 178, 2726–2739.

Strle, K., Shin, J.J., Glickstein, L.J. and Steere, A.C. (2012) Association of a Toll-like receptor 1 polymorphism with heightened Th1 inflammatory responses and antibiotic-refractory Lyme arthritis. *Arthritis and Rheumatism* 64, 1497–1507.

Strnad, M., Hönig, V., Růžek, D., Grubhoffer, L. and Rego, R.O.M. (2017) Europe-wide meta-analysis of *Borrelia burgdorferi* sensu lato prevalence in questing *Ixodes ricinus* ticks. *Applied and Environmental Microbiology* 83(15). pii: e00609–17. DOI: 10.1128/AEM.00609-17.

Stupica, D., Lusa, L., Cerar, T., Ružić-Sabljić, E. and Strle F. (2011) Comparison of post-Lyme borreliosis symptoms in erythema migrans patients with positive and negative *Borrelia burgdorferi* sensu lato skin culture. *Vector-Borne and Zoonotic Diseases* 11, 883–889.

Stupica, D., Lusa, L., Ružić-Sabljić, E., Cerar, T. and Strle, F. (2012) Treatment of erythema migrans with doxycycline for 10 days versus 15 days. *Clinical Infectious Diseases* 55, 343–350.

Sykes, R.A. and Makiello, P. (2017) An estimate of Lyme borreliosis incidence in western Europe. *Journal of Public Health – Oxford Academic* 39(1), 74–81. DOI: 10.1093/pubmed/fdw017.

Thyresson, N. (1949) The penicillin treatment of acrodermatitis chronica atrophicans (Herxheimer). *Acta Dermato-Venereologica (Stockholm)* 29, 572–621.

Tibbles, C.D. and Edlow, J.A. (2007) Does this patient have erythema migrans? *JAMA* 297, 2617–2627.

van den Wijngaard, C.C., Hofhuis, A., Simões, M., Rood, E., van Pelt, W., Zeller, H. and van Bortel, W. (2017) Surveillance perspective on Lyme borreliosis across the European Union and European Economic Area. *Eurosurveillance* 22(27), pii: 30569. DOI: 10.2807/1560-7917.ES.2017.22.27.30569.

Vandenesch, A., Turbelin, C., Couturier, E. et al. (2014) Incidence and hospitalisation rates of Lyme borreliosis, France, 2004 to 2012. *Eurosurveillance* 19(20883). Available at: http://dx.doi.org/10.2807/1560-7917.ES2014.19.34.20883 (accessed 5 July 2017).

Vasiliu, V., Herzer, P., Rossler, D., Lehnert, G. and Wilske, B. (1998) Heterogeneity of *Borrelia burgdorferi* sensu lato demonstrated by an ospA-type-specific PCR in synovial fluid from patients with Lyme arthritis. *Medical Microbiology and Immunology* 187, 97–102.

Viljanen, M.K., Oksi, J., Salomaa, P., Skurnik, M., Peltonen, R. and Kalimo, H. (1992) Cultivation of *Borrelia burgdorferi* from the blood and a subcutaneous lesion of a patient with relapsing febrile nodular nonsuppurative panniculitis. *Journal of Infectious Diseases* 165, 596–597.

Waton, J., Pinault, A.L., Pouaha, J. and Truchetet, F. (2007) [Lyme disease could mimic dermatomyositis]. *La Revue de Medecine Interne* 28, 343–345.

Weber, K. (1974) Erythema chronicum migrans meningitis – eine bakterielle Infektionskrankheit? *Munchener Medizinische Wochenschrift* 116, 1993–1998.

Wei-Gang, Q. and Martin, C.L. (2014) Evolutionary genomics of *Borrelia burgdorferi* sensu lato: findings, hypotheses, and the rise of hybrids. *Infection, Genetics and Evolution* 27, 576–593.

Wilking, H. and Stark, K. (2014) Trends in surveillance data of human Lyme borreliosis from six federal states in eastern Germany, 2009–2012. *Ticks and Tick-borne Diseases* 5, 219–224.

Wilske, B., Preac-Mursic, V. and Schierz, G. (1985) Antigenic heterogeneity of European *Borrelia burgdorferi* strains isolated from patients and ticks. *Lancet* 1(8437), 1099.

Wilske, B., Preac-Mursic, V., Göbel, U.B., Graf, B., Jauris, S., Soutschek, E., Schwab, E. and Zumstein, G. (1993) An OspA serotyping system for *Borrelia burgdorferi* based on reactivity with monoclonal antibodies and OspA sequence analysis. *Journal of Clinical Microbiology* 31, 340–350.

Wilske, B., Zöller, L., Brade, V., Eiffert, H., Göbel, U.B. and Stanek, G. (2000) *Quality Standards for the Microbiological Diagnosis of Infectious Diseases, MIQ 12/2000 Lyme Borreliosis*. Urban & Fischer Verlag, Munich, Jena, p. 59.

Wormser, G.P. and Wormser, V. (2016) Did Garin and Bujadoux actually report a case of Lyme radiculoneuritis? *Open Forum Infectious Diseases* 3. DOI: 10.1093/ofid/ofw085.

Wormser, G.P., Dattwyler, R.J., Shapiro, E.D. *et al.* (2006) The clinical assessment, treatment, and prevention of Lyme disease, human granulocytic anaplasmosis, and babesiosis: clinical practice guidelines by the Infectious Diseases Society of America. *Clinical Infectious Diseases* 43, 1089–1134.

Wormser, G.P., Tang, A.T., Schimmoeller, N.R., Bittker, S., Cooper, D., Visintainer, P., Aguero-Rosenfeld, M.E., Ogrinc, K., Strle, F. and Stanek G. (2014) Utility of serodiagnostics designed for use in the United States for detection of Lyme borreliosis acquired in Europe and vice versa. *Medical Microbiology and Immunology* 203, 65–71.

Zore, A., Ružić-Sabljić, E., Maraspin, V., Cimperman, J., Lotric-Furlan, S., Pikelj, A., Jurca, T., Logar, M. and Strle, F. (2002) Sensitivity of culture and polymerase chain reaction for the etiologic diagnosis of erythema migrans. *Wiener klinische Wochenschrift* 114, 606–609.

8 Lyme Neuroborreliosis: A European Perspective

Rick Dersch
Department of Neurology, Medical Center – University of Freiburg, Freiburg, Germany

8.1 Introduction

Lyme disease is a tick-borne infectious disease caused by the spirochete bacterium *Borrelia burgdorferi* sensu lato. Its main vectors in Europe are hard-bodied ticks of the species *Ixodes ricinus*. In North America the main vectors are ticks of the species *Ixodes scapularis* and *Ixodes pacificus*.

Lyme disease can be caused by several genospecies of *Borrelia burgdorferi* sensu lato (Bbsl). Genospecies with human pathogenic potential that are prevalent in Europe are *B. afzelii*, *B. garinii*, *B. burgdorferi* sensu stricto (Bbss), *B. bavariensis* and *B. spielmanii* (Nadelman and Wormser, 1998). In North America Bbss is the principle genospecies of Bbsl with human pathogenic potential (Nadelman and Wormser, 1998; Clark *et al.*, 2014), several cases with a novel pathogen, *B. mayonii*, have been described recently (Pritt *et al.*, 2016).

All these genospecies can cause Lyme disease. However, there are differences in specific disease manifestations, as some genospecies cause certain organ manifestations more frequently than others, referred to as organotropism. Erythema migrans, the most common manifestation of Lyme disease, can be caused by all five species with human pathogenic potential.

In Europe, *B. garinii* and *B. bavariensis* are most likely to cause neurological manifestations of Lyme disease in infected patients (Ornstein *et al.*, 2001; Stanek and Strle, 2003). To a lesser degree, these can also be seen in patients infected with *B. afzelii* and Bbss (Ornstein *et al.*, 2001; Stanek and Strle, 2003). North American patients infected with Bbss develop similar neurologic involvement (Koedel *et al.*, 2015).

Bbss, the most important borrelial genospecies in North America, is closely associated with Lyme arthritis (Stanek and Strle, 2003). *Borrelia afzelii* seems to be associated with acrodermatitis chronica atrophicans, a late dermatologic manifestation of Lyme disease (van Dam *et al.*, 1993; Wienecke *et al.*, 1994). To date *B. spielmanii* has only been found in patients with erythema migrans (Fingerle *et al.*, 2008).

The incidence of Lyme disease in Europe shows regional differences. Reported incidences of Lyme disease are shown in Table 8.1.

Diverging methods in assessing incidence in different countries may partly account for differences in reported incidences. Reporting of cases of Lyme disease or at least some manifestations of Lyme disease is mandatory in some European countries, while in other countries (e.g. Germany) no reporting system exists and prevalence rates are derived from epidemiological enquiries. Overall 3–12% of all patients with Lyme disease in both Europe and the USA have neurological manifestations (Bacon *et al.*, 2008).

Manifestations of Lyme neuroborreliosis are categorized as early and late, depending on the respective incubation period. Early manifestations are polyradiculoneuritis (Bannwarth's

Table 8.1. Incidence of Lyme disease in different European countries.

	Lyme disease (all manifestations)	Lyme neuroborreliosis
Germany (Huppertz et al., 1999; Robert Koch Institut, 2015)	49–111/100,000	1/100,000
Netherlands (Hofhuis et al., 2015)	132/100,000 (erythema migrans)	2.2/100,000
Norway (Eliassen et al., 2017a)	148/100,000 (erythema migrans) 5.5/100,000 (disseminated Lyme disease)	
Slovenia (Strle, 1999)	155/100,000	n.a.

syndrome) and meningitis. Bannwarth's syndrome consists of a painful polyradiculoneuritis, typically with nocturnal worsening, followed by paresthesias and motor disturbances in the same dermatomes. Fifty percent of these patients also show a cranial nerve disorder, in >90% a facial nerve paresis (Pfister et al., 1987). Bilateral facial nerve paresis is common in Lyme neuroborreliosis (Pfister et al., 1987). Isolated cranial nerve disorders can be the only symptom of Lyme neuroborreliosis. The neurological symptoms are in most cases located at the site where the initial tick bite or the initial erythema migrans was located, but can also be located in different anatomic regions (Ogrinc et al., 2016). Severity of symptoms is not dependent on whether the site of neurological symptoms and the site of an erythema migrans match (Ogrinc et al., 2016). Bannwarth's syndrome is the second most common manifestation of Lyme disease in Germany after erythema migrans (Huppertz et al., 1999).

Meningitis is another early manifestation of Lyme neuroborreliosis. Meningitis due to *B. burgdorferi* is more often seen in children than in adults (Pfister et al., 1987). Symptoms are headache, nausea and a stiff neck. Symptoms are usually less severe compared to a bacterial meningitis caused by other pathogens (e.g. meningitis due to *Neisseria meningitidis* or *Streptococcus pneumoniae*).

More than 90% of patients with Lyme neuroborreliosis have early manifestations like polyradiculoneuritis or meningitis. Late manifestations involve the central nervous system, usually an encephalomyelitis. This condition is rarely seen. Patients show symptoms of spastic gait disturbance, pareses, micturition disorder and rarely cortical symptoms like aphasia, apraxia or epileptic seizures. Peripheral polyneuropathy caused by *B. burgdorferi* is a manifestation that is, in Europe, only described in combination with acrodermatitis chronica atrophicans, a late dermatologic manifestation of Lyme disease (Hopf, 1975; Halperin, 2017).

Another neurological manifestation of Lyme disease that is very rarely seen but can have devastating consequences for affected patients is *Borrelia*-associated cerebral vasculitis, which can lead to cerebral ischemia. Patients show symptoms according to the cerebral territories of the affected vessels. Vasculitic changes can be detected by digital subtraction angiography, magnetic resonance angiography or transcranial Doppler ultrasound. The posterior circulation is more often affected than the anterior circulation (Back et al., 2013). These patients show signs of inflammation in cerebrospinal fluid analysis that are typical for Lyme neuroborreliosis (pleocytosis, signs of blood–brain barrier disruption, intrathecal synthesis of immunoglobulins). As these patients with *Borrelia*-associated cerebral vasculitis develop cerebral ischemia with persistent tissue damage to the central nervous system, they often suffer from residual symptoms despite treatment.

8.2 Principles of Evidence-based Medicine

Evidence-based medicine describes an approach to making decisions in the care of individual patients by using the best evidence currently available (Sackett et al., 1996). By applying this approach, clinicians can ensure that decisions in the care of individual patients rely on the currently available knowledge. To retrieve all available evidence regarding a specific topic, systematic literature searches are needed. If applicable, the available evidence can be synthesized by statistical methods, usually meta-analysis, to provide combined estimates to evaluate the effects of different treatments or accuracy of diagnostic tools. Such comprehensive literature searches with an assessment of the available evidence are performed in systematic reviews.

Methodological flaws in clinical studies can influence reported outcomes, leading to low confidence in the results. Therefore, the literature retrieved from a systematic search has to be assessed for methodological quality to evaluate the retrieved estimates (Higgins and Green, 2011).

The Cochrane Collaboration has developed an excellent formal methodology for performing systematic reviews. Different statistical methods have to be applied when different aspects (interventions or diagnostic tools) are studied (Higgins and Green, 2011). Systematic reviews should be performed in a transparent way, so that users can understand how recommendations for clinical practice are derived from the available literature, how relevant literature was searched, how it was evaluated and how it was synthesized. Transparency regarding search strategies and assessment of the available evidence is particularly crucial when addressing questions where high quality evidence is scarce.

Different sources of evidence may be appropriate to address different clinical questions. Questions about efficacy and safety of certain treatments can best be answered by randomized controlled trials (RCTs). When addressing questions about treatment in clinical trials, baseline differences in patient groups receiving different kinds of treatment can lead to confounding and may influence apparent treatment effects.

In RCTs, risk of such confounding is minimized for both known and unknown influencing factors by applying a random allocation of treatments.

Other study designs may be better suited for questions regarding accuracy of diagnostic tools (Sackett et al., 1996). Case control studies are commonly used to assess diagnostic tools comparing a group of patients with a certain medical condition to a group of healthy controls or to patients with other medical conditions. However, such designs tend to overestimate sensitivity and specificity of a diagnostic tool, usually because of spectrum bias. This design typically investigates an artificial situation not reflective of clinical practice. Study designs better suited to assess diagnostic test accuracy are prospective cross-sectional studies. In these, a series of representative patients, equally suspected of having a specific medical condition (e.g. presenting with certain specific symptoms) undergo both the diagnostic test that is to be assessed (the 'index text') and another test, regarded as a reference for this condition (Knottnerus and Muris, 2003). Such a design better resembles clinical practice and the retrieved estimates for sensitivity and specificity can better be translated in clinical practice.

For questions of prognosis and course of a specific disease, follow-up studies of patients with a well-established diagnosis, assessed at a uniform, early time point, using well defined outcome parameters are best suited (Sackett et al., 1996).

8.3 Diagnosis of Lyme Neuroborreliosis – European Federation of Neurological Societies Criteria

To provide guidance on how diagnosis of Lyme neuroborreliosis can be established in a particular patient, an expert committee of the European Federation of Neurological Societies (EFNS) developed case definitions (Mygland et al., 2010). These case definitions help to evaluate the likelihood of a diagnosis of Lyme neuroborreliosis based on the clinical and diagnostic findings in a particular patient (Table 8.2). As seroprevalence of anti-*Borrelia* antibodies is high in the general population, a positive serology in patients with neurological symptoms has a very low positive predictive value and is not sufficient to state the diagnosis of Lyme neuroborreliosis. Whenever possible, cerebrospinal fluid analysis should be performed when Lyme neuroborreliosis is suspected. Cerebrospinal fluid analysis is crucial for the diagnosis and investigation of an acute or ongoing infection of the central nervous system.

The EFNS provides diagnostic criteria for possible and definite Lyme neuroborreliosis. The detection of intrathecal synthesis of anti-*Borrelia* antibodies is considered necessary for the diagnosis. For the diagnosis of definite Lyme neuroborreliosis, three criteria have to be fulfilled: a clinical syndrome suggestive of Lyme neuroborreliosis without other obvious reasons; cerebrospinal

Table 8.2. Case definitions of Lyme neuroborreliosis according to the available diagnostic results. (From Kaiser, 1998; Rauer, 2012.)

Possible Lyme neuroborreliosis	Probable Lyme neuroborreliosis	Definite Lyme neuroborreliosis
Compatible neurological symptoms + Antibodies against Bb in serum	Compatible neurological symptoms + CSF pleocytosis + Intrathecal IgG-synthesis + Antibodies against Bb in serum	Compatible neurological symptoms + CSF pleocytosis + Intrathecal IgG-synthesis + Positive anti-*Borrelia* antibody specificity index (AI) + Antibodies against Bb in serum

B.b., *Borrelia burgdorferi* sensu lato.

fluid pleocytosis; and intrathecal synthesis of anti-*Borrelia* antibodies with a positive antibody index (AI). For the diagnosis of possible Lyme neuroborreliosis, only two of the mentioned criteria have to be fulfilled, with the expectation that if no intrathecal anti-*Borrelia* antibodies are detected, at least serum anti-*Borrelia* antibodies will be evident in patients with symptom duration of 6 weeks or more. These criteria apply to all neurological manifestations of Lyme neuroborreliosis except for polyneuropathy associated with acrodermatitis chronica atrophicans (ACA), where the following criteria should be applied for a definite diagnosis: peripheral neuropathy; dermatological evidence of ACA; and positive anti-*Borrelia* antibodies in serum.

Clinical syndromes suggestive of Lyme neuroborreliosis are meningoradiculitis (Bannwarth's syndrome), cranial nerve palsies, meningitis, encephalomyelitis and cerebral vasculitis.

However, as the sensitivity of the AI may be low, and positive anti-*Borrelia* antibodies in serum are not incorporated in the case definitions, some European authors have proposed more detailed case definitions (Kaiser, 1998).

These case definitions are used in the current German guidelines for diagnosis and treatment of Lyme neuroborreliosis (Rauer, 2012, 2018). 'Definite Lyme neuroborreliosis', the case definition with the highest likelihood of a diagnosis of Lyme neuroborreliosis, requires a compatible clinical syndrome (polyradiculoneuritis, meningitis, cranial nerve disorders or encephalomyelitis), a cerebrospinal fluid pleocytosis, evidence of intrathecal IgG-synthesis and evidence for intrathecal synthesis of specific anti-*Borrelia* antibodies in cerebrospinal fluid. To evaluate intrathecal synthesis of specific anti-*Borrelia* antibodies in cerebrospinal fluid, the AI is calculated.

AI values >2 are regarded as indicative of intrathecal synthesis of specific antibodies.

Cerebrospinal fluid culture and polymerase chain reaction (PCR) for *Borrelia* DNA only have limited sensitivity (10–30%), so these methods are of minor value in clinical practice (Wilske *et al.*, 2007).

8.4 Cerebrospinal Fluid Analysis in Lyme Neuroborreliosis

As stated before, a cerebrospinal fluid analysis should be performed when Lyme neuroborreliosis is suspected in a patient. Cerebrospinal fluid analysis is crucial for the diagnosis and investigation of an acute or ongoing infection of the central nervous system. Typical findings from cerebrospinal fluid analysis from patients with Lyme neuroborreliosis are pleocytosis (elevation of white blood cells in cerebrospinal fluid), elevated protein concentration, disruption of the blood–brain barrier, intrathecal synthesis of immunoglobulins and intrathecal synthesis of anti-*Borrelia* antibodies.

Intrathecal synthesis of immunoglobulins is frequently detected in cerebrospinal fluid of patients with Lyme neuroborreliosis. Intrathecal synthesis of IgM-antibodies predominates in cerebrospinal fluid of patients with early manifestations, while intrathecal synthesis of IgG antibodies can be found to a lesser degree. A profound intrathecal synthesis of IgG and IgA antibodies in cerebrospinal fluid is typical for late manifestations of Lyme neuroborreliosis (Kaiser, 1994; Djukic *et al.*, 2012). Pleocytosis (elevated white blood cell count in cerebrospinal fluid) is a marker of disease activity of Lyme neuroborreliosis.

Without evidence of a pleocytosis in cerebrospinal fluid analysis, a diagnosis of Lyme neuroborreliosis remains doubtful (except for the rarely seen peripheral neuropathy associated with acrodermatitis atrophicans mentioned earlier, where cerebrospinal fluid analysis may be unremarkable). Cerebrospinal fluid from patients with Lyme neuroborreliosis usually shows a lymphocytic pleocytosis with cell counts between the range of 10–1000/mm^3, with 60% of the patients showing cell counts between 30 and 300 cells/mm^3 (Djukic et al., 2012). Typically activated lymphocytes and plasma cells can be observed in cytologic specimens from cerebrospinal fluid in Lyme neuroborreliosis. After antibiotic treatment, pleocytosis declines slowly over the course of weeks (Hansen and Lebech, 1992).

Assessing the AI, determining ongoing intrathecal synthesis of anti-*Borrelia* antibodies (Reiber and Lange, 1991), is essential in proving central nervous system infection, as this indicates autochthonous active production of anti-*Borrelia* antibodies in the central nervous system, in response to ongoing infection within the central nervous system.

The AI is estimated by calculating the ratio between the cerebrospinal fluid/serum quotients for specific antibodies (Qspec, in this case anti-*Borrelia* antibodies) and total IgG (QIgG). However, a positive AI may persist after treatment of Lyme neuroborreliosis. The AI may even rise alongside the reconstitution of the blood–brain barrier. An elevated AI value (>2) is therefore no sign of an ongoing infection without concurrent cerebrospinal fluid pleocytosis.

A recently discussed marker for Lyme neuroborreliosis is the cytokine CXCL13. The cytokine CXCL13 is produced by antigen-presenting cells in cerebrospinal fluid and promotes migration of lymphocytes into the cerebrospinal fluid compartment. In patients with Lyme neuroborreliosis, concentrations of CXCL13 are highly elevated compared to other neuroinfectious or neuroimmunological diseases. After antibiotic treatment, concentrations of CXCL13 in cerebrospinal fluid decline during the first 2 weeks alongside cerebrospinal fluid pleocytosis, providing a possible marker of disease activity (Senel et al., 2010).

A recent study on diagnostic accuracy investigated CXCL13 in patients where Lyme neuroborreliosis was considered in the differential diagnosis. Diagnosis of Lyme neuroborreliosis was then examined according to the previously stated case definitions with serological testing and cerebrospinal fluid analysis. Concentrations of CXCL13 were compared to the definite diagnoses of these patients. Overall 18 patients with definite Lyme neuroborreliosis were compared to 161 patients with a variety of other diseases. A cut-off of 250 pg/ml in cerebrospinal fluid was applied diagnosing Lyme neuroborreliosis. CXCL13 showed a sensitivity of 100%, a specificity of 99%, a positive predictive value of 88% and a remarkably high negative predictive value of 100% (Rupprecht et al., 2014). The control group in this study consisted of relevant differential diagnoses (like facial palsy) as well as syndromes that are often confused with Lyme neuroborreliosis like so-called post-treatment Lyme disease syndrome or chronic fatigue syndrome.

However, the cut-off for diagnosing Lyme neuroborreliosis varies in the available literature and across individual laboratories due to different assays and different validation cohorts (Schmidt et al., 2011; Rupprecht et al., 2014). Several other studies investigating the diagnostic accuracy of CXCL13 in patients with Lyme disease compared to patients with other neuroinfectious or neuroimmunological diseases show similar results with sensitivity of 96.4–100% and a specificity of 93.3–99.7%, albeit using different cut-off values (Senel et al., 2010; Schmidt et al., 2011; Hytönen et al., 2014).

However, other diseases with subacute course, like neurosyphilis show similar CXCL13 concentrations as in Lyme neuroborreliosis (Dersch et al., 2015b).

The mentioned studies show very promising results regarding the diagnostic test accuracy of CXCL13. However, as these studies suffer from a limited sample size, these results should be investigated in a larger prospective trial investigating course of disease and the performance of CXCL13 in late manifestations of Lyme neuroborreliosis as well.

Up to now, CXCL13 is not part of official case definitions for diagnosing Lyme neuroborreliosis. With its remarkably high negative predictive value, CXCL13 seems very useful in ruling out suspected Lyme neuroborreliosis or in calming patients who fear having Lyme neuroborreliosis and are suspicious of serological testing.

8.5 Evidence-based Approach to the Diagnosis of Lyme Neuroborreliosis

8.5.1 Diagnostic test accuracy of serologic tests in Lyme disease

Seroprevalence for *Borrelia* antibodies is high in Europe. Large differences exist among different regions and among populations with different tick exposure. In Germany, seroprevalence among males is about 13%, in females about 6% and rises with age (Wilking *et al.*, 2015). In groups with high tick exposure (e.g. occupational or leisure activities), seroprevalence can be as high as 34% (Oehme *et al.*, 2002). A positive anti-*Borrelia* serology alone, without compatible neurological symptoms, is therefore in no way sufficient to state a diagnosis of Lyme disease or the necessity to start antibiotic treatment. As positive anti-*Borrelia* serology nonetheless remains an important component for the diagnosis of Lyme neuroborreliosis, knowing about its diagnostic accuracy is important when faced with treatment decisions.

Leeflang *et al.* conducted an elaborate systematic review to assess the diagnostic test accuracy of serologic tests for Lyme disease in Europe. Overall, 75 studies evaluating serologic tests for Lyme disease could be assessed (Leeflang *et al.*, 2016). To assess diagnostic test accuracy, a test being assessed (the 'index test') must be compared to another, preferably with sensitivity and specificity close to 100% (the 'reference test' or 'gold standard'). As no diagnostic method exists to state a diagnosis of Lyme disease with 100% accuracy, these studies lack a valid reference test. In most studies, the results from serologic testing were compared with a 'clinical diagnosis' provided by the physicians involved as a reference standard. While this may reflect the clinical reality, from a methodological point of view this lack of a clearly defined reference standard introduces an unquantifiable amount of bias to these results. However, as the validity of serologic testing is much criticized, especially by patient advocacy groups, it remains very helpful to assess the available literature on serologic testing in Lyme disease.

In early manifestations of Lyme disease, for example, erythema migrans, sensitivity is low (54% for enzyme linked immunosorbent assay (ELISA), 58% for immunoblot), while specificity is rather high (93% for ELISA, 86% for immunoblot). As an erythema migrans represents an indication for antibiotic treatment in itself, this rather low sensitivity in this specific setting does not decrease the value of serologic testing in other settings.

Regarding Lyme neuroborreliosis, several different scenarios have been investigated. Again, as no reference standard exists for the diagnosis of Lyme neuroborreliosis, the diagnostic test accuracy of serologic testing was compared to a 'clinical diagnosis' provided by the physicians involved in the primary studies. For serologic testing for Lyme neuroborreliosis in serum only, sensitivity and specificity are about 78%. For combined test results from serum and cerebrospinal fluid, testing by calculating an AI for anti-*Borrelia* antibodies, sensitivity stays at about 79%, whereas specificity rises to a striking 96%. By adding the calculation of an AI to the diagnostic work up, specificity rises without lowering sensitivity.

Over time, methods for serological testing for Lyme disease have improved. At first, antigens were derived from whole cell sonicates, then assays moved to purified antigens. Current tests predominantly use recombinant antigens. As serologic test methodology has improved, so has their diagnostic test accuracy. Serological tests using antigens from whole cell sonicates achieved a sensitivity of 72% and a specificity of 90% for Lyme neuroborreliosis; tests with recombinant antigens show a remarkable diagnostic test accuracy with a sensitivity of 84% and a specificity of 93% (Leeflang *et al.*, 2016). Statements that serological testing for Lyme disease is flawed are certainly not true for newer generation tests using recombinant antigens.

Sensitivity of serological testing for Lyme disease is closely linked to the debate on 'seronegativity' in Lyme disease. Advocacy groups state that sensitivity of serological testing for Lyme disease is low and that therefore a large number of 'seronegative' patients may exist and may be underdiagnosed and undertreated. As stated above, sensitivity of serological testing in the setting of erythema migrans is about 54–58%. However, the clinical manifestation of an erythema migrans needs no serological confirmation, as erythema migrans is a visual diagnosis and is in itself an indication to start antibiotic treatment. In other manifestations of Lyme disease, especially Lyme neuroborreliosis, sensitivity is much higher. In patients with Lyme disease of >2–3 months' duration, serologic testing in serum is positive in almost 100% of cases (Wilske et al., 2007). A statement that almost 50% of patients with Lyme disease are 'seronegative' and are therefore misdiagnosed is an inappropriate generalization of sensitivity in erythema migrans, something that occurs very early in infection, and therefore an example of fabricated 'fake news' in the controversy around Lyme disease.

8.6 Evidence-based Treatment of Lyme Neuroborreliosis

Different guideline recommendations exist regarding the treatment of Lyme neuroborreliosis. The main difference lies between guidelines from patient advocacy groups and guidelines from scientific societies. Whereas guidelines from scientific societies (EFNS, American Academy of Neurology (AAN), Infectious Diseases Society of America (IDSA)) recommend antibiotic treatment with doxycycline or beta-lactam antibiotics over 10–21 days (Mygland et al., 2010), guidelines from patient advocacy groups (International Lyme and Associated Diseases Society (ILADS), Deutsche Borreliose Gesellschaft (German Borreliosis Society; DBG)) recommend treatment for several months, and recommend antibiotics such as carbapenems, metronidazole or antimalarials like hydroxychloroquine. Importantly, some of these antibiotics are regarded as reserve antibiotics, meaning they are usually reserved for severe life-threatening infections like sepsis (carbapenems, azithromycin).

A systematic review assessed the available literature on antibiotic treatment of Lyme neuroborreliosis (Dersch et al., 2015a). Overall data from 16 studies could be extracted. Of these, eight were RCTs, two were prospective cohort studies and six were retrospective cohort studies (non-randomized studies, NRS). All studies were performed in Europe. Data on neurological symptoms after treatment and on adverse events were extracted. Data from studies comparing doxycycline to beta-lactam antibiotics (ceftriaxone, penicillin G) were pooled in a meta-analysis.

Doxycycline and beta-lactam antibiotics were similar regarding efficacy for neurological symptoms, with no statistically significant difference between doxycycline and beta-lactam antibiotics. Regarding safety, no statistically significant difference was found between treatment with doxycycline or beta-lactam antibiotics. Doxycycline is taken orally in contrast to beta-lactam antibiotics, which are, in the context of Lyme neuroborreliosis, administered intravenously. According to the available evidence, oral treatment with doxycycline and intravenous beta-lactam antibiotics can be regarded as equivalent in the treatment of Lyme neuroborreliosis.

The majority of patients in the included studies suffered from early manifestations of Lyme neuroborreliosis (polyradiculoneuritis or meningitis), but some had late manifestations (encephalomyelitis). The studies included too few patients with late neuroborreliosis to assess this subgroup separately. However, there was no indication that treatment effects were different among early and late manifestations.

No studies were found that assessed treatment with carbapenem antibiotics or antimalarial drugs in Lyme neuroborreliosis. Therefore, guideline recommendations for the use of these drugs lack a rationale based on evidence from clinical studies.

Regarding Lyme neuroborreliosis, no studies were found that compare different lengths of treatment. However, there is indirect evidence regarding this. Oksi et al. performed a study on different treatment lengths for 145 patients suffering from Lyme disease in Finland (Oksi et al., 2007). While most included patients ($n = 115$) were suffering from Lyme neuroborreliosis, others were included as well, including Lyme arthritis ($n = 45$) or dermatological manifestations ($n = 5$). All patients received a course of ceftriaxone intravenously over 21 days and were then randomized to receive either amoxicillin 1 g twice daily or a placebo over 100 days. Patients were then assessed for up to 12 months following treatment. Clinical outcome was assessed using a visual analogue scale. Unfortunately, outcomes were not reported separately for different manifestations of Lyme disease. However, the main outcome showed no statistically significant difference between the group treated with amoxicillin and the group treated with placebo. Adverse events (diarrhea) were more frequent in the amoxicillin group. As the majority of included patients suffered from Lyme neuroborreliosis, this study provides valuable indirect evidence that antibiotic treatment courses exceeding 21 days show no better clinical outcome compared to shorter treatment courses.

The results from systematic reviews on pharmacological treatment of Lyme neuroborreliosis are in line with the recommendations already given in guidelines from scientific societies (EFNS, AAN, IDSA) (Wormser *et al.*, 2006; Halperin *et al.*, 2007; Mygland *et al.*, 2010). On the other hand, no evidence supporting diverging recommendations, like extended treatment durations or combination of antibiotics, as are recommended by guidelines from patient advocacy groups, could be found (Cameron *et al.*, 2004). Antibiotic treatment should be used reasonably and on the basis of evidence-based recommendations, as excessive use adds to the rising problem of multi-resistant pathogens. In Lyme neuroborreliosis, this means following the recommendations from guidelines provided by scientific societies (EFNS, AAN, IDSA) (Wormser *et al.*, 2006; Halperin *et al.*, 2007; Mygland *et al.*, 2010).

8.7 Course of Disease and Prognosis for Lyme Neuroborreliosis in the Light of Evidence-based Medicine

The course of Lyme neuroborreliosis is subject to intense controversy. Some authors report debilitating fatigue and cognitive impairment with tremendous impact on the quality of life that would affect a considerable proportion of patients with Lyme disease. Sometimes this symptom complex is called post-treatment Lyme disease syndrome (Koedel *et al.*, 2015). Some authors and patient support groups state that these patients suffer from a chronic *Borrelia* infection and should therefore be treated with extensive antibiotic courses over several months. However, as stated in the previous section, extended antibiotic treatment shows no advantage regarding clinical outcome, but rather more adverse events.

This uncertainty and perceived severity of residual symptoms leads to anxiety and possible distrust in affected patients. As contradictory statements exist on the matter of prognosis and cause of disease for Lyme neuroborreliosis, an assessment of all the available literature on this topic may overcome different biased attitudes. A summary of all the available literature can provide an unbiased view according to which statements can be established on reliable evidence. A systematic review assessed the prevalence and spectrum of residual symptoms reported for patients with Lyme neuroborreliosis in studies evaluating antibiotic treatment (Dersch *et al.*, 2016).

Forty-four studies were assessed: 8 RCTs, 17 cohort studies, 2 case control studies and 17 case series. From 38 of these studies, data on the prevalence of residual symptoms could be extracted, 31 studies provided data on the spectrum of residual symptoms. The patients in the single studies were categorized according to the case definition of Lyme neuroborreliosis, as defined by the EFNS (see above). Prevalence and spectrum of residual symptoms were pooled among these studies in a meta-analysis. Prevalence and spectrum of residual symptoms according to these case definitions then were assessed in a subgroup analysis.

In these studies assessing antibiotic treatment in patients with Lyme neuroborreliosis, prevalence of residual symptoms was approximately 28%. When considering this figure, one has to bear in mind that this number contains no information regarding severity of the reported residual symptoms, as this was not reported in the primary studies. Also, as these studies focus on treatment effects, residual symptoms may be overreported.

When the case definition of the included patients in single studies is considered, the differences between the case definition 'possible Lyme neuroborreliosis' on the one hand, and the definitions 'probable' and 'definite Lyme neuroborreliosis' have to be considered. The case definitions 'probable' and 'definite Lyme neuroborreliosis' both show evidence of inflammatory changes in cerebrospinal fluid (pleocytosis, intrathecal IgG-synthesis), whereas the case definition of 'possible Lyme neuroborreliosis' lacks confirmation by cerebrospinal fluid analysis. Therefore, the latter case definition is much more prone to false positive diagnoses of conditions that are not responsive to antibiotic treatment (e.g. multiple sclerosis).

Thirteen studies included patients according to the case definition of 'probable/definite Lyme neuroborreliosis', while 31 studies included patients according to the case definition of 'possible Lyme neuroborreliosis'. Interestingly, prevalence of residual symptoms differed between studies that had patients fulfilling the criteria for 'probable/definite Lyme neuroborreliosis' and studies of patients fulfilling the criteria for 'possible Lyme neuroborreliosis'. Studies that included patients without confirmation by cerebrospinal fluid analysis had statistically significantly higher rates of residual symptoms (31%) compared to studies with patients with confirmation by cerebrospinal fluid analysis (24%). This difference could be due to the inclusion of patients diagnosed with Lyme neuroborreliosis without cerebrospinal fluid confirmation, who were actually suffering from other conditions. Since these conditions were less likely to be antibiotic responsive, the higher rate of residual symptoms reported by these patients after treatment would not be surprising.

Reports of debilitating courses of Lyme neuroborreliosis with fatigue and cognitive impairment after treatment could therefore be an artifact of inaccurate diagnoses, without confirmation from cerebrospinal fluid analysis, leading to inclusion of patients with other diseases.

Not only did primary studies apply different inclusion criteria to their patients, they also differed in the spectrum of residual symptoms (Table 8.3).

Patients with residual symptoms, such as cranial neuropathy, pain, paresis, cognitive disturbances, headache, fatigue and diverse unspecific symptoms, were statistically significantly fewer in studies using the case definition of 'probable/definite Lyme neuroborreliosis' compared to the case definition of 'possible Lyme neuroborreliosis' (Table 8.2). Remarkably, in studies limited to 'probable/definite Lyme neuroborreliosis' and reporting residual symptoms in detail, there were no reports of patients with residual fatigue at all.

Regarding the spectrum of residual symptoms after therapy provided in Table 8.3, the frequency of residual symptoms seems lower than the prevalence of residual symptoms mentioned earlier. However, the data on the spectrum of residual symptoms are likely more accurate, as studies reporting the spectrum of residual symptoms provided more detail on their patients than those only summarizing their patients' residual symptoms. Studies providing more details regarding residual symptoms suggest they occur infrequently, so the overall prognosis of Lyme neuroborreliosis can be regarded as quite favorable.

8.8 So-called Post-Lyme Disease Symptoms

Another way of investigating reports of debilitating fatigue, cognitive impairment, depression and other long-term sequelae occurring in patients who have been diagnosed with Lyme disease, often called post-treatment Lyme disease syndrome, is to assess the long-term follow-up of patients with Lyme neuroborreliosis and compare them to healthy controls not suffering from Lyme disease.

Table 8.3. Proportion of patients with residual symptoms after therapy (%) in eligible studies. Last column shows comparison of studies using different case definitions. *$P < 0.0055$ (level of significance adjusted via Bonferroni correction). (From Dersch et al., 2016.)

Residual symptom	All studies (%) (n = 1311)	Probable/definite Lyme neuroborreliosis (%) (n = 687)	Possible Lyme neuroborreliosis (%) (n = 624)	P value
Cranial neuropathy	9.84	3.6	14.59	<0.0001*
Sensory disturbances	6.48	5.24	7.85	0.1483
Pain	10.37	2.77	18.75	<0.0001*
Paresis	5.57	2.33	9.13	<0.0001*
Unsteadiness/ataxia/vertigo	2.29	2.62	1.92	0.4329
Cognitive disturbances	8.77	1.6	16.67	<0.0001*
Headache	4.88	1.75	8.33	<0.0001*
Neurasthenia/fatigue	2.44	0	5.13	<0.0001*
Diverse	7.55	3.64	12.02	<0.0001*

Some authors argue that the cited symptoms of post-treatment Lyme disease syndrome are rather non-specific and that they exist as 'background symptoms' with no identifiable cause in the general population as well (Auwaerter et al., 2011). According to this point of view, post-treatment Lyme disease syndrome therefore could derive from a false attribution of these background symptoms to an episode of Lyme disease, representing a 'post hoc ergo propter hoc' fallacy. The issue of patients being falsely labeled as having Lyme disease by only having a positive serology and a non-specific complex of symptoms adds to this problem (Sigal, 1990; Cottle et al., 2012; Coumou et al., 2015).

Longitudinal studies explicitly assessing the long-term outcome of patients diagnosed with Lyme neuroborreliosis and confirmed by cerebrospinal fluid analysis, show a low rate of residual symptoms at follow-up (Hansen and Lebech, 1992; Kaiser, 2004; Dersch et al., 2015a; Ogrinc et al., 2016). The respective outcome is dependent on the manifestation of Lyme neuroborreliosis (Table 8.4).

Patients with early Lyme neuroborreliosis (polyradiculoneuritis, meningitis) show a favorable course (Ogrinc et al., 2016). Across all of the presented longitudinal studies, only 12% of patients with Lyme neuroborreliosis with early manifestations had residual symptoms at long-term follow-up (Hansen and Lebech, 1992; Kaiser, 2004; Dersch et al., 2015a; Ogrinc et al., 2016). These residual symptoms mostly consist of alleviated symptoms that were also present at the initial manifestation of Lyme neuroborreliosis like a residual facial weakness after a facial nerve palsy or a residual numbness after a polyradiculoneuritis.

In patients with late manifestations (encephalomyelitis), residual symptoms were reported much more frequently, in approximately 50% of cases (Kaiser, 2004; Dersch et al., 2015a). Again, these reported residual symptoms consist of neurological deficits that were present at initial presentation but ameliorated during treatment, like residual paraparesis or micturition disorder. Patients with late manifestations suffer from more severe symptoms with parenchymal damage that can only partially be influenced by antibiotic therapy. Therefore, a higher frequency of residual symptoms in these patients is not surprising.

Non-specific symptoms like fatigue are seldom reported in follow-up studies of Lyme neuroborreliosis (Dersch et al., 2015a). Patients experiencing fatigue all had the very rare late manifestations of Lyme neuroborreliosis consisting of encephalomyelitis with severe parenchymal involvement. These symptoms are a consequence of the parenchymal central nervous system damage and are neither responsive to antibiotic treatment nor a sign of ongoing 'chronic' infection. In such cases, fatigue is not a symptom specific or unique to Lyme disease but occurs in other disorders that cause permanent central nervous system damage, like stroke, multiple sclerosis, systemic lupus erythematosis or viral encephalitis (Bakshi, 2003; Schmeding and Schneider, 2013; Acciarresi et al., 2014; Veje et al., 2016).

Several studies have compared residual symptoms, fatigue and cognitive impairment in patients with Lyme neuroborreliosis to healthy controls. With this design, the hypothesis that symptoms attributed to post-treatment Lyme disease syndrome consist merely of background symptoms, frequently found in the general population, can be investigated.

Patients with central nervous system disease can develop cognitive impairment; fatigue or depression are much less specific in central nervous system disorders. Should pronounced neurocognitive deficits after Lyme disease exist, these symptoms should therefore be more pronounced in patients who suffered from Lyme neuroborreliosis compared to patients suffering from non-neurological manifestations of Lyme disease.

One study from Germany compared 30 patients with Lyme neuroborreliosis with confirmation by cerebrospinal fluid analysis with 35 healthy controls. Estimates of fatigue, quality of life, depression, verbal memory and cognition were similar in patients with Lyme neuroborreliosis and healthy controls, and showed no statistically significant difference (Dersch et al., 2015c). A study from Kalish et al. published in 2001 with a remarkably long follow-up period of 10–20 years compared 31 patients with Lyme neuroborreliosis with 30 healthy controls. This study even included patients that were not treated with antibiotics at all. No statistically significant difference could be found for the investigated items: quality of

Table 8.4. Residual symptoms in patients with Lyme neuroborreliosis at long-term follow-up.

Patients' characteristics	Therapy	Residual symptoms overall	Single residual symptoms
Ogrinc et al., 2016			
Overall: $n = 77$ Early manifestations: $n = 77$ (Bannwarth's syndrome) Follow-up period: 1 year	Ceftriaxone, doxycycline	9 (12%)	Unspecific symptoms, facial palsy, other palsies (frequency not stated)
Dersch et al., 2015c			
Overall: $n = 30$ Early manifestations: $n = 22$ Late manifestations: $n = 8$ Follow-up period: 4.9 years (SD 2.7 years) No statistically significant difference regarding depression, fatigue, quality of life, cognition and verbal memory between patients with Lyme neuroborreliosis and healthy controls	Ceftriaxone, doxycycline	17 (57%) Early manifestations: $n = 10$ Late manifestations: $n = 7$	Pain: $n = 6$ Ataxia: $n = 6$ Sensory disturbances: $n = 4$ Cranial neuropathy: $n = 2$ Spastic gait disorder: $n = 2$ Fatigue: $n = 2$ Micturition disorder: $n = 1$
Kaiser, 2004			
Overall: $n = 101$ Early manifestations: $n = 86$ Late manifestations: $n = 15$ Follow-up period: 1 year	Ceftriaxone	9 (9%) Early manifestations: $n = 4$ Late manifestations: $n = 5$	Discrete facial palsy: $n = 4$ Ataxia: $n = 4$ Restless legs: $n = 2$ Micturition disorder: $n = 3$ Paraparesis: $n = 1$
Hansen and Lebech, 1992			
Overall: $n = 187$ Early manifestations: $n = 169$ Late manifestations: $n = 18$ Follow-up period: 4–72 months, median 33 months	Penicillin G, ceftriaxone, Doxycycline, penicillin G + ceftriaxone, Chloramphenicole, cefotaxime, cefuroxime	18 (10%)	Sensory disturbances: $n = 14$ Radicular pain: $n = 3$ Arthralgia: $n = 1$

life, depression, verbal memory and cognitive impairment (Kalish *et al.*, 2001).

However, Eikeland *et al.* report lower quality of life, more fatigue and more difficulties in verbal memory tests in patients with Lyme neuroborreliosis compared to healthy controls (Eikeland *et al.*, 2011; 2012; updated in Chapter 9 of this volume). The authors of these studies report that most patients with Lyme neuroborreliosis performed comparably with healthy controls, while a small subset had more difficulties, accounting for the overall statistically significant result. Although this study shows some differences, it mainly shows that a few patients with more severe initial neurological symptoms (and therefore presumably more parenchymal damage to the central nervous system) have remaining residual symptoms with impairments in daily life, while most patients with Lyme neuroborreliosis have a favorable prognosis and quality of life in general is not compromised.

Other studies focus not only on patients with Lyme neuroborreliosis but rather on more frequent manifestations of Lyme disease, like erythema migrans (Cerar *et al.*, 2010; Wormser *et al.*, 2015). One study from Cerar *et al.* from Slovenia followed 194 patients with erythema migrans (Cerar *et al.*, 2010). Concomitant with enrollment into this study, healthy controls without signs of Lyme disease were included for follow-up. Patients with erythema migrans were treated with either doxycycline or cefuroxime. After 6 and 12 months, patients and controls were again assessed for frequency and severity of clinical symptoms. None of the assessed symptoms was statistically significantly more frequent in patients with erythema migrans than in healthy controls. Symptoms like fatigue were actually more frequent in healthy controls than in patients with erythema migrans. Eliassen *et al.* followed 188 patients from Norway with erythema migrans for 1 year after treatment (Eliassen *et al.*, 2017b). After this year, symptom load in these patients was similar to the general population. A long-term study assessed quality of life after a remarkably long follow-up period of 11–20 years after an initial episode with erythema migrans (in patients from the United States) (Wormser *et al.*, 2015). Health-related quality of life was assessed in 100 patients, results were compared to the general population. The results for the health-related quality of life from the patients were similar to those from the general population.

Again, these studies from patients with the most frequent manifestation of Lyme disease, erythema migrans, support the view that most residual symptoms after Lyme disease are, in fact, 'background symptoms' that can also be observed in the general population in similar frequencies. Attributing such symptoms to an episode of Lyme disease could therefore, as stated above, represent a 'post hoc ergo propter hoc' fallacy.

References

Acciarresi, M., Bogousslavsky, J. and Paciaroni, M. (2014) Post-stroke fatigue: epidemiology, clinical characteristics and treatment. *European Neurology* 72, 255–261.

Auwaerter, P.G., Bakken, J.S., Dattwyler, R.J. *et al.* (2011) Antiscience and ethical concerns associated with advocacy of Lyme disease. *Lancet Infectious Diseases* 11, 713–719.

Back, T., Grünig, S., Winter, Y., Bodechtel, U., Guthke, K., Khati, D. and von Kummer, R. (2013) Neuroborreliosis-associated cerebral vasculitis: long-term outcome and health-related quality of life. *Journal of Neurology* 260, 1569–1575.

Bacon, R.M., Kugeler, K.J., Mead, P.S. and Centers for Disease Control and Prevention (CDC) (2008) Surveillance for Lyme disease – United States, 1992–2006. *Morbidity and Mortality Weekly Report Surveillance Summaries*. Washington DC 2002 57, 1–9.

Bakshi, R. (2003) Fatigue associated with multiple sclerosis: diagnosis, impact and management. *Multiple Sclerosis* 9, 219–227.

Cameron, D., Gaito, A., Harris, N. *et al.* (2004) Evidence-based guidelines for the management of Lyme disease. *Expert Review of Anti-infective Therapy* 2, S1–13.

Cerar, D., Cerar, T., Ružić-Sabljić, E., Wormser, G.P. and Strle, F. (2010) Subjective symptoms after treatment of early Lyme disease. *American Journal of Medicine* 123, 79–86.

Clark, K.L., Leydet, B.F. and Threlkeld, C. (2014) Geographical and genospecies distribution of *Borrelia burgdorferi* sensu lato DNA detected in humans in the USA. *Journal of Medical Microbiology* 63, 674–684.

Cottle, L.E., Mekonnen, E., Beadsworth, M.B.J., Miller, A.R.O. and Beeching, N.J. (2012) Lyme disease in a British referral clinic. *QJM – Monthly Journal of the Association of Physicians* 105, 537–543.

Coumou, J., Herkes, E.A., Brouwer, M.C. *et al*. (2015) Ticking the right boxes: classification of patients suspected of Lyme borreliosis at an academic referral center in the Netherlands. *Clinical Microbiology and Infection: The Official Publication of the European Society of Clinical Microbiology and Infectious Diseases* 21(368), e11–e20.

Dersch, R., Freitag, M.H., Schmidt, S., Sommer, H., Rauer, S. and Meerpohl, J.J. (2015a) Efficacy and safety of pharmacological treatments for acute Lyme neuroborreliosis – a systematic review. *European Journal of Neurology* 22, 1249–1259.

Dersch, R., Hottenrott, T., Senel, M., Lehmensiek, V., Tumani, H., Rauer, S. and Stich, O. (2015b) The chemokine CXCL13 is elevated in the cerebrospinal fluid of patients with neurosyphilis. *Fluids and Barriers of the CNS* 12, 12.

Dersch, R., Sarnes, A.A., Maul, M., Hottenrott, T., Baumgartner, A., Rauer, S. and Stich, O. (2015c) Quality of life, fatigue, depression and cognitive impairment in Lyme neuroborreliosis. *Journal of Neurology* 262, 2572–2577.

Dersch, R., Sommer, H., Rauer, S. and Meerpohl, J.J. (2016) Prevalence and spectrum of residual symptoms in Lyme neuroborreliosis after pharmacological treatment: a systematic review. *Journal of Neurology* 263, 17–24.

Djukic, M., Schmidt-Samoa, C., Lange, P., Spreer, A., Neubieser, K., Eiffert, H., Nau, R. and Schmidt, H. (2012) Cerebrospinal fluid findings in adults with acute Lyme neuroborreliosis. *Journal of Neurology* 259, 630–636.

Eikeland, R., Mygland, Å., Herlofson, K. and Ljøstad, U. (2011) European neuroborreliosis: quality of life 30 months after treatment. *Acta Neurologica Scandinavica* 124, 349–354.

Eikeland, R., Ljøstad, U., Mygland, Å., Herlofson, K. and Løhaugen, G.C. (2012) European neuroborreliosis: neuropsychological findings 30 months post-treatment. *European Journal of Neurology* 19, 480–487.

Eliassen, K.E., Berild, D., Reiso, H., Grude, N., Christophersen, K.S., Finckenhagen, C. and Lindbæk, M. (2017a) Incidence and antibiotic treatment of erythema migrans in Norway 2005–2009. *Ticks and Tick-borne Diseases* 8, 1–8.

Eliassen, K.E., Hjetland, R., Reiso, H., Lindbæk, M. and Tschudi-Madsen, H. (2017b) Symptom load and general function among patients with erythema migrans: a prospective study with a 1-year follow-up after antibiotic treatment in Norwegian general practice. *Scandinavian Journal of Primary Health Care* 35, 75–83.

Fingerle, V., Schulte-Spechtel, U.C., Ružić-Sabljić, E., Leonhard, S., Hofmann, H., Weber, K., Pfister, K., Strle, F. and Wilske, B. (2008) Epidemiological aspects and molecular characterization of *Borrelia burgdorferi* s.l. from southern Germany with special respect to the new species *Borrelia spielmanii* sp. nov. *Indian Journal of Medical Microbiology* 298, 279–290.

Halperin, J. (2017) A critical appraisal of the mild axonal peripheral neuropathy of late neurologic Lyme disease. *Diagnostic Microbiology and Infectious Disease* 88(1), 107.

Halperin, J.J., Shapiro, E.D., Logigian, E., Belman, A.L., Dotevall, L., Wormser, G.P., Krupp, L., Gronseth, G., Bever, C.T. and Quality Standards Subcommittee of the American Academy of Neurology (2007) Practice parameter: treatment of nervous system Lyme disease (an evidence-based review): report of the quality standards subcommittee of the American Academy of Neurology. *Neurology* 69, 91–102.

Hansen, K. and Lebech, A.M. (1992) The clinical and epidemiological profile of Lyme neuroborreliosis in Denmark 1985–1990. A prospective study of 187 patients with *Borrelia burgdorferi* specific intrathecal antibody production. *Brain Journal of Neurology* 115(2), 399–423.

Higgins, J. and Green, S. (2011) *Cochrane Handbook for Systematic Reviews of Interventions Version 5.1.0* [updated March 2011]. The Cochrane Collaboration. Available at: http://handbook-5-1.cochrane.org/ (accessed 3 May 2018).

Hofhuis, A., Harms, M., Bennema, S., van den Wijngaard, C.C. and van Pelt, W. (2015) Physician reported incidence of early and late Lyme borreliosis. *Parasites and Vectors* 8, 161.

Hopf, H.C. (1975) Peripheral neuropathy in acrodermatitis chronica atrophicans (Herxheimer). *Journal of Neurology, Neurosurgery, and Psychiatry* 38, 452–458.

Huppertz, H.I., Böhme, M., Standaert, S.M., Karch, H. and Plotkin, S.A. (1999) Incidence of Lyme borreliosis in the Würzburg region of Germany. *European Journal of Clinical Microbiology and Infectious Diseases: Official Publication of the European Society of Clinical Microbiology* 18, 697–703.

Hytönen, J., Kortela, E., Waris, M., Puustinen, J., Salo, J. and Oksi, J. (2014) CXCL13 and neopterin concentrations in cerebrospinal fluid of patients with Lyme neuroborreliosis and other diseases that cause neuroinflammation. *Journal of Neuroinflammation* 11, 103.

Kaiser, R. (1994) Variable CSF findings in early and late Lyme neuroborreliosis: a follow-up study in 47 patients. *Journal of Neurology* 242, 26–36.

Kaiser, R. (1998) Neuroborreliosis. *Journal of Neurology* 245, 247–255.

Kaiser, R. (2004) [Clinical courses of acute and chronic neuroborreliosis following treatment with ceftriaxone]. *Nervenarzt* 75, 553–557.

Kalish, R.A., Kaplan, R.F., Taylor, E., Jones-Woodward, L., Workman, K. and Steere, A.C. (2001) Evaluation of study patients with Lyme disease, 10–20-year follow-up. *Journal of Infectious Diseases* 183, 453–460.

Knottnerus, J.A. and Muris, J.W. (2003) Assessment of the accuracy of diagnostic tests: the cross-sectional study. *Journal of Clinical Epidemiology* 56, 1118–1128.

Koedel, U., Fingerle, V. and Pfister, H.-W. (2015) Lyme neuroborreliosis – epidemiology, diagnosis and management. *Nature Reviews Neurology* 11, 446–456.

Leeflang, M.M.G., Ang, C.W., Berkhout, J. *et al.* (2016) The diagnostic accuracy of serological tests for Lyme borreliosis in Europe: a systematic review and meta-analysis. *BMC Infectious Diseases* 16, 140.

Mygland, A., Ljøstad, U., Fingerle, V., Rupprecht, T., Schmutzhard, E., Steiner, I. and European Federation of Neurological Societies (2010) EFNS guidelines on the diagnosis and management of European Lyme neuroborreliosis. *European Journal of Neurology* 17(8–16), e1–e4.

Nadelman, R.B. and Wormser, G.P. (1998) Lyme borreliosis. *The Lancet* 352, 557–565.

Oehme, R., Hartelt, K., Backe, H., Brockmann, S. and Kimmig, P. (2002) Foci of tick-borne diseases in southwest Germany. *International Journal of Medical Microbiology* 291(33), 22–29.

Ogrinc, K., Lusa, L., Lotrič-Furlan, S., Bogovič, P., Stupica, D., Cerar, T., Ružić-Sabljić, E. and Strle, F. (2016) Course and outcome of early European Lyme neuroborreliosis (Bannwarth syndrome): clinical and laboratory findings. *Clinical Infectious Diseases* 63, 346–353.

Oksi, J., Nikoskelainen, J., Hiekkanen, H., Lauhio, A., Peltomaa, M., Pitkäranta, A., Nyman, D., Granlund, H., Carlsson, S.-A., Seppälä, I., Valtonen, V. and Viljanen, M. (2007) Duration of antibiotic treatment in disseminated Lyme borreliosis: a double-blind, randomized, placebo-controlled, multicenter clinical study. *European Journal of Clinical Microbiology and Infectious Diseases* 26, 571–581.

Ornstein, K., Berglund, J., Nilsson, I., Norrby, R. and Bergström, S. (2001) Characterization of Lyme borreliosis isolates from patients with erythema migrans and neuroborreliosis in southern Sweden. *Journal of Clinical Microbiology* 39, 1294–1298.

Pfister, H.W., Einhäupl, K.M., Wilske, B. and Preac-Mursic, V. (1987) Bannwarth's syndrome and the enlarged neurological spectrum of arthropod-borne borreliosis. *Zentralblatt für Bakteriologie, Mikrobiologie und Hygiene. Series A: Medical Microbiology, Infectious Diseases, Virology, Parasitology* 263, 343–347.

Pritt, B.S., Respicio-Kingry, L.B., Sloan, L.M. *et al.* (2016) *Borrelia mayonii* sp. nov., a member of the *Borrelia burgdorferi* sensu lato complex, detected in patients and ticks in the upper midwestern United States. *International Journal of Systematic and Evolutionary Microbiology* 66, 4878–4880.

Rauer, S. (2012) S1 *Leitlinie Neuroborreliose*. In: *Leitlinien Für Diagnostik Und Therapie in Der Neurologie*. Thieme Verlag, Stuttgart, Germany.

Rauer, S., Kastenbauer, S. *et al.* (2018) S3 *Leitlinie Neuroborreliose*. In: *Deutsche Gesellschaft für Neurologie* (Hrsg.), Leitlinien für Diagnostik und Therapie in der Neurologie.

Reiber, H. and Lange, P. (1991) Quantification of virus-specific antibodies in cerebrospinal fluid and serum: sensitive and specific detection of antibody synthesis in brain. *Clinical Chemistry* 37, 1153–1160.

Robert Koch Institut (2015) Meldepflicht für Lyme-Borreliose in Bayern – eine erste Bilanz. *Epidemiology Bulletin* 8/2015.

Rupprecht, T.A., Lechner, C., Tumani, H. and Fingerle, V. (2014) [CXCL13: a biomarker for acute Lyme neuroborreliosis: investigation of the predictive value in the clinical routine]. *Nervenarzt* 85, 459–464.

Sackett, D.L., Rosenberg, W.M., Gray, J.A., Haynes, R.B. and Richardson, W.S. (1996) Evidence based medicine: what it is and what it isn't. *BMJ* 312, 71–72.

Schmeding, A. and Schneider, M. (2013) Fatigue, health-related quality of life and other patient-reported outcomes in systemic lupus erythematosus. *Best Practice and Research: Clinical Rheumatology* 27, 363–375.

Schmidt, C., Plate, A., Angele, B., Pfister, H.-W., Wick, M., Koedel, U. and Rupprecht, T.A. (2011) A prospective study on the role of CXCL13 in Lyme neuroborreliosis. *Neurology* 76, 1051–1058.

Senel, M., Rupprecht, T.A., Tumani, H., Pfister, H.W., Ludolph, A.C. and Brettschneider, J. (2010) The chemokine CXCL13 in acute neuroborreliosis. *Journal of Neurology, Neurosurgery, and Psychiatry* 81, 929–933.

Sigal, L.H. (1990) Summary of the first 100 patients seen at a Lyme disease referral center. *The American Journal of Medicine* 88, 577–581.

Stanek, G. and Strle, F. (2003) Lyme borreliosis. *The Lancet* 362, 1639–1647.

Strle, F. (1999) Lyme borreliosis in Slovenia. Zentralblatt Bakteriol. *International Journal of Medical Microbiology* 289, 643–652.

van Dam, A.P., Kuiper, H., Vos, K., Widjojokusumo, A., de Jongh, B.M., Spanjaard, L., Ramselaar, A.C., Kramer, M.D. and Dankert, J. (1993) Different genospecies of *Borrelia burgdorferi* are associated with distinct clinical manifestations of Lyme borreliosis. *Clinical Infectious Diseases* 17, 708–717.

Veje, M., Nolskog, P., Petzold, M., Bergström, T., Lindén, T., Peker, Y. and Studahl, M. (2016) Tick-borne encephalitis sequelae at long-term follow-up: a self-reported case-control study. *Acta Neurologica Scandinavica* 134, 434–441.

Wienecke, R., Zöchling, N., Neubert, U., Schlüpen, E.M., Meurer, M. and Volkenandt, M. (1994) Molecular subtyping of *Borrelia burgdorferi* in erythema migrans and acrodermatitis chronica atrophicans. *Journal of Investigative Dermatology* 103, 19–22.

Wilking, H., Fingerle, V., Klier, C., Thamm, M. and Stark, K. (2015) Antibodies against *Borrelia burgdorferi* sensu lato among adults, Germany, 2008–2011. *Emerging Infectious Diseases* 21, 107–110.

Wilske, B., Fingerle, V. and Schulte-Spechtel, U. (2007) Microbiological and serological diagnosis of Lyme borreliosis. *FEMS Immunology and Medical Microbiology* 49, 13–21.

Wormser, G.P., Dattwyler, R.J., Shapiro, E.D., Halperin, J.J., Steere, A.C., Klempner, M.S., Krause, P.J., Bakken, J.S., Strle, F., Stanek, G., Bockenstedt, L., Fish, D., Dumler, J.S. and Nadelman, R.B. (2006) The clinical assessment, treatment, and prevention of Lyme disease, human granulocytic anaplasmosis, and babesiosis: clinical practice guidelines by the Infectious Diseases Society of America. *Clinical Infectious Diseases* 43, 1089–1134.

Wormser, G.P., Weitzner, E., McKenna, D., Nadelman, R.B., Scavarda, C., Molla, I., Dornbush, R., Visintainer, P. and Nowakowski, J. (2015) Long-term assessment of health-related quality of life in patients with culture-confirmed early Lyme disease. *Clinical Infectious Diseases* 61, 244–247.

9 Medically Unexplained Symptoms and Lyme Neuroborreliosis – Not the Same: A Study in an Endemic Area of Norway

Erlend Roaldsnes,[1] Randi Eikeland[2] and Dag Berild[3]

[1]Oslo University Hospital, Faculty of Medicine, University of Oslo, Oslo, Norway; [2]National Advisory Unit for Tick-borne Diseases, Department of Neurology, Hospital of Southern Norway, Sørlandet, Norway; [3]Department of Infectious Diseases, Oslo University Hospital, Faculty of Medicine, University of Oslo, and Faculty of Health Science, Oslo Metropolitan University Oslo, Norway

9.1 Introduction

Norway has approximately 300–400 cases of disseminated Lyme borreliosis (LB) each year, which yields an incidence of 7/100,000 inhabitants/year. This includes all types of disseminated LB, but since reporting of disseminated borreliosis in Norway is mandatory, we know that neuroborreliosis (LNB) accounts for 60% of the cases (Ocampo, 2016). The incidence of erythema migrans is 148/100,000 inhabitants/year (Eliassen et al., 2017). In earlier years ticks were found only in the southern part of Norway, but they have spread north to the arctic circle and also into the highlands, mainly because of climate change (Jore et al., 2011). It is especially the coastal region of southern Norway that is considered an endemic area, with around 30% of all ticks being carriers of *Borreliella* species. The leading genotypes are *B. afzelii* (61%), *B. garinii* (23%) and *B. burgdorferi* sensu stricto (11%) (Kjelland et al., 2010). In Norway, definite and possible LNB are diagnosed on the basis of European guidelines (Mygland et al., 2010), which require neurological symptoms consistent with LNB, a lumbar puncture with cerebrospinal fluid pleocytosis and a positive antibody index as evidence of intrathecal production of antibodies against *Borreliella*. A Norwegian National Advisory Unit on Tick-borne Diseases was established in 2014 for the purpose of providing evidence-based advice and up to date information to doctors and the general population.

9.2 Background for the Study

There has been an increasing perception that medically unexplained symptoms might be due to LNB. Some groups of doctors are advocating that LNB should be diagnosed on the basis of symptoms alone, including chronic non-specific symptoms, without a lumbar puncture and with the use of non-validated tests (Cameron et al., 2004; Feder et al., 2007). These opinions are regarded as controversial in the academic community (Feder et al., 2007). A Norwegian study showed that persons who are exposed to *Borreliella* and become seropositive for *Borreliella* antibodies do not suffer from more health problems compared to the rest of the population (Hjetland et al., 2015). Other studies have shown that as many as 50% of LNB-treated patients suffer from health problems 30 months post-treatment, especially fatigue, neuropsychological symptoms and reduced quality of life (Eikeland et al., 2011;

2012). Primary care physicians find themselves in the middle of this controversy when seeing patients who are frustrated because they are suffering from unexplained health complaints and are concerned that it could be caused by Lyme disease. The Hospital of Southern Norway has experienced a rise in referrals for suspected LNB so we examined these patients' symptoms and final diagnoses to learn more about the presentation of LNB in Norway. We searched the medical records of all patients who were referred for lumbar puncture for possible LNB at the hospital in 2013 (Roaldsnes et al., 2017). Further we grouped the patients, based on their symptoms, into two groups to compare:

1. Patients with symptoms typical for LNB: radiculitis, peripheral cranial nerve palsy or other symptoms suggestive of central nervous system involvement.
2. Patients with non-specific symptoms: fatigue, dizziness, difficulty concentrating, non-specific paresthesia and headaches.

Finally we compared the clinical presentations of patients diagnosed with LNB to those who did not meet the criteria for a LNB diagnosis.

9.3 Observations

We found 140 patients who were examined with a lumbar puncture, and had LNB as their initial tentative diagnosis. Thirty had typical LNB symptoms and 110 had non-specific symptoms (Table 9.1). Out of the 110 with non-specific symptoms only one was diagnosed with *possible* LNB. Of the 30 patients with symptoms typical of LNB, six were diagnosed with definite LNB, and one possible LNB. None of the patients diagnosed with LNB had symptom duration over 6 months, and four of six had symptom duration of less than 1 month (Table 9.2). The most common symptom of LNB was peripheral facial nerve palsy: 24% of those evaluated for LNB because of acquired peripheral facial nerve palsy had LNB. A total of 66% of all 140 patients had positive serology for antibodies against *Borreliella*: IgM, IgG or both. All the patients who were diagnosed with *definite* LNB had high titers of *Borreliella* IgG antibodies with levels above 650% from cut-off.

Table 9.1. Patients meeting diagnostic criteria for Lyme neuroborreliosis (LNB) with Lyme-specific neuroborreliosis symptoms vs. non-specific symptoms.

	Negative for LNB	Possible LNB	Definite LNB	Total
Typical symptoms	23	1	6	30
Non-specific neurological symptoms	109	1	0	110
Total	132	2	6	140

Table 9.2. Various symptoms among patients with Lyme neuroborreliosis vs. not.

Symptoms	Definite or possible LNB (n = 8)	No LNB (n = 132)
Cranial nerve deficit	5 (63)	16 (12)
Radiculitis	4 (50)	11 (8)
Paresthesias	4 (50)	55 (42)
Myalgias	3 (38)	69 (52)
Tension-type headache	3 (38)	45 (34)
Tick bite within last 3 months	2 (25)	8 (6)
Tiredness	1 (13)	57 (43)
Dizziness	1 (13)	39 (30)
Meningitis symptoms	0	1 (1)
Difficulty concentrating	0	28 (21)
Erythema migrans	0	6 (5)
Symptom duration:		
<1 month	4 (50)	36 (27)
1–3 months	2 (25)	23 (17)
3–6 months	1 (13)	10 (8)
6–12 months	0	15 (11)
>12 months	0	40 (30)
Unknown	1 (17)	8 (6)
Total:	132 (100)	8 (100)

9.4 Discussion

Out of the 140 patients referred to the hospital with possible LNB 79% did not have symptoms typical of LNB. This group had low probability of abnormalities in their cerebrospinal fluid and a diagnosis of LNB, especially if they had symptoms of more than 6 months' duration. The patient with low suspicion of LNB who was diagnosed with possible LNB was a 73-year-old woman with 2 weeks of paresthesia, headache and myalgia. There was no history of tick bite or erythema migrans; she had a positive serum *Borreliella* IgG and negative IgM. Her CSF showed 9×10^6 cells/l with a positive antibody index as evidence of intrathecal production of *Borreliella* antibodies. She had previously been treated for LNB, but at an unknown time. The current symptoms could have been a reinfection or traces of an old infection. This case exemplifies how difficult it can be to diagnose LNB when we know that patients can be seropositive and have a positive antibody index for many years after exposure (Hammers-Berggren *et al.*, 1993).

The reason so many persons were referred to the hospital with the question of LNB, despite the absence of typical symptoms of the condition, is unclear. However, this might relate to the media's focus on concerns about underdiagnosing tick-borne diseases, something also seen in social media. Importantly, in our county 18% of healthy individuals have positive titers for *Borreliella* antibodies in serum (Mygland *et al.*, 2006), and of the 140 referred with the question of LNB, 66% had positive *Borreliella* antibodies. Several patients with non-specific health complaints might have been tested for *Borreliella* antibodies by their general practitioner and because of a positive test have been referred to the hospital for a lumbar puncture that could have been avoided.

9.5 Conclusion

LNB is an unlikely explanation for long-lasting subjective health complaints, even in individuals with positive *Borreliella* serology. People with new onset of peripheral cranial nerve palsy should be examined with a lumbar puncture for LNB in an endemic area.

References

Cameron, D., Gaito, A., Harris, N. *et al.* (2004) Evidence-based guidelines for the management of Lyme disease. *Expert Review of Anti-infective Therapy* 2, S1–S13.

Eikeland, R., Mygland, A., Herlofson, K. and Ljostad, U. (2011) European neuroborreliosis: quality of life 30 months after treatment. *Acta Neurologica Scandinavica* 124, 349–354.

Eikeland, R., Ljostad, U., Mygland, A., Herlofson, K. and Lohaugen, G.C. (2012) European neuroborreliosis: neuropsychological findings 30 months post-treatment. *European Journal of Neurology* 19, 480–487.

Eliassen, K.E., Berild, D., Reiso, H., Grude, N., Christophersen, K.S., Finckenhagen, C. and Lindbaek, M. (2017) Incidence and antibiotic treatment of erythema migrans in Norway 2005–2009. *Ticks and Tick-borne Diseases* 8, 1–8.

Feder Jr, H.M., Johnson, B.J., O'Connell, S. *et al.* (2007) A critical appraisal of 'chronic Lyme disease'. *New England Journal of Medicine* 357, 1422–1430.

Hammers-Berggren, S., Hansen, K., Lebech, A.M. and Karlsson, M. (1993) *Borrelia burgdorferi*-specific intrathecal antibody production in neuroborreliosis: a follow-up study. *Neurology* 43, 169–175.

Hjetland, R., Reiso, H., Ihlebaek, C., Nilsen, R.M., Grude, N. and Ulvestad, E. (2015) Subjective health complaints are not associated with tick bites or antibodies to *Borrelia burgdorferi* sensu lato in blood donors in western Norway: a cross-sectional study. *BMC Public Health* 15, 657.

Jore, S., Viljugrein, H., Hofshagen, M., Brun-Hansen, H., Kristoffersen, A.B., Nygard, K., Brun, E., Ottesen, P., Saevik, B.K. and Ytrehus, B. (2011) Multi-source analysis reveals latitudinal and altitudinal shifts in range of *Ixodes ricinus* at its northern distribution limit. *Parasites and Vectors* 4, 84.

Kjelland, V., Stuen, S., Skarpaas, T. and Slettan, A. (2010) Prevalence and genotypes of *Borrelia burgdorferi* sensu lato infection in *Ixodes ricinus* ticks in southern Norway. *Scandinavian Journal of Infectious Diseases* 42, 579–585.

Mygland, A., Skarpaas, T. and Ljostad, U. (2006) Chronic polyneuropathy and Lyme disease. *European Journal of Neurology* 13, 1213–1215.

Mygland, A., Ljostad, U., Fingerle, V., Rupprecht, T., Schmutzhard, E. and Steiner, I. (2010) EFNS guidelines on the diagnosis and management of European Lyme neuroborreliosis. *European Journal of Neurology* 17(8–16), e1–e4.

Ocampo, J.M.F., Vold, I.J.S. *et al.* (2016) Årsrapport flått og flåttbårne sykdommer i 2015. *Norwegian Institute of Public Health*.

Roaldsnes, E., Eikeland, R. and Berild, D. (2017) Lyme neuroborreliosis in cases of non-specific neurological symptoms. *Journal of the Norwegian Medical Association* 137, 101–104.

10 Erythema Migrans

Robert B. Nadelman[1] and Linden Hu[2]
[1]*Department of Medicine, New York Medical College, Valhalla, New York, USA;*
[2]*Tufts University School of Medicine, Boston, Massachusetts, USA*

10.1 Introduction

Erythema migrans (EM) (previously known as erythema chronicum migrans) is an expanding erythematous rash that develops at the site of the bite of certain *Ixodes* ticks within days to weeks (Steere *et al.*, 1983b; 1985; Åsbrink and Olsson, 1985; Nadelman and Wormser, 1995, 2002). It is the most common objective manifestation of Lyme disease, accounting for about 90% of cases (Gerber *et al.*, 1996; Krause *et al.*, 1996; Nadelman and Wormser, 1998; 2002). The dramatic and distinctive 'bull's eye' appearance of the rash and its occurrence in the late spring and summer enabled the recognition of Lyme disease as a vector-borne infection years before the discovery of the causative pathogen, *Borreliella burgdorferi* sensu lato, and the development of the first diagnostic laboratory assays. Nevertheless, it is now evident that the 'classic' EM presentation with central clearing accounts for a minority of cases of early Lyme disease in the United States (Nadelman *et al.*, 1996; Nadelman and Wormser, 2002; Smith *et al.*, 2002, Schutzer *et al.*, 2013). Furthermore, the rash alone cannot be said to be pathognomonic for infection with *B. burgdorferi* because of the virtually indistinguishable appearance of certain other entities, in particular, southern tick-associated rash illness (STARI) (see Section 10.2.8) (Kirkland *et al.*, 1997; Masters *et al.*, 1998; Wormser *et al.*, 2005c).

10.2 Clinical Diagnosis

EM is an expanding erythematous skin lesion, usually round or oval, that develops 7–14 days (range 1–36 days) following the detachment of certain *Ixodes* ticks at the site of inoculation of *B. burgdorferi* (Steere *et al.*, 1983b; Berger, 1989; Malane *et al.*, 1991; Nadelman and Wormser, 1995; Nadelman *et al.*, 1996) (Figs 10.1–10.4). EM must be distinguished from localized and transient inflammatory reactions to the bite of an arthropod that are not associated with infection (Fig. 10.5). The latter resolve spontaneously within a day or two (Feder and Whitaker, 1995; Nadelman and Wormser, 1995; Wormser, 2006; Wormser *et al.*, 2006). In order to increase the specificity of the diagnosis of EM by limiting confusion with such localized reactions, the Centers for Disease Control and Prevention (CDC) has designated 5 cm in largest diameter as a minimum size for EM lesions in the case definition of Lyme disease (Bacon *et al.*, 2008). Although useful for increasing accuracy in the clinical diagnosis of Lyme disease, particularly, in clinical and epidemiologic studies, the size limitation should not be used alone to exclude the diagnosis of EM in individual patients with clinical and epidemiologic features that are otherwise suggestive (Krause *et al.*, 2006; Wormser *et al.*, 2006; Bacon *et al.*, 2008).

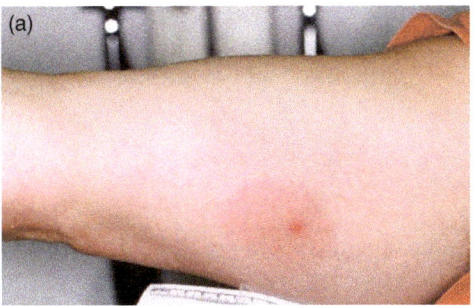
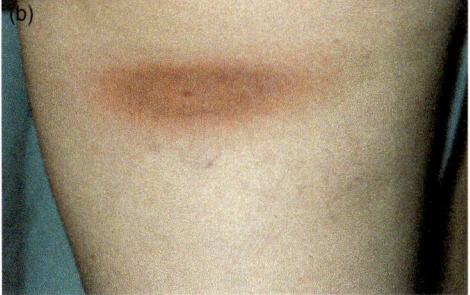

Fig. 10.1. (a) Erythema migrans lesions with raised punctum (arm). (b) Erythema migrans lesion with depressed punctum (leg).

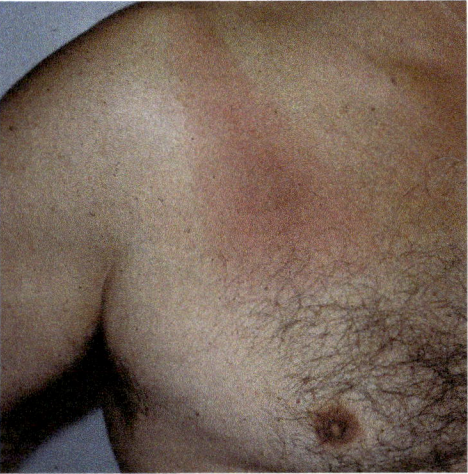

Fig. 10.2. Triangular EM lesion. (Reprinted by permission of Elsevier, Infectious Disease Clinics of North America.)

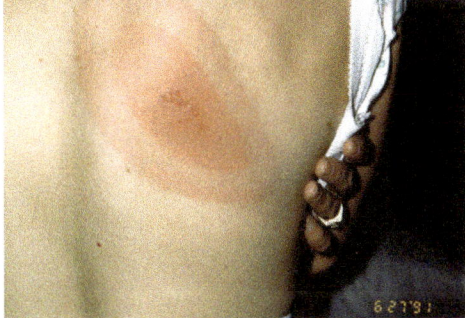

Fig. 10.3. Vesicular erythema migrans lesion.

10.2.1 Epidemiology

More than 90% of the 28,000 cases of Lyme disease reported to the CDC in 2015 originated from ten states in New England, the middle Atlantic, and north central regions (CDC, 2016). Although not required for diagnosis of EM in an endemic area (see Section 10.2.10), isolation in culture of *B. burgdorferi* sensu lato from clinical specimens has confirmed the diagnosis in patients from endemic areas in the US as well as much of Europe and parts of Asia where *B. afzelii* and *B. garinii* are the most common etiologic genospecies (Kuiper *et al.*, 1994; Hashimoto *et al.*, 1995; Busch *et al.*, 1996; Strle *et al.*, 1996a; 1996b; 1999; Ornstein *et al.*, 2001; Antoni-Bach *et al.*, 2002; Lipsker *et al.*, 2002; Logar *et al.*, 2004; Masuzawa, 2004; Cerar *et al.*, 2010; Strle *et al.*, 2011). Reports of Lyme disease associated with EM from non-endemic regions in the US and elsewhere (Sharma *et al.*, 2010) without culture isolation of *B. burgdorferi* sensu lato from human specimens or vector ticks should be viewed with some skepticism since the clinical appearance of a rash and serologic testing have a low positive predictive value for *B. burgdorferi* infection in this setting.

EM is commonly said to occur in approximately 70% of patients with Lyme disease in the US (Bacon *et al.*, 2008), but this is likely to be an underestimate for several reasons. This skin lesion may go unrecognized when it occurs at body sites such as the buttocks that are not easily visualized, or when it is associated with minimal or no systemic or local symptoms (Nadelman and Wormser, 1995; 1998; Gerber *et al.*, 1996; Krause *et al.*, 1996; Wormser *et al.*, 2006). In addition, case reporting is biased toward detecting later manifestations of Lyme disease such as

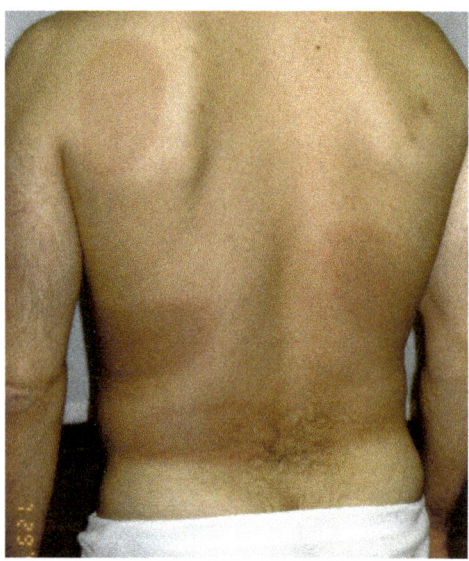

Fig. 10.4. Multiple erythema migrans lesions.

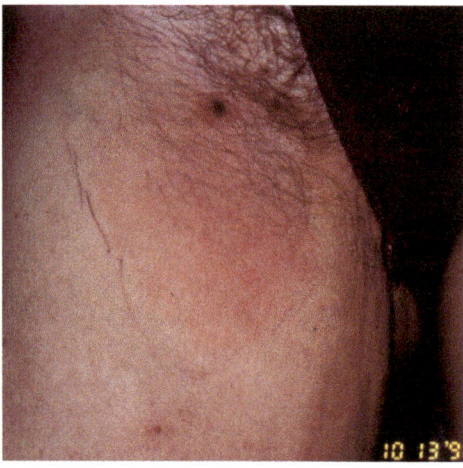

Fig. 10.5. A probable hypersensitivity reaction to a tick bite mimicking erythema migrans. The rash (well over 5 cm and thus technically fulfilling CDC criteria for a diagnosis of erythema migrans) was noted at the time an adult *Ixodes scapularis* tick was removed, a few hours prior to taking this photograph. The patient experienced intense pruritus at the site, which she had noted in the past with tick bites. There were no associated systemic symptoms. The rash resolved within approximately 48 h without treatment. The patient remained well and serology for antibodies to *Borreliella burgdorferi*, performed after approximately 3 months, was negative.

arthritis. The reason for this is that serologic tests are reportable and tabulated in some states if positive, as they often are in extracutaneous Lyme disease. In contrast, no such laboratory reporting occurs if the tests are negative, as they often are in patients with EM (see Section 10.2.10) (Aguero-Rosenfeld *et al.*, 1993; 2005; Wormser *et al.*, 2006).

There are two peaks in the age distribution for EM, occurring at 5–14 years old and 45–54 years old. Almost all cases of EM occur in late spring or summer (Falco *et al.*, 1999; Krause *et al.*, 2006) following bites of nymphal (rather than adult) *I. scapularis* ticks, which are most active from May through July (Fish, 1995; Falco *et al.*, 1999). This immature tick stage is more numerous than adult stage ticks. Nymphs are also much smaller than adult ticks and thus less likely to be noticed and removed before transmission of infection can occur (Nadelman *et al.*, 2001; Wormser *et al.*, 2006). In addition, humans are more likely to come into contact with ticks with increased outdoor activity during the warmer months (Fish, 1995).

10.2.2 Characteristics of EM

EM begins as a small macule or papule at the site of a bite by certain *Ixodes* ticks that have fed and detached a median of 7–14 days (range of 1–36 days) previously (Steere *et al.*, 1983b; Berger, 1989; Nadelman *et al.*, 1996; Nadelman and Wormser, 1998). European patients with EM are much more likely than US patients to recall a prior tick bite (Strle *et al.*, 1999, Strle *et al.*, 2011), perhaps because of more intense local reaction to the bite or faster transmission of infection. Only a minority (14–32%) (Nadelman *et al.*, 1996; Smith *et al.*, 2002; Wormser *et al.*, 2006) of US patients recall the bite that transmitted infection, in part because the vector nymphal stage ticks are only about the size of a poppy seed, and their bites are not associated with significant pruritus or pain (Nadelman and Wormser, 1995; Nadelman *et al.*, 2001; Wormser *et al.*, 2006). In addition, tick bites that ultimately result in infection typically occur at body sites where the tick can feed unvisualized for days, such as the buttocks in adults or the hairline of children (Nadelman and Wormser, 1995; Nadelman *et al.*, 1996;

Tibbles and Edlow, 2007). The likelihood of transmission of *B. burgdorferi* from an infected tick to a mammalian host is correlated with duration of attachment of the tick. Experimental infections in animal models indicate that ticks that are visualized and removed within 24–48 h of attachment are less likely to transmit disease (Falco *et al.*, 1996; Piesman *et al.*, 1987; Piesman, 1993). Selected features of EM, including the location of primary lesions in one study of 119 US patients whose infection was culture-confirmed, is depicted in Table 10.1 (Strle *et al.*, 1999). EM lesions do not occur on mucous membranes, palms or soles (Steere *et al.*, 1983b).

Within days of the appearance of the initial macule or papule, a slowly enlarging erythematous patch develops (Steere *et al.*, 1983b; Berger, 1989; Malane *et al.*, 1991; Habif, 2004), sometimes with a depressed or raised area (punctum) at the center of the lesion at the site of tick detachment (Berger, 1989; Malane *et al.*, 1991; Melski *et al.*, 1993; Nadelman and Wormser, 2007) (Fig. 10.1). An annular or 'bull's eye' appearance may develop when central or paracentral clearing occurs as the lesion expands over days to weeks. The skin lesion remains flat, blanches with pressure and usually does not desquamate or vesiculate at the periphery (Steere *et al.*, 1983b; Malane *et al.*, 1991; Nadelman and Wormser, 1995; Nadelman *et al.*, 1996; Smith *et al.*, 2002; Habif, 2004). The median diameter in each of five studies comprising a total of more than 500 US patients was between 10 and 16 cm but lesions may exceed 70 cm (Steere *et al.*, 1983b; Malane *et al.*, 1991; Nadelman *et al.*, 1996; Strle *et al.*, 1999; Smith *et al.*, 2002; Nowakowski *et al.*, 2003). EM size usually appears to be a function of its duration (Åsbrink and Olsson, 1985; Berger, 1989; Nadelman *et al.*, 1996; Strle *et al.*, 1999), varying in a linear fashion with a correlation coefficient of 0.7 (Nadelman *et al.*, 1996). Early EM lesions grow at a rate of 20 cm^2/day presumably related to the migration of spirochetes away from the inoculation site (Berger, 1989). *Borreliella burgdorferi* can be isolated from the center and leading margin of EM lesions, and from normal skin surrounding the lesion (Berger *et al.*, 1992; Kuiper *et al.*, 1994; Nadelman and Wormser, 1995; Nadelman *et al.*, 1996; Jurca *et al.*, 1998; Smith *et al.*, 2002).

It is incorrectly assumed by many practitioners and patients that EM usually has central clearing. This feature occurred in only 37% and 9% of cases, respectively, in two large studies conducted in the northeastern USA, involving nearly 200 patients with culture-confirmed EM (Nadelman *et al.*, 1996; Smith *et al.*, 2002). The reason for the discrepancy is related to early descriptions of Lyme disease from Europe and from the US in the days before effective antibiotic treatment was recognized. Since central clearing appears to be a function of duration of EM (Åsbrink and Olsson, 1985; Berger, 1989; Strle *et al.*, 1999) an annular appearance was emphasized in early descriptions of the longstanding rashes (i.e. erythema chronicum migrans (ECM)) that were seen in untreated patients. In addition, European cases, which comprised many of the first reports of Lyme disease, are most often associated with *B. afzelii*, which is responsible for a somewhat different clinical course and appearance of EM than disease related to *B. burgdorferi* sensu stricto in North America (Åsbrink and Olsson, 1985; Berger *et al.*, 1992; Kuiper *et al.*, 1994; Strle *et al.*, 1999; Lipsker *et al.*, 2002; Logar *et al.*, 2004). In one early Swedish study, 80% of cases had central clearing, associated with EM of 5–6 weeks' duration (Åsbrink and Olsson, 1985). This contrasts with US experience over the past two decades, where EM has been diagnosed and treated within 1–2 weeks of onset and usually lacks central or paracentral clearing at the time of presentation (Nadelman and Wormser, 1995; 2002; Nadelman *et al.*, 1996;

Table 10.1. Selected characteristics of 119 patients with culture-confirmed erythema migrans seen in Westchester County, New York. (Strle *et al.*, 1999.)

Characteristic	No. (%)
Recall of prior tick bite at site	30 (25)
Median duration of rash at presentation (days)	4 (range 1–39)
Median size of primary lesion (cm)	14 (range 5–73)
Multiple lesions	16 (13)
Location of primary lesion	
Trunk and abdomen[a]	60 (50)
Leg	40 (34)
Arm and shoulder	17 (14)
Head and neck	2 (2)
Central clearing of primary lesion	36 (35)

[a]Includes axilla, flank, groin

Smith et al., 2002). However, it is likely that additional factors besides rash duration influence whether central clearing occurs. In one study, Slovenian patients infected with B. garinii were nearly twice as likely as US patients infected with B. burgdorferi to have EM with central clearing despite similar durations of rash (Strle et al., 2011). Furthermore, there was no difference in duration of EM associated with B. garinii in the European patients who had central clearing compared with those who did not (Strle et al., 2011).

EM lesions are usually oval or circular, with the shape partially influenced by the pre-existing lines of skin tension (Berger 1989; Malane et al., 1991; Melski et al., 1993; Nadelman and Wormser, 1995). For example, groin lesions are generally oval along the horizontal axis (Malane et al., 1991; Melski et al., 1993; Nadelman and Wormser, 1995). Unusual configurations such as triangles may occur (Berger, 1989; Malane et al., 1991) (Fig. 10.2). EM margins are usually regular and are not raised compared with the interior. Central vesicles were present in 8% of lesions in one study (Fig. 10.3) (Goldberg et al., 1992), which may lead to confusion with spider bites, contact dermatitis, or even herpes simplex or varicella zoster virus infection.

Scaling is uncommon in EM lesions, occurring primarily at the tick bite site (punctum), in fading rashes of long duration or after antimicrobial treatment (Nadelman and Wormser, 1995). Use of topical steroids may also lead to scaling, in addition to conferring an uncharacteristic pallor (Nadelman and Wormser, 1995). EM lesions display a degree of erythema from faint pink to dark red. Lesions on the lower extremities may acquire a bluish tint (Berger, 1989; Malane et al., 1991). Lesions are warmer than surrounding normal appearing skin. Pruritus or pain may be present at the site of EM but is almost always mild in severity (Åsbrink and Olsson, 1985; Malane et al., 1991; Nadelman et al., 1996; Strle et al., 1996a; 1996b; Logar et al., 2004). A minority of patients, more often in Europe, experience transient numbness or tingling at the site of EM (Steere et al., 1983b; Åsbrink and Olsson, 1985; Malane et al., 1991; Kuiper et al., 1994; Nadelman et al., 1996; Smith et al., 2002; Logar et al., 2004). In some patients, secondary lesions may arise as the result of spirochetemia (see Section 10.2.5)

10.2.3 Associated systemic symptoms

As many as 80% of US patients with EM have related systemic complaints that may precede, accompany or follow resolution of the EM (Steere et al., 1983b; Berger, 1989; Nadelman and Wormser, 1995). The most common systemic complaints in more than 600 US patients enrolled in four large prospective studies were malaise (10–80%), headache (28–64%), fever and chills (31–59%), and myalgias and arthralgias (35–48%), with nausea, anorexia, dizziness and difficulty concentrating reported less frequently (Steere et al., 1983b; Berger, 1989; Nadelman et al., 1996; Smith et al., 2002). Neither diarrhea nor respiratory symptoms are characteristic of Lyme disease and, if present, should raise the possibility of a different diagnosis or an additional co-existing process that is unrelated.

Systemic symptoms are less frequent in European than in US patients with EM, reported in 23–50% of more than 800 patients in representative prospective studies from five different European countries (Åsbrink and Olsson, 1985; Weber et al., 1988; 1990; Kuiper et al., 1994; Strle et al., 1996a; 1996b; 1999; Lipsker et al., 2002; Logar et al., 2004). The disparity between US and European disease is probably largely attributable to the lower virulence of European genospecies compared with B. burgdorferi sensu stricto, the only genospecies that has been implicated as causing human disease in the US (Nadelman and Wormser, 1998; Strle et al., 1999, Strle et al., 2011; Antoni-Bach et al., 2002; Logar et al., 2004; Cerar et al., 2010). Borreliella afzelii (the major cause of EM in Europe) appears to be less virulent than B. garinii, a European genospecies that also appears to be the most neurotropic (Logar et al., 2004). Patients with EM caused by B. garinii tended to have more frequent myalgia and chills, more often had local symptoms and abnormal liver function tests, were more frequently seropositive, and had a shorter incubation period and faster evolution of EM, when compared with patients having EM associated with B. afzelii (Logar et al., 2004). EM caused by either of these species in Slovenian patients was associated with significantly less systemic symptomatology than occurs in US patients infected with B. burgdorferi sensu stricto (Strle et al., 1999; 2011). These differences may be partially attributable to a greater ability of

B. burgdorferi sensu stricto to stimulate macrophages to secrete higher levels of chemokines and cytokines and to activate both innate and adaptive immune responses compared with European genospecies (Strle *et al.*, 2009).

A new species of *B. burgdorferi* sensu lato, provisionally designated *B. mayonii*, has been identified in patients in the upper Midwestern United States. Although only a few patients have been described to date, there appear to be potential differences in the frequency of spirochetemia and, possibly related, the incidence of multiple EM lesions; however, the number of patients described with *B. mayonii* remains too low to draw definitive conclusions (Pritt *et al.*, 2016).

10.2.4 Associated findings on physical examination

The most common objective physical findings at the time of diagnosis of EM in US patients are regional lymphadenopathy (23–41%), fever (14–31%) and pain on neck flexion (5–20%) (Steere *et al.*, 1983b; Nadelman *et al.*, 1996; Smith *et al.*, 2002; Nowakowski *et al.*, 2003). One to six percent of patients have concomitant cranial nerve palsies (usually facial nerve) (Steere *et al.*, 1983b; Nadelman *et al.*, 1996; Smith *et al.*, 2002; Nowakowski *et al.*, 2003). Abnormal physical findings were much more common in patients with EM from New York State infected with *B. burgdorferi* sensu stricto than in patients from Slovenia with either *B. afzelii* or *B. garinii* infection (Strle *et al.*, 1999; 2011). Regional lymphadenopathy, found in 7.2% of 316 patients from two prospective studies was the most common finding in Slovenian patients (Strle *et al.*, 1996a; 1996b; 1999).

10.2.5 Multiple erythema migrans and spirochetemia

Half of 314 patients with EM in an observational study conducted in Connecticut from 1976 though 1982 developed multiple annular secondary lesions (Steere *et al.*, 1983b), with 13% of patients having more than 20 lesions, including two patients with more than 100 (Fig. 10.4). Secondary lesions are similar in morphology to the initial (i.e. primary) lesion with which most patients present but are typically smaller (usually 2–3 cm) (Steere *et al.*, 1983b; Malane *et al.*, 1991; Melski *et al.*, 1993). Like primary lesions, they are not present on mucous membranes, palms or soles. Since secondary lesions, the result of hematogenous dissemination of spirochetes to new sites, are not at the site of tick bites, they lack a punctum, vesiculation, local pruritus and tenderness. Viable spirochetes may be recovered from a biopsy of the lesion or from blood using special culture media (Melski *et al.*, 1993; Wormser *et al.*, 2005a). Secondary lesions may be fleeting, emerging and vanishing suddenly during examination (Steere *et al.*, 1983b). Such evanescent lesions were described in one series as a separate entity, appearing for several weeks in untreated patients after resolution of primary and secondary lesions (Steere *et al.*, 1983b).

Up to half of US patients with EM have detectable spirochetemia at the time of presentation when blood is cultured with high volume ($\geq$9 ml) samples (Wormser *et al.*, 2005a). The percentage of positive blood cultures can be increased to 70% with the addition of quantitative polymerase chain reaction (PCR) of the incubating cultures (Liveris *et al.*, 2011). The duration of spirochetemia is unknown, but in one study blood cultures were positive in one-third to one-half of untreated patients seen at presentation at various time intervals ranging from 1–37 days after appearance of EM (Wormser *et al.*, 2005a). Systemic symptoms are more frequent in patients with spirochetemia than in those with negative blood cultures, and spirochetemic patients also have more symptoms as well as a higher cumulative symptom severity score (Wormser *et al.*, 2005a). Chills (but not fever), headaches, stiff neck, multiple EM lesions (40%) and regional lymphadenopathy are significantly more likely to be present in this group (Wormser *et al.*, 2005a). However, no single characteristic or combination of variables had enough specificity and sensitivity (>80%) to predict spirochetemia (Wormser *et al.*, 2005a).

10.2.6 Influence of strain differences on clinical manifestations

Hematogenous dissemination of *B. burgdorferi* from the initial site of the primary EM lesion is believed to be responsible for the occurrence of multiple EM lesions and the objective extracutaneous manifestations of Lyme disease (e.g. facial nerve palsy, meningitis, carditis and arthritis). *Borreliella burgdorferi* sensu stricto can be classified into subtypes, using restriction fragment length polymorphism (RFLP) to determine the 16S–23S ribosome intergenic spacer type (RST) of *B. burgdorferi* (Liveris *et al.*, 1999), or based on genotyping of the outer surface protein (Osp) C gene (Seinost *et al.*, 1999; Grimm *et al.*, 2004). Certain subtypes of *B. burgdorferi* have been linked to disseminated disease, while others appear less likely to circulate in the blood (Liveris *et al.*, 1999; Seinost *et al.*, 1999; Wormser *et al.*, 2005a), perhaps accounting for the observation in one study that 20% of 55 untreated patients with EM remained symptom free after a median of 6 (range 3–8) years. In general, patients infected with RST 1, RST 2 and *OspC* types A, B, I and K are more likely to have multiple EM lesions and spirochetemia (Liveris *et al.*, 1999; Seinost *et al.*, 1999). However, some patients with solitary EM lesions and less invasive subtypes may have significant systemic complaints, implying that other factors (e.g. host factors (Wormser *et al.*, 2005d) or cytokine production) may contribute to these symptoms. Preliminary results of a study of patients with EM indicated that patients infected with RST 1 strains had more symptoms and greater cytokine levels including IFN-γ, IFN-γ-inducible chemokines, CXCL9 and CXCL10 (Strle *et al.*, 2010). In addition, in this report, peripheral blood mononuclear cells from healthy humans secreted significantly higher levels of IFN-α, IFN-γ and CXCL10 when stimulated with RST 1 isolates compared with RST 2 or RST 3 strains (Strle *et al.*, 2010).

10.2.7 Differential diagnosis

The most important but too often ignored key to recognizing EM is to perform an examination of the entire body with all clothes removed in order to evaluate areas poorly visualized by the patient. It is not uncommon to identify an EM previously unrecognized by a patient with an otherwise non-specific acute illness. The diagnosis of EM should be considered especially in patients from endemic areas who present with new unexplained complaints of headache, myalgia, arthralgia and fever during the late spring and summer, even if a rash is initially not reported (Nadelman and Wormser, 1995; Nadelman *et al.*, 1997). The diagnosis of EM should also be considered in patients with unexplained atrioventricular heart block, since carditis due to *B. burgdorferi* has been reported in 2–9% of untreated patients with EM (the higher incidence was observed in early studies predating recognition of effective antimicrobial therapy for Lyme disease) (Steere *et al.*, 1983b; Rubin *et al.*, 1992; Haddad and Nadelman, 2003).

One report investigated the diagnostic value of clinical history and physical examination in the assessment of rashes consistent with EM (Tibbles and Edlow, 2007). The authors reviewed more than 50 European and US studies that enrolled more than 8000 patients but were unable to identify a single element in the history or physical examination that was alone highly sensitive for the diagnosis of EM. In view of the wide variability in the clinical presentation, the authors cited the need for an algorithm combining specific signs or symptoms to improve diagnostic sensitivity (Tibbles and Edlow, 2007).

EM as a manifestation of Lyme disease only occurs in areas where vector ticks (*Ixodes scapularis* or *I. pacificus* in the US, *I. ricinis* in Europe and *I. persulcatus* in Eurasia) are infected with *B. burgdorferi* sensu lato. In other parts of the world where infected vectors are not present (Sharma *et al.*, 2010) or infrequently bite humans (Felz *et al.*, 1996), rashes that are target-like or have other features resembling EM are not likely to be associated with Lyme disease (i.e. *B. burgdorferi* infection). Instead, other entities should be considered.

Perhaps the most important alternative diagnosis to consider is a hypersensitivity reaction to the bite of an arthropod. An erythematous lesion surrounding a bite site while a tick is still attached, or within 48 h of detachment, is most likely a hypersensitivity reaction to the tick bite, and is not an indication of infection (Nadelman and Wormser, 1995; Wormser, 2006; Wormser *et al.*, 2006; Feder and Whitaker, 1995) (Table 10.2). Despite education efforts, there continues to be significant misclassification of hypersensitivity reactions as EM lesions by primary care practitioners, with over 60% of cases of Lyme disease in one series attributed to misdiagnosed hypersensitivity reactions (Gasmi *et al.*,

Table 10.2. Differentiating erythema migrans from hypersensitivity reaction to an arthropod bite. (Adapted from Nadelman and Wormser, 1995. Reprinted by permission of Elsevier, Infectious Disease Clinics of North America.)

Characteristic	Erythema migrans	Arthropod bite hypersensitivity reaction
Recall of bite at site	~20%	Variable
Tick present at time of rash	No	Yes (or detached within prior 24 h); also may occur after other arthropod (e.g. mosquito) bites
Time interval between bite and rash	Median 7–10 days (range 1–36 days)[a]	Hours
Location	Intertriginous areas, border of tight fitting clothing	Same; also can occur on exposed areas such as face or forearm
Local symptoms	Rare; minimal if present	Pruritus
Evolution	Expands over days to weeks	Expands over hours
Resolution	Days to weeks (median 4 weeks if untreated)[b]	Less than 48 h
Size	≥5 cm (can be smaller)	<5 cm (can be larger)
Systemic symptoms	Up to 80%	Absent
Fever	16% documented, 39% subjective[c]	Absent

[a]Steere et al. (1983b); Berger (1989); Nadelman and Wormser (1995); Nadelman et al. (1996).
[b]Steere et al. (1983b).
[c]Nadelman et al. (1996).

2017). Hypersensitivity lesions may be associated with significant pruritus (atypical for EM), and generally fade spontaneously within 24–48 h. In contrast, an EM lesion typically increases progressively in size over this time frame. Although local bite reactions are usually less than 5 cm in the largest diameter, they may expand (usually over hours rather than days, in contrast to EM) to a much larger size before spontaneously fading. More than half of patients with EM seen in the US also have accompanying systemic symptoms, unlike those with local tick bite hypersensitivity reactions. In cases of uncertainty in the diagnosis, it may be helpful for the health care practitioner to mark the contours of the rash with ink and observe over 1–2 days without treatment. If the rash expands or systemic symptoms develop antimicrobial treatment should be initiated, whereas if the rash resolves within 48 h, no treatment is necessary (Nadelman and Wormser, 1995; Wormser et al., 2006) (Fig. 10.5).

Although arthropod bites unassociated with EM occur during the late spring and summer when EM is most prevalent, other processes do not have a seasonal variation. Staphylococcal and streptococcal cellulitis tend to develop rapidly, evolving over hours with a band-like rather than oval or circular shape, and are usually painful. They are commonly associated with high fever, leukocytosis and often a toxic-appearing patient, all which are uncommon with EM. Cellulitis caused by pyogenic organisms usually occurs on the distal lower extremities, sometimes after trauma, and often in a person with underlying vascular disease (e.g. venous stasis) or with a history of prior surgery that adversely affected venous or lymphatic flow (e.g. saphenous vein harvesting for coronary artery bypass surgery or mastectomy) (Nadelman and Wormser, 1995). Conversely, the location of an erythematous rash at locations unusual for bacterial cellulitis (e.g. buttocks, groin, axilla, popliteal fossa) should significantly raise the suspicion for EM.

Patients with EM lesions having vesicular centers often present with the complaint of an unwitnessed 'spider bite' (Fig. 10.3). This scenario should raise the suspicion for atypical EM in most areas of the US endemic for Lyme disease since there is little overlap with the geographic range of the brown recluse spider (which extends from southeastern Nebraska to southern Ohio) (Vetter and Bush, 2002; Frithsen et al., 2007). EM lesions with vesicular centers may also be confused with herpes simplex or varicella zoster infections, but, unlike the latter viral exanthem, lack a dermatomal distribution.

Although vesicular EM lesions may be somewhat more tender than those without vesiculation, pain is very prominent in herpetic lesions.

Tinea infection may resemble EM with an erythematous border and central clearing. However, tinea rashes evolve much more slowly than EM (weeks to months rather than days to weeks) and systemic symptoms are absent. Scaling and thin irregular raised borders should suggest tinea. Characteristics of some skin disorders that may be confused with EM are summarized in Table 10.3.

10.2.8 Southern tick-associated rash infection (STARI)

A rash resembling EM that occurs in many patients residing in the southern US must be distinguished from EM caused by *B. burgdorferi* (Kirkland et al., 1997; Masters et al., 1998; Wormser et al., 2005c). Similarities with EM include rash appearance (including occasional multiple lesions), peak incidence in summer and similar incubation period after a tick bite. However, in contrast to patients with Lyme disease, efforts to culture *B. burgdorferi* in Barbour–Stoenner–Kelly (BSK) media from biopsied skin lesions from patients with EM-like lesions in the southern USA have been consistently unsuccessful (in contrast to EM associated with Lyme disease where biopsy cultures have been positive in 50–86% of US patients (Berger et al., 1992; Nowakowski et al., 2001)). Acute and convalescent phase serologic assays are almost always negative for antibodies to *B. burgdorferi* in patients with EM-like rashes in the southern US (Wormser et al., 2005b; 2005c). In addition, *I. scapularis* ticks, the usual vector for Lyme disease, are rarely infected with *B. burgdorferi* in the southern US (<0.5%) and infrequently bite humans (Felz et al., 1996). The tick vector for this rash in patients in the south appears to be *Amblyomma americanum*, which is not believed to be a competent vector for *B. burgdorferi* (Piesman and Sinsky, 1988). Therefore, it has been concluded that this rash does not represent Lyme disease; instead it is known as STARI, or Masters' disease (after a key investigator) (Masters et al., 1998, Wormser et al., 2005b; 2005c). Although a new *Borrelia* genospecies, *B. lonestarii*, was postulated to be the pathogen (Barbour et al., 1996), a subsequent study of 19 patients with STARI failed to detect this organism (Wormser et al., 2005b), and the etiology remains unknown. Patients with STARI have clinical characteristics somewhat distinct from EM patients with *B. burgdorferi* infection (Wormser et al., 2005c). In a prospective clinical evaluation of patients from Missouri with STARI and patients from New York with EM, the Missouri patients were significantly more likely to recall a tick bite, and had a shorter time to onset of rash than the New York patients. EM-like lesions in the Missouri patients were more circular and smaller in size, but more likely to have central clearing. The New York patients were more likely to be symptomatic, and were more likely to have multiple skin lesions. The Missouri patients recovered more rapidly than the New York patients (Wormser et al., 2005c).

The range of *Amblyomma* ticks has been expanding in recent years and now extends up the eastern coast into Maine as well as in the Midwestern US where *B. burgdorferi* is present. Cases of STARI occurring in Lyme endemic areas have been reported (Feder et al.,2011). Distinguishing between STARI and EM lesions in Lyme endemic areas is difficult and current recommendations are to treat these rashes as EM in patients with exposure in these areas unless the tick has been identified (Sanchez et al., 2016).

10.2.9 Co-infection

Patients with EM may also be co-infected with other tick-borne pathogens, since *I. scapularis*, the vector tick for *B. burgdorferi*, may transmit the protozoan *Babesia microti* causing babesiosis, a malaria-like infection (Krause et al., 1996; Steere et al., 2003; Wormser et al., 2006); the bacterium, *Anaplasma phagocytophilum*, the agent of human granulocytic anaplasmosis (HGA) (formerly known as human granulocytic ehrlichiosis (he)) (Nadelman et al., 1997; Belongia et al., 1999; Steere et al., 2003; Wormser et al., 2006); or *Borrelia miyamotoi*, a relapsing fever like spirochete (Platanov et al., 2011; Chowdri et al., 2013; Krause et al., 2015; Molloy et al., 2015; Sinski et al., 2016). In Eurasia, *I. ricinus* and *I. persulcatus*, the vector ticks for *B. burgdorferi* sensu lato, may also transmit the flavivirus causing tick-borne encephalitis (Mansfield et al.,

Table 10.3. Differential diagnosis of erythema migrans. (Adapted from Feder and Whitaker, 1995 and Tibbles and Edlow, 2007. Reprinted by permission of Elsevier, Infectious Disease Clinics of North America and JAMA.)[a]

Diagnosis	Appearance	Body site	Size	Progression	Seasonal tendency	Miscellaneous
Tinea (ringworm)	Ring shape, with satellite lesions; scaling at periphery	Variable; exposed skin	1–10 cm	Days to weeks	No	Pruritus; pet exposure
Bacterial cellulitis	Homogenous erythema; band-like appearance; warm and tender, lymphangitic streaking; tender regional lymphadenopathy	Distal extremities; site of prior trauma	Rarely large except on lower extremities	More rapid than EM (hours to days)	No	Pain, fever, leukocytosis; history of prior trauma, vascular disease or surgery
Contact dermatitis	Shape related to contact; vesicles and bullae may be present	Variable	Variable	Variable (often slow progression)	No	Pruritus often severe; history of contact with inciting substance (e.g., poison ivy)
Urticaria	Raised, multiple lesions	Variable	Variable	Waxes and wanes over hours	No	Pruritus
Fixed drug eruption	Deep, well demarcated violaceous plaque	Fixed, often involves genitals	Variable	Fixed in size	No	Burning
Brown recluse spider bite	Necrotic; red white and blue sign	Extremities	Variable	Spreads centrifugally	Yes (mates May to September)	May be painful; uncommon in northeastern US
Herpes simplex/varicella zoster	Vesicles on erythematous base	Dermatomal distribution	Variable	May progress rapidly (days)	No	Prodrome may occur; pain (sometimes severe); pruritus, fever
Nummular eczema	Circular red lesions	Variable	Variable	Slow progression, slow resolution	No	Can often be pruritic; plaque-like lesions
STARI	Circular lesions emanating from a tick bite site	Variable	Typically 6–10 cm	Onset within 7 days of tick bite. Spontaneous resolution	Seasonal with tick feeding	Multiple lesions less common than with Lyme

[a] See Table 10.2 for distinguishing erythema migrans from a hypersensitivity reaction to an arthropod bite.

2009). In the US, *I. scapularis* may transmit related viruses, such as deer tick virus (DTV), that can cause encephalitis (El Khoury, 2013). Since *B. burgdorferi* infection does not cause cytopenias, the occurrence of leukopenia, thrombocytopenia or anemia in a patient with Lyme disease should suggest co-infection (Nadelman et al., 1997; 1999; Belongia et al., 1999). Abnormal transaminases and other liver enzymes may be present in patients with Lyme disease but are particularly common in patients with HGA (Steere et al., 1983b; Nadelman et al., 1996) and *B. miyamotoi* infection. Co-infection should be strongly considered in a patient without a rapid improvement (48 h) after receiving either amoxicillin or cefuroxime axetil (which have no activity against HGA, unlike doxycycline), particularly if fever persists (Wormser, 2006; Wormser et al., 2006). A toxic appearance or an illness requiring intensive care in a patient with EM should initiate a prompt assessment for babesiosis (especially in an immunocompromised or asplenic patient (Krause et al., 2008)) or HGA (Bakken and Dumler, 2006) since these illnesses may be fatal.

10.2.10 Laboratory diagnosis

The diagnosis of EM is made on clinical grounds based upon the characteristic appearance of the skin lesion in a patient with the appropriate epidemiologic and exposure history. Routine laboratory tests such as complete blood counts and liver enzyme assays may, if abnormal, point to co-infection with *A. phagocytophilum* or *Babesia microti* (see Section 10.2.9) but are usually unremarkable, as is sedimentation rate. However, support for the clinical diagnosis can be made through specific laboratory testing, with isolation of *B. burgdorferi* in culture from skin and/or blood being the gold standard for accurate identification.

Although the sensitivity of blood and skin biopsy cultures in EM (as high as 50% (Wormser et al., 2000) and 86% (Berger et al., 1992), respectively), is actually greater than that for cellulitis caused by pyogenic bacteria (Sigurdsson and Gudmundsson, 1989), these techniques are of limited value in clinical practice. This is because of the invasive (although minimally so) biopsy procedure and special isolation media required, the delay in detecting growth of *B. burgdorferi* until an average of approximately 2 weeks (although 90% of cultures that will turn positive do so within 1 week), the added cost and, most importantly, the straightforward *clinical* diagnosis of EM in endemic areas rendering laboratory testing superfluous in most cases. However, laboratory tests may help validate the diagnosis when a rash is atypical or the exposure history uncertain, especially in an investigational setting (i.e. treatment trials or epidemiologic studies). Besides culture, the diagnosis of infection with *B. burgdorferi* may be supported by serology (acute and convalescent phase), and PCR (nested and quantitative reverse transcription (RT) PCR from skin). These tests were compared in 47 patients with EM (Table 10.4) (Nowakowski et al., 2001).

The most practical laboratory method available to the clinician is serologic testing for antibodies to *B. burgdorferi* using a two-tier system (usually polyvalent enzyme-linked immunosorbent assay (ELISA) followed by IgM and IgG immunoblots if the first step test is positive or equivocal) (CDC, 1995; Aguero-Rosenfeld et al., 2005; Wormser et al., 2006; Sanchez et al., 2016). However, serology lacks sensitivity in early Lyme disease; half of patients with EM have negative results on initial antibody testing (Aguero-Rosenfeld et al., 1993; 2005; Nowakowski et al., 2001). The probability of seroreactivity increases significantly with increased duration

Table 10.4. Comparison of diagnostic tests for 47 adult patients with erythema migrans. (From Nowakowski et al., 2001. Reprinted by permission of the University of Chicago Press, Clinical Infectious Diseases.)

Diagnostic method	No (%) positive result
Skin culture	24 (51.1)
Blood culture (18 ml)	21 (44.7)
Any culture	31 (66)
Nested PCR	30 (63.8)
Quantitative PCR	38 (80.9)
Any PCR	38 (80.9)
Acute phase serology	19 (40.4)
Convalescent phase serology	31 (66)
Any serology	32 (68.1)
Any test positive	44 (93.6)
All tests negative	3 (6.4)

of EM (Aguero-Rosenfeld et al., 1993; 2005). In one report, all 14 patients presenting with an EM duration of ≥2 weeks had positive ELISA and IgM immunoblot at study entry (Aguero-Rosenfeld et al., 1993). A further increase in the sensitivity of serologic testing can be accomplished by including convalescent phase testing (Aguero-Rosenfeld et al., 2005; Wormser et al., 2006). Recently, the use of a C6 ELISA, based on a peptide (C6) with the amino acid sequence of a conserved, immunodominant region of the VlsE protein of B. burgdorferi, has been proposed to replace immunoblotting in two-tiered testing with little loss of sensitivity or specificity, especially in patients with EM (Branda et al., 2011; Molins et al., 2016). However, one caveat is that this strategy cannot differentiate B. miyamotoi infection from B. burgdorferi as serum from patients infected with B. miyamotoi can cross react with both the EIA and C6 (Sudhindra et al., 2016).

In summary, the routine use of laboratory testing is not presently recommended for patients with EM because the clinical identification of EM is usually clear-cut, and since serology often yields false negative results (Wormser et al., 2006). Diagnostic testing in patients with EM should generally be reserved for problematic cases (e.g. difficulty in distinguishing between EM and a hypersensitivity reaction to an arthropod bite, or an EM-like rash in a non-endemic region), or for those in clinical trials or epidemiologic studies for whom a definitive diagnosis is essential. Use of the laboratory in the diagnosis of Lyme disease is discussed in more detail in Chapter 4.

10.3 Treatment

10.3.1 Long-term outcome of untreated patients

Untreated EM resolves spontaneously, within a median of 4 weeks (Steere et al., 1983b; 1987). Prior to the recognition that antimicrobial treatment was effective in both hastening resolution of EM and associated symptoms and preventing extracutaneous complications, a group of 55 patients was followed prospectively for a median duration of 6 years without receiving antimicrobial therapy (Steere et al., 1987). All EM lesions resolved spontaneously but after 1–14 months, 9% had experienced recurrent EM at the site of the primary lesion, 5% had recurrence of secondary lesions and 7% had recurrence of both. Evanescent lesions returned in 5% including two children whose frequent episodes occurred over more than 3 years. In 12 patients, other manifestations of Lyme disease accompanied the recurrent skin lesions (Steere et al., 1983b). Eighty percent of those enrolled had joint symptoms ranging from arthralgias to intermittent episodes of arthritis, to chronic synovitis. Fourteen percent of these 44 patients with joint symptoms also developed neurologic abnormalities while 4% also had cardiac abnormalities. 51% of patients experienced intermittent attacks of monoarticular or oligoarticular arthritis of large joints (almost always involving the knee), beginning months after the initial infection (Steere et al., 1987). Many patients experienced repeated attacks of arthritis for years, but the number of recurrences decreased each year by 10 to 20% (Steere et al., 1987). Severity of symptoms at onset of illness predicted development of late disease (arthritis) (Steere et al., 1987). However, over a median of 6 years (range 3–8 years) follow-up, 20% of the 55 patients originally enrolled with EM had no subsequent manifestations of Lyme disease.

10.3.2 Treatment trials

The first randomized prospective trial in the US to study treatment for EM compared 10-day courses of tetracycline, penicillin or erythromycin in 112 patients (Steere et al., 1983a). EM and associated symptoms improved more rapidly in patients receiving penicillin or tetracycline compared with those receiving erythromycin. An intensification of fever, rash or pain in the first 24 h after initiation of antimicrobial therapy, experienced by 15%, was considered to constitute a Jarisch–Hexheimer-like reaction. Patients treated with tetracycline or penicillin were less likely than those receiving erythromycin to develop objective extracutaneous complications such as meningitis, carditis and arthritis (Steere et al., 1983a). No additional benefit was experienced by those who completed 20, as opposed to 10 days of tetracycline (Steere et al., 1983a). In two subsequent smaller studies, rapid resolution of EM and associated symptoms, and a satisfactory outcome at 6 months were observed in nearly all patients who were randomized to receive either doxycycline or amoxicillin (to which probenecid was added to increase drug levels) (Dattwyler et al., 1990; Massarotti et al., 1992). Patients receiving azithromycin in a third treatment arm in one of these studies had a similar favorable outcome (Massarotti et al., 1992).

Oral cefuroxime axetil 500 mg twice daily and doxycycline 100 mg three times daily, for 20 days (rather than the usual twice daily dose), were compared in two randomized multicenter investigator-blinded prospective controlled studies including 364 patients (from New York, New Jersey and Connecticut) with EM (Nadelman et al., 1992; Luger et al., 1995). A satisfactory clinical outcome (defined as resolution of EM by day 5 post-treatment completion with resolution or improvement of associated signs and symptoms at 1 month post-treatment) was observed in 93% and 90% of the cefuroxime axetil groups and in 88% and 95% of the doxycycline groups in the two respective studies (Nadelman et al., 1992; Luger et al., 1995). Of those who were evaluable one year after treatment, satisfactory outcomes were observed in 90% and 95% of patients receiving cefuroxime axetil and in 92% and 100% of those treated with doxycycline, in the two respective studies (Nadelman et al., 1992; Luger et al., 1995). Patients with unsatisfactory outcomes principally had subjective symptoms including musculoskeletal complaints, headache, paresthesias, malaise and fatigue; several patients developed objective arthritis, although this was in some cases considered by the investigators to be unrelated to B. burgdorferi infection (Nadelman et al., 1992; Luger et al., 1995). Patients receiving cefuroxime axetil experienced diarrhea significantly more often, while those treated with doxycycline were significantly more likely to experience photosensitivity reactions. Most adverse effects were mild and did not result in patients stopping treatment (Nadelman et al., 1992; Luger et al., 1995). In summary, cefuroxime axetil and doxycycline were equally well tolerated, and equally effective in treatment of early Lyme disease and prevention of extracutaneous disease at 1 year of follow-up (Nadelman et al., 1992; Luger et al., 1995).

An additional prospective (but unblinded) controlled multicenter clinical trial evaluated the efficacy of oral doxycycline vs. parenteral ceftriaxone for treatment of adult and pediatric patients with EM and disseminated Lyme disease (defined as ≥2 erythema migrans lesions; carditis manifested by heart block; neurologic abnormalities [seventh cranial nerve palsy or radiculitis of less than 3 months' duration]; and acute large joint arthritis) (Dattwyler et al., 1997). Patients with meningitis were excluded from the study. Of 140 patients with EM and disseminated disease, 133 (95%) had multiple EM lesions at enrollment, 9 (6%) had carditis, 10 (7%) had facial nerve palsy and 9 (6%) had joint swelling. Adult patients received either 21 days of oral doxycycline (100 mg twice daily) or 14 days of parenteral ceftriaxone (2 g daily, intravenously or intramuscularly, at the discretion of the treating physician). Doses for children were adjusted for weight. Resolution of symptoms and prevention of complications were comparable in the two treatment groups (85% and 88% cured in the ceftriaxone and doxycycline groups, respectively, with most of the remainder unevaluable due to inadequate follow-up or withdrawal from the study) (Dattwyler et al., 1997). Only two patients were felt to have failed treatment, one with facial nerve palsy that persisted despite an additional 5-week course of ceftriaxone, and another patient who developed arthritis that ultimately resolved after treatment with a 3-week course of ceftriaxone.

Azithromycin (500 mg daily for 7 days) was compared with amoxicillin (500 mg three times daily for 20 days) in a multicenter prospective controlled randomized trial enrolling 246 patients (from two areas of New York, Connecticut, Missouri, Wisconsin, New Jersey, Minnesota, California and Rhode Island) (Luft et al., 1996). (It is probable that the patients from Missouri, a non-endemic area for Lyme disease, had STARI rather than EM.) Amoxicillin was significantly more effective than azithromycin in bringing about the resolution of EM and accompanying symptoms, and in preventing objective evidence of relapse at 6 months (Luft et al., 1996). It is unclear whether the worse outcomes associated with azithromycin were related to the relatively short duration of treatment, to low achievable levels in blood or other body compartments, or to other factors.

Azithromycin appeared to be more effective in European studies of early Lyme disease. Azithromycin showed comparable efficacy to phenoxymethylpenicillin and to doxycycline, possibly resulting in more rapid resolution of symptoms in prospective randomized trials from Slovenia and Germany (Strle et al., 1992; 1996a; 1996b; Weber et al., 1993). A Scandinavian clinical trial of patients with uncomplicated EM compared phenoxymethylpenicillin to roxithromycin, a semi-synthetic macrolide with promising *in vitro* activity against *B. burgdorferi* (Hansen et al., 1992). The study had to be terminated prematurely because of treatment failure in 5 out of 19 patients receiving roxithromycin, including 1 patient who developed neuroborreliosis and 2 patients whose persistent EM was confirmed through isolation in culture of *B. burgdorferi* sensu lato. This compared with no failures among 10 patients randomized to receive phenoxymethylpenicillin (Hansen et al., 1992).

Ten-day courses of tetracyclines have been shown to have comparable efficacy to longer courses (Steere et al., 1983a; Nowakowski et al., 1995; Wormser et al., 2003; Kowalski et al., 2010). A prospective randomized double blind controlled trial in Westchester County, New York, compared 10 days of oral doxycycline twice daily with or without a single 2-g IV dose of ceftriaxone, to 20 days of oral doxycycline twice daily (Wormser et al., 2003). The rate of complete response was similar for the three treatment groups at all assessment times over 30 months. Regardless of the regimen, objective evidence of treatment failure was extremely rare (Wormser et al., 2003). It was concluded that extending the course of doxycycline from 10 to 20 days, or adding one dose of ceftriaxone IV at the beginning of a 10-day course of doxycycline did not enhance therapeutic efficacy in patients with EM (Wormser et al., 2003). A retrospective study of 607 adult patients with early Lyme disease from Wisconsin evaluated outcomes a mean of 2.9 years after initiation of treatment with ≤10 days, 11–15 days or ≥16 days of antimicrobials (93% doxycycline, 4% amoxicillin and the remainder with other or unknown medication) (Kowalski et al., 2010). Two-thirds of patients (404 of 607) had EM including 275 (45%) with single and 129 (21%) with multiple EM lesions. A small percentage (4%) of patients with EM received retreatment for 'possible treatment failure', related to subjective symptoms and/or positive serologic tests. Only four patients (1%) with EM were considered to have had objective treatment failure. One of these patients developed facial nerve palsy on the 12th day of doxycycline. In two others who developed facial nerve palsy 1 year and 3 years after treatment, reinfection could not be ruled out. The last patient developed facial nerve palsy and lymphocytic meningitis after being treated with cefadroxil, a first-generation cephalosporin without significant activity against *B. burgdorferi* (Agger et al., 1992). His illness promptly responded to doxycycline. In summary, the overall outcome, regardless of treatment duration was excellent (Kowalski et al., 2010).

10.3.3 Treatment recommendations

A low incidence of serious adverse effects has been observed in treatment trials for early Lyme disease. Doxycycline has the advantage of good oral absorption, twice daily dosing and efficacy against *A. phagocytophilum*, with which patients may be co-infected when compared to other agents. Recent studies have also shown that oral doxycycline is as effective as intravenous ceftriaxone for treatment of CNS infection (Karlsson et al., 1994; Dotevall and Hagberg, 1999; Borg et al., 2005; Ljostad et al., 2008; Bremell and Dotevall, 2014). However, doxycycline may cause photosensitivity, a serious concern since EM usually occurs in late spring or summer. Patients receiving doxycycline should accordingly be counseled regarding avoiding strong sunlight, and using sun block. In addition, since doxycycline has been associated with esophagitis, patients should be advised to drink a full 8 oz (227 ml) of fluid with this medication, and should avoid a recumbent position for 1 h afterwards. Doxycycline has been considered relatively contraindicated in children <8 years old and in pregnant and breastfeeding women but this is being reconsidered, at least for rickettsial diseases (Biggs et al., 2016). Amoxicillin and cefuroxime axetil have been associated with rash, diarrhea and other adverse effects. Ceftriaxone has no advantage over oral agents in the treatment of EM, and should be reserved for patients with EM associated with more severe disease such as meningitis and advanced heart block (Wormser et al., 2006). Macrolides such as azithromycin should be reserved for patients who cannot tolerate other more effective agents (Wormser et al.,

2006). First-generation cephalosporins (e.g. cephalexin and cefadroxil), fluoroquinolones, metronidazole and sulfonamides have no appreciable activity against *B. burgdorferi* and should not be used to treat patients with Lyme disease (Nowakowski et al., 2000; Wormser et al., 2006). Guidelines from the Infectious Diseases Society of America (IDSA) for the treatment of EM are summarized in Table 10.5.

10.3.4 Treatment of children

Previously, doxycycline has been avoided in children <8 years of age due to concerns about staining of developing teeth by tetracyclines (Lochary et al., 1998). However, more recent data have shown that doxycycline, which is structurally different than tetracycline and does not have the same affinity for calcium, is not associated with teeth staining (Todd et al., 2015; Biggs et al., 2016). Two alternative antimicrobial agents were compared in a prospective randomized unblinded study of 43 children aged 6 months to 12 years who received one of two different dosing schedules of cefuroxime axetil (20 mg/kg/day or 30 mg/kg/day) or amoxicillin (50 mg/kg/day) (Eppes and Childs, 2002). EM and associated symptoms resolved in all patients with no long-term problems attributable to Lyme disease; minimal adverse effects were observed (Eppes and Childs, 2002). Both amoxicillin and cefuroxime axetil have been recommended as the preferred regimen for pediatric patients <8 years old (Wormser et al., 2006). Treatment recommendations for Lyme disease in children are summarized in Table 10.5 and discussed in detail in Chapters 6 and 14 of this book.

10.3.5 Long-term outcome after treatment

The long-term prognosis for patients with EM who receive timely and appropriate therapy is excellent (Nadelman et al., 1992; Luger et al., 1995; Smith et al., 2002; Nowakowski et al., 2003; Wormser et al., 2003; Wormser, 2006;

Table 10.5. Infectious Diseases Society of America (IDSA) recommendations for treatment of patients with erythema migrans.[a] (Wormser et al., 2006. Reprinted by permission of the University of Chicago Press, Clinical Infectious Diseases.)

Drug	Dosage for adults	Dosage for children
Preferred[b]		
Amoxicillin	500 mg three times per day	50 mg/kg per day in three divided doses (maximum 500 mg per dose)
Doxycycline	100 mg twice per day. Relatively contraindicated in pregnant or lactating women	Not recommended for children <8 years. For children ≥8 years, 4 mg/kg per day, in two divided doses (maximum 100 mg per dose)[c]
Cefuroxime axetil	500 mg twice per day	30 mg/kg per day in two divided doses (maximum 500 mg per dose)
Alternative[d]		
Azithromycin	500 mg per day for 7–10 days	10 mg/kg per day (maximum 500 mg per day)
Clarithromycin	500 mg twice per day for 14–21 days. Relatively contraindicated in pregnant women	7.5 mg/kg twice per day (maximum 500 mg per dose)
Erythromycin	500 mg four times per day for 14–21 days	12.5 mg/kg four times per day (maximum 500 mg per dose)

[a]In patients suspected of having co-infection with human granulocytic anaplasmosis (HGA), doxycycline is preferred if not contraindicated.
[b]Recommended duration is 14 days (10–21 for doxycycline or 14–21 days for amoxicillin and cefuroxime axetil).
[c]Recommendations on the use of doxycycline in children are changing and it is likely to be endorsed for children > 2 months of age.
[d]Because of their lower efficacy, macrolides are reserved for patients who are unable to take or who are intolerant of tetracyclines, penicillins and cephalosporins; patients treated with macrolides should be closely observed to ensure resolution of clinical symptoms.

Cerar et al., 2010; Kowalski et al., 2010). Two US cohorts of culture-confirmed cases offer the best opportunity to study outcome because of the certainty of the diagnosis of EM. A multicenter observational study conducted in ten endemic states evaluated 118 patients seen with culture-confirmed EM (from the LYMErix vaccine trial (Steere et al., 1998)), almost all of whom were treated with oral doxycycline or amoxicillin (Smith et al., 2002). Associated extracutaneous signs and symptoms persisted for more than 30 days after treatment in 11%, decreasing to 4% at 60 days (Smith et al., 2002). All of these patients had only subjective complaints (e.g. headache, fatigue and arthralgias) except for two patients who manifested seventh cranial nerve palsy with residual weakness. All but one patient had completely recovered by follow-up at 20 months (Smith et al., 2002).

In another prospective study, 99 patients seen in Westchester County, New York, with culture-confirmed EM were followed for a mean of 4.9 ± 2.9 years (Nowakowski et al., 2003). After antimicrobial treatment, EM resolved within 3 weeks in all cases, and no patient developed objective extracutaneous manifestations of late Lyme disease. Almost all patients (90%) were enrolled in treatment trials; although a few patients received a 7-day course of azithromycin (9%) or a course of intravenous ceftriaxone, the overwhelming majority of patients received doxycycline, amoxicillin or cefuroxime axetil for 10–21 days. Improvement was documented in all but the two patients (2%) who failed to return after the baseline visit. From 3 months onwards 84% to 92% of patients were asymptomatic or had symptoms consistent with their health status prior to Lyme disease (Nowakowski et al., 2003). Some asymptomatic patients developed subjective symptoms at a subsequent visit. Only 8 (10%) of the 81 patients followed for ≥1 year were symptomatic at their last visit, a mean of 5.6 ± 2.6 years into follow-up. Their symptoms were usually mild and intermittent, with only three patients (4%) consistently symptomatic at each follow-up visit. Two patients were re-treated for continuing symptoms, one at 3 and 6 months and the other at 6 years but neither had a significant clinical response. Patients with a greater number and severity of symptoms at study enrollment, and those with multiple EM were more likely to report symptoms at follow-up visits (Nowakowski et al., 2003). Repeat tick bites were reported by 47% of patients and repeated episodes of EM occurred in 15% of patients (see Section 10.4) emphasizing the need for education on preventing tick bites.

Patients with EM treated with currently recommended regimens (Wormser et al., 2006) almost never develop objective evidence of late disease (Nadelman et al., 1992; Luger et al., 1995; Luft et al., 1996; Dattwyler et al., 1997; Wormser et al., 2003, Cerar et al., 2010). Some patients who developed objective neurologic disease after treatment for EM, had, in retrospect, findings suggesting subtle CNS involvement at the time oral antimicrobials were initiated (Massarotti et al., 1992). Approximately 10% of patients report subjective complaints such as fatigue, myalgias and arthralgias, and vague 'neurologic symptoms' after completion of treatment for EM (Nadelman et al., 1992; Luger et al., 1995; Luft et al., 1996; Nowakowski et al., 2003; Wormser et al., 2003, Feder et al., 2007). Prolonged antimicrobial treatment for these patients has been ineffective in achieving sustained improvement and can be harmful (Nadelman et al., 1991; Ettestad et al., 1995; Patel et al., 2000; Klempner et al., 2001; Krupp et al., 2003; Wormser et al., 2006; Fallon et al., 2008; Halperin, 2008; Holzbauer et al., 2010; Kullberg et al., 2016).

Subjective background complaints are quite common in the general 'healthy' population, and may account for some of the symptoms that patients experience after treatment (Barsky and Borus, 1999; Seltzer et al., 2000). Ninety percent of the general population describes one or more somatic symptoms in a given 2–4-week period and 30% report current musculoskeletal symptoms (Barsky and Borus, 1999). Significant fatigue is experienced by 20% of adults, and more than 75% of healthy college students report at least one symptom in a 3-day period (Barsky and Borus, 1999).

One recently published report assessed subjective complaints in Slovenian patients with solitary EM after treatment with either doxycycline or cefuroxime axetil for 15 days (Cerar et al., 2010). A novel feature of the study was the selection by the patient of a control at baseline consisting of a spouse, family member or friend who did not have a history of prior Lyme disease and was within 5 years of the patient's age. Patients and controls were evaluated at baseline,

6 and 12 months using identical questionnaires to assess symptoms. At the final visit, patients were somewhat *less likely* than controls to have subjective complaints (5/230 (2%) vs. 21/224 (9%); $P = 0.002$). None of the symptoms experienced by patients was of sufficient severity to be functionally disabling (Cerar et al., 2010). These findings suggest that some of the subjective complaints experienced after treatment may be unrelated to infection. However, this conclusion may be somewhat limited because the study excluded patients with early disseminated Lyme disease, including those with multiple EM skin lesions who might have a greater likelihood of developing post-treatment Lyme disease symptoms. It is also uncertain whether similar findings would be applicable to disease in US patients who are infected with *B. burgdorferi* sensu stricto rather than *B. afzelii*.

Fourteen (10.9%) of 128 patients with culture-confirmed EM, followed for 15 years (range 11–20 years) were felt to have possible post-treatment Lyme disease syndrome (PTLDS), but only 6 (4.7%) had PTLDS documented at their last study visit. Most had only a single symptom and no patient with PTLDS at the last visit was considered to be functionally impaired by the symptom(s) (Weitzner et al., 2015). Fibromyalgia and fatigue due to Lyme disease were very uncommon (1 and 3%, respectively) in 100 patients followed for 15 years after culture-confirmed EM (Weitzner et al., 2015). Health-related quality of life, evaluated using the 36-Item Short Form General Health Survey version 2 (SF-36v2) questionnaire at 11–20 years after diagnosis, was similar to that of the general population (Wormser et al., 2015a; 2015b).

Excellent outcomes in European patients treated for EM have been observed at short- and long-term follow-up (up to 3 years) (Weber et al., 1990; 1993; Strle et al., 1992; 1996a; 1996b; Kuiper et al., 1994; Hulshof et al., 1997; Lipsker et al., 2002; Cerar et al., 2010). European EM is discussed in more detail in Chapter 7.

10.3.6 Outcome in special patient groups: pregnancy and immunocompromised hosts

Epidemiologic studies have failed to confirm an early report (Markowitz et al., 1986) of 19 patients with adverse pregnancy outcomes initially attributed to *B. burgdorferi* infection during pregnancy (Strobino et al., 1993; 1999; Williams et al., 1995). Furthermore, a survey of 162 pediatric neurologists in Connecticut (the state with the highest incidence of Lyme disease at that time (Bacon et al., 2008)) failed to identify a single child with a neurologic problem believed to be related to Lyme disease during pregnancy (Gerber and Zalneraitis, 1994). In a prospective Slovenian study, 93/105 (88.6%) pregnant women with EM had excellent outcomes after treatment with intravenous beta-lactam antimicrobials; adverse outcomes (abortion; preterm birth; syndactyly and urologic anomalies) were not clearly linked to Lyme disease (Maraspin et al., 1999b). There have been no treatment trials comparing intravenous vs. oral antibiotics for pregnant women with EM. However, there are no data to support treating pregnant patients with EM differently than non-pregnant patients with EM, aside from avoiding doxycycline (Wormser et al., 2006).

Controlled studies comparing presentation and outcome of immunocompromised patients with EM with those having normal immune function are rare (Maraspin et al. 1999a; Fürst et al., 2006; Maraspin et al., 2015). Early disseminated disease and objective and subjective 'treatment failure' prompting repeat courses of antimicrobials were reported to be more common in 67 Slovenian patients with a variety of causes of immunosuppression, when compared with the control group (Maraspin et al., 1999a). However, favorable outcomes were seen in both groups at 1-year follow-up (Maraspin et al., 1999a). A retrospective study from Austria found that 33 immunosuppressed patients with EM had similar clinical presentations, rates of seropositivity, and favorable response to therapy when compared with controls with EM who had normal immune function (Fürst et al., 2006). In a preliminary report, 35 Slovenian patients with hematologic malignancies had similar clinical presentations compared with 70 immunocompetent patients, but were more likely to have leukocytosis or leukopenia, and were more often re-treated (one patient each with subjective symptoms, persistence of EM or development of multiple EM vs. zero immunocompetent patients) (Maraspin et al., 2010). In an uncontrolled observational report from Slovenia, six patients with a history of prior organ transplant had excellent outcomes after treatment for EM (Maraspin et al., 2006).

10.4 Reinfection

Repeat episodes of EM are not uncommon in endemic areas. As many as 15% of patients with EM followed in several prospective studies in the US had more than one episode, with repeat episodes averaging 1.2 to 3.1% per year over 1–5 years (Smith et al., 2002; Nowakowski et al., 2003; Wormser et al., 2003, Nadelman et al., 2012). This incidence is actually 20–50 times that for Lyme disease in the general population living in the same community (Nadelman and Wormser, 2007). Patients may experience a second and occasionally more episodes of Lyme disease after the first episode has resolved. These subsequent occurrences, nearly invariably associated with EM, are almost always the result of reinfection rather than relapse (Nadelman and Wormser, 2007). Reinfection may be defined as a new infection that occurs after successful antimicrobial treatment of a prior episode of Lyme disease (Nadelman and Wormser, 2007).

The most likely explanation for recurrent EM is that repeat tick bites are quite common in endemic areas. In Westchester County, New York, in a study of doxycycline prophylaxis after a recognized tick bite, 17% of 335 subjects sustained new tick bites over the 6 weeks following enrollment, despite receiving specific oral and written instructions on ways to reduce the risk of tick bite (Nadelman et al., 2001). Many people in endemic areas acquire tick bites and Lyme disease on their own property (Falco and Fish, 1988).

The normal human immune response is insufficiently protective against reinfection. One reason for this may be that there are at least 17 OspC genotypes of B. burgdorferi causing clinical disease in the US (Ivanova et al., 2009). Evidence that reinfection with a new strain of B. burgdorferi accounts in part for repeat episodes of EM was obtained from 17 patients who had 22 consecutive episodes of culture-confirmed EM occurring up to 15 years apart (Nadelman et al., 2012). No two consecutive episodes were caused by the same OspC genotype, suggesting that these were new infections rather than incompletely treated infections that relapsed. This conclusion is supported by an animal experiment (Probert et al., 1997). Mice were immune to challenge with an OspC genotype to which they had previously been immunized, but were susceptible to infection with a different OspC genotype (Probert et al., 1997).

Published information is limited concerning the clinical manifestations in patients with repeat episodes of EM. None of the 28 patients seen in Rhode Island with recurrent EM was believed to have an immunodeficiency, and almost all cases occurred in the summer, paralleling the peak questing period of I. scapularis nymphal ticks, consistent with reinfection rather than relapse (Krause et al., 2006). The signs, symptoms and demographics of patients with recurrent EM appear generally similar to those associated with the initial episode (Nadelman et al., 2002; Krause et al., 2006; Nadelman and Wormser, 2007). A Swedish finding that women are more likely than men to have a second bout of EM (Jarefors et al., 2006) differs from the experience reported in the US to date where the gender distribution is similar at first and second episodes (Nadelman et al., 2002; Krause et al., 2006; Nadelman and Wormser, 2007). In 22 patients there appeared to be a trend (not statistically significant) for multiple EM lesions to occur less frequently in recurrences than in initial episodes (3/11 (14%) vs. 7/11 (32%); $P = 0.15$) (Nadelman et al., 2002; Nadelman and Wormser, 2007). This observation, if confirmed in a larger study, might be compatible with the acquisition of partial immunity aborting hematogenous spread of spirochetes during the second episode (Nadelman and Wormser, 2007). Consistent with this hypothesis is the finding in a separate report that spirochetemia was significantly less likely in patients with a previous history of Lyme disease, compared with those experiencing their first episode (OR = 2.5 (CI = 1.1–5.7); $P = 0.03$) (Wormser et al., 2005a).

Relapse of B. burgdorferi infection due to persistence of the organism after recommended courses of treatment is not well documented in the US (Krause et al., 2006; Nadelman and Wormser, 2007). However, relapse has been well documented in patients who were treated with antibiotics *not* recommended for Lyme disease (e.g. cephalexin) (Nowakowski et al., 2000) and has been reported in patients receiving macrolides (Luft et al., 1996).

10.5 Summary

EM, the most common objective manifestation of Lyme disease, is associated with infection with *B. burgdorferi* sensu stricto in the US as well as other genospecies causing Lyme disease (often referred to as Lyme borreliosis) in Europe and Asia (Kuiper *et al.*, 1994; Hashimoto *et al.*, 1995; Busch *et al.*, 1996; Strle *et al.*, 1996a; 1996b; 1999, Ornstein *et al.*, 2001; Antoni-Bach *et al.*, 2002; Lipsker *et al.*, 2002; Logar *et al.*, 2004; Cerar *et al.*, 2016). Despite their characteristic appearance, EM-like lesions should not be considered pathognomonic for Lyme disease, because other skin lesions may appear indistinguishable, including localized tick bite reactions and STARI, neither of which is associated with *B. burgdorferi* infection (Masters *et al.*, 1998; Nadelman and Wormser, 2002; Wormser *et al.*, 2005b; 2005c; Tibbles and Edlow, 2007).

EM is associated with excellent outcome after appropriate treatment with oral antibiotics; objective treatment failures are exceedingly rare (Dattwyler *et al.*, 1990; 1997; Massarotti *et al.*, 1992; Nadelman *et al.*, 1992; Strle *et al.*, 1992; 1996a; 1996b; Weber *et al.*, 1993; Luger *et al.*, 1995; Luft *et al.*, 1996; Eppes and Childs, 2002; Smith *et al.*, 2002; Wormser *et al.*, 2003; 2006; Wormser, 2006; Cerar *et al.*, 2010). Although *B. burgdorferi* may be isolated in culture from a biopsy taken from a sample of the skin lesion (Berger *et al.*, 1992; Kuiper *et al.*, 1994; Busch *et al.*, 1996; Nadelman *et al.*, 1996; Strle *et al.*, 1996a; 1996b; 1999; Antoni-Bach *et al.*, 2002; Smith *et al.*, 2002; Logar *et al.*, 2004) or blood (Wormser *et al.*, 2000; 2005a) laboratory diagnosis, including use of serology, is generally neither helpful nor necessary (Aguero-Rosenfeld *et al.*, 1993; 2005; CDC, 1995; Wormser *et al.*, 2006). For the practitioner, EM remains a clinical diagnosis (Nadelman and Wormser, 1998; 2002; Wormser *et al.*, 2006).

References

Agger, W.A., Callister, S.M. and Jobe, D.A. (1992) In vitro susceptibilities of *Borrelia burgdorferi* to five oral cephalosporins and ceftriaxone. *Antimicrobial Agents Chemotherapy* 36, 1788–1790.

Aguero-Rosenfeld, M.E., Nowakowski, J., McKenna, D., Carbonaro, C.A. and Wormser, G.P. (1993) Serodiagnosis in early Lyme disease. *Journal of Clinical Microbiology* 31, 3090–3095.

Aguero-Rosenfeld, M.E., Wang, G., Schwartz, I. and Wormser, G.P. (2005) Diagnosis of Lyme borreliosis. *Clinical Microbiology Reviews* 18, 484–509.

Antoni-Bach, N., Jaulhac, B., Hansmann, Y., Limbach, F. and Lipsker, D. (2002) Borrelia strains that cause erythema migrans in Alsace, France. *Annals of Dermatology and Venereology* 129, 15–18.

Åsbrink, E. and Olsson, I. (1985) Clinical manifestations of erythema chronicum migrans afzelius in 161 patients. *Acta Dermatology and Venereology* 65, 43–52.

Bacon, R.M., Kugeler, K.J. and Mead, P.S. (2008) Centers for Disease Control and Prevention (CDC). Surveillance for Lyme disease – United States, 1992–2006. *MMWR Surveillance Summary* 57, 1–9.

Bakken, J.S. and Dumler, J.S. (2006) Clinical diagnosis and treatment of human granulocytotropic anaplasmosis. *Annals of the New York Academy of Sciences* 1078, 236–247.

Barbour, A.G., Maupin, G.O., Teltow, G.J., Carter, C.J. and Piesman, J. (1996) Identification of an uncultivable *Borrelia* species in the hard tick *Amblyomma americanum*: possible agent of a Lyme disease-like illness. *Journal of Infectious Diseases* 173, 403–409.

Barsky, A.J. and Borus, J.F. (1999) Functional somatic syndromes. *Annals of Internal Medicine* 130, 910–921.

Belongia, E.A., Reed, K.D., Mitchell, P.D., Chyou, P.H., Mueller-Rizner, N., Finkel, M.F. and Schriefer, M.E. (1999) Clinical and epidemiological features of early Lyme disease and human granulocytic ehrlichiosis in Wisconsin. *Clinical Infectious Diseases* 29, 1472–1477.

Berger, B.W. (1989) Dermatologic manifestations of Lyme disease. *Reviews of Infectious Diseases* 11 (Suppl 6), S1475–S1481.

Berger, B.W., Johnson, R.C., Kodner, C. and Coleman, L. (1992) Cultivation *of Borrelia burgdorferi* from erythema migrans lesions and perilesional skin. *Journal of Clinical Microbiology* 30, 359–361.

Biggs, H.M., Behravesh, C.B., Bradley, K.K. *et al.* (2016) Diagnosis and management of tickborne rickettsial diseases: Rocky Mountain spotted fever and other spotted fever group rickettsioses, ehrlichioses, and anaplasmosis – United States. *MMWR Recommendations and Reports* 65(2), 1–44.

Borg, R., Dotevall, L., Hagberg, L., Maraspin, V., Lotric-Furlan, S., Cimperman, J. and Strle, F. (2005) Intravenous ceftriaxone compared with oral doxycycline for the treatment of Lyme neuroborreliosis. *Scandinavian Journal of Infectious Diseases* 37(6–7), 449–454.

Branda, J.A., Linskey, K., Kim, Y.A., Steere, A.C. and Ferraro, M.J. (2011) Two-tiered antibody testing for Lyme disease with use of 2 enzyme immunoassays, a whole-cell sonicate enzyme immunoassay followed by a VlsE C6 peptide enzyme immunoassay. *Clinical Infectious Diseases* 53(6), 541–547.

Bremell, D. and Dotevall, L. (2014). Oral doxycycline for Lyme neuroborreliosis with symptoms of encephalitis, myelitis, vasculitis or intracranial hypertension. *European Journal of Neurology* 21(9), 1162–1167.

Busch, U., Hizo-Teufel, C., Böhmer, R., Fingerle, V., Rössler, D., Wilske, B., Preac-Mursic, V. (1996) *Borrelia burgdorferi* sensu lato strains isolated from cutaneous Lyme borreliosis biopsies differentiated by pulsed-field gel electrophoresis. *Scandinavian Journal of Infectious Diseases* 28, 583–589.

Centers for Disease Control and Prevention (CDC) (1995) Recommendations for test performance and interpretation from the second national conference on serologic diagnosis of Lyme disease. *Morbidity and Mortality Weekly Report* 44, 590–591.

Centers for Disease Control and Prevention (CDC) (2016) Lyme Disease Data Tables, Available at: https://www.cdc.gov/lyme/stats/tables.html (accessed 7 August 2017).

Cerar, D., Cerar, T., Ružić-Sabljić, E., Wormser, G.P. and Strle, F. (2010) Subjective symptoms after treatment of early Lyme disease. *American Journal of Medicine* 123, 79–86.

Cerar, T., Strle, F., Stupica, D. et al. (2016). Differences in Genotype, Clinical Features, and Inflammatory Potential of *Borrelia burgdorferi* sensu stricto Strains from Europe and the United States. *Emerging Infectious Diseases* 22(5), 818–827.

Chowdri, H.R., Gugliotta, J.L., Berardi, V.P., Goethert, H.K., Molloy, P.J., Sterling, S.L. et al. (2013) *Borrelia miyamotoi* infection presenting as human granulocytic anaplasmosis: a case report. *Annals of Internal Medicine* 159(1), 21–27.

Dattwyler, R.J., Volkman, D.J., Conaty, S.M., Platkin, S.P. and Luft, B.J. (1990) Amoxicillin plus probenecid versus doxycycline for treatment of erythema migrans borreliosis. *Lancet* 336, 1404–1406.

Dattwyler, R.J., Luft, B.J., Kunkel, M.J., Finkel, M.F., Wormser, G.P., Rush, T.J., Grunwaldt, E., Agger, W.A., Franklin, M., Oswald, D., Cockey, L. and Maladorno, D. (1997) Ceftriaxone compared with doxycycline for the treatment of acute disseminated Lyme disease. *New England Journal of Medicine* 337, 289–294.

Dotevall, L. and Hagberg, L. (1999). Successful oral doxycycline treatment of Lyme disease-associated facial palsy and meningitis. *Clinical Infectious Diseases* 28(3), 569–574.

El Khoury, M.Y., Camargo, J.F., White, J.L., Backenson, B.P., Dupuis, A.P., 2nd, Escuyer, K.L. et al. (2013) Potential role of deer tick virus in Powassan encephalitis cases in Lyme disease-endemic areas of New York, U.S.A. *Emerging Infectious Diseases* 19(12),1926–1933.

Eppes, S.C. and Childs, J.A. (2002) Comparative study of cefuroxime axetil versus amoxicillin in children with early Lyme disease. *Pediatrics* 109, 1173–1177.

Ettestad, P.J., Campbell, G.L., Welbel, S.F., Genese, C.A., Spitalny, K.C., Marchetti, C.M. and Dennis, D.T. (1995) Biliary complications in the treatment of unsubstantiated Lyme disease. *Journal of Infectious Diseases* 171, 356–361.

Falco, R.C. and Fish, D. (1988) Prevalence of *Ixodes dammini* near the homes of Lyme disease patients in Westchester County, New York. *American Journal of Epidemiology* 127, 826–830.

Falco, R.C., Fish, D. and Piesman, J. (1996) Duration of tick bites in a Lyme disease-endemic area. *American Journal of Epidemiology* 143(2),187–192.

Falco, R.C., McKenna, D.F., Daniels, T.J., Nadelman, R.B., Nowakowski, J., Fish, D. and Wormser, G.P. (1999) Temporal relation between *Ixodes scapularis* abundance and risk for Lyme disease associated with erythema migrans. *American Journal of Epidemiology* 149, 771–776.

Fallon, B.A., Keilp, J.G., Corbera, K.M. et al. (2008) A randomized, placebo-controlled trial of repeated IV antibiotic therapy for Lyme encephalopathy. *Neurology* 70, 992–1003.

Feder, H.M. and Whitaker, D.L. (1995) Misdiagnosis of erythema migrans. *American Journal of Medicine* 99, 412–419.

Feder, H.M. Jr, Johnson, B.J., O'Connell, S. et al. (2007) A critical appraisal of 'chronic Lyme disease'. *New England Journal of Medicine* 357, 1422–1430.

Feder, H.M., Jr, Hoss, D.M., Zemel, L., Telford, S.R. III, Dias, F. and Wormser, G.P. (2011) Southern tick-associated rash illness (STARI) in the north: STARI following a tick bite in Long Island, New York. *Clinical Infectious Diseases* 53(10), e142–146.

Felz, M.W., Durden, L.A. and Oliver, J.H. Jr (1996) Ticks parasitizing humans in Georgia and South Carolina. *Journal of Parasitology* 82, 505–508.
Fish, D. (1995) Environmental risk and prevention of Lyme disease. *American Journal of Medicine* 98, 2S–8S.
Frithsen, I.L., Vetter, R.S. and Stocks, I.C. (2007) Reports of envenomation by brown recluse spiders exceed verified specimens of Loxosceles spiders in South Carolina. *Journal of the American Board of Family Medicine* 20, 483–488.
Fürst, B., Glatz, M., Kerl, H. and Müllegger, R.R. (2006) The impact of immunosuppression on erythema migrans. A retrospective study of clinical presentation, response to treatment and production of *Borrelia* antibodies in 33 patients. *Clinical and Experimental Dermatology* 31, 509–514. Erratum in: *Clinical and Experimental Dermatology* (2006) 31, 751.
Gasmi, S., Ogden, N.H., Leighton, P.A. *et al.* (2017) Practices of Lyme disease diagnosis and treatment by general practitioners in Quebec, 2008–2015. *BMC Family Practice* 18(1), 65.
Gerber, M.A. and Zalneraitis, E.L. (1994) Childhood neurologic disorders and Lyme disease during pregnancy. *Pediatric Neurology* 11, 41–43.
Gerber, M.A., Shapiro, E.D., Burke, G.S., Parcells, V.J. and Bell, G.L. (1996) Lyme disease in children in southeastern Connecticut. Pediatric Lyme Disease Study Group. *New England Journal of Medicine* 335, 1270–1274.
Goldberg, N.S., Forseter, G., Nadelman, R.B., Schwartz, I., Jorde, U., McKenna, D., Holmgren, D., Bittker, S., Montecalvo, M. and Wormser, G.P. (1992) Vesicular erythema migrans. *Archives of Dermatology* 128, 1495–1498.
Grimm, D., Tilly, K., Byram, R., Stewart, P.E., Krum, J.G., Bueschel, D.M., Schwan, T.G., Policastro, P.F., Elias, A.F. and Rosa, P.A. (2004) Outer surface protein C of the Lyme disease spirochete: a protein induced in ticks for infection in mammals. *Proceedings of the National Academy of Sciences of the United States of America* 101, 3142–3147.
Habif, T.P. (2004) Infestations and bites. In: Habif, T.P. (ed.) *Clinical Dermatology*, 4th edn. Mosby Inc, St Louis, Missouri, pp. 497–546.
Haddad, F.A. and Nadelman, R.B. (2003) Lyme disease and the heart. *Frontiers in Bioscience* 8, s769–s782.
Halperin, J.J. (2008) Prolonged Lyme disease treatment: enough is enough. *Neurology* 70, 986–987.
Hansen, K., Hovmark, A., Lebech, A.M., Lebech, K., Olsson, I., Halkier-Sørensen, L., Olsson, E. and Asbrink, E. (1992) Roxithromycin in Lyme borreliosis: discrepant results of an *in vitro* and *in vivo* animal susceptibility study and a clinical trial in patients with erythema migrans. *Acta Dermato-Venereologica* 72, 297–300.
Hashimoto, Y., Kawagishi, N., Sakai, H., Takahashi, H., Matsuo, S., Nakao, M., Miyamoto, K. and Iizuka, H. (1995) Lyme disease in Japan. Analysis of Borrelia species using rRNA gene restriction fragment length polymorphism. *Dermatology* 191, 193–198.
Holzbauer, S.M., Kemperman, M.M. and Lynfield, R. (2010) Death due to community-associated *Clostridium difficile* in a woman receiving prolonged antibiotic therapy for suspected Lyme disease. *Clinical Infectious Diseases* 51, 369–370.
Hulshof, M.M., Vandenbroucke, J.P., Nohlmans, L.M., Spanjaard, L., Bavinck, J.N. and Dijkmans, B.A. (1997) Long-term prognosis in patients treated for erythema chronicum migrans and acrodermatitis chronica atrophicans. *Archives of Dermatology* 133, 33–37.
Ivanova, L., Christova, I., Neves, V., Aroso, M., Meirelles, L., Brisson, D. and Gomes-Solecki, M. (2009) Comprehensive seroprofiling of sixteen *B. burgdorferi* OspC: implications for Lyme disease diagnostics design. *Journal of Clinical Immunology* 132, 393–400.
Jarefors, S., Bennet, L., You, E., Forsberg, P., Ekerfelt, C., Berglund, J. and Ernerudh, J. (2006) Lyme borreliosis reinfection: might it be explained by a gender difference in immune response? *Immunology* 118, 224–232.
Jurca, T., Ružić-Sabljić, E., Lotric-Furlan, S., Maraspin, V., Cimperman, J., Picken, R.N., Strle, F. (1998) Comparison of peripheral and central biopsy sites for the isolation of *Borrelia burgdorferi* sensu lato from erythema migrans skin lesions. *Clinical Infectious Diseases* 27, 636–638.
Karlsson, M., Hammers-Berggren, S., Lindquist, L., Stiernstedt, G. and Svenungsson, B. (1994). Comparison of intravenous penicillin G and oral doxycycline for treatment of Lyme neuroborreliosis. *Neurology* 44(7), 1203–1207.
Kirkland, K.B., Klimko, T.B., Meriwether, R.A., Schriefer, M., Levin, M., Levine, J., MacKenzie, W.R. and Dennis, D.T. (1997) Erythema migrans-like rash illness at a camp in North Carolina: a new tick-borne disease? *Archives of Internal Medicine* 157, 2635–2641.

Klempner, M.S., Hu, L.T., Evans, J. et al. (2001) Two controlled trials of antibiotic treatment in patients with persistent symptoms and a history of Lyme disease. *New England Journal of Medicine* 345, 85–92.

Kowalski, T.J., Tata, S., Berth, W., Mathiason, M.A. and Agger, W.A. (2010) Antibiotic treatment duration and long-term outcomes of patients with early Lyme disease from a Lyme disease-hyperendemic area. *Clinical Infectious Diseases* 50, 512–520.

Krause, P.J., Telford, S.R. III, Spielman, A., Sikand, V., Ryan, R., Christianson, D., Burke, G., Brassard, P., Pollack, R., Peck, J. and Persing, D.H. (1996) Concurrent Lyme disease and babesiosis. Evidence for increased severity and duration of illness. *JAMA* 275, 1657–1660.

Krause, P.J., Foley, D.T., Burke, G.S., Christianson, D., Closter, L., Spielman, A., Tick-Borne Disease Study Group (2006) Reinfection and relapse in early Lyme disease. *American Journal of Tropical Medicine and Hygiene* 75, 1090–1094.

Krause, P.J., Gewurz, B.E., Hill, D. et al. (2008) Persistent and relapsing babesiosis in immunocompromised patients. *Clinical Infectious Diseases* 46, 370–376.

Krause, P.J., Fish, D., Narasimhan, S. and Barbour, A.G. (2015) *Borrelia miyamotoi* infection in nature and in humans. *Clinical Microbiology and Infection* 21(7), 631–639.

Krupp, L.B., Hyman, L.G., Grimson, R., Coyle, P.K., Melville, P., Ahnn, S., Dattwyler, R., Chandler, B. (2003) Study and treatment of post Lyme disease (STOP-LD): a randomized double masked clinical trial. *Neurology* 60, 1923–1930.

Kuiper, H., Cairo, I., Van Dam, A., De Jongh, B., Ramselaar, T., Spanjaard, L., Dankert, J. (1994) Solitary erythema migrans: a clinical, laboratory and epidemiological study of 77 Dutch patients. *British Journal of Dermatology* 130, 466–472.

Kullberg, B.J., Berende, A., Evers, A.W. (2016) Longer-term therapy for symptoms attributed to Lyme disease. *New England Journal of Medicine* 375(10), 998.

Lipsker, D., Antoni-Bach, N., Hansmann, Y. and Jaulhac, B. (2002) Long-term prognosis of patients treated for erythema migrans in France. *British Journal of Dermatology* 146, 872–876.

Liveris, D., Varde, S., Iyer, R., Koenig, S., Bittker, S., Cooper, D., McKenna, D., Nowakowski, J., Nadelman, R.B., Wormser, G.P. and Schwartz, I. (1999) Genetic diversity of *Borrelia burgdorferi* in Lyme disease patients as determined by culture versus direct PCR with clinical specimens. *Journal of Clinical Microbiology* 37, 565–569.

Liveris, D., Schwartz, I., Bittker, S., Cooper, D., Iyer, R., Cox, M.E. et al. (2011) Improving the yield of blood cultures from patients with early Lyme disease. *Journal of Clinical Microbiology* 49(6), 2166–2168.

Ljostad, U., Skogvoll, E., Eikeland, R., Midgard, R., Skarpaas, T., Berg, A. and Mygland, A. (2008) Oral doxycycline versus intravenous ceftriaxone for European Lyme neuroborreliosis: a multicentre, non-inferiority, double-blind, randomised trial. *Lancet Neurology* 7(8), 690–695.

Lochary, M.E., Lockhart, P.B. and Williams, W.T. Jr (1998) Doxycycline and staining of permanent teeth. *Pediatric Infectious Disease Journal* 17, 429–431.

Logar, M., Ružić-Sabljić, E., Maraspin, V., Lotric-Furlan, S., Cimperman, J., Jurca, T. and Strle, F. (2004) Comparison of erythema migrans caused by *Borrelia afzelii* and *Borrelia garinii*. *Infection* 32, 15–19.

Luft, B.J., Dattwyler, R.J., Johnson, R.C., Luger, S.W., Bosler, E.M., Rahn, D.W., Masters, E.J., Grunwaldt, E. and Gadgil, S.D. (1996) Azithromycin compared with amoxicillin in the treatment of erythema migrans: a double blind, randomized, controlled trial. *Annals of Internal Medicine* 124, 785–791.

Luger, S.W., Paparone, P., Wormser, G.P., Nadelman, R.B., Grunwaldt, E., Gomez, G., Wisniewski, M. and Collins, J.J. (1995) Comparison of cefuroxime axetil and doxycycline in treatment of patients with early Lyme disease associated with erythema migrans. *Antimicrobial Agents and Chemotherapy* 39, 661–667.

Malane, M.S., Grant-Kels, J.M., Feder, H.M. Jr and Luger, S.W. (1991) Diagnosis of Lyme disease based on dermatologic manifestations. *Annals of Internal Medicine* 114, 490–498.

Mansfield, K.L., Johnson, N., Phipps, L.P., Stephenson, J.R., Fooks, A.R. and Solomon, T. (2009) Tick-borne encephalitis virus – a review of an emerging zoonosis. *Generation Joshua* 90, 1781–1794.

Maraspin, V., Lotric-Furlan, S., Cimperman, J., Ružić-Sabljić, E. and Strle, F. (1999a) Erythema migrans in the immunocompromised host. *Wiener klinische Wochenschrift* 111, 923–932.

Maraspin, V., Cimperman, J., Lotric-Furlan, S., Pleterski-Rigler, D. and Strle, F. (1999b) Erythema migrans in pregnancy. *Wiener klinische Wochenschrift* 111, 933–940.

Maraspin, V., Cimperman, J., Lotric-Furlan, S., Logar, M., Ružić-Sabljić, E. and Strle, F. (2006) Erythema migrans in solid organ transplant recipients. *Clinical Infectious Diseases* 42, 1751–1754.

Maraspin, V., Cimperman, C., Lotrič-Furlan, C., Ružić-Sabljić, E. and Strle, F. (2010) Course and outcome of erythema migrans in patients with haematological malignancies. *Program and Abstracts of the*

12th International Conference on Lyme Borreliosis and other Tick-Borne Diseases (Ljubljana, Slovenia), 26–29 September. Abstract P12, page 41.

Maraspin, V., Ružić-Sabljić, E., Lusa, L. and Strle, F. (2015) Course and outcome of early Lyme borreliosis in patients with hematological malignancies. *Clinical Infectious Diseases* 61(3), 427–431.

Markowitz, L.E., Steere, A.C., Benach, J.L., Slade, J.D. and Broome, C.V. (1986) Lyme disease during pregnancy. *JAMA* 255, 3394–3396.

Massarotti, E.M., Luger, S.W., Rahn, D.W., Messner, R.P., Wong, J.B., Johnson, R.C. and Steere, A.C. (1992) Treatment of early Lyme disease. *American Journal of Medicine* 92, 396–403.

Masters, E., Granter, S., Duray, P. and Cordes P. (1998) Physician-diagnosed erythema migrans and erythema migrans-like rashes following lone star tick bites. *Archives of Dermatology* 134, 955–960.

Masuzawa, T. (2004) Terrestrial distribution of the Lyme borreliosis agent *Borrelia burgdorferi* sensu lato in east Asia. *Japanese Journal of Infectious Diseases* 57, 229–235.

Melski, J.W., Reed, K.D., Mitchell, P.D., Barth, G.D. (1993) Primary and secondary erythema migrans in central Wisconsin. *Archives of Dermatology* 129, 709–716.

Molins, C.R., Delorey, M.J., Sexton, C. and Schriefer, M.E., (2016) Lyme borreliosis serology: performance of several commonly used laboratory diagnostic tests and a large resource panel of well-characterized patient samples. *Journal of Clinical Microbiology* 54(11), 2726–2734.

Molloy, P.J., Telford, S.R. III, Chowdri, H.R., Lepore, T.J., Gugliotta, J.L., Weeks, K.E. *et al*. (2015) Borrelia miyamotoi disease in the northeastern United States: a case series. *Annals of Internal Medicine* 163(2), 91–98.

Nadelman, R.B. and Wormser, G.P. (1995) Erythema migrans and early Lyme disease. *American Journal of Medicine* 98, 15S–23S.

Nadelman, R.B. and Wormser, G.P. (1998) Lyme borreliosis. *Lancet* 352, 557–565.

Nadelman, R.B. and Wormser, G.P. (2002) Recognition and treatment of erythema migrans: are we off target? *Annals of Internal Medicine* 136, 477–479.

Nadelman, R.B. and Wormser, G.P. (2007) Reinfection in patients with Lyme disease. *Clinical Infectious Diseases* 45, 1032–1038.

Nadelman, R.B., Arlin, Z. and Wormser, G.P. (1991) Life-threatening complications of empiric ceftriaxone therapy for 'seronegative Lyme disease'. *Southern Medical Journal* 84, 1263–1265.

Nadelman, R.B., Luger, S.W., Frank, E., Wisniewski, M., Collins, J.J. and Wormser, G.P. (1992) Comparison of cefuroxime axetil and doxycycline in the treatment of early Lyme disease. *Annals of Internal Medicine* 117, 273–280.

Nadelman, R.B., Nowakowski, J., Forseter, G., Goldberg, N.S., Bittker, S., Cooper, D., Aguero-Rosenfeld, M. and Wormser, G.P. (1996) The clinical spectrum of early Lyme borreliosis in patients with culture-confirmed erythema migrans. *American Journal of Medicine* 100, 502–508.

Nadelman, R.B., Horowitz, H.W., Hsieh, T.-C., Wu, J.M., Aguero-Rosenfeld, M.E., Schwartz, I., Nowakowski, J., Varde, S. and Wormser, G.P. (1997) Simultaneous human granulocytic ehrlichiosis and Lyme borreliosis. *New England Journal of Medicine* 337, 27–30.

Nadelman, R.B., Nowakowski, J., Horowitz, H.W., Strle, F. and Wormser, G.P. (1999) Thrombocytopenia and *Borrelia burgdorferi*: an association remains unproven. *Clinical Infectious Diseases* 29, 1603–1605.

Nadelman, R.B., Nowakowski, J., Fish, D., Falco, R.C., Freeman, K., McKenna, D., Welch, P., Marcus, R., Agüero-Rosenfeld, M.E., Dennis, D.T., Wormser, G.P., Tick Bite Study Group (2001) Prophylaxis with single-dose doxycycline for the prevention of Lyme disease after an *Ixodes scapularis* tick bite. *New England Journal of Medicine* 345, 79–84.

Nadelman, R.B., Gaidici, A.T., McKenna, D. *et al*. (2002) Comparison of clinical manifestations of 1st and 2nd episodes of erythema migrans (EM). In: *Program and abstracts of the 9th International conference on Lyme borreliosis and other tick-borne diseases* (New York), Abstract P-51.

Nadelman, R.B., Hanincová, K., Mukherjee, P., Liveris, D., Nowakowski, J., McKenna, D., Brisson, D., Cooper, D., Bittker, S., Madison, G., Holmgren, D., Schwartz, I., Wormser, G.P. (2012) Differentiation of reinfection from relapse in recurrent Lyme disease. *New England Journal of Medicine* 367(20), 1883–1890.

Nowakowski, J., Nadelman, R.B., Forester, G., McKenna, D. and Wormser, G.P. (1995) Doxycycline versus tetracycline therapy for Lyme disease associated with erythema migrans. *Journal of the American Academy of Dermatology* 32, 223–227.

Nowakowski, J., McKenna, D., Nadelman, R.B., Cooper, D., Bittker, S., Holmgren, D., Pavia, C., Johnson, R.C. and Wormser, G.P. (2000) Failure of treatment with cephalexin for Lyme disease. *Archives of Family Medicine* 9, 563–567.

Nowakowski, J., Schwartz, I., Liveris, D., Wang, G., Aguero-Rosenfeld, M.E., Girao, G., McKenna, D., Nadelman, R.B., Cavaliere, L.F., Wormser, G.P., Lyme Disease Study Group (2001) Laboratory diagnostic techniques for patients with early Lyme disease associated with erythema migrans: a comparison of different techniques. *Clinical Infectious Diseases* 33, 2023–2027.

Nowakowski, J., Nadelman, R.B., Sell, R., McKenna, D., Cavaliere, L.F., Holmgren, D., Gaidici, A., Wormser, G.P. (2003) Long-term follow-up of patients with culture-confirmed Lyme disease. *American Journal of Medicine* 115, 91–96.

Ornstein, K., Berglund, J., Nilsson, I., Norrby, R. and Bergström, S. (2001) Characterization of Lyme borreliosis isolates from patients with erythema migrans and neuroborreliosis in southern Sweden. *Journal of Clinical Microbiology* 39, 1294–1298.

Patel, R., Grogg, K.L., Edwards, W.D., Wright, A.J. and Schwenk, N.M. (2000) Death from inappropriate therapy for Lyme disease. *Clinical Infectious Diseases* 31, 1107–1109.

Piesman, J. (1993) Dynamics of *Borrelia burgdorferi* transmission by nymphal *Ixodes dammini* ticks. *Journal of Infectious Disease* 167(5), 1082–1085.

Piesman, J. and Sinsky, R.J. (1988) Ability of *Ixodes scapularis*, *Dermacentor variabilis* and *Amblyomma americanum* to acquire, maintain and transmit Lyme disease spirochetes. *Journal of Medical Entomology* 25, 336–339.

Piesman, J., Mather, T.N., Sinsky, R.J. and Spielman, A. (1987) Duration of tick attachment and *Borrelia burgdorferi* transmission. *Journal of Clinical Microbiology* 25(3), 557–558.

Platonov, A.E., Karan, L.S., Kolyasnikova, N.M., Makhneva, N.A., Toporkova, M.G., Maleev, V.V. *et al.* (2011) Humans infected with relapsing fever spirochete *Borrelia miyamotoi*, Russia. *Emerging Infectious Diseases* 17(10), 1816–1823.

Pritt, B.S., Mead, P.S., Johnson, D.K.H. *et al.* (2016) Identification of a novel pathogenic Borrelia species causing Lyme borreliosis with unusually high spirochaetaemia: a descriptive study. *Lancet Infectious Diseases* 16(5), 556–564.

Probert, W.S., Crawford, M., Cadiz, R.B. and LeFebvre, R.B. (1997) Immunization with outer surface protein (Osp) A but not OspC provides cross-protection of mice challenged with North American isolates of *Borrelia burgdorferi*. *Journal of Infectious Diseases* 175, 400–405.

Rubin, D.A., Sorbera, C., Nikitin, P., McAllister, A., Wormser, G.P. and Nadelman, R.B. (1992) Prospective evaluation of heart block complicating early Lyme disease. *Pacing and Clinical Electrophysiology* 15, 252–255.

Sanchez, E., Vannier, E., Wormser, G.P. and Hu, L.T. (2016) Diagnosis, treatment, and prevention of Lyme disease, human granulocytic anaplasmosis, and babesiosis: a review. *JAMA* 315(16), 1767–1777.

Schutzer, S., Berger, B.W., Krueger, J.G., Eshoo, M.W., Ecker, D.J. and Aucott, J.N. (2013) Atypical erythema migrans in patients with PCR-positive Lyme disease. *Emerging Infectious Diseases* 19(5), 815–816.

Seinost, G., Dykhuizen, D.E., Dattwyler, R.J., Golde, W.T., Dunn, J.J., Wang, I.N., Wormser, G.P., Schriefer, M.E. and Luft, B.J. (1999) Four clones of *Borrelia burgdorferi* sensu stricto cause invasive infections in humans. *Infection and Immunity* 67, 3518–3524.

Seltzer, E.G., Gerber, M.A., Cartter, M.L., Freudigman, K. and Shapiro, E.D. (2000) Long-term outcomes of persons with Lyme disease. *JAMA* 283, 609–616.

Sharma, A., Jaimungal, S., Basdeo-Maharaj, K., Chalapathi Rao, A.V. and Teelucksingh, S. (2010) Erythema migrans-like illness among Caribbean islanders. *Emerging Infectious Diseases* 16, 1615–1617.

Sigurdsson, A.F. and Gudmundsson, S. (1989) The etiology of bacterial cellulitis as determined by fine-needle aspiration. *Scandinavian Journal of Infectious Diseases* 21, 537–542.

Sinski, E., Welc-Faleciak, R. and Zajkowska, J. (2016) *Borrelia miyamotoi*: a human tick-borne relapsing fever spirochete in Europe and its potential impact on public health. *Advances in Medical Sciences* 61(2), 255–260.

Smith, R.P., Schoen, R.T., Rahn, D.W., Sikand, V.K., Nowakowski, J., Parenti, D.L., Holman, M.S., Persing, D.H. and Steere, A.C. (2002) Clinical characteristics and treatment outcome of early Lyme disease in patients with microbiologically confirmed erythema migrans. *Annals of Internal Medicine* 136, 421–428.

Steere, A.C., Hutchinson, G.J., Rahn, D.W., Sigal, L.H., Craft, J.E., DeSanna, E.T. and Malawista, S.E. (1983a) Treatment of the early manifestations of Lyme disease. *Annals of Internal Medicine* 99, 22–26.

Steere, A.C., Bartenhagen, N.H., Craft, J.E., Hutchinson, G.J., Newman, J.H., Rahn, D.W., Sigal L.H., Spieler, P.N., Stenn, K.S. and Malawista, S.E. (1983b) The early clinical manifestations of Lyme disease. *Annals of Internal Medicine* 99, 76–82.

Steere, A.C., Snydman, D., Murray, P., Mensch, J., Main, A.J. Jr, Wallis, R.C., Shope, R.E. and Malawista, S.E. (1985) Historical perspectives. In: Lyme borreliosis. *Proceedings of the Second International Symposium on Lyme Disease and Related Disorders*, Vienna, pp. 3–6.

Steere, A.C., Schoen, R.T. and Taylor, E. (1987) The clinical evolution of Lyme arthritis. *Annals of Internal Medicine* 107, 725–731.

Steere, A.C., Sikand, V.K., Meurice, F., Parenti, D.L., Fikrig, E., Schoen, R.T., Nowakowski, J., Schmid, C.H., Laukamp, S., Buscarino, C. and Krause, D.S. (1998) Vaccination against Lyme disease with recombinant *Borrelia burgdorferi* outer-surface lipoprotein A with adjuvant. Lyme Disease Vaccine Study Group. *New England Journal of Medicine* 339, 209–215.

Steere, A.C., McHugh, G., Suarez, C., Hoitt, J., Damle, N. and Sikand, V.K. (2003) Prospective study of coinfection in patients with erythema migrans. *Clinical Infectious Diseases* 36, 1078–1081.

Strle, F., Ruzic, E. and Cimperman, J. (1992) Erythema migrans: comparison of treatment with azithromycin, doxycycline and phenoxymethylpenicillin. *Journal of Antimicrobial Chemotherapy* 30, 543–550.

Strle, F., Maraspin, V., Lotric-Furlan, S., Ružić-Sabljić, E. and Cimperman, J. (1996a) Azithromycin and doxycycline for treatment of *Borrelia* culture-proven erythema migrans. *Infection* 24, 64–68.

Strle, F., Nelson, J.A., Ružić-Sabljić, E., Cimperman, J., Maraspin, V., Lotric-Furlan, S., Cheng, Y., Picken, M.M., Trenholme, G.M. and Picken, R.N. (1996b) European Lyme Borreliosis: 231 culture-confirmed cases involving patients with erythema migrans. *Clinical Infectious Diseases* 23, 61–65.

Strle, F., Nadelman, R.B., Cimperman, J., Nowakowski, J., Picken, R.N., Schwartz, I., Maraspin, V., Aguero-Rosenfeld, M.E., Varde, S., Lotric-Furlan, S. and Wormser, G.P. (1999) Comparison of culture-confirmed erythema migrans caused by *Borrelia burgdorferi* sensu stricto in New York and by *Borrelia afzelii* in Slovenia. *Annals of Internal Medicine* 130, 32–36.

Strle, K., Drouin, E.E., Shen, S., Khoury, J.E., McHugh, G., Ružić-Sabljić, E., Strle, F. and Steere, A.C. (2009) *Borrelia burgdorferi* stimulates macrophages to secrete higher levels of cytokines and chemokines than *Borrelia afzelii* or *Borrelia garinii*. *Journal of Infectious Diseases* 200, 1936–1943.

Strle, K., Jones, K., Drouin, E., Li, X. and Steere, A.C. (2010) Greater inflammatory potential of *Borrelia burgdorferi* RST1 (OspC Type A) isolates in cell culture and in patients with erythema migrans or Lyme arthritis. In: *Program and Abstracts of the 12th International Conference on Lyme Borreliosis and other Tick-Borne Diseases* (Ljubljana, Slovenia) 26–29 September. Abstract 8, page 9.

Strle, F., Ružić-Sabljić, E., Logar, M., Maraspin, V., Lotrić-Furlan, S., Cimperman, J., Ogrinc, K., Stupica, D., Nadelman, R.B., Nowakowski, J. and Wormser, G.P. (2011) Comparison of erythema migrans caused by *Borrelia burgdorferi* and *Borrelia garini*. *Vector-Borne and Zoonotic Diseases* 9, 1253–1258.

Strobino, B.A., Williams, C.L., Abid, S., Chalson, R. and Spierling, P. (1993) Lyme disease and pregnancy outcome: a prospective study of two thousand prenatal patients. *American Journal of Obstetrics and Gynecology* 169, 367–374.

Strobino, B., Abid, S. and Gewitz, M. (1999) Maternal Lyme disease and congenital heart disease: a case-control study in an endemic area. *American Journal of Obstetrics and Gynecology* 180, 711–716.

Sudhindra, P., Wang, G., Schriefer, M.E., McKenna, D., Zhuge, J., Krause, P.J., Marques, A.R. and Wormser, G.P. (2016) Insights into *Borrelia miyamotoi* infection from an untreated case demonstrating relapsing fever, monocytosis and a positive C6 Lyme serology. *Diagnostic Microbiology and Infectious Disease* 86(1), 93–96.

Tibbles, C.D. and Edlow, J.A. (2007) Does this patient have erythema migrans? *JAMA* 297, 2617–2627.

Todd, S.R., Dahlgren, F.S., Traeger, M.S., Beltrán-Aguilar, E.D., Marianos, D.W., Hamilton, C., McQuiston, J.H. and Regan, J.J. (2015) No visible dental staining in children treated with doxycycline for suspected Rocky Mountain spotted fever. *Journal of Pediatrics* 166(5), 1246–1251.

Vetter, R.S. and Bush, S.P. (2002) Reports of presumptive brown recluse spider bites reinforce improbable diagnosis in regions of North America where the spider is not endemic. *Clinical Infectious Diseases* 35, 442–445.

Weber, K., Preac-Mursic, V., Neubert, U., Thurmayr, R., Herzer, P., Wilske, B., Schierz, G. and Marget, W. (1988) Antibiotic therapy of early European Lyme borreliosis and acrodermatitis chronica atrophicans. *Annals of the New York Academy of Sciences* 539, 324–345.

Weber, K., Preac-Mursic, V., Wilske, B., Thurmayr, R., Neubert, U. and Scherwitz, C. (1990) A randomized trial of ceftriaxone versus oral penicillin for the treatment of early European Lyme borreliosis. *Infection* 18, 91–96.

Weber, K., Wilske, B., Preac-Mursic, V. and Thurmayr, R. (1993) Azithromycin versus penicillin V for the treatment of early Lyme borreliosis. *Infection* 21, 367–372.

Weitzner, E., McKenna, D., Nowakowski, J., Scavarda, C., Dornbush, R., Bittker, S., Cooper, D., Nadelman, R.B., Visintainer, P., Schwartz, I. and Wormser, G.P. (2015) Long-term assessment of post-treatment symptoms in patients with culture-confirmed early Lyme disease. *Clinical Infectious Diseases* 61(12), 1800–1806.

Williams, C.L., Strobino, B., Weinstein, A., Spierling, P. and Medici, F. (1995) Maternal Lyme disease and congenital malformation: a cord blood serosurvey in endemic and control areas. *Paediatric and Perinatal Epidemiology* 9, 320–330.

Wormser, G.P. (2006) Early Lyme disease. *New England Journal of Medicine* 354, 2794–2801.

Wormser, G.P., Bittker, S., Cooper, D., Nowakowski, J., Nadelman, R.B. and Pavia, C. (2000) Comparison of the yields of blood cultures using serum or plasma from patients with early Lyme disease. *Journal of Clinical Microbiology* 38, 1648–1650.

Wormser, G.P., Ramanathan, R., Nowakowski, J., McKenna, D., Holmgren, D., Visintainer, P., Dornbush, R., Singh, B. and Nadelman, R.B. (2003) Duration of antibiotic therapy for early Lyme disease. *Annals of Internal Medicine* 138, 697–704.

Wormser, G.P., McKenna, D., Carlin, J., Nadelman, R.B., Cavaliere, L.F., Holmgren, D., Byrne, D.W. and Nowakowski, J. (2005a) Brief communication: hematogenous dissemination in early Lyme disease. *Annals of Internal Medicine* 142, 751–755.

Wormser, G.P., Masters, E., Liveris, D., Nowakowski, J., Nadelman, R.B., Holmgren, D., Bittker, S., Cooper, D., Wang, G. and Schwartz, I. (2005b) Microbiologic evaluation of patients from Missouri with erythema migrans. *Clinical Infectious Diseases* 40, 423–428.

Wormser, G.P., Masters, E., Nowakowski, J., McKenna, D., Holmgren, D., Ma, K., Ihde, L., Cavaliere, L.F. and Nadelman, R.B. (2005c) Prospective clinical evaluation of patients from Missouri and New York with erythema migrans-like skin lesions. *Clinical Infectious Diseases* 41, 958–465.

Wormser, G.P., Kaslow, R., Tang, J., Wade, K., Liveris, D., Schwartz, I. and Klempner, M. (2005d) Association between human leukocyte antigen class II alleles and genotype of *Borrelia burgdorferi* in patients with early Lyme disease. *Journal of Infectious Diseases* 192, 2020–2026.

Wormser, G.P., Dattwyler, R.J., Shapiro, E.D. *et al.* (2006) The clinical assessment, treatment, and prevention of Lyme disease, human granulocytic anaplasmosis, and babesiosis: clinical practice guidelines by the Infectious Diseases Society of America. *Clinical Infectious Diseases* 43, 1089–1134. Erratum in: *Clinical Infectious Diseases* (2007) 45, 941.

Wormser, G.P., Weitzner, E., McKenna, D., Nadelman, R.B., Scavarda, C. and Nowakowski, J. (2015a) Long-term assessment of fatigue in patients with culture-confirmed Lyme disease. *American Journal of Medicine* 128(2), 181–184.

Wormser, G.P., Weitzner, E., McKenna, D., Nadelman, R.B., Scavarda, C., Molla, I., Dornbush, R., Visintainer, P. and Nowakowski, J. (2015b) Long-term assessment of health-related quality of life in patients with culture-confirmed early Lyme disease. *Clinical Infectious Diseases* 61(2), 244–247.

11 Lyme Carditis

Jonathan R. Salik and David M. Dudzinski
Massachusetts General Hospital, Boston, Massachusetts, USA

11.1 Introduction

First described in 1977, the cardiac complications of Lyme disease – termed 'Lyme carditis' – present during the early disseminated phase of infection by *Borreliella burgdorferi*, usually 3 weeks to 3 months after initial inoculation (Steere *et al.*, 1977; 1980). The clinical manifestations of Lyme carditis are typically self-limited and almost always involve the heart's conduction system at the level of the atrioventricular node, although occasionally other cardiac manifestations, such as myocarditis and pericarditis, may be seen. The epidemiology, pathogenesis, clinical manifestations, diagnosis, treatment and prognosis of Lyme carditis will be reviewed in this chapter.

11.2 Epidemiology

In the initial surveillance studies conducted in the United States on Lyme disease, Lyme carditis was reported to occur in as many as 4–10% of patients with serologically confirmed Lyme disease (Schmid *et al.*, 1985; Ciesielski *et al.*, 1989; McAlister *et al.*, 1989). However, these studies, published in the mid-1980s, did not employ a standardized definition of Lyme carditis. As such, the majority of reported cases consisted of patients with symptomatic palpitations alone in the absence of other, more objective findings of conduction disease, thereby calling into question the validity of the data.

To that end, in 1990, the Centers for Disease Control and Prevention (CDC) established a uniform definition of Lyme carditis in order to improve the accuracy of reported data. In its statement, the CDC defined Lyme carditis as the:

> acute onset of high-grade (second- or third-degree) atrioventricular conduction defects that resolve in days to weeks and are sometimes associated with myocarditis. (Wharton *et al.*, 1990)

Using this stricter definition of Lyme carditis, updated surveillance data suggest that the incidence of Lyme carditis among patients with Lyme disease in the United States is in fact closer to 1%, which better aligns with case rates quoted in European studies (Cimmino, 1998; Forrester *et al.*, 2014; CDC, 2016) (Fig. 11.1).

Interestingly, although the gender distribution of Lyme disease is divided almost evenly between men and women, Lyme carditis is two to three times more common in men; 65% of cases reported to the CDC between 2001 and 2010 occurred in male patients, and other studies have reported the ratio of male to female patients with Lyme carditis to be roughly three to one (Vlay *et al.*, 1991; Forrester *et al.*, 2014). The development of third-degree (i.e. complete)

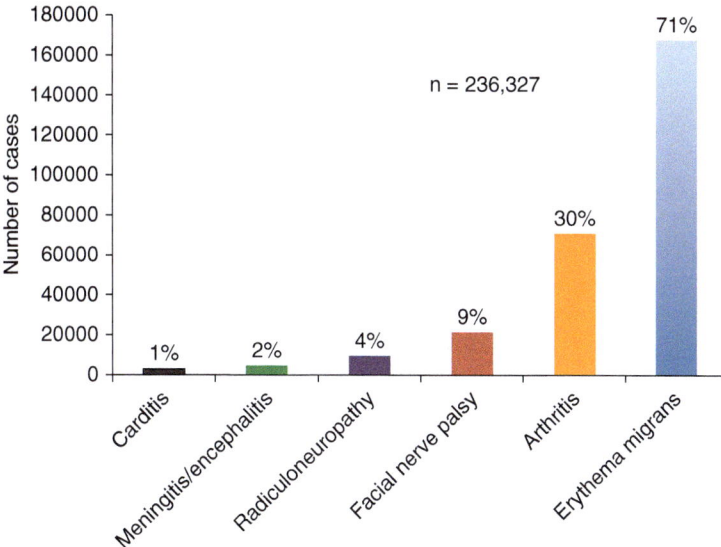

Fig. 11.1. Clinical manifestations of Lyme disease in the United States, 2001–2010. This figure outlines the most common clinical manifestations of serologically confirmed Lyme disease reported to the Centers for Disease Control and Prevention (CDC) between 2001 and 2010. Cardiac symptoms were present in 1% of cases.

atrioventricular block is particularly associated with male gender; in a case series of 45 patients with Lyme carditis and third-degree atrioventricular block, 84% of cases occurred in men (Forrester and Mead, 2014).

The incidence of Lyme carditis in children is less well studied; in one study investigating 207 children with early disseminated Lyme disease, 16% were found to have evidence of Lyme carditis, well above the case rate reported in adults (Costello et al., 2009).

11.3 Pathogenesis

Three potential mechanisms are implicated in the pathogenesis of Lyme carditis: (i) direct spirochetal infiltration of cardiac tissue; (ii) maladaptive secondary inflammatory response within the myocardium in the absence of direct invasion; and (iii) molecular mimicry. Of note, these mechanisms have been elucidated primarily through the use of murine models since the vast majority of patients with Lyme carditis improve without the need for endomyocardial biopsy, thereby precluding extensive study of affected human tissue.

11.3.1 Direct spirochetal infiltration

Multiple studies have demonstrated the ability of *B. burgdorferi* to directly invade all three layers of the heart wall (epicardium, myocardium and endocardium) as well as the aortic adventitia (Armstrong et al., 1992; Barthold et al., 1993; Ruderman et al., 1995). The myocardial interstitium may represent a particularly hospitable site for *B. burgdorferi* infection because the spirochete is able to interact with proteins in the extracellular matrix, specifically decorin, heparan sulfate and dermatan sulfate, to promote self-adhesion. Moreover, these extracellular matrix proteins are also thought to play a critical role in the spirochete's ability to evade the host immune system, although the mechanism by which this occurs has yet to be fully delineated (Saba et al., 2001; Cabello et al., 2007; Imai et al., 2013).

11.3.2 Maladaptive secondary inflammatory response

Unlike Lyme arthritis, which is characterized by an infiltration of neutrophils into joint tissue, Lyme carditis is characterized by an infiltration of macrophages (Ruderman *et al.*, 1995; Cadavid *et al.*, 2004). In particular, the inflammatory response within the myocardium is mediated by macrophage chemoattractant protein 1 (MCP-1), a chemokine produced by cardiac myocytes whose expression is induced by *B. burgdorferi*. In addition, cytokines manufactured by macrophages themselves, such as CXCL1, have been shown to promote sustained inflammation in models of Lyme arthritis and may be implicated in the pathogenesis of Lyme carditis, as well (Guerau-de-Arrelano *et al.*, 2005; De Filippo *et al.*, 2013).

In contrast, lymphocytes may play a protective role against the development of Lyme carditis. Multiple murine models, for example, have demonstrated a correlation between T- and B-cell immunodeficiencies – specifically severe combined immunodeficiency – and the severity of Lyme carditis. Moreover, deficiencies in the production of invariant natural killer T cells have also been correlated with increased severity of Lyme carditis, a response thought to be mediated by the resultant lack of interferon-gamma normally manufactured by these cells (Schaible *et al.*, 1989; 1990; Zimmer *et al.*, 1990; Museteanu *et al.*, 1991; Barthold *et al.*, 1992; Brown *et al.*, 2006; Olson *et al.*, 2009).

11.3.3 Molecular mimicry

Molecular mimicry, a form of autoimmunity in which a foreign antigen stimulates the production of cross-reactive antibodies against a self-antigen, may also be involved in the pathogenesis of Lyme carditis. This association is possibly mediated by outer-surface protein A (OspA), a protein on the surface of *B. burgdorferi* that shares epitopes with cardiac myosin (Raveche *et al.*, 2005). Though more research is needed to fully articulate the role of molecular mimicry in the development of Lyme carditis, the presence of structural similarities between OspA and cardiac myosin is a hypothesis-generating finding.

11.4 Clinical Manifestations

Lyme carditis presents during the early disseminated phase of Lyme disease, typically 3 weeks to 3 months after initial inoculation with *B. burgdorferi*. The hallmark cardiac manifestation is conduction disease, usually located at the level of the atrioventricular node, although myocarditis and pericarditis may also be seen. Other cardiac abnormalities, including valvular regurgitation, coronary artery aneurysm and endocarditis, are rare and have been described in case reports only. Lyme carditis is ordinarily self-limited in nature, and usually resolves within 6 weeks of onset. Of note, though several studies have suggested a causal relationship between Lyme carditis and the development of chronic dilated cardiomyopathy; this association remains controversial and not well validated.

11.4.1 Conduction disease

Conduction disease is by far the most common manifestation of Lyme carditis, occurring in up to 87% of cases (McAlister *et al.*, 1989). Symptoms are varied and include lightheadedness, dizziness, syncope, palpitations, dyspnea, chest pain and fatigue (Fish *et al.*, 2008). Patients almost exclusively present with atrioventricular block, although other types of conduction defects, including sinoatrial nodal exit block, intra-atrial block, bundle branch block, fascicular block, QTc prolongation, ventricular arrhythmias and atrial fibrillation, may occasionally be seen (Reznick *et al.*, 1986; van der Linde *et al.*, 1989; 1990; McAlister *et al.*, 1989; Seslar *et al.*, 2006; Welsh *et al.*, 2012; Koene *et al.*, 2012; Wenger *et al.*, 2012).

Though rarely performed, electrophysiologic studies in patients with Lyme-associated conduction disease typically demonstrate a prolonged atrial–His interval, representing delayed conduction at or above the level of the atrioventricular node. In contrast, prolongation of the His–ventricular interval, representing delayed conduction below the level of the atrioventricular node, is less common (van der Linde, 1991).

While patients with Lyme carditis may exhibit any degree of atrioventricular block, episodes of third-degree atrioventricular block are particularly common, occurring in 40–50% of cases (Goldings and Jericho, 1986; van der Linde, 1991; Fish *et al.*, 2008; Lelovas *et al.*, 2008; Forrester and Mead, 2014; Robinson *et al.*, 2015). Often, third-degree atrioventricular block presents as the initial conduction disturbance, followed by a gradual resolution to second- and then first-degree atrioventricular block; however, rapid alternation between first-, second- and third-degree atrioventricular block may also be seen (Steere et al., 1980; McAlister et al., 1989; Fish et al., 2008). Of note, in patients with fluctuating degrees of atrioventricular block, the strongest predictor of progression from first- to third-degree atrioventricular block is a PR interval greater than 300 ms (compared to a normal interval of 120–200 ms) (Steere et al., 1980).

Lyme-associated conduction disease is usually transient and almost always resolves within 6 weeks of initial presentation. Third-degree atrioventricular block is particularly short-lived, typically converting to a lesser degree of atrioventricular block within 6 days (McAlister et al., 1989; Forrester and Mead, 2014). In rare instances Lyme-associated conduction disease persists beyond 6 weeks; permanent conduction disease is extremely uncommon and has been described in only a handful of known cases (McAlister et al., 1989; van der Linde et al., 1990; Mayer et al., 1990; Artigao et al., 1991).

Rarely, sudden cardiac death may occur in the setting of Lyme carditis. In the majority of reported cases, at least some degree of underlying cardiovascular disease was identified on autopsy, including two cases of Wolf–Parkinson–White syndrome (Marcus et al., 1985; Cary et al., 1990; Tavora et al., 2008; CDC, 2013; Muehlenbachs et al., 2016).

11.4.2 Myocarditis and pericarditis

Myocarditis is an uncommon manifestation in Lyme carditis, occurring in approximately 10–15% of cases (Ciesielski et al., 1989; Fish et al., 2008). Typically, Lyme-associated myocarditis presents with diffuse, non-specific ST-segment and T-wave changes on electrocardiogram, although reduced left ventricular ejection fraction and signs and symptoms of congestive heart failure may also be seen. As with conduction disease, Lyme-associated myocarditis is generally mild and self-limited in nature; severe complications such as biventricular heart failure, cardiogenic shock and death are extremely rare (Steere et al., 1980; Horowitz and Belkin, 1995; Koene et al., 2012; Maher et al., 2012; Yoon et al., 2015).

Pericarditis is another uncommon manifestation of Lyme carditis, occurring in approximately 2–16% of cases (Lorcerie, et al., 1987; Ciesielski et al., 1989; Fish et al., 2008). While patients with Lyme-associated pericarditis may develop pericardial effusions, only one case of cardiac tamponade has been described (Steere et al., 1980; Bruyn et al., 1994).

11.4.3 Other cardiac manifestations

Several other cardiac abnormalities have been rarely reported to occur in patients with Lyme carditis, including coronary artery aneurysm and acute mitral regurgitation (Gasser et al., 1994; 1998; Canver et al., 2000; Cuisset et al., 2008). Additionally, though B. burgdorferi itself has never been isolated as a source of endocarditis, two cases of endocarditis caused by B. bissettii and B. afzelii – strains endemic to Europe – have been identified from samples of explanted valve tissue taken from patients in the Czech Republic and France, respectively (Rudenko et al., 2008; Hidri et al., 2012).

11.4.4 Chronic dilated cardiomyopathy

Though multiple studies have implicated Lyme carditis as a cause of chronic dilated cardiomyopathy, this association remains controversial. The first putative case of Lyme-associated cardiomyopathy was detailed in a 1990 Austrian case report describing a patient with dilated cardiomyopathy of unknown cause who was found to have positive IgG serologies against B. burgdorferi and widespread spirochetal infiltration on endomyocardial biopsy (Stanek et al., 1990). In a subsequent case series by the same Austrian group, 19 of 72 patients with idiopathic dilated cardiomyopathy were shown to be seropositive for IgG antibodies against B. burgdorferi, compared to only seven of 55 patients with known ischemic cardiomyopathy. Several other European studies from this time period uncovered similar results; in fact, a non-controlled case series by Gasser et al. (1992) investigating nine Austrian patients with idiopathic dilated cardiomyopathy and positive Lyme serologies suggested that treatment with 2 weeks of intravenous ceftriaxone led to the complete normalization of ventricular function in six cases (Klein et al., 1991; Stanek et al., 1991; Lardieri et al., 1993).

Although these initial studies are provocative, their external validity is dubious. For one, the data are derived exclusively from observational case reports that are neither randomized nor matched to normal controls, thereby limiting the strength of the conclusions. In addition, the majority of these studies do not indicate the type of serology testing performed; as such, it is unclear if patients tested positive for IgG antibodies alone, or for both IgM and IgG antibodies, which could suggest a more acute cause of cardiomyopathy. Finally, and perhaps most importantly, 20 years of subsequent investigations in both Europe and North America have failed to consistently reproduce these findings.

In a study of 175 patients with dilated cardiomyopathy in Minnesota, for example, the rate of *B. burgdorferi* IgG seropositivity did not differ significantly between patients with known ischemic cardiomyopathy and those with idiopathic cardiomyopathy (9.6% vs. 7.8%, $P = 0.07$). Moreover, though six of the seropositive patients were treated with an empiric course of antibiotics against *B. burgdorferi* (three with intravenous ceftriaxone for 2 weeks and three with oral doxycycline for 1 month), none demonstrated an improvement in left ventricle ejection fraction after completion of therapy (Sonnesyn et al., 1995). In a subsequent study investigating endomyocardial biopsy samples taken from 68 patients with idiopathic dilated cardiomyopathy from an endemic area of Germany, polymerase chain reaction (PCR) testing for *B. burgdorferi* DNA was negative in all 68 cases (Suedkamp et al., 1999).

In total, since the initial European case reports were published in the early 1990s, at least four studies from both Europe and North America have failed to demonstrate an association between Lyme borreliosis and chronic dilated cardiomyopathy (Rees et al., 1994; Sonnesyn et al., 1995; Suedkamp et al., 1999; Karatolios et al., 2015). As such, any causative relationship between the two remains speculative.

11.5 Diagnosis

No single definitive test for Lyme carditis exists; rather, the diagnosis of Lyme carditis is based upon a combination of serologic, electrocardiographic and echocardiographic data in conjunction with compatible epidemiologic and clinical findings.

In assessing a patient with possible Lyme carditis, consideration of the epidemiologic risk for acquisition of *B. burgdorferi* is paramount; in patients who have not traveled to a Lyme-endemic area within the past 3–6 months, the diagnosis of Lyme carditis can essentially be excluded (Robinson et al., 2015).

A careful history should be taken to assess for symptoms of Lyme carditis, including lightheadedness, dizziness, syncope, palpitations, dyspnea, chest pain and fatigue. Physical examination may reveal the presence of a tick bite, although erythema migrans is generally absent (Fish et al., 2008). In addition, other manifestations of early disseminated Lyme disease, such as neurologic Lyme borreliosis, often co-exist and may manifest with lymphocytic meningitis, cranial neuropathy (especially involving the facial nerve), sensorimotor radiculopathy (Bannwarth syndrome) or encephalitis.

Two-tier serologic testing – a screening enzyme linked immunosorbent assay (ELISA) followed by a confirmatory protein immunoblot (Western blot) analysis – is essential to perform in all patients with suspected Lyme carditis (Robinson et al., 2015). Since cardiac involvement reflects early dissemination of infection, the vast majority of affected patients exhibit positive serologic testing for both IgM and IgG antibodies. However, it is critical to note that negative serologies are not sufficiently sensitive to exclude the diagnosis of Lyme carditis because both antibodies may be negative for the first 3-6 weeks after initial infection (Fish et al., 2008; Steere et al., 2008).

Electrocardiography (EKG) should be obtained in all patients exhibiting signs or symptoms of Lyme carditis or other forms of early disseminated disease. The EKG typically reveals various degrees of atrioventricular block, although other abnormalities, such as ST-segment changes, T-wave flattening or inversions, QTc prolongation, ventricular arrhythmias and atrial fibrillation, may also be seen (Figs 11.2–11.4) (Steere et al., 1980; Dolbec et al., 2010; Robinson et al., 2015; Afari et al., 2016). In patients with evidence of myocarditis or pericarditis, echocardiography should promptly be obtained

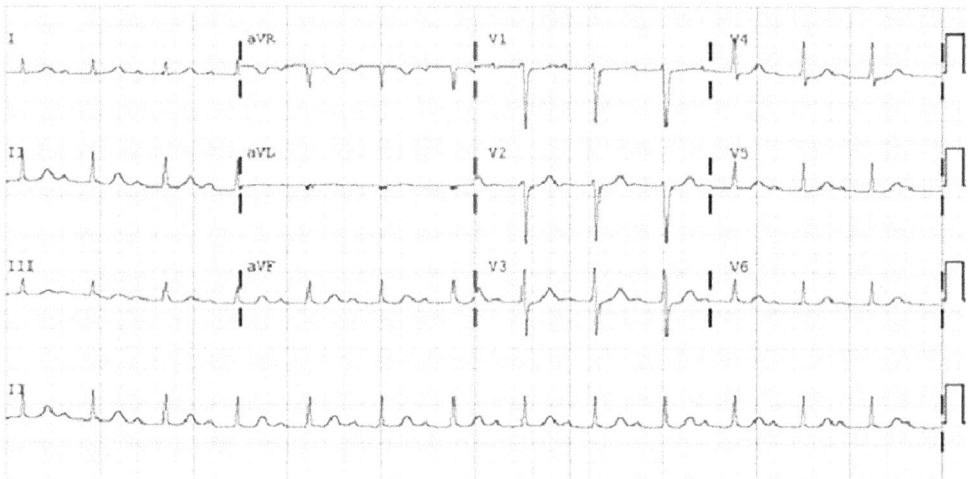

Fig. 11.2. Lyme carditis with first-degree atrioventricular block. This electrocardiogram from a patient with Lyme carditis demonstrates first-degree atrioventricular block with a PR interval of 320 ms. (From Afari et al., 2016.)

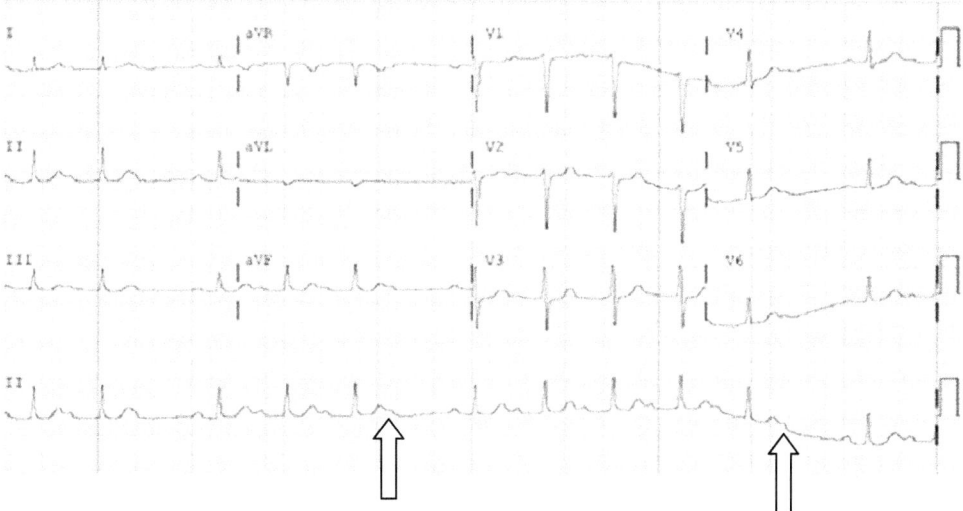

Fig. 11.3. Lyme carditis with Mobitz Type I (Wenckebach) second-degree atrioventricular block. This electrocardiogram from a patient with Lyme carditis demonstrates Mobitz Type I (Wenckebach) second-degree atrioventricular block, with cycles of progressive prolongation of the PR interval followed by a non-conducted P wave (arrows). (From Afari et al., 2016.)

to evaluate for reduced left ventricular ejection fraction, global or regional ventricular wall hypokinesis, cardiac chamber enlargement or pericardial effusion (Robinson et al., 2015).

Additional imaging modalities, such as cardiac magnetic resonance imaging, gallium-67 myocardial scintigraphy, and indium-111 antimyosin scintigraphy, may reveal myocardial inflammation, thereby supporting a diagnosis of carditis. Of note, however, gallium- and indium-based imaging studies are usually obtained for research purposes only and are not commonly

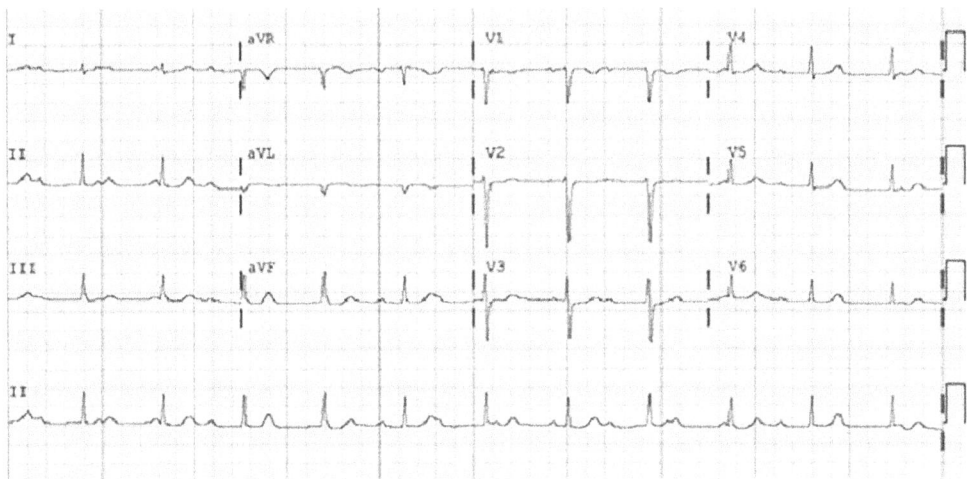

Fig. 11.4. Lyme carditis with third-degree (complete) atrioventricular block. This electrocardiogram from a patient with Lyme carditis demonstrates third-degree (complete) atrioventricular block. Third-degree atrioventricular block is characterized by lack of conduction between the atria and the ventricles, manifested by lack of relationship between the P waves and QRS complex on the electrocardiogram ('atrioventricular dissociation'). The QRS complex is narrow, suggesting a junctional escape rhythm. (From Afari et al., 2016.)

available in clinical practice (Jacobs et al., 1984; Alpert et al., 1985; Bergler-Klein et al., 1993; Munk et al., 2007; Maher et al., 2012).

Finally, while endomyocardial biopsy may allow for the direct isolation of B. burgdorferi from cardiac tissue, such invasive testing is not recommended in routine clinical practice given the self-limited nature of Lyme carditis and the risk of myocardial perforation associated with the procedure (Wu et al., 2001; Fish et al., 2008).

11.6 Treatment

The mainstay of treatment for Lyme carditis is antibiotic therapy, which may be administered orally or intravenously in accordance with guidelines established by the Infectious Diseases Society of America (IDSA). Anti-inflammatory agents have unclear benefit and are not routinely recommended. For patients with symptomatic or hemodynamically unstable atrioventricular block, temporary cardiac pacing is indicated. In contrast, placement of a permanent cardiac pacemaker is not indicated given the self-limited nature of the disease and the anticipation of complete cardiac recovery.

11.6.1 Antibiotic therapy

Hospitalization and initiation of intravenous antibiotic therapy are indicated for patients with significant symptoms (e.g. syncope), second- or third-degree atrioventricular block or first-degree atrioventricular block with a PR interval greater than 300 ms. The parenteral antibiotic of choice is ceftriaxone 2 g daily; alternative agents include cefotaxime 2 g every 8 h or penicillin G 3–4 million units every 4 h (Wormser et al., 2006; Fish et al., 2008; Robinson et al., 2015). Intravenous antibiotics are typically continued until resolution of the above indications, at which time the patient may be transitioned to oral antibiotics.

Outpatient therapy with oral antibiotics may be pursued in asymptomatic patients with first-degree atrioventricular block and a PR interval less than 300 ms. The preferred enteral agent is doxycycline 100 mg twice per day; other acceptable regimens include amoxicillin 500 mg three times per day or cefuroxime 500 mg twice per day. Of note, doxycycline should not be administered to pregnant women; its use in children under 8 years of age while avoided in the past, is currently under review (see Chapters 6 and 14 in this volume)

(Wormser et al., 2006; Fish et al., 2008; Robinson et al., 2015).

The optimal duration of antibiotic therapy is unknown. Based on expert opinion, antibiotic treatment – whether oral or intravenous – is recommended for at least 14 to 21 days, although some studies have advocated for up to 28 days of therapy (Olson et al., 1986; Wormser et al., 2006; Fish et al., 2008; Robinson et al., 2015).

Patients treated for Lyme carditis may rarely experience the Jarisch–Herxheimer reaction, an acute immunologic reaction that occurs after initiation of antibiotic therapy in patients with certain infections, most commonly syphilis. The hallmark symptom is fever, which usually occurs within hours of antibiotic administration; additional symptoms include headache, myalgias, rigors and hypotension (Moore, 1987; Maloy et al., 1998). More significant symptoms, such as ventricular tachycardia and acute myocarditis, have been described in a single case report only (Koene et al., 2012).

11.6.2 Anti-inflammatory agents

Although several studies have investigated the benefits of anti-inflammatory agents – specifically aspirin and glucocorticoids – in the management of refractory Lyme carditis, there is no high-quality evidence supporting their use (McAlister et al., 1989; Koene et al., 2012). In fact, one study demonstrated a paradoxical worsening of neurologic and rheumatologic symptoms upon withdrawal of short-term glucocorticoid therapy after initial administration (Cox and Krajden, 1991; Fish et al., 2008). As such, neither medication is recommended for use in routine clinical practice.

11.6.3 Cardiac pacing

All patients hospitalized with Lyme carditis should be monitored on cardiac telemetry. For patients with asymptomatic or hemodynamically stable atrioventricular block, management is expectant and no additional treatment is necessary. For patients with symptomatic or hemodynamically unstable first-degree or Mobitz Type I second-degree atrioventricular block, intravenous atropine 0.5 mg should be administered every 3–5 min in accordance with advanced cardiac life support guidelines (maximum total dose 3 g). In contrast, for patients with symptomatic or hemodynamically unstable Mobitz Type II second-degree or third-degree atrioventricular block, the anti-cholinergic effects of atropine are unlikely to be effective since the location of the block is usually below the level of the atrioventricular node. In such cases, treatment is with beta-adrenergic agonists such as dopamine, epinephrine or isoproterenol (Neumar et al., 2015).

The primary indication for temporary cardiac pacing is the development of symptomatic or hemodynamically unstable atrioventricular block refractory to medical management (Gammage, 2000; Robinson et al., 2015). Temporary cardiac pacing may be initiated through either a transvenous or transcutaneous approach and should be maintained until complete resolution of symptoms or hemodynamic instability. Importantly, while the presence of a PR interval greater than 300 ms predicts progression to third-degree atrioventricular block, it is not an indication for temporary cardiac pacing itself (Goldings and Jericho, 1986; van der Linde, 1991; Pinto, 2002; Lelovas et al., 2008; Forrester and Mead, 2014; Robinson et al., 2015).

Placement of a permanent cardiac pacemaker in patients with Lyme carditis is not recommended since the associated conduction disease is self-limited and resolves without expectation of recurrence or long-term cardiac dysfunction (Epstein et al., 2008). In the rare circumstance that a patient with Lyme carditis does, in fact, develop chronic conduction disease, placement of a permanent cardiac pacemaker may then be considered, but this has been described in an extremely small number of isolated case reports (van der Linde et al., 1990; Mayer et al., 1990; Artigao et al., 1991).

11.7 Prognosis

The prognosis of Lyme carditis is generally excellent. Symptoms usually resolve within 6 weeks of onset, and well over 90% of patients make a complete recovery even in the absence of antibiotic therapy (Lelovas et al., 2008). As discussed in Section 11.4.1, permanent conduction disease and life-threatening complications such as sudden cardiac death are rare and have developed in only a handful of known cases.

11.8 Further Directions for Research

Unfortunately, given the relative rarity of Lyme carditis, no randomized trials have been conducted evaluating the efficacy of various diagnostic or treatment strategies. Current recommendations guiding clinical practice are therefore based solely on expert opinion. As such, more high-quality evidence is needed to help answer a number of outstanding clinical questions, including: the most appropriate choice, route and duration of antibiotic therapy; the role of aspirin and glucocorticoids in the management of refractory Lyme carditis; the role of biomarkers including erythrocyte sedimentation rate (ESR) and C-reactive protein (CRP) in the diagnosis of Lyme carditis; and the utility of screening electrocardiograms in individuals diagnosed with other forms of Lyme disease.

11.9 Summary

Lyme carditis occurs in approximately 1% of patients with Lyme disease and presents within the early disseminated phase of infection with *B. burgdorferi*. Multiple mechanisms are possibly involved in the pathogenesis of Lyme carditis, including direct spirochetal infiltration of cardiac tissue, maladaptive secondary inflammatory response in the absence of direct invasion and molecular mimicry. The most common clinical manifestation of Lyme carditis is conduction disease at the level of the atrioventricular node, although myocarditis and pericarditis may also be seen. Chronic dilated cardiomyopathy is a speculative long-term sequela of Lyme carditis, but further research is needed to assess this association. Diagnosis of Lyme carditis is based on a combination of clinical, laboratory, electrocardiographic and echocardiographic data. Treatment consists of oral or intravenous antibiotics for at least 14–21 days along with temporary cardiac pacing in select circumstances. Prognosis is excellent as almost all patients make a complete recovery without persistence of conduction disease or myocardial dysfunction.

References

Afari, M.E., Marmoush, F., Rehman, M.U., Gorsi, U. and Yammine, J.F. (2016) Lyme carditis: an interesting trip to third-degree heart block and back. *Case Reports in Cardiology* 2016, 1–3.

Alpert, L.I., Welch, P. and Fisher, N (1985) Gallium-positive Lyme disease myocarditis. *Clinical Nuclear Medicine* 10, 617.

Armstrong, A.L., Barthold, S.W., Persing, D.H. and Beck, D.S. (1992) Carditis in Lyme disease susceptible and resistant strains of laboratory mice infected with *Borrelia burgdorferi*. *American Journal of Tropical Medicine and Hygiene* 47, 249–258.

Artigao, R., Torres, G., Guerrero, A., Jimenez-Mena, M. and Bayas Paredes, M. (1991) Irreversible complete heart block in Lyme disease. *American Journal of Medicine* 90, 531–533.

Barthold, S.W., Sidman, C.L. and Smith, A.L. (1992) Lyme borreliosis in genetically resistant and susceptible mice with severe combined immunodeficiency. *American Journal of Tropical Medicine and Hygiene* 47, 605–613.

Barthold, S.W., De Souza, M.S., Janotka, J.L., Smith, A.L. and Pershing, D.H. (1993) Chronic Lyme borreliosis in the laboratory mouse. *American Journal of Pathology* 143, 959–971.

Bergler-Klein, J., Sochor, H., Stanek G., Globits, S., Ullrich, R. and Glogar, D. (1993) Indium 111-monoclonal antimyosin antibody and magnetic resonance imaging in the diagnosis of acute Lyme myopericarditis. *Archives of Internal Medicine* 153, 2696–2700.

Brown, C.R., Blaho, V.A., Fritsche, K.L. and Loiacono, C.M. (2006) Stat1 deficiency exacerbates carditis but not arthritis during experimental Lyme borreliosis. *Journal of Interferon and Cytokine Research* 26, 390–399.

Bruyn, G.A., De Koning, J., Reijsoo, F.J., Houtman, P.M. and Hoogkamp-Korstanje, J.A.A. (1994) Lyme pericarditis leading to tamponade. *Rheumatology* 9, 862–866.

Cabello, F.C., Godfrey, H.P. and Newman, S.A. (2007) Hidden in plain sight: *Borrelia burgdorferi* and the extracellular matrix. *Trends in Microbiology* 15, 350–354.

Cadavid, D., Bai, Y., Hodzic, E., Narayan, K., Barthold, S.W. and Pachner, A.R. (2004) Cardiac involvement in non-human primates infected with the Lyme disease spirochete *Borrelia burgdorferi*. *Laboratory Investigation* 84, 1439–1450.

Canver, C.C., Chanda, J., DeBellis, D.M. and Kelley, J.M. (2000) Possible relationship between degenerative cardiac valvular pathology and Lyme disease. *Annals of Thoracic Surgery* 70, 283–285.

Cary, N.R., Fox, B., Wright, D.J., Cutler, S.J., Shapiro, L.M. and Grace, A.A. (1990) Fatal Lyme carditis and endodermal heterotopia of the atrioventricular node. *Postgraduate Medical Journal* 66, 134–136.

Centers for Disease Control and Prevention (CDC) (2013) Three sudden cardiac deaths associated with Lyme carditis – United States, November 2012–July 2013. *Morbidity and Mortality Weekly Report* 62, 993–996.

Centers for Disease Control and Prevention (CDC) (2016) Lyme Disease Cases by Symptoms. Available at: www.cdc.gov/lyme/stats/graphs.html (accessed 28 March 2017).

Ciesielski, C.A., Markowitz, L.E., Horsley, R., Hightower, A.W., Russell, H. and Broome, C.V. (1989) Lyme disease surveillance in the United States, 1983–1986. *Clinical Infectious Diseases* 11, S1435–S1441.

Cimmino, M.A. (1998) Relative frequency of Lyme borreliosis and of its clinical manifestations in Europe: European community concerted action on risk assessment in Lyme borreliosis. *Infection* 26, 298–300.

Costello, J.M., Alexander, M.E., Greco, K.M., Perez-Atayde, A.R. and Laussen, P.C. (2009) Lyme carditis in children: presentation, predictive factors, and clinical course. *Pediatrics* 123, e835–e841.

Cox, J. and Krajden, M. (1991) Cardiovascular manifestations of Lyme disease. *American Heart Journal* 122(5), 1449–1555.

Cuisset, T., Hamilos, M. and Vanderheyden, M. (2008) Coronary aneurysm in Lyme disease: treatment by covered stent. *International Journal of Cardiology* 128, e72–e73.

De Filippo, K., Dudeck, A., Hasenberg, M., Nye, E., van Rooijen, N., Hartmann, K., Gunzer, M., Roers, A. and Hogg, N. (2013) Mast cell and macrophage chemokines CXCL1/CXCL2 control the early stage of neutrophil recruitment during tissue inflammation. *Blood* 121, 4930–4937.

Dolbec, K.W.D., Higgins, G.L. and Saucier, J.R. (2010) Lyme carditis with transient complete heart block. *Western Journal of Emergency Medicine* 11, 211–212.

Epstein, A.E., DiMarco, J.P., Ellenbogen, K.A. et al. (2008) ACC/AHA/HRS 2008 guidelines for device-based therapy of cardiac rhythm abnormalities. *Circulation* 117, e350–e408.

Fish, A.E., Pride, Y.B. and Pinto, D.S. (2008) Lyme carditis. *Infectious Disease Clinics of North America* 22, 275–288.

Forrester, J.D. and Mead, P. (2014) Third-degree heart block associated with Lyme carditis: review of published cases. *Clinical Infectious Diseases* 59, 996–1000.

Forrester, J.D., Meiman, J., Mullins, J. et al. (2014) Notes from the field: update on Lyme carditis, groups at high risk, and frequency of associated sudden cardiac death – United States. *Morbidity and Mortality Weekly Report* 63, 982–983.

Gammage, M.D. (2000) Temporary cardiac pacing. *Heart* 83, 725–720.

Gasser, R., Dusleag, J., Reisinger, E., Stauber, R., Feigl, B., Pongratz, S., Klein, W., Furian, C. and Pierer, K. (1992) Reversal by ceftriaxone of dilated cardiomyopathy *Borrelia burgdorferi* infection. *Lancet* 339, 1174–1175.

Gasser, R., Watzinger, N., Eber, B., Luha, O., Reisinger, E., Seinost, G. and Klein, W. (1994) Coronary artery aneurysm in two patients with long-standing Lyme borreliosis. *Lancet* 344, 1300–1301.

Gasser, R., Horn, S., Reisinger, E., Fischer, L., Pokan, R., Wendelin, I. and Klein, W. (1998) First description of recurrent pericardial effusion associated with *Borrelia burgdorferi* infection. *International Journal of Cardiology* 64, 309–310.

Goldings, E.A. and Jericho, J. (1986) Lyme disease. *Clinics in Rheumatic Diseases* 12, 343–367.

Guerau-de-Arrelano, M., Alroy, J. and Huber, B.T. (2005) β2 integrins control the severity of murine Lyme carditis. *Infection and Immunity* 73, 3242–3250.

Hidri, N., Barraud, O., de Martino, S., Garnier, F., Paraf, F, Martin, C., Sekkal, S., Laskar, M., Jaulhac, B. and Ploy, M.C. (2012) Lyme endocarditis. *Clinical Microbiology and Infection* 18, e531–e532.

Horowitz, H.W. and Belkin, R.N. (1995) Acute myopericarditis resulting from Lyme disease. *American Heart Journal* 130, 176–178.

Imai, D.M., Feng, S., Hodzic, E. and Barthold, S.W. (2013) Dynamics of connective-tissue localization during chronic *Borrelia burgdorferi* infection. *Laboratory Investigation* 93, 900–910.

Jacobs, J.C., Rosen, J.M. and Szer, I.S. (1984) Lyme myocarditis diagnosed by gallium scan. *Journal of Pediatrics* 105, 950–952.

Karatolios, K., Maisch, B. and Pankuweit, S. (2015) Suspected inflammatory cardiomyopathy: prevalence of *Borrelia burgdorferi* in endomyocardial biopsies with positive serological evidence. *Herz* 40, 91–95.

Klein, J., Stanek, G., Bittner, R., Horvat, R., Holzinger, C. and Glogar, D. (1991) Lyme borreliosis as a cause of myocarditis and heart muscle disease. *European Heart Journal* 12, 73–75.

Koene, R., Boulware, D.R., Kemperman, M., Konety, S.H., Groth, M., Jessurun, J. and Eckman, P.M. (2012) Acute heart failure from Lyme carditis. *Circulation Heart Failure* 5, e24–e26.

Lardieri, G., Salvi, A., Camerini, F., Cinco, M. and Trevisan, G. (1993) Isolation of *Borrelia burgdorferi* from myocardium. *Lancet* 8869, 490.

Lelovas, P., Dontas, I., Bassiakou, E. and Xanthos, T. (2008) Cardiac implications of Lyme disease, diagnosis and therapeutic approach. *International Journal of Cardiology* 129, 15–21.

Lorcerie, B., Boutron, M.C., Portier, H., Beuriat, P., Ravisy, J. and Martin, F. (1987) [Pericardial manifestations of Lyme disease.] *Annales de Medecine Interne* 138, 601–603.

Maher, B., Murday, D. and Harden, S.P. (2012) Cardiac MRI of Lyme disease myocarditis. *Heart* 98, 264.

Maloy, A.L., Black, R.D. and Segurola, R.J. (1998) Lyme disease complicated by the Jarisch-Herxheimer reaction. *Journal of Emergency Medicine* 16, 437–438.

Marcus, L.C., Steere, A.C., Duray, P.H., Anderson, A.E. and Mahoney, E.B. (1985) Fatal pancarditis in a patient with coexistent Lyme disease and babesiosis: demonstration of spirochetes in the myocardium. *Annals of Internal Medicine* 103, 374–376.

Mayer, W., Kleber, F.X., Wilske, B., Preac-Mursic, V., Maciejewski, W., Sigl, H., Holzer, E. and Doering, W. (1990) Persistent atrioventricular block in Lyme borreliosis. *Klinische Wochenschrift* 68, 431–435.

McAlister, H.F., Klementowicz, P.T., Andrews, C., Fisher, J.D., Feld, M. and Furman, S. (1989) Lyme carditis: an important cause of reversible heart block. *Annals of Internal Medicine* 110, 339–345.

Moore, J.A. (1987) Jarisch-Herxheimer reaction in Lyme disease. *Cutis* 39, 397–398.

Muehlenbachs, A., Bollweg, B.C., Schulz, T.J. et al. (2016) Cardiac tropism of *Borrelia burgdorferi*: an autopsy study of sudden cardiac death associated with Lyme carditis. *American Journal of Pathology* 186, 1195–1205.

Munk, P.S., Orn, S. and Larsen, A.I. (2007) Lyme carditis: persistent local delayed enhancement by cardiac magnetic resonance imaging. *International Journal of Cardiology* 115, e108–e110.

Museteanu, C., Schaible, U.E., Stehle, T., Kramer, M.D. and Simon, M.M. (1991) Myositis in mice inoculated with *Borrelia burgdorferi*. *American Journal of Pathology* 139, 1267–1271.

Neumar, R.W., Otto, C.W., Link, M.S. et al. (2015) Part 8: adult advanced cardiovascular life support. 2010 American Heart Association guidelines for cardiopulmonary resuscitation and emergency cardiovascular care. *Circulation* 122, S729–S767.

Olson, L.J., Okafor, E.C. and Clements, I.P. (1986) Cardiac involvement in Lyme disease: manifestations and management. *Mayo Clinic Proceedings* 61, 745–749.

Olson, C.M., Bates, T.C., Izadi, H., Radolf, J.D., Huber, S.A., Boyson, J.E. and Anguita, J. (2009) Local production of IFN-gamma by invariant NKT cells modulates acute Lyme carditis. *Journal of Immunology* 182, 3728–3734.

Pinto, D.S. (2002) Cardiac manifestations of Lyme disease. *Medical Clinics of North America* 86, 285–296.

Raveche, E.S., Schutzer, S.E., Fernandes, H., Bateman, H., McCarthy, B.A., Nickell, S.P. and Cunningham, M.W. (2005) Evidence of *Borrelia* autoimmunity-induced component of Lyme carditis and arthritis. *Journal of Clinical Microbiology* 43, 850–856.

Rees, D.H.E., Keeling, P.J., McKenna, W.J. and Axford, J.S. (1994) No evidence to implicate *Borrelia burgdorferi* in the pathogenesis of dilated cardiomyopathy in the United Kingdom. *British Heart Journal* 71, 459–461.

Reznick, J.W., Braunstein, D.B., Walsh, R.L., Smith, C.R., Wolfson, P.M., Gierke, L.W., Gorelkin, L. and Chandler, F.W. (1986) Lyme carditis: electrophysiologic and histopathologic study. *American Journal of Medicine* 81, 923–927.

Robinson, M.L., Kobayashi, T., Higgins, Y., Calkins, H. and Melia, M.T. (2015) Lyme carditis. *Infectious Disease Clinics of North America* 29, 255–268.

Rudenko, N., Golovchenko, M., Mokracek, A., Piskunova, N., Ruzek, D., Mallatova, N. and Grubhoffer, L. (2008) Detection of *Borrelia bissettii* in cardiac valve tissue of a patient with endocarditis and aortic valve stenosis in the Czech Republic. *Journal of Clinical Microbiology* 46, 3540–3543.

Ruderman, E.M., Kerr, J.S., Telford, S.R. III, Spielman, A., Glimcher, L.H. and Gravallese, E.M. (1995) Early murine Lyme carditis has a macrophage predominance and is independent of major histocompatibility complex class II-CD4+ T cell interactions. *Journal of Infectious Diseases* 171, 362–370.

Saba, S., Vanderbrink, B.A., Perides, G., Glickstein, L.J., Link, M.S., Homoud, M.K., Bronson, R.T., Estes, M. III and Wang, P.J. (2001) Cardiac conduction abnormalities in a mouse model of Lyme borreliosis. *Journal of Interventional Cardiac Electrophysiology* 5, 137–143.

Schaible, U.E., Kramer, M.D., Museteanu, C., Zimmer, G., Mossmann, H. and Simon, M.M. (1989) The severe combined immunodeficiency (SCID) mouse: a laboratory model for the analysis of Lyme arthritis and carditis. *Journal of Experimental Medicine* 170, 1427–1432.

Schaible, U.E., Gay, S., Museteanu, C., Kramer, M.D., Zimmer, G., Eichmann, K., Museteanu, U. and Simon, M.M. (1990) Lyme borreliosis in the severe combined immunodeficiency (SCID) mouse manifests predominantly in the joints, hearts, and liver. *American Journal of Pathology* 137, 811–820.

Schmid, G.P., Horsley, R., Steere, A.C., Hanrahan, J.P., Davis, J.P., Bowen, G.S., Osterholm, M.T., Weisfeld, J.S., Hightower, A.W. and Broome, C.V. (1985) Surveillance of Lyme disease in the United States, 1982. *Journal of Infectious Diseases* 151, 1144–1149.

Seslar, S.P., Berul, C.I., Burklow, T.R., Cecchin, F., and Alexander, M.E. (2006) Transient prolonged corrected QT interval in Lyme disease. *Journal of Pediatrics* 148, 692–697.

Sonnesyn, S.W., Diehl, S.C., Johnson, R.C., Kubo, S.H. and Goodman, J.L. (1995) A prospective study of the seroprevalence of *Borrelia burgdorferi* infection in patients with severe heart failure. *American Journal of Cardiology* 76, 97–100.

Stanek, G., Klein, J., Bittner, R. and Glogar, D. (1990) Isolation of *Borrelia burgdorferi* from the myocardium of a patient with longstanding cardiomyopathy. *New England Journal of Medicine* 322, 249–252.

Stanek, G., Klein, J., Bittner, R. and Glogar, D. (1991) *Borrelia burgdorferi* as an etiologic agent in chronic heart failure? *Scandinavian Journal of Infectious Diseases* 23, 85–87.

Steere, A.C., Malawista, S.E., Hardin, J.A., Ruddy, S., Askenase, W., and Andiman, W.A. (1977) Erythema chronicum migrans and Lyme arthritis: the enlarging clinical spectrum. *Annals of Internal Medicine* 86, 685–698.

Steere, A.C., Batsford, W.P., Weinberg, M., Alexander, J., Berger, J.J., Wolfson, S. and Malawista, S.E. (1980) Lyme carditis: cardiac abnormalities of Lyme disease. *Annals of Internal Medicine* 93, 8–16.

Steere, A.C., McHugh, G., Damle, N. and Sikand, V.K. (2008) Prospective study of serologic tests for Lyme disease. *Clinical Infectious Diseases* 47, 188–195.

Suedkamp, M., Lissel, C., Eiffert, H., Flesch, M., Boehm, M., Mehlhorn, U., Thomssen, R. and Rainer de Vivie, E. (1999) Cardiac myocytes of hearts from patients with end-stage dilated cardiomyopathy do not contain *Borrelia burgdorferi* DNA. *American Heart Journal* 138, 269–272.

Tavora, F., Burke, A., Li, L., Franks, T.J. and Virmani, R. (2008) Postmortem confirmation of Lyme carditis with polymerase chain reaction. *Cardiovascular Pathology* 17, 103–107.

van der Linde, M.R. (1991) Lyme carditis: clinical characteristics of 105 cases. *Scandinavian Journal of Infectious Diseases* 77, 81–84.

van der Linde, M.R., Crijns, H.J. and Lie, K.I. (1989) Transient complete AV block in Lyme disease: electrophysiologic observations. *Chest* 96, 219–221.

van der Linde, M.R., Crijns, H.J., de Koning, J., Hoogkamp-Korstanje, J.A., de Graaf, J.J., Piers, D.A., van der Galien, A. and Lie, K.I. (1990) Range of atrioventricular conduction disturbances in Lyme borreliosis: a report of four cases and review of other published reports. *British Heart Journal* 63, 162–168.

Vlay, S.C., Dervan, J.P., Elias, J., Kane, P.P. and Dattwyler, R. (1991) Ventricular tachycardia associated with Lyme carditis. *American Heart Journal* 121, 1558–1560.

Welsh, E.J., Cohn, K.A., Nigrovic, L.E., Thompson, A.D., Hines, E.M., Lyons, T.W., Glatz, A.C. and Shah, S.S. (2012) Electrocardiograph abnormalities in children with Lyme meningitis. *Journal of the Pediatric Infectious Diseases Society* 1, 293–298.

Wenger, N., Pellaton, C., Bruchez, P. and Schlapfer, J. (2012) Atrial fibrillation, complete atrioventricular block and escape rhythm with bundle-branch block morphologies: an exceptional presentation of Lyme carditis. *International Journal of Cardiology* 160, e12–e14.

Wharton, M., Chorba, T.L., Vogt, R.L., Morse, D.L. and Buehler, J.W. (1990) Case definitions for public health surveillance. *Morbidity and Mortality Weekly Report* 39, 1–43.

Wormser, G.P., Dattwyler, R.J., Shapiro, E.D. *et al.* (2006) The clinical assessment, treatment, and prevention of Lyme disease, human granulocytic anaplasmosis, and babesosis: clinical practice guidelines by the Infectious Diseases Society of America. *Clinical Infectious Diseases* 43, 1089–1134.

Wu, L.A., Lapeyre, A.C. III and Cooper, L.T. (2001) Current role of endomyocardial biopsy in the management of dilated cardiomyopathy and myocarditis. *Mayo Clinic Proceedings* 76, 1030–1038.

Yoon, E.C., Vail, E., Kleinman, G., Lento, P.A., Li, S., Wang, G., Limberger, R. and Fallon, J.T. (2015) Lyme disease: a case report of a 17-year-old male with fatal Lyme carditis. *Cardiovascular Pathology* 24, 317–321.

Zimmer, G., Schaible, U.E., Kramer, M.D., Mall, G., Museteanu, C. and Simon, M.M. (1990) Lyme carditis in immunodeficient mice during experimental infection of *Borrelia burgdorferi*. *Virchows Archiv* 417, 129–135.

12 The Musculoskeletal Manifestations of Lyme Disease (Infection with *Borrelia burgdorferi*)

Leonard H. Sigal
Department of Medicine, Division of Rheumatology, RUTGERS – Robert Wood Johnson Medical School, Stockbridge, Massachusetts, USA

12.1 Introduction

The first description of the syndrome that came to be known as 'Lyme disease' began with the investigation of a group of patients living in three towns along the Connecticut River (Steere *et al.*, 1977c), who experienced mono-arthritis resembling juvenile rheumatoid arthritis (JRA). As the researchers noted, JRA does not occur in geographic, familial or temporal clusters. The initial sero-epidemiologic exploration identified no pathogen, although the pattern of case distribution suggested an arthropod-borne infection (Steere *et al.*, 1977c). Many patients recalled a preceding tick bite and/or an expanding erythematous rash, consistent with erythema chronicum migrans (ECM) (Steere *et al.*, 1978) – a rash initially described in Sweden by Afzelius in 1909 (Afzelius, 1910) and first noted in the United States in 1970 by Scrimenti in Wisconsin (Scrimenti, 1970). Recently, Lyme arthritis may have been present on eastern Long Island and along the New England coast for many years prior to the identification of Lyme disease; residents of eastern Long Island recall cases of 'Montauk knee' occurring as early as the 19th century. Of note, studies of Otzi, the frozen hunter of the Swiss Alps entombed 5300 years ago, suggest he may have had musculoskeletal features of Lyme disease (Steere, 2001). Thus, arthritis, that is, inflammation of one or more joints (synovitis), was the first noted consequence of Lyme borreliosis in the US and may have been present in Europe millennia before the initial identification of ECM or arthritis. However, true arthritis is only one of the many musculoskeletal consequences of this infection (Puius and Kalish, 2008; Kean *et al.*, 2013). A recent review of the many mechanisms at the disposal of *Borrelia burgdorferi* describes how the organism escapes the inoculation site and disseminates to cause inflammation elsewhere (Hyde, 2017). Bockenstedt and Wormser have recently published a concise review of Lyme disease (Bockenstedt and Wormser, 2014).

Once Lyme arthritis was identified, other clinical findings of Lyme disease were soon described (Steere *et al.*, 1977b). Prior to the identification of the pathogenic organism, ECM, now more commonly referred to as erythema migrans (EM), in Europe (Hollstrom, 1951) and the US (Steere *et al.*, 1980; 1983b), was found to respond to antibiotics. A trial of intravenous penicillin for Lyme arthritis showed success in the majority of patients (Steere *et al.*, 1985). A spirochete, isolated from patient and tick sources, was found to be the underlying organism of Lyme disease and was named *Borrelia burgdorferi* (Steere *et al.*, 1983a). European Lyme borreliosis and Lyme disease in the US have many similarities, although differences in the causative agents and the ambient immunogenetics of those affected may contribute to differences in clinical features of infection (Sigal, 1988; 1997).

This chapter will be divided into three sections:

- musculoskeletal consequences of Lyme borreliosis;
  - arthralgias/migratory polyarthralgias/myalgias;
  - mono-arthritis/oligoarthritis;
  - patellofemoral joint dysfunction;
  - persisting musculoskeletal pain following antibiotic therapy; and
  - fibromyalgia-like syndromes;
- hypothesized pathogenesis of these clinical manifestations;
  - local presence of organism, dead or alive;
  - pro-inflammatory molecule release;
  - autonomous self-perpetuating immune/inflammatory reaction;
  - molecular mimicry; and
  - the dulling of Ockham's razor – the presence of a second pathogenetic process unrelated to *B. burgdorferi* infection;
- proposed treatments for each of these clinical consequences.

12.2 Musculoskeletal Consequences of Lyme Borreliosis

Diagnosing a patient with possible Lyme disease requires the clinician to make proper use of historical findings and physical examination and then fully understand the proper use of serological studies: when to order serologies in the first place; how to interpret the immunoglobulin isotype (class) enzyme linked immunosorbent assay (ELISA) reactivities typically reported (IgG and IgM (some laboratories also offer IgA testing)); when to obtain Western blot (immunoblot) confirmation of ELISA reactivity; and how to interpret IgG and IgM Western blot reactivity, especially in endemic areas where past, perhaps inapparent infections, may be common. It is also very important to know when *not* to order serologies. A positive test in a patient with a very low *a priori* likelihood of Lyme disease has a very low positive predictive value, that is, a positive result is likely to be of no consequence and may cause confusion, anxiety and incorrect conclusions, whereas a negative result should be taken as very firm evidence that infection with *B. burgdorferi* is not present. Likewise, it is important to be wary of new testing technologies – these may be flawed by technique and/or interpretation, each must be validated by rigorous comparative testing with established techniques and none is as valuable in confirming the diagnosis of Lyme arthritis as taking a detailed history and doing a complete physical examination. Thus, as noted, it is also very important to know when *not* to order other tests. The term 'Lyme disease test' is an unfortunate misnomer, often used and potentially quite misleading. Serological tests merely detect antibodies that bind to *B. burgdorferi*. No test can determine categorically that the current clinical findings are due to *B. burgdorferi*; no currently available test is diagnostic of active infection, that is, current infection with *B. burgdorferi*. When interpreted appropriately, in a clinical setting suggestive of Lyme disease, serological tests can offer substantiation of that clinical impression. Do not invest in a diagnosis of Lyme arthritis unless there is explicit evidence suggesting the diagnosis, including objective evidence on physical examination or specific historical features. Do not diagnose Lyme disease based merely on time of year, geographic location, family or neighborhood history, family pressure, local enthusiasm, anxiety or personal bias.

12.2.1 Arthralgias/migratory polyarthralgias/myalgias

The musculoskeletal system is commonly affected in early Lyme disease (Sigal, 1988) with symptoms including arthralgias – joint pain without inflammation – and true arthritis – joint inflammation, manifested by the classic signs as originally described by Aulus Cornelius Celsus in the first century CE: heat, erythema, pain, swelling and loss of function (*calor, rubor, dolor, tumor and functio laesa*). The cause of the typically migratory polyarthralgias noted by many patients with early Lyme disease is unclear, but there is no evidence that there are live *B. burgdorferi* within the affected joints.

In the largest reported series of untreated patients with EM (patients accrued from 1976 to 1979) (Steere *et al.*, 1987), 80% (44/55) developed some sort of musculoskeletal manifestation of

Lyme disease. Non-inflammatory musculoskeletal pain occurred in 18% (10/55), including arthralgias and myalgias, as well as pain in tendons, bursae, entheses (insertion of ligament or tendon into bone) and bones. These were typically brief episodes of migratory mild to moderate pain with no signs of inflammation, usually beginning a mean of 2 weeks (range 1 day to 8 weeks) following the EM rash. Symptoms recurred for as long as 6 years, often with accompanying fatigue.

Myalgias and arthralgias are common features of early Lyme disease. If they occur in the presence of EM or other findings explicitly suggestive of the diagnosis of Lyme disease, serologic confirmation of the diagnosis may not be necessary. On the other hand, these *non-specific* complaints may be a relatively early finding of *B. burgdorferi* infection, often a harbinger of other clinical findings of Lyme disease, and may occur in the absence of EM or any other evidence of *B. burgdorferi* infection. Serologies at this early stage are often negative: watchful waiting is in order rather than laboratory testing. A strongly positive serological test in such a patient would be unexpected, as this is early disease – such a result may be reactivity related to a prior infection or a false positive test. Of greater concern is that the patient does not now have Lyme disease and the result is a false positive. Non-specific complaints in a patient from an endemic area may result in an incorrect diagnosis of Lyme disease, exposing the patient to the dual risks of unnecessary antibiotics and the possibility that another underlying disorder, perhaps one more serious than Lyme disease (perhaps life-threatening), will not be considered.

12.2.1.1 Differential diagnosis

Migratory polyarthralgia can occur in the setting of many viral infections and early in the evolution of inflammatory rheumatologic syndromes, for example, rheumatoid arthritis, systemic lupus erythematosus, juvenile idiopathic arthritis, giant cell arteritis/polymyalgia rheumatica, seronegative spondyloarthropathies and sarcoidosis. It is crucial not to jump to the diagnosis of early Lyme disease in the absence of objective evidence specifically supporting this diagnosis.

12.2.2 Mono-arthritis/oligoarthritis

The best known inflammatory joint feature of Lyme disease is mono-arthritis, usually affecting one knee. Clinical findings are typically (although not always) remarkable swelling, with effusions of over 100 cc common. Of note, the knee is often more stiff and difficult to move than painful – pain may be entirely absent, a pattern that should make one consider the diagnosis of Lyme arthritis. Many adult patients with Lyme arthritis have no prior history of EM or other features of Lyme disease, but a history of prior findings suggestive of Lyme disease, for example, EM, aseptic meningitis, carditis, cranial or peripheral neuropathy, should be sought. Prior or current 'flu-like symptoms' is not a helpful finding as these are non-specific, usually occurring only in early disease, and most often due to other processes, especially if associated with upper respiratory tract or gastrointestinal complaints. Physical examination to seek evidence of other features of Lyme disease is mandatory, but often not fruitful. Laboratory evaluation focuses on blood and synovial fluid.

IgG anti-*B. burgdorferi* serologies should be positive when Lyme arthritis is active – if the test is negative the diagnosis of Lyme arthritis should be very much in doubt. A recent study from the north of France demonstrates that there is no added value in doing routine anti-*B. burgdorferi* serologies for patients with the new onset of arthritis (Guellec et al., 2016), the message being that if there is a low *a priori* likelihood that the new onset of arthritis is a feature of Lyme disease adding these serologies to the work-up is not helpful (in fact, a weakly reactive serology may be a red herring, leading to useless antibiotics and a missed true diagnosis). The corroborative Western blot should reveal a broad spectrum of reactivity, but no pattern is diagnostic, nor is there a pattern that predicts outcome. This is the currently recommended two-tiered testing algorithm (occasionally abbreviated as 'TTTA'). Antibody levels should not be expected to fall with antibiotic therapy and therefore levels should not be followed post-therapy. Persisting antibody levels are not a poor prognostic marker. The only serological technique shown to correlate with disease activity is the presence of serum immune complexes containing specific anti-*B. burgdorferi* antibodies within the isolated complexes (Brunner et al.,

1998; Brunner and Sigal, 2000, 2001). Immune complexes are formed only when there are live *B. burgdorferi* liberating antigens to be bound by the antibodies. This technique is not commercially available. These immune complexes are not to be confused with the cryoglobulins found in samples from patients with Lyme disease, an immune phenomenon that correlates with the presence of arthritis (Steere *et al.*, 1977a, 1979; Hardin *et al.*, 1979). New seroconfirmatory techniques have recently been summarized (Theel, 2016).

Synovial fluid should be analyzed for cell count, chemistries, routine culture and crystal analysis (in adults). A moderately elevated white blood cell count with a neutrophilic predominance is expected; typical counts are 20,000–25,000 cells/μl, although higher counts have been reported. The protein is elevated, the mean being 4.5 g/dl (Kean *et al.*, 2013). There is nothing in the routine fluid analysis uniquely diagnostic or even suggestive of the specific diagnosis of Lyme disease. A report of immunoblotting of synovial fluid in ten patients who were misdiagnosed on the basis of a 'positive blot' found that none of the ten patients diagnosed in this manner had a clinical response to previously received antibiotics (mean duration of therapy was 72 days) (Barclay *et al.*, 2012).

Concentration of immune reactivity is found within the synovial space, both antigen-specific antibodies and mononuclear cells (Steere, *et al.*, 1985; 1987; Sigal, 1997). However, neither technology is easily available, or clinically practical, due to lack of technique standardization (both) and the need to deliver viable, fresh cells to the testing laboratory immediately (the latter).

Culture of synovial fluid has very low yield, and is not recommended in clinical practice, as anything but the extremely rare positive cannot be interpreted. Over 20 years ago a novel growth medium based on Detroit city tap water was reported as growing *B. burgdorferi* in a very high proportion of samples. These results were never replicated and remain unexplained, but do not offer hope that culture can be a useful tool in clinical practice.

Polymerase chain reaction (PCR) has become more easily available from reputable laboratories, but is not recommended as a routine diagnostic tool. Historical and clinical findings supplemented by judiciously obtained and interpreted serological results should be sufficient to make the diagnosis of Lyme arthritis. PCR can detect *B. burgdorferi* in a variety of clinical specimens, including synovial fluid and tissue (the latter is likely to have a better yield than the former, since *B. burgdorferi* tends to bind to tissue rather than remain in suspension). The yield in some studies has been as high as 80–85% (Nishio *et al.*, 1993; Nocton *et al.*, 1994). It has been suggested that PCR might be useful in determining if sufficient antibiotic therapy has been given. Recent reports suggest that targeting certain *B. burgdorferi* plasmids may improve the sensitivity of PCR in early disease (Weiner *et al.*, 2015). PCR has been reported to become negative after receipt of 1–2 months of antibiotics (Carlson *et al.*, 1999). However, while persisting PCR positivity may indicate ongoing infection, dead organisms can also give a positive PCR result (Sigal, 2001). Thus, PCR cannot be used as a 'gold standard': a positive test may not mean active infection – it could be due to the presence of dead or dying spirochetes – and a negative test may not equate with cure, since inflammation may not depend upon the presence of organism. Especially in inexperienced hands the test may be falsely negative if there are very few organisms present in the sample. The use of PCR outside of the experimental realm is clearly not warranted except perhaps in the skin (van Dam, 2011).

There are other potentially available tests, oftentimes advocated by Lyme disease activists (many of whom are called 'Lyme literate doctors'), that are not of proven value or reliability (Auwaerter, 2011). These include:

- urinary antigen test (Lyme urinary antigen test (LUAT));
- urine dot blot;
- urine reverse Western blot;
- CD57 lymphocyte cell count;
- flow cytometry;
- immunofluorescence for L-forms of *B. burgdorferi*;
- peripheral blood mononuclear cell proliferation assay; and
- concentration of immune reactivity in synovial fluid.

12.2.2.1 Differential diagnosis

The immediate differential diagnosis of a monoarthritis is the triad: sepsis; crystal-induced; and trauma.

Although Lyme arthritis is due to an infection, at least early in its course, its presentation is not as abrupt and its magnitude not as severe as arthritides caused by pyogenic organisms, for example Staph. and Strep. species. Joint infections can also be caused by less virulent organisms, especially in immune-compromised patients, in whom the degree of inflammation from such infections may mimic Lyme arthritis. All fluids aspirated from a possibly infected joint must be sent for Gram stain, cell count, chemistries and, always, culture. Infections typically cause a moderate to severely inflammatory fluid, with 20,000–100,000 cells/µl, depending on the organism, with neutrophilic predominance. Gram stain may reveal organisms. Clinical clues suggesting gonococcal infection can be obtained from history (gonococcal mono-arthritis may be preceded by migratory polyarthralgias) and physical examination (e.g. cutaneous pustules or other lesions, genital discharge). A recent study retrospectively reviewed 189 patients with knee effusions (23 with culture-positive septic arthritis, 26 with culture-negative septic arthritis and 140 with Lyme disease), all under the age of 18 who had arthrocentesis. The study was prompted by the occasional similarity between septic and Lyme arthritis and the need to differentiate. The independent predictive factors for septic arthritis included 'pain with short arc motion, history of fever reported by the patient or a family member, C-reactive protein of >4 mg/L, and age younger than 2 years'. The authors' model defined the risk of septic arthritis with no factors present as 2%, with one factor 18%, two factors was 45%, three factors as 84% and with all four at 100% (Baldwin et al., 2016, p. 726). Thus, even if Lyme disease is strongly anticipated as the diagnosis, a full evaluation of the joint fluid as noted above must be done.

A patient with periprosthetic joint infection due to *B. burgdorferi* was recently reported, so that Lyme arthritis should be a consideration in late prosthetic joint infection in the proper setting (Wright and Oliverio, 2016).

Gout (monosodium urate crystal-induced disease) and 'pseudo-gout' (calcium pyrophosphate dihydrate crystal-induced disease) usually present with an abrupt and more rapidly evolving severe mono-arthritis, although occasionally the severity may mimic that of Lyme arthritis. Patients with gout are typically older males, usually have an elevated serum uric acid level (although paradoxically the uric acid concentration may drop during an attack of gout) and may have a past history of such events or tophi and/or of features of the cardiac dysmetabolic syndrome (this is not to say that females and younger patients cannot experience gout). The joint is typically very swollen and invariably intensely painful, with prominent surrounding erythema the norm. Desquamation over the affected joint can be seen in gout as the inflammation wanes, a sign never described in Lyme arthritis. Fluid analysis reveals moderately to severely inflammatory fluid, with 20,000 to often more than 100,000 cells/µl. Polarizing microscopy may reveal crystals within cells; finding a single crystal within a cell is diagnostic. Radiographic findings may include chondrocalcinosis, which is not diagnostic of crystal-induced disease.

Recent knee trauma may be blatant or subtle and a history of even trivial trauma should be sought. Knee effusions may appear overnight in the setting of 'internal knee derangement', for example, torn meniscus or cartilage, and are due to a mechanical synovitis. The amount of intra-articular fluid build-up is usually less than seen in Lyme arthritis. Another difference is that mechanical synovitis is usually painful, especially on weight bearing and movements that stress the damaged structure. Synovial fluid analysis typically reveals at most a mildly inflammatory fluid, usually 50 to 3000 cells/µl. Finding blood in all tubes collected is evidence of a recently torn internal structure. Prior injury, for example, damaged meniscus or ligaments, with chronic low level mechanical synovitis can also cause intermittent, although usually small, knee effusions with mildly inflammatory fluid.

Osteoarthritis may be the cause of a bland effusion in older patients, that is, modestly elevated protein and cell count. History and physical examination will be helpful in establishing this diagnosis, as there is often evidence of osteoarthritis elsewhere, for example, interphalangeal joints, hips. However, the finding of a virtually ubiquitous disorder like osteoarthritis should not be taken as definitive evidence that the mono-arthritis being evaluated is not Lyme disease – a proper evaluation should proceed to its logical outcome.

12.2.3 Patellofemoral joint dysfunction

Osteoarthritis of the patellofemoral joint (also called by its histopathological name 'chondromalacia patella') is a common cause of knee pain, regardless of age, and can cause small to moderate knee effusions of bland to mildly inflammatory fluid. Patellofemoral joint dysfunction is caused by malalignment of the patella in the femoral groove due to imbalance of the four muscle bellies that come together in the quadriceps femoris muscle (anterior thigh). The result is pain localized to the front of the knee or described as being immediately behind the patella. Any form of knee inflammation, trauma or damage, even of a relatively trivial nature, may cause reactive quadriceps muscle atrophy resulting in such an imbalance. Patellofemoral joint dysfunction is quite common and should be considered as a cause of knee pain with a modest effusion. Treatment is physical therapy to strengthen the quadriceps in order to re-align the patella within the femoral groove. Even though the cause of the muscle atrophy may have been prior Lyme arthritis, in such a patient ongoing modest knee pain and effusion may be caused by patellofemoral joint dysfunction, not ongoing infection or inflammation. The correct diagnosis dictates the proper therapy.

Isolated mono-arthritis or oligoarthritis may be the presenting feature of rheumatoid arthritis, reactive arthritis or psoriatic arthritis, with evolution into polyarthritis (usually the case in rheumatoid arthritis) or oligoarthritis (usually the case in psoriatic arthritis or reactive arthritis). The passage of time will reveal the evolution of these chronic inflammatory diseases.

Asymmetric oligo- or polyarthritis may represent emerging psoriatic or reactive arthritis (the former affecting the upper more than the lower extremities, with the reverse pattern typical of the latter). Current or prior evidence of integumentary features of psoriasis (nails, extensor surface of the arms, scalp, peri-umbilicus, intergluteal fold), family history of psoriasis and/or psoriatic arthritis, eye inflammation, dactylitis, enthesitis and spondylitis may allow the proper diagnosis of psoriatic arthritis to be made definitively. Reactive arthritis is more likely with recent exposure to culpable enteric or genitourinary pathogens. The full differential diagnosis of oligo-arthritis is beyond the scope of this chapter (the interested reader is referred to Pinals, 2001).

Erythema overlying a joint may be due to a cellulitis, an infection of the skin, which will not penetrate the intact joint capsule. In patients with cellulitis, painless passive flexion and extension of the joint is maintained, in marked contrast to the pain experienced on passive range of motion in a patient with arthritis. As noted, Lyme arthritis may be less painful than the other inflammatory arthropathies noted.

Unless there is explicit evidence suggesting that the arthritis is due to Lyme disease, that is, the *a priori* likelihood of the diagnosis is great, screening serological studies should not be done. In areas with endemic Lyme disease, prior, even inapparent, *B. burgdorferi* infection may be the cause of a persisting positive test that may be unrelated to the current arthritis. Thus, a positive test may not be evidence that the current synovitis is really related to active *B. burgdorferi* infection in the joint or elsewhere. Plausible exposure should be considered, for example, a man who lives in an endemic area who takes walks with his golden retriever in the fields and along deer paths is at risk, whereas an elderly woman who lives in an endemic area but never leaves her house except to get the mail and go shopping is not. Even in patients with no evidence of *B. burgdorferi* of any sort, false positive test results can lead to a false diagnosis, for, as Bayes said, if the *a priori* likelihood of a test is low the positive predictive value of a positive result will also be low.

Fixed polyarthritis (inflammation of multiple joints, as opposed to the migratory polyarthralgias relatively common in early disseminated Lyme disease) is a rare feature of Lyme disease (the author has seen this twice in antibiotic-untreated patients in a long consultation career). Most patients with true polyarthritis after an episode of Lyme disease, even if the initial diagnosis of Lyme disease was correct (and misdiagnosis must be a consideration), have another cause of the active polysynovitis. Arvikar *et al.* (2017, p. 199) collected a series of 30 patients in a 13-year period who experienced a 'new onset systemic autoimmune joint disorder, a median of 4 months after Lyme disease'. Of these 30 patients, 15 had rheumatoid arthritis, 13 had psoriatic arthritis and two had a peripheral spondyloarthritis. Most of these patients had measurable IgG anti-*B. burgdorferi* antibodies, but at significantly lower titer and a lower likelihood to have 'Lyme disease-associated autoantibodies' (directed at matrix metalloproteinase – 10 (MMP-10), endothelial cell growth factor (ECGF) and apolipoprotein (Apo)-B100) than control patients with documented Lyme arthritis (Lochhead et al., 2017). Antibodies to ECGF have been implicated in the pathogenesis of the obliterative microvascular disease seen in Lyme arthritis synovial tissue (Londoño et al., 2004): recall the endarteritis obliterans seen in another spirochetal infection – syphilis. The authors offer three potential explanations for this association: pure coincidence; induction by a non-specific adjuvant effect of the infection; or a specific *B. burgdorferi*-induced autoimmune reaction, with any being plausible. However, the authors caution that the appropriate treatment for a systemic autoimmune joint disease following Lyme disease should be disease-modifying anti-rheumatic drugs (DMARDs) rather than more and/or prolonged antibiotics. Additional causes might include systemic lupus erythematosus and a viral syndrome. The diagnosis of Lyme disease in such a setting must be a diagnosis based on explicit evidence, but also one of exclusion. The exclusionary process must be pursued aggressively and without *a priori* bias in favor of the diagnosis of Lyme disease.

Bursitis and tendonitis have been reported by many patients with Lyme disease, but there is no proof of the presence of the organism at the site of inflammation.

There have been isolated cases reported of *B. burgdorferi* present in biopsies taken from patients with fasciitis, myositis and dermatomyositis-like syndromes.

12.2.4 Persisting musculoskeletal pain following antibiotic therapy of Lyme disease

Following appropriate antibiotic therapy some patients with Lyme disease have persistence of some or all their initial complaints, which may include diffuse musculoskeletal pain (Sigal, 1994). So long as the complaints are not increasing in severity or expanding in location, and/or no new non-musculoskeletal complaints compatible with Lyme disease emerge, there is no reason to suspect ongoing infection; a pattern of slow but steady improvement is expected. Such persisting but slowly improving symptoms should not cause concern about ongoing *B. burgdorferi* infection, and further antibiotic therapy is not warranted. The appearance of new complaints, especially if accompanied by objective evidence of new inflammation or new organ system dysfunction, may represent ongoing infection, a new infection or the consequences of another independent pathologic process, for example, rheumatoid arthritis developing following (not because of) Lyme disease (Arvikar et al., 2017). Such a change should elicit a diligent search for objective evidence of infection or another process. As noted, patellofemoral joint pain may represent prior Lyme arthritis having induced muscle atrophy with subsequent mechanical damage causing symptoms and a mild synovitis. This should be treated with physical therapy, not further antibiotics.

12.2.5 Fibromyalgia-like syndromes

Fibromyalgia is a relatively common non-inflammatory musculoskeletal pain syndrome, often related to sleep disturbance/deprivation and muscle deconditioning. Presenting complaints include widespread non-inflammatory pain, usually not solely localized to the joints; fatigue, with difficulty falling or staying asleep (these patients often need daytime naps); and cognitive, concentration and memory difficulties. Of note, some patients with early Lyme disease experience sleep disturbance, which can rarely persist even after adequate antibiotic-induced eradication of infection. Patients presenting to Lyme disease clinics may have fibromyalgia, either full-blown or as a *forme fruste* (Sigal, 1990; Hsu et al., 1993; Sigal and Patella, 1992). Some may have been appropriately diagnosed and treated for Lyme disease previously, whereas in others that diagnosis was fallacious. In some patients the musculoskeletal complaints of fibromyalgia have been mistaken for the polyarthralgia of early Lyme disease. In some, Lyme disease (whether the correct diagnosis or not) may have interrupted the regular exercise patterns that the patient had adopted, which had been holding their diffuse pain syndrome at bay. In others, the non-inflammatory process had been misclassified as polyarthritis and treated as if a manifestation of ongoing active infection. Many such diagnoses are based on speculation (by the patient or clinician) and/or misuse of laboratory testing (either established or esoteric).

Initial improvement of these vague complaints coincident with antibiotic therapy is often viewed (incorrectly) as proof of the diagnosis of Lyme disease, often with the institution of further (often long-term) antibiotic therapy. Inevitably the antibiotics are ineffective and the patient suffers (Lightfoot et al., 1993).

In whatever manner an incorrect diagnosis was made, many such patients have been subjected to repeated courses of inappropriate antibiotics. A review of recent developments in the pathogenesis and treatment of fibromyalgia is beyond the scope of this chapter (the interested reader is referred to detailed reviews of the management of fibromyalgia; Goldenberg, 2017).

12.3 Hypothesized Pathogenesis of These Clinical Manifestations

Central to determining appropriate therapies for disease processes is identifying the pathogenesis of the disease's various manifestations (Steere et al., 1983b). Borrelia burgdorferi interacts with the host's immune system in a number of different ways. In the mouse (and probably universally), B. burgdorferi does not produce or release toxins. The damage to infected organs – that is, clinical disease – is determined by the host's immune response to the organism, with release of pro-inflammatory molecules a part of that response. Peromyscus leucopus (the white-footed field mouse), a reservoir host, does not get sick despite persistent carriage of the organism. The white-footed field mouse has an immune system that essentially ignores B. burgdorferi and there is no reason to believe the mouse is any the worse for this immunologic lacuna.

Any pathogenic organism elicits a range of both non-specific and antigen-specific immune responses, which can cause the variety of inflammatory manifestations occurring with that infection. Non-specific responses mediated by the innate immune system include complement fixation, with binding by C-reactive protein or other scavengers, engagement by Toll-like receptors (TLRs) or nucleotide-binding oligomerization domains (NODs), or being recognized by other innate immune receptors. Borrelial antigens are taken up by antigen-presenting cells (APCs), resulting in cytokine release and the initiation of antigen-specific T cell activation. B cells, the other cells capable of producing an antigen-specific immune response, bind borrelial antigens without APC help. When activated they are producers of anti-inflammatory cytokines and antibodies through antigen-specific immune activation.

An infection may cause clinical signs and symptoms due to:

- local inflammation due to the organism's presence (live or dead, i.e. debris) and the attendant immune response to it;
- toxins released by the organism (some organisms produce toxins that cause tissue damage, e.g. Clostridium difficile, Staphylococcus aureus, but no such toxin has been identified in or on B. burgdorferi);
- production of pro-inflammatory substances during the immune response to the organism;
- poorly regulated local immune reaction with a shift to an autonomous, independent and unregulated inflammatory condition; and
- poorly regulated immune response to the organism resulting in autoimmune reactivity, for example, molecular mimicry.

This model, that 'disease is due to the immune/inflammatory response to the organism' (Steere et al., 1983a, p. 737), provides a logical framework for understanding B. burgdorferi infection (Sigal, 1996), permits a better understanding of its various manifestations and informs the choice of potential appropriate therapies.

12.3.1 Local presence of organism, dead or alive

There is ample evidence that B. burgdorferi is present at a number of sites of inflammation and organ dysfunction: the skin (EM and acrodermatitis chronicum atrophicans), the heart (myocardium-cardiomyopathy and conduction system-conduction defects), the brain (meninges, spinal fluid – meningitis – and brain – encephalitis) and the joints (synovitis). It is not clear why the organism has the common tropisms it demonstrates, but all organisms regardless of where they are found (except EM) are there due to hematogenous spread. Despite the fact that active and viable spirochetes can be found in biopsies of EM, no viable forms were found in synovial fluid, despite the finding of DNA by PCR (Li et al., 2011). It is reasonable to assume that the immune/inflammatory reaction to the organism is the cause of organ or dysfunction at each site, there being no evidence of pathogenic organ-specific autoimmunity, in Lyme disease (anti-neuronal seroreactivity in patients with neurologic features of Lyme disease will be discussed in Section 12.3.4). Thus, in each of these clinical circumstances one should expect appropriate antibiotic therapy will eradicate the organism with resolution of the signs and symptoms resulting from local infection. No isolate of *B. burgdorferi* has ever been found to be resistant to the standard antibiotics recommended in the Infectious Disease Society of America (IDSA) guidelines (Sigal and Hassett, 2002; Hunfeld et al., 2005). As noted, there is no evidence that this organism produces any toxins itself. The only toxic substances present at the site of inflammation are those produced by the host.

Were there to be inflammation focused on debris of dead/dying organisms one might expect a delay in resolution of symptoms until the debris is cleared. Bockenstedt and colleagues identified persisting spirochetal antigens following antibiotic treatment near cartilage in a murine model of Lyme disease; no viable spirochetes were identified, but the remaining material was capable of eliciting an IgG anti-*B. burgdorferi* antibody response when injected into naive mice (Bockenstedt et al., 2012). Were this persistence to occur in human patients, it might explain persistence of some symptoms in Lyme disease (Steere et al., 1983b). The ultimate response will not be accelerated by further antibiotics. Such a phenomenon has been termed 'the amber hypothesis': 'non-viable spirochetes or more likely spirochetal debris enmeshed in a host-derived fibrinous or collagenous matrix' acting as a focus of immune assault and inflammatory reaction (Wormser et al., 2012, p. 989).

Some have theorized that live, but dormant or otherwise 'alternative lifestyle' *B. burgdorferi* (e.g. 'L-forms') persist within the synovial space, thereby causing ongoing inflammation; some have postulated the existence of L-forms, resistant to antibiotics and theoretically capable of reverting to an infectious morphology. So-called 'persisters' (Sharma et al., 2015) have been produced *in vitro*, but the relevance of such forms to the pathogenesis of disease is unclear. If they bear the antigens of the organism they should be subject to immune attack and if they revert to normal form they should be susceptible to other antibiotics. If a persisting organism is contained within a host cell, it is unlikely to be the source of ongoing inflammation. Intracellular organisms usually do their best to avoid immune activation within the cell serving as host, as inflammation will likely lead to the organism's death. In the case of a dormant or hiding organism causing disease, the adaptive immune response would recognize it (the infection is not in an immunologically inaccessible location) and attack it, in concert with the antibiotics given to such patients. The lack of response and the usual lack of true inflammation in such cases make the claim of ongoing infection lose much of its plausibility.

12.3.2 Pro-inflammatory molecule release

Many of the inflammatory and non-inflammatory features of Lyme disease are due to the immune reaction to the organism (Steere et al., 1983a). This can include release of certain cytokines, for example, interleukin (IL)-1 and tumor necrosis factor-α (TNFα) (which can cause fatigue, cognitive dysfunction and widespread musculoskeletal symptoms) as well as other pro-inflammatory molecules (Shin et al., 2007). Recent reports have documented release of both Type I and Type II interferons, the former via interaction of *B. burgdorferi* with TLRs 7 and 9 (Olson et al., 2009; Petzke et al., 2009). The interaction of *B. burgdorferi* (more vigorous when using live rather than heat-killed organisms) with TLR 7 and 9 also caused peripheral blood mononuclear cells (PBMC) to produce an array of NF-κB-associated cytokines and chemokines, including TNFα, IL-1, IL-6, IL-8, IL-10 and IL-12 (Petzke et al., 2009).

A single polymorphism in TLR1 (TLR1-1805GG) causes patients infected with a specific strain of *B. burgdorferi* (16s–23s rRNA intergenic spacer type (RST) genotype 1) to have stronger Th1-like inflammatory responses. The authors speculate that this may render these patients more susceptible to antibiotic-refractory arthritis

(Shin et al., 2010). Upregulation of TLR2 induced by the presence of B. burgdorferi may activate bystander T-cells, thereby causing inflammation (Whiteside et al., 2018). A B. burgdorferi virulence factor, NapA (neutrophil-activating protein A) binds to TLR2 on monocytes, with release of IL-1, IL-6, IL-17, IL-23 and transforming growth factor β (TGFβ), suggesting that NapA is a potent activator of Th17 cells, which have been implicated in the chronic inflammation of rheumatoid arthritis. Th17 cells produce large amounts of IL-17 (hence their name), an inducer of cytokine release by stromal cells, synoviocytes, chondrocytes, fibroblasts and macrophages, and a potent recruiter and activator of neutrophils (Codolo et al., 2008). Apparently, Th17 cells may have two roles in B. burgdorferi infection: a pronounced Th17 cell response early in infection, which may help control infection, but a later excessive response that may contribute to damage with autoimmune responses associated with antibiotic-refractory LA (Strle et al., 2017). A recent study of the balance between proinflammatory IL-17 and the suppressive effects of IL-10 on murine Lyme arthritis also showed that exogenous anti-IL-17 antibody can suppress the arthritis (Hansen et al., 2013). Borrelia burgdorferi stimulates peripheral blood mononuclear cells or CD14+ monocytes/macrophages directly to secrete the chemokine CCL4, but spirochetal stimulation of other cells in the mixed PBMC population is required to induce CD14+ cells to secrete CCL2, CXCL9 and CXCL10 (Shin et al., 2010). Natural killer (NK) cells and NK T cells both play a role in host defenses early in Lyme disease, but their persistence in large numbers in patients with antibiotic-refractory disease suggests they may play a role in the ongoing inflammation and tissue damage (Katchar et al., 2013). Thus, there is ample evidence of the ability of B. burgdorferi to activate innate immune mechanisms that effectively drive inflammation.

It is clear there are many components of B. burgdorferi that are immunogenic, eliciting antigen-specific immune responses. The organism is also capable of causing non-antigen-specific activation of many B cells, a phenomenon known as 'polyclonal B cell activation' (Sigal et al., 1988). There is no evidence that this feature of B. burgdorferi is involved in the immunopathogenesis of disease. There is no evidence that B. burgdorferi contains a T cell-superantigen, which would cause non-antigen-specific activation of multiple T cell families. The consequence of the resulting abrupt release of large quantities of T cell-derived cytokines would be similar to toxic shock syndrome, caused by a Staphylococcal super-antigen – something never reported to occur as a manifestation of or in association with Lyme disease.

A recent paper by Lochhead et al. reports on the types of microRNA expressed in the synovial fluid of patients with Lyme arthritis, before and following antibiotic therapy. MicroRNA-223 (miR-223) was found during active infection, but following antibiotics inflammatory (miR-146a and miR-155), wound repair (mi-142) and proliferative (miR-17-92) microRNA were expressed, the levels rising with the duration of the arthritis. Levels of miR-146a, miR-155, miR-142, miR-223 and miR-17-92 were also found in synovial tissue in patients with post-antibiotic-therapy arthritis. This pattern of microRNA expression is similar to that seen in rheumatoid arthritis; as noted above, there has been a report of patients developing rheumatoid arthritis following Lyme arthritis (Lochhead et al., 2015). MiR-155 may play a role in the pathogenesis of both arthritis and carditis. It is suppressed by IL-10, a potent anti-inflammatory cytokine. In a murine model of Lyme disease, IL-10 and pro-inflammatory miR-155 have opposite effects on the development of carditis, although both were required for the suppression of carditis. This study found that miR-155 had little effect on arthritis (Lochhead et al., 2015).

The 'flu-like syndrome' of early Lyme disease is likely due to release of IL-1 and other inflammatory mediators, known to cause 'flu-like symptoms' in viral infections. The recurrent and often intermittent flu-like symptoms reported by some later in the course of 'chronic Lyme disease' are likely non-specific, and not of an immunologic etiology, since intermittent cytokine release, for example, IL-1, interferon γ, with no immune stimulus is unlikely.

As noted, production of these pro-inflammatory cytokines may also be due to stimulation of immune cells by debris derived from dead organisms, which could drive such an inflammatory process (Bockenstedt et al., 2012). The persistence within certain joints of non-viable organism-related material or live organisms may drive the inflammatory process in reactive arthritis (usually oligoarthritis following certain genitourinary or gastrointestinal infections; Petersel and Sigal, 2005). The fact that early antibiotic therapy may prevent the establishment of chronic synovitis is in keeping with the premise that early synovitis is due to active local infection, but later antibiotic-refractory synovitis may not represent ongoing infection.

12.3.3 Autonomous self-perpetuating immune/inflammatory reaction

Early in the investigation of the immunopathogenesis of Lyme arthritis studies suggested that the primary driver of the inflammation was a Th1 cell response to borrelial antigens, with interferon γ the most prominent modulator of the process (Yssel et al., 1991). More recent work has called this view into question. Evidence is now pointing to a fundamental role for Th17 cells. One aspect of Th17 activation has already been briefly described in this chapter. A good summary of the potential role of Th17 cells in the immunopathogenesis of Lyme arthritis is found in the review by Nardelli, Callister and Schell (Nardelli et al., 2008a). The autonomous activation of Th17 independent of further antigen-specific mechanisms may be an explanation for ongoing self-perpetuating inflammation independent of ongoing infection in antibiotic-refractory Lyme arthritis (Nardelli et al., 2008b; Nardelli and Schell, 2009), perhaps in a manner similar to, but different from, rheumatoid arthritis. IL-23 has also been implicated in the mouse model of Lyme arthritis (Kotloski et al., 2008). Dysfunction of regulatory T cells (Treg; CD4 + CD25 + T cells) might be implicated in Lyme arthritis (Nardelli et al., 2004; 2005). Tregs are involved in resolution of inflammation in both murine and human disease. A paucity of these cells may be the reason that some patients' arthritis does not resolve (Shen et al., 2010). Singh and Girschick (2004) describe means by which B. burgdorferi might cause a self-perpetuating disease.

12.3.4 Molecular mimicry

Molecular mimicry is a condition in which an invading organism contains a molecule, an immunogen, which, as determined by the host's immune system's identifying skills, resembles a host molecule. When the organism-derived immunogen is recognized by the host's immune system the pathogen is attacked, but so too is the host molecule that the immune system recognizes as looking like that particular organism's immunogen, a concept known as 'cross-reacting'. Recognition of the cross-reacting host molecule leads to subsequent damage to the host. Examples of this phenomenon include Chagas disease (*Trypanosoma cruzi* components cross-react with human cardiac muscle and peripheral nerve, causing Chagasic cardiomyopathy and neuropathy) and rheumatic fever (the M proteins of certain Group A β hemolytic Streptococci cross-react with human cardiac myosin, causing rheumatic carditis). A similar breakdown of immunologic tolerance can occur when antigens that have been sequestered, that is, not available to the immune system previously, are suddenly liberated. The immune response to these antigens then can cause an organ-specific autoimmune disease, such as post-traumatic sympathetic ophthalmitis and post-pericardiotomy (Dressler's) syndrome.

One proposed explanation for the development of antibiotic-refractory Lyme arthritis has been molecular mimicry, the presence of cross-reactivity between *B. burgdorferi* and synovial antigens. Steere and colleagues found that lymphocyte function associated antigen 1 (LFA-1; also known as αLβ2 integrin and CD11a/CD18) contained an epitope that cross-reacts with an epitope on outer-surface protein A (OspA) (Gross et al., 1998); both epitopes are presented by the same HLA-DR molecule, HLA-DR4, on the surface of APCs. HLA-DR4 has been associated with antibiotic-refractory Lyme arthritis and implicated as a risk factor. The same group found that antibiotic-refractory Lyme arthritis was associated with T cell responses to certain epitopes of OspA (notably, not the same as the cross-reacting epitope noted above; Chen et al., 1999; Steere et al., 2003). This and further work were viewed as suggesting that molecular mimicry, leading to an organ-specific autoimmunity, was at the root of antibiotic-refractory Lyme arthritis (Steere et al., 2001; Ball et al., 2009; Iliopoulou et al., 2009; Jones et al., 2009). Kalish et al. (2003) found no such association between clinical status and T cell responses to OspA or LFA-1. Maier and colleagues (2000, p. 455) found that OspA-specific T cells recognized many epitopes on many other human proteins, causing the authors to conclude '…the existence of cross-reactive epitopes alone does not imply molecular mimicry-mediated pathology and autoimmunity'. Of note, OspA vaccination in a relevant murine strain and in humans was not associated with arthritis (Steere et al., 2001). LFA-1 is a ubiquitous protein; thus, autoimmunity would be expected to be a more systemic phenomenon were cross-reactivity to be etiologically relevant (Steere et al., 2001). Instead, there is a postulated autoimmune process affecting a single organ system, in fact a single joint. One might then speculate that the cross-reacting immune principle was active only in the joint, either because the specific LFA-1 epitope is available only in the synovium or that the immune reactivity is somehow isolated to the synovial space of a single joint. Neither of these theories is supportable by scientific evidence and in fact the latter is illogical.

An additional example of molecular mimicry is found between linear epitopes of *B. burgdorferi*'s flagellin (p41) and human heat shock protein 60 (the latter epitope exposed only in cytoplasmic, not mitochondrial, HSP60; Sigal and Tatum, 1988a; 1988b; Dai et al., 1993; Fikrig et al., 1993; Sigal, 1993; Maier, et al., 2000; Steere et al., 2001; 2011; Kalish et al., 2003; Iliopoulou et al., 2009; Jones et al., 2009). A single monoclonal antibody to flagellin, H9724, binds to these two epitopes. Sera from patients with neurologic manifestations of Lyme disease also bound these epitopes. When added to cultures of neuroblastoma cells, H9724 penetrated living neuroblastoma cells, profoundly suppressing outgrowth of dendrites. Alteration of axonal/neuronal function due to this mechanism is unlikely to be a cause of the patchy peripheral neuropathy of Lyme disease; to this point, no clinical role for these cross-reacting antibodies has been proven. Of note, neuropathy is an antibiotic-sensitive manifestation of Lyme disease, implicating active infection, rather than molecular mimicry, as the cause.

Thus, although there are two examples of molecular mimicry of theoretical interest in our understanding of the immunopathogenesis of different aspects of Lyme disease, neither has been demonstrated to be clinically relevant. In any event, were these mechanisms to be germane to the immunopathogenesis of antibiotic-refractory Lyme arthritis (or any other feature of Lyme disease) there would be no role for further antibiotics. Archimedes is said to have noted that given a long enough lever arm he could move the world; using computerized searches, one can often find high stringency cross-reactivity between a pathogen-related protein and many proteins in data banks, of human, mammalian and other sources. One must separate the wheat from the chaff.

12.3.5 The dulling of Ockham's razor – the presence of a second pathogenetic process unrelated to *Borrelia burgdorferi* infection

From early in medical training we are drilled with the importance of Ockham's razor, in the words of William of Ockham (William Seach, a 14th-century Franciscan friar) variously: *Entia non sunt multiplicanda praeter necessitatem* [Entities should not be multiplied unnecessarily]; *numquam ponenda est pluralitas sine necessitate* [Plurality must never be posited without necessity], *frustra fit per plura quod potest fieri per pauciora* [It is futile to do with more things that which can be done with fewer]. In the late 20th century this was adapted directly from the Latin to the more direct and pithy aphorism: 'keep it simple, stupid'.

However, sometimes the hoof beats we hear are from an additional species. Some patients with prior established Lyme disease may have, develop or become symptomatic with other illnesses. One might predict the incidence of rheumatoid arthritis, ankylosing spondylitis or other autoimmune and non-autoimmune disorders to be that of society at large, regardless of prior exposure to *B. burgdorferi*. Thus, as noted previously, a second, unrelated disorder can afflict a patient who has, or has been previously exposed to, Lyme disease (Arvikar et al., 2017). As described above, the second ailment might be related to Lyme disease without being directly attributable to ongoing infection *per se*, for example, patellofemoral joint dysfunction; the treatment for such a second affliction is likely not to be antibiotics.

12.4 Proposed Treatments for Each of These Clinical Consequences

Many different forms of therapy have been proposed for Lyme disease. Antibiotics, intravenous or oral, depending on the manifestations of disease and prior treatment history, are effective in most patients with musculoskeletal features of Lyme disease. As noted, however, many patients with persisting musculoskeletal symptomatology do not have evidence of active infection with *B. burgdorferi*, and many have evidence suggesting the presence of another disease. It is far beyond the scope of this chapter to discuss therapies for the many non-Lyme disease causes of musculoskeletal symptoms in such patients, a list that includes fibromyalgia, patellofemoral joint dysfunction, rheumatoid arthritis, lupus, the seronegative spondyloarthropathies (ankylosing spondylitis, psoriatic arthritis, reactive arthritis) and osteoarthritis (Sigal, 1990; 1996; Sigal and Patella, 1992; Hsu et al., 1993; Lightfoot et al., 1993; Goldenberg, 2017).

Antibiotic therapy has been a topic of heated debate, with no sign of abatement. Nonetheless, a recent review of the 2006 IDSA therapeutic guidelines (Wormser et al., 2006) by an independent panel, formed as a result of a lawsuit in Connecticut, unanimously found no reason to change these guidelines, based on the best evidence available. Thus, the antibiotic doses and durations suggested in this chapter are identical to those of the guidelines. An update of the guidelines is underway, but no substantial revision in therapeutic recommendations is envisioned at this time.

Persisting symptoms, mistakenly interpreted as indicative of ongoing infection, have led some clinicians to innovative, albeit flawed, approaches to try to eradicate the suspected ongoing infection. The approach of 'antibiotic treatment until cessation of symptoms' is fundamentally flawed, potentially dangerous (both medically and psychologically) (Sigal and Hassett, 2002) and has no place in informed, evidence-based practice.

'Creative' therapies have included some that might be considered bizarre. In the 1970s and 1980s patients were taken to a foreign country and given malaria, in an attempt to replicate a form of fever therapy used for syphilis (Heimlich, 1990); this form of therapy has never been subjected to scientific study for either syphilis or Lyme disease, and apparently was ineffective.

Hyperbaric therapy was, and is, occasionally used: a therapeutic strategy apparently based on the aversion of *B. burgdorferi* for oxygen *in vitro* (Taylor and Simpson, 2005; Stricker et al., 2006). Despite mention in these two reviews, this approach has never been subjected to scientific scrutiny and remains a highly speculative approach in the repertoire of certain 'Lyme disease experts' (also known as 'Lyme literate doctors') only. Its use is seemingly based more on the availability of the hyperbaric chamber than on proof of efficacy.

Cholestyramine has been suggested as a means of removing a toxin that certain clinicians believe is produced by *B. burgdorferi*; the claim is that this toxin causes some of the symptoms of chronic Lyme disease (Shoemaker et al., 2006). This toxin has never been identified and there is no evidence that it exists. There is no proof that cholestyramine has any effect on Lyme disease.

Hydroxychloroquine is an effective form of treatment for some patients with rheumatoid arthritis or lupus, and may have an effect on the chronic synovitis of Lyme arthritis (Steere and Angelis, 2006). There is no clinical proof of the assertion by 'Lyme literate doctors' that hydroxychloroquine may enhance the efficacy of antibiotics by allowing better entry of antibiotics into cells, a refuge serving as an occult site of infection, or by any innate antimicrobial activity.

Some clinicians continue to use very prolonged therapy (in the author's experience, 9 years of nearly continuous therapy is the record), combinations of oral and/or intravenous antibiotics, 'cycling' through various antibiotics and the addition of hydroxychloroquine to antibiotics (Sigal, 1994; 1996). None of these therapies has established validity and, thus, these and other therapies discussed and rejected by the IDSA panel should be eschewed (Wormser et al., 2006). None of these therapies has ever been subjected to rigorous scientific study and found to be effective. In fact, Klempner et al. addressed the issue of long-term therapy and found it without merit (Klempner et al., 2001), although some have disputed this conclusion because the duration of therapy was insufficient. Berende and colleagues in a larger study also gave 12 weeks of antibiotic therapy with no effect seen (Stricker, 2007). Scientifically valid studies supporting prolonged therapy have not been forthcoming. There have been claims that long-term therapy is of value (Shoemaker et al., 2006), but these assertions are not based on scientific study. Furthermore, such therapy is not without potential harm (Marzec et al., 2017), related to toxicity of antibiotics and indwelling catheters. Nonetheless, some clinicians think long-term therapy is warranted, the treatment ended when the symptoms have abated. This is not evidence-based practice, but rather is based on speculation and hearsay, and does not serve the patient well.

A recent review found over 30 different types of alternative treatments, categorized as: oxygen and reactive oxygen therapies; energy and radiation-based therapies; nutritional therapies; chelation and heavy metal therapies; and biological (including immunoglobulin) and pharmacological therapies, which ranged from the use of a variety of medications without recognized benefit in *B. burgdorferi* infection to stem cell transplantation (Lantos *et al*., 2015).

A word of caution when treating Lyme disease – one must have patience. The organism does not die immediately. Borrelial debris does not get cleared immediately. Cytokine production does not decrease to baseline levels immediately.

In the words of the Danish poet, mathematician and city planner Piet Hein:

> Put up in a place where it is easy to see
> The cryptic admonishment 'TTT'
> When you feel how depressingly slowly you climb
> It is well to remember that 'Things Take Time'
>   (Hein, 1966, p. 5)

Early in the course of Lyme disease, when EM is present (or recently resolved) or other objective features of early Lyme disease are noted, musculoskeletal features are usually not the most prominent feature. Nonetheless, in Steere's classic description of the musculoskeletal features of Lyme disease (Steere, *et al.*, 1985), 62% of patients with early Lyme disease (34/55 patients with untreated early Lyme disease) experienced musculoskeletal complaints, including arthralgias and myalgias. The former may include pain in a single joint (monoarthralgia), pain in multiple joints (polyarthralgia), migratory joint pains (migratory polyarthralgia) or in peri-articular structures, for example, enthesis. Symptomatic therapy is in order, for example, acetaminophen or non-steroidal anti-inflammatory agents at recommended doses, in addition to the appropriate antibiotic therapy. True arthritis, that is, joint inflammation, is uncommon in early Lyme disease. Its presence should suggest a second underlying disorder, as noted above. According to the IDSA guidelines (Wormser *et al.*, 2006), the recommended antibiotic therapy for early Lyme disease is doxycycline (100 mg PO bid) or amoxicillin (500 mg PO tid) or cefuroxime axetil (500 mg PO bid) for 14 days (10–21 days for doxycycline and 14–21 days for the latter two agents). First-generation cephalosporins are ineffective in the treatment of Lyme disease and therefore have no role. Other antibiotics are not of proven efficacy.

Many patients experience persistence of non-specific complaints, often including arthralgias. Further therapy for these ongoing issues should be symptomatic, there being no evidence that further antibiotic therapy is warranted. As long as these complaints are not worsening and no new manifestations of Lyme disease occur, no further antibiotics should be given. It is crucial to evaluate all new complaints thoroughly. Thus, a patient with early Lyme disease and arthralgias given appropriate oral therapy who then develops central nervous system features of Lyme disease or true joint inflammation may require antibiotic therapy, whereas a patient whose joints continue to hurt with the same or diminishing intensity should complete the oral therapy at the initially prescribed dose and duration.

Enthesitis is a common feature of the seronegative spondyloarthropathies, which include ankylosing spondylitis, psoriatic arthritis, reactive arthritis and inflammatory joint disease in the presence of inflammatory bowel disease. A single report by Weyand and Goronzy (1989) has suggested that *B. burgdorferi* infection might be the cause of reactive arthritis and there is a separate case report of sacroiliitis in a patient with Lyme disease (Kinigadner *et al.*, 1991). There have been no further reports to substantiate this association and nothing to link any features of Lyme disease to HLA-B27, the genetic marker for susceptibility to reactive arthritis and ankylosing spondylitis. Thus, there is no proof that sacroiliitis and/or spondylitis are features of Lyme disease, regardless of the presence of HLA-B27. Patients with enthesitis and/or dactylitis as part of their 'Lyme disease' should be treated symptomatically, with antibiotics as appropriate for the primary features of their disease, and evaluated for an underlying seronegative spondyloarthropathy.

Later in disease, arthritis, that is, true inflammatory joint disease, may occur, most often as a mono-arthritis or an asymmetric oligoarthritis.

As noted, large knee effusions are common and an important part of therapy is removal of fluid to decrease the concentration of inflammatory cytokines perpetuating the synovitis and to decrease discomfort and prevent stretching of the surrounding connective tissues. Removal of synovial fluid from the knee (the most commonly affected joint), shoulder, ankle, elbow and some of the small joints of the hands and feet (the next most commonly affected joints, in decreasing frequency) is an office procedure and can give instant and significant symptomatic relief. Fluid removal from the hip is a more difficult procedure, usually requiring radiographic targeting. Fluid should be sent for analysis as described earlier. Samples should *not* be sent to try to grow *B. burgdorferi*.

Intra-articular steroids may give relatively rapid relief when injected into an evacuated joint. There is still speculation that such injections may predispose to persistence of inflammation in the injected joint. This is based entirely on *post hoc* analysis of patients with Lyme arthritis (Steere et al., 1985) and subsequent case reports. In all likelihood, the patients who received the intra-articular injections had more severe arthritis and a poorer prognosis than patients who did not – thus, selection bias is probably at work and there is probably no contra-indication to judicious use of intra-articular steroids.

Antibiotic therapy for Lyme arthritis, as recommended by the IDSA (Wormser et al., 2006), is 28 days of doxycycline, amoxicillin or cefuroxime axetil, at the daily doses noted previously. Some clinicians give these oral agents for up to 6 weeks, but there is no scientific evidence favoring the claim that longer therapy is any more efficacious.

In some patients, initial oral therapy for Lyme arthritis will be ineffective, in which case either a repeat course of oral therapy (recommended, which can be extended in duration – an approach not endorsed by the IDSA) or intravenous therapy for 21 days can be given. However, it is important to define 'ineffective' very carefully. As noted, inflammation due to initial *B. burgdorferi* infection may be slow to resolve totally. One should not judge slow but steady diminution in inflammation as a failure or 'ineffective' therapy. Clearly, if there is the appearance of arthritis in new joints, one must consider the possibility that the preceding therapy was ineffective. However, it is also possible that the initial diagnosis was incorrect.

A recent recommendation from Dr Steere's group is that patients are usually treated with 2–3 months of oral and intravenous antibiotics, with follow-on DMARD therapy for post-infectious persisting arthritis (Arvikar and Steere, 2015).

Outcomes in pediatric Lyme arthritis have been reviewed by Tory, Surakowski and Sundel from Yale (Tory et al., 2010). In reviewing 10 years of records at a tertiary care center, 99 children with Lyme arthritis were identified, of whom 76 had full recovery in response to antibiotics. The authors could not predict response based on their clinical or laboratory data. A definition of joint involvement lasting at least 3 months after antibiotic therapy yielded 23 patients with antibiotic-refractory Lyme arthritis. Of these, the majority were successfully treated with non-steroidal anti-inflammatory drugs (six patients), intra-articular injections of corticosteroids (four patients) or disease-modifying antirheumatic drugs (two patients); five additional patients were lost to follow-up. None of the patients available for follow-up evaluation had chronic arthritis, joint deformities or recurrence of the infection. In a review of 506 pediatric patients with joint effusions 51 had culture-positive septic arthritis. Fever (>101.5°F; >40.6°C) at the time of presentation, refusal to bear weight, elevated peripheral and joint fluid white blood cell counts were higher in the septic group. The erythrocyte sedimentation rate and the C-reactive protein level were not significantly different between the two cohorts. Refusal to bear weight was the strongest predictor of the diagnosis of septic arthritis. Overall the prevalence of Lyme arthritis was 31%, 45% if there was a knee effusion (Daikh et al., 2013). A recent review of pediatric Lyme arthritis was written by S. Sood (2015). A comparison of adult and pediatric Lyme arthritis found that in the 29 adults and 52 children reviewed, children were more likely to present acutely and had a higher mean peripheral blood and synovial fluid white cell count, but there was no difference in hospitalization or surgical intervention. Adults were treated with more courses of antibiotics and were more likely to have intravenous therapy subsequently. Children were often returned to normal function within a 4-week follow-up after antibiotics (Milewski et al., 2011).

A lack of response to appropriate antibiotics should raise consideration that the diagnosis of Lyme arthritis was incorrect. Mono-arthritis may represent psoriatic arthritis, atypical rheumatoid arthritis, or another 'idiopathic inflammatory joint disease' unrelated to but coincident with or following Lyme disease. If this is the case, there is *nothing* to suggest causality, no immunopathogenetic mechanism to link *B. burgdorferi* with these inflammatory joint diseases (*post hoc, ergo propter hoc* does not make for good medical practice).

In the rare case where Lyme arthritis does not resolve despite two or three adequate courses of appropriate antibiotics, one must reconsider the initial diagnosis of Lyme arthritis. If this diagnosis seems secure, and the synovitis has persisted for more than 6 months unabated, despite antibiotics and appropriate use of non-steroidal anti-inflammatory agents, therapeutic options are few and largely unproven.

Arthroscopic synovectomy (Schoen *et al.*, 1991) is often effective, although if the synovectomy is not complete (i.e. there is residual synovium remaining within the joint), there may be a return of inflammation (the synovium grows back and a self-perpetuating inflammatory process re-emerges). In cases refractory to synovectomy or where synovectomy is not considered an option, therapies analogous to those used for rheumatoid arthritis have been adopted. These unstudied and therefore unapproved medical therapies for refractory Lyme arthritis include:

- Hydroxychloroquine (200 mg PO bid or 400 mg PO qd). This requires monitoring for retinal toxicity with retinal examination every 6 months and use of the Amsler grid for home monitoring of retinal toxicity (the Amsler grid is no longer routinely used and its veracity has recently been questioned; reference to local ophthalmologic care is suggested). The serum CPK should be checked every 6 months. This drug can take 8 weeks or longer to start working. The dose should not be increased and, in fact, should be decreased for small patients, to no more than 7 mg/kg. The use of hydroxychloroquine is based on its efficacy in the chronic synovitis seen in rheumatoid arthritis or lupus, to treat what has become a self-perpetuating synovitis. This is in marked contrast to the unproven and purely speculative use of hydroxychloroquine to enhance entry of antibiotics into cells putatively infected with dormant or live *B. burgdorferi*.
- Methotrexate, used for patients with rheumatoid arthritis, has been suggested for use in patients with the chronic, self-perpetuating synovitis, seen rarely after *B. burgdorferi* infection. Methotrexate is started at 7.5 or 10 mg given once a week. If an adequate response has not been attained after 6 weeks at a given dose level, the dose can be increased by 2.5 mg weekly, until toxicity limits further increases. The maximum should be 25 mg once a week. The clinician must monitor for oral ulcers, bone marrow and hepatic toxicities and, rarely, interstitial pulmonary fibrosis, which presents as a dry, non-productive cough. Folic acid 1 mg/day every day of the week is mandatory co-therapy to diminish the likelihood of toxicity related to folic acid deficiency – methotrexate inhibits metabolism and activation of folic acid, so folic acid 'prophylaxis' is necessary to achieve healthy levels of the active metabolite tetrahydofolate crucial in the synthesis of purines and pyrimidines. In addition, methotrexate forms polyglutamates that inhibit the enzyme 5-aminoimidazole-4-carboxamidoribonucleotide (AICAR) transformylase. Excess AICAR, the substrate for this transformylase, accumulates as the result of this enzymatic blockade, leading to adenosine release extracellularly. Adenosine then binds to anti-inflammatory receptors on a variety of immune cells, for example, lymphocytes and macrophages, leading to a lessening of inflammation.
- The use of molecular biologic therapies targeting TNFα or interleukin (IL)-1 in patients with refractory Lyme arthritis has never been formally studied. Given the immune response to the organism, this sort of therapy has face validity but does not represent an approved use of these agents. Intra-articular infusion of an IL-1 antagonist into a single refractory Lyme arthritis joint has been discussed by some thought leaders informally but has never been studied and is certainly not an approved use. A patient with antibiotic-resistant Lyme arthritis initially was recently reported as having had a

partial response to the tumor necrosis factor (TNF)-α blockade compound etanercept, but then had long-term remission with subsequent tocilizumab (Hirsch et al., 2016). Although not proof-positive that this patient had an immune-mediated, rather than infection-association, synovitis, the clinical response does suggest that *B. burgdorferi* was not the cause of the persisting arthritis.

Arthritis may cause overlying muscles to either atrophy or shorten ('flexion contracture'). In either event, subsequent joint dysfunction may occur. Physical therapy is warranted for patients recovering from long-term synovitis, in order to assure return to normal function. In the case of the knee, chronic arthritis often causes atrophy of the overlying quadriceps femoris muscle mechanism, with subsequent patellofemoral joint dysfunction. This may cause pain, swelling and redness of the knee – in essence this is a mechanical synovitis, but it is not evidence of a newly reactivated infection and should not be treated as such. In such cases, aspiration of the fluid will serve two purposes: decrease pain and substantiate the diagnosis, as the fluid will be only minimally inflammatory (500–2000 cells/μl). Thus, it is imperative that the default diagnosis in a patient with the recurrence of knee arthritis after adequate antibiotic therapy not be recurrent Lyme arthritis.

Some patients with prior documented *B. burgdorferi* infection (and some with an unsubstantiated diagnosis of Lyme disease) develop a syndrome compatible with the diagnosis of fibromyalgia; some may have features of 'chronic fatigue syndrome'. There is no evidence that the fibromyalgia or chronic fatigue syndromes are in any way due to active infection with *B. burgdorferi*. Patients with these chronic and debilitating afflictions do not benefit from antibiotic therapy. In fact, we believe that the very insistence by their clinicians that they have 'chronic Lyme disease', an allegedly chronic, incurable infection that will never resolve, makes these patients worse. The sense of having no path forward, known as 'aporia', is very much part of the psychopathogenesis of these afflictions in these patients. It is crucial that these patients be disabused of the diagnosis of 'chronic Lyme disease' and be informed that such treatment is not in accord with evidence-based medical practice. Emotional support of these fragile individuals, listening to them and never dismissing their symptoms and suffering, is critical. They are oftentimes demanding and needy, but much of this is due to fear and anxiety and a sense of helplessness that medications do not cure (Sigal and Hassett, 2002). This issue and the therapeutic approaches that can be tried are dealt with in more detail in the chapter in this volume by Hassett and Sigal (Chapter 15).

References

Afzelius, A. (1910) *Verhandlungen der dermatologischen Gesellschaft zu Stockholm*. Archiv für Dermatologie und Syphilis, Berlin 101, 104.

Arvikar, S.L. and Steere, A.C. (2015) Diagnosis and treatment of Lyme arthritis. *Infectious Disease Clinics of North America* 29, 269–280.

Arvikar, S.L., Crowley, J.T., Sulka, K.B. and Steere, A.C. (2017) Autoimmune arthritides, rheumatoid arthritis, psoriatic arthritis, or peripheral spondyloarthritis following Lyme disease. *Arthritis and Rheumatology* 69(1), 194–202.

Auwaerter, P.G., Bakken, J.S., Dattwyler, R.J. et al. (2011) Antiscience and ethical concerns associated with advocacy of Lyme disease. *The Lancet – Infectious Diseases* 11, 713–719.

Baldwin, K.D., Brusalis, C.M., Nduaguba, A.M. and Sankar, W.N. (2016) Predictive factors for differentiating between septic arthritis and Lyme disease of the knee in children. *Journal of Bone and Joint Surgery. American Volume* 98(9), 721–728. DOI: 10.2106/JBJS.14.01331.

Ball, R., Shadomy, S.V., Meyer, A. et al. (2009) HLA type and immune response to *Borrelia burgdorferi* outer surface A protein in people in whom arthritis developed after Lyme disease vaccination. *Arthritis and Rheumatism* 60, 1179–1186.

Barclay, S.S., Melia, M.T. and Auwaerter, P.G. (2012) Misdiagnosis of late-onset Lyme arthritis by inappropriate use of *Borrelia burgdorferi* immunoblot testing with synovial fluid. *Clinical and Vaccine Immunology* 19(11), 1806–1809. DOI: 10.1128/CVI.00383-12 PMCID: PMC3491552.

Berende, A., ter Hofstede, H.J., Vos, F.J., van Middendorp, H., Vogelaar, M.L., Tromp, M., van den Hoogen, F.H., Donders, A.R., Evers, A.W. and Kullberg, B.J. (2016) Randomized trial of longer-term therapy for symptoms attributed to Lyme disease. *New England Journal of Medicine* 374(13), 1209–1220. DOI: 10.1056/NEJMoa1505425.

Bockenstedt, L.K., Gonzalez, D.G., Haberman, A.M. and Belperron, A.A. (2012) Spirochete antigens persist near cartilage after murine Lyme borreliosis therapy. *Journal of Clinical Investigation* 122(7), 2652–2660.

Bockenstedt, L.K. and Wormser, G.P. (2014) Unraveling Lyme disease. *Arthritis and Rheumatology* 66(9), 2313–2323. DOI: 10.1002/art.38756.

Brunner, M. and Sigal, L.H. (2000) Immune complexes from Lyme disease sera contain *Borrelia burgdorferi* antigen and antigen-specific antibodies: potential use for improved testing. *Journal of Infectious Diseases* 182, 534–539.

Brunner, M. and Sigal, L.H. (2001) Use of serum immune complexes in a new test that accurately confirms early Lyme disease and active infection with *Borrelia burgdorferi*. *Journal of Clinical Microbiology* 39, 3213–3221.

Brunner, M., Stein, S., Mitchell, P.D. and Sigal, L.H. (1998) IgM capture assay for the serologic confirmation of early Lyme disease: analyzing immune complexes with biotinylated *Borrelia burgdorferi* sonicate enhanced with flagellin peptide epitope. *Journal of Clinical Microbiology* 36, 1074–1080.

Carlson, D., Hernandez, J., Bloom, B.J. *et al.* (1999) Lack of *Borrelia burgdorferi* DNA in synovial fluid samples from patients with antibiotic-resistant Lyme arthritis. *Arthritis and Rheumatism* 42, 2705–2709.

Chen, J., Field, J.A., Glickstein, L., Molloy, P.J., Huber, B.T. and Steere, A.C. (1999) Association of antibiotic treatment-resistant Lyme arthritis with T cell responses to dominant epitopes of outer surface protein A of *Borrelia burgdorferi*. *Arthritis and Rheumatism* 42, 1813–1822.

Codolo, G., Amedei, A., Steere, A.C. *et al.* (2008) *Borrelia burgdorferi* NapA-driven Th17 cell inflammation in Lyme arthritis. *Arthritis and Rheumatism* 58, 3609–3617.

Dai, Z.Z., Lackland, H., Stein, S., Li, Q., Radziewicz, R., Williams, S. and Sigal, L.H. (1993) Molecular mimicry in Lyme disease: monoclonal antibody H9724 to *Borrelia burgdorferi* flagellin specifically detects chaperonin-HSP60. *Biochimica et Biophysica Acta* 1181, 97–100.

Daikh, B.E., Emerson, F.E., Smith, R.P., Lucas, F.L. and McCarthy, C.A. (2013) Lyme arthritis: a comparison of presentation, synovial fluid analysis, and treatment course in children and adults. *Arthritis Care and Research* (Hoboken) 65(12), 1986–1990. DOI: 10.1002/acr.22086.

Fikrig, E., Berland, R., Chen, M., Williams, S., Sigal, L.H. and Flavell, R. (1993) Fine mapping of the serologic response to the *Borrelia burgdorferi* flagellin demonstrates an epitope common to neural tissue. *Proceedings of the National Academy of Sciences of the USA* 90, 183–187.

Goldenberg, D. (2017) 'Initial treatment of fibromyalgia in adults' and 'Treatment of fibromyalgia in adults not responsive to initial therapies'. May 2017. UpToDate, Wolters Kluwer. Available at: https://www.uptodate.com/contents/initial-treatment-of-fibromyalgia-in-adults#! and https://www.uptodate.com/contents/treatment-of-fibromyalgia-in-adults-not-responsive-to-initial-therapies (accessed 3 May 2018).

Gross, D.M., Forsthuber, T., Tary-Lehmann, M., Etling, C., Ito, K., Nagy, Z.A., Field, J.A., Steere, A.C. and Huber, B.T. (1998) Identification of LFA-1 as a candidate autoantigen in treatment-resistant Lyme arthritis. *Science* 281, 703–706.

Guellec, D., Narbonne, V., Cornec, D., Marhadour, T., Varache, S., Dougados, M., Daurès, J.P., Jousse-Joulin, S., Devauchelle-Pensec, V. and Saraux, A. (2016) Diagnostic impact of routine Lyme serology in recent-onset arthritis: results from the ESPOIR cohort. *Rheumatic and Musculoskeletal Diseases Open* 2(1), e000120. DOI: 10.1136/rmdopen-2015-000120. eCollection 2016.

Hansen, E.S., Medić, V., Kuo, J., Warner, T.F., Schell, R.F. and Nardelli, D.T. (2013) Interleukin-10 (IL-10) inhibits Borrelia burgdorferi-induced IL-17 production and attenuates IL-17-mediated Lyme arthritis. *Infection and Immunity* 81(12), 4421–4430. DOI: 10.1128/IAI.01129-13. Epub 16 September 2013.

Hardin, J.A., Steere, A.C. and Malawista, S.E. (1979) Immune complexes and the evolution of Lyme arthritis. Dissemination and localization of abnormal C1q binding activity. *New England Journal of Medicine* 301(25), 1358–1363.

Hardin, J.A., Walker, L.C., Steere, A.C., Trumble, T.C., Tung, K.S., Williams Jr, R.C., Ruddy, S. and Malawista, S.E. (1979) Circulating immune complexes in Lyme arthritis. Detection by the 125I-C1q binding, C1q solid phase, and Raji cell assays. *Journal of Clinical Investigation* 63(3), 468–477.

Heimlich, H.J. (1990) Should we try malariotherapy for Lyme disease? *New England Journal of Medicine* 322(17), 1234–1235.

Hein, P. (1966) *Grooks*. The MIT Press, Cambridge, Massachusetts.

Hirsch, J., Rosner, I., Rimar, D., Kaly, L., Rozenbaum, M., Boulman, N. and Slobodin, G. (2016) Tocilizumab efficacy in a patient with positive anti-CCP chronic Lyme arthritis. *North American Journal of Medical Sciences* 8(4), 194–196. DOI: 10.4103/1947-2714.179960.

Hollstrom, E. (1951) Successful treatment of erythema migrans Afzelius. *Acta Dermato-Venereologica* 31(2), 235–243.

Hsu, V., Patella, S.J. and Sigal, L.H. (1993) 'Chronic Lyme disease' as the incorrect diagnosis in patients with fibromyalgia. *Arthritis and Rheumatism* 36, 1493–1500.

Hunfeld, K.P., Ružić-Sabljić, E., Norris D.E., Kraiczy, P. and Strle, F. (2005) In vitro susceptibility testing of *Borrelia burgdorferi* sensu lato isolates cultured from patients with erythema migrans before and after antimicrobial chemotherapy. *Antimicrobial Agents and Chemotherapy* 49(4), 1294–1301.

Hyde, J.A. (2017) *Borrelia burgdorferi* keeps moving and carries on: a review of borrelial dissemination and invasion. *Frontiers in Immunology* 8, 114. DOI: 10.3389/fimmu.2017.00114 PMCID: PMC5318424.

Iliopoulou, B.P., Guerau-de-Arellano, M. and Huber, B.T. (2009) HLA-DR alleles determine responsiveness to *Borrelia burgdorferi* antigens in a mouse model of self-perpetuating arthritis. *Arthritis and Rheumatism* 60, 3831–3840.

Jones, K.L., McHugh, G.A., Glickstein, L.J. and Steere, A.C. (2009) Analysis of *Borrelia burgdorferi* genotypes in patients with Lyme arthritis. *Arthritis and Rheumatism* 60(7), 2174–2182.

Kalish, R.S., Wood, J.A., Golde, W., Bernard, R., Davis, L.E., Grimson, R.C., Coyle, P.K. and Luft, B.J. (2003) Human T lymphocyte response to *Borrelia burgdorferi* infection: no correlation between human leukocyte function antigen type 1 peptide response and clinical status. *Journal of Infectious Diseases* 187, 102–108.

Katchar, K., Drouin, E.E. and Steere, A.C. (2013) Natural killer cells and natural killer T cells in Lyme arthritis. *Arthritis Research and Therapy* 15, R183.

Kean, W.F., Tocchio, S., Kean, M. and Rainsford, K.D. (2013) The musculoskeletal abnormalities of the Similaun Iceman ('ÖTZI'): clues to chronic pain and possible treatments. *Inflammopharmacology* 21(1), 11–20. DOI: 10.1007/s10787-012-0153-5. Epub 25 October 2012.

Kinigadner, U., Mur, E., Möst, J., Frank, R. and Stanek, G. (1991) Borrelia infection as a possible cause of HLA-B27 negative sacroiliitis. *Journal of Rheumatology* 18(3), 484–485.

Klempner, M.S., Hu, L.T., Evans, J., Schmid, C.H., Johnson, G.M., Trevino, R.P., Norton, D., Levy, L., Wall, D., McCall, J., Kosinski, M. and Weinstein, A. (2001) Two controlled trials of antibiotic treatment in patients with persistent symptoms and a history of Lyme disease. *New England Journal of Medicine* 345(2), 85–92.

Kotloski, N.J., Nardelli, D.T., Peterson, S.H., Torrealba, J.R., Warner, T.F., Callister, S.M. and Schell, R.F. (2008) Interleukin-23 is required for development of arthritis in mice vaccinated and challenged with *Borrelia* species. *Clinical and Vaccine Immunology* 15(8), 1199–1207.

Lantos, P.M., Shapiro, E.D., Auwaerter, P.G., Baker, P.J., Halperin, J.J., McSweegan, E. and Wormser, G.P. (2015) Unorthodox alternative therapies marketed to treat Lyme disease. *Clinical Infectious Diseases* 60(12), 1776–1782. DOI: 10.1093/cid/civ186. Epub 6 April 2015.

Li, X., McHugh, G.A., Damle, N., Sikind, V.K., Glickstein, L. and Steere, A.C. (2011) Burden and viability of *Borrelia burgdorferi* in skin and joints of patients with erythema migrans and Lyme arthritis. *Arthritis and Rheumatism* 63(8), 2238–2247.

Lightfoot Jr, R.W., Luft, B.J., Rahn, D.W., Steere, A.C., Sigal, L.H., Zoschke, D.C., Gardner, P., Britton, M.C. and Kaufman, R.L. (1993) Empiric parenteral antibiotic treatment of patients with fibromyalgia and fatigue and a positive serologic result for Lyme disease. A cost-effectiveness analysis. *Annals of Internal Medicine* 119, 503–509.

Lochhead, R.B., Zachary, J.F., Dalla Rosa, L., Ma, Y., Weis, J.H., O'Connell, R.M. and Weis, J.J. (2015) Antagonistic interplay between MicroRNA-155 and IL-10 during Lyme carditis and arthritis. *PLoS One* 10(8), e0135142. DOI: 10.1371/journal.pone.0135142. eCollection 2015.

Lochhead, R.B., Strle, K., Kim, N.D., Kohler, M.J., Arvikar, S.L., Aversa, J.M. and Steere A.C. (2017) MicroRNA expression shows inflammatory dysregulation and tumor-like proliferative response in joints of patients with postinfectious Lyme arthritis. *Arthritis and Rheumatology* 69(5), 1100–1110. DOI: 10.1002/art.40039.

Londoño, D., Cadavid, D., Drouin, E.E., Strle, K., McHugh, G., Aversa J. and Steere A.C. (2014) Microvascular lesions in synovia of patients with antibiotic refractory Lyme arthritis. *Arthritis and Rhematology* 66(8), 2124–2133. DOI: 10.1002/art.38618.

Maier, B., Molinger, M., Cope, A.P., Fugger, L., Schneider-Mergener, J., Sønderstrup, G., Kamradt, T. and Kramer, A. (2000) Multiple cross-reactive self-ligands for *Borrelia burgdorferi*-specific HLA-DR4-restricted T cells. *European Journal of Immunology* 30(2), 448–457.

Marzec, N.S., Nelson, C., Waldron, P.R., Blackburn, B.G., Hosain, S., Greenhow, T., Green, G.M., Lomen-Hoerth, C., Golden, M. and Mead, P.S. (2017) Serious bacterial infections acquired during treatment of patients given a diagnosis of chronic Lyme disease – United States. *Morbidity and Mortality Weekly Report (MMWR)* 66(23), 607–609.

Milewski, M.D., Cruz Jr, A.I., Miller, C.P., Peterson, A.T. and Smith, B.G. (2011) Lyme arthritis in children presenting with joint effusions. *Journal of Bone and Joint Surgery. American Volume* 93(3), 252–260. DOI: 10.2106/JBJS.I.01776. Erratum in *Journal of Bone and Joint Surgery. American Volume* 2011 93(3), e11.

Nardelli, D.T. and Schell, R.D. (2009) Expanded role for interleukin-17 in Lyme arthritis: comment on article by Codolo, et al. *Arthritis and Rheumatism* 60, 1202.

Nardelli, D.T., Burchill, M.A., England, D.M., Torrealba, J., Callister, S.M. and Schell, R.F. (2004) Association of CD4+ CD25+ T cells with prevention of severe destructive arthritis in *Borrelia burgdorferi*-vaccinated and challenged gamma interferon-deficient mice treated with anti-interleukin-17 antibody. *Clinical and Diagnostic Laboratory Immunology* 11(6), 1075–1084.

Nardelli, D.T., Cloute, J.P., Luk, K.H.K., Torrealba, J., Warner, T.F., Callister, S.M. and Schell, R.F. (2005) CD4+ CD25+ T cells prevent arthritis associated with *Borrelia* vaccination and infection. *Clinical and Diagnostic Laboratory Immunology* 12(6), 786–792.

Nardelli, D.T., Callister, S.M. and Schell, R.F. (2008a) Lyme arthritis: current concepts and a change in paradigm. *Clinical and Vaccine Immunology* 15(1), 21–34.

Nardelli, D.T., Luk, K.H.K., Kotloski, N.J., Warner, T.F., Torrealba, J.R., Callister, S.M. and Schell, R.F. (2008b) Role of interleukin-17, transforming growth factor-β, and IL-6 in the development of arthritis and production of anti-outer surface protein A borreliacidal antibodies in *Borrelia*-vaccinated and -challenged mice. *FEMS Immunology and Medical Microbiology* 53, 265–274.

Nishio, M.J., Liebling, M.R., Rodrigues, A., Sigal, L.H. and Louie, J.S. (1993) Identification of *Borrelia burgdorferi* using interrupted polymerase chain reaction. *Arthritis and Rheumatism* 36, 665–675.

Nocton, J.J., Dressler, F., Rutledge, B.J., Rys, P.N., Persing, D.H. and Steere A.C. (1994) Detection of *Borrelia burgdorferi* DNA by polymerase chain reaction in synovial fluid from patients with Lyme arthritis. *New England Journal of Medicine* 330(4), 229–234.

Olson Jr, C.M., Bates, T.C., Izadi, H., Radolf, J.D., Huber, S.A., Boyson, J.E. and Anguita, J. (2009) Local production of IFN-gamma by invariant NKT cells modulates acute Lyme carditis. *Journal of Immunology* 182(6), 3728–3734.

Petersel, D. and Sigal, L.H. (2005) Reactive arthritis, in infectious arthritis. In: Ross, R. and Moellering Jr, R.C. (eds) *Infectious Disease Clinics of North America: Update on Musculoskeletal Infections* 19. W.B. Saunders – Division of Elsevier, Philadelphia, Pennsylvania, pp. 863–883.

Petzke, M.M., Brooks, A., Krupna, M.A., Mordue, D. and Schwartz, I. (2009) Recognition of *Borrelia burgdorferi*, the Lyme disease spirochete, by TLR7 and TLR9 induces a type I IFN response by human immune cells. *Journal of Immunology* 183, 5279–5292.

Pinals, R.S. (2001) Musculoskeletal signs and symptoms: a monoarticular joint disease. In: Klippel, J.H., Crofford, L.J., Stone, J.H. and Weyand, C.M. (eds) *Primer on Rheumatic Diseases*, fifth edn. Arthritis Foundation, Atlanta, Georgia.

Puius, Y.A. and Kalish, R.A. (2008) Lyme arthritis: pathogenesis, clinical presentation, and management. *Infectious Disease Clinics of North America* 22, 289–300.

Schoen, R.T., Aversa, J.M., Rahn, D.W. et al. (1991) Treatment of refractory chronic Lyme arthritis with arthroscopic synovectomy. *Arthritis Rheumatism* 34, 1056–1060.

Scrimenti, R.J. (1970) Erythema chronicum migrans. *Archives of Dermatology* 102(1), 104–105.

Sharma, B., Brown, A.V., Matluck, N.E., Hu, L.T. and Lewis, K. (2015) *Borrelia burgdorferi*, the causative agent of Lyme disease, forms drug-tolerant persister cells. *Antimicrobial Agents and Chemotherapy* 59(8), 4616–4624. DOI: 10.1128/AAC.00864-15. Epub 26 May 2015.

Shen, S., Shin, J.J., Strle, K., McHugh, G., Li, X., Glickstein, L.J., Drouin, E.E. and Steere, A.C. (2010) T regulatory cell numbers and function in patients with antibiotic-refractory or antibiotic-responsive Lyme arthritis. *Arthritis and Rheumatism* 62(7), 2127–2137. DOI: 10.1002/art.27468.

Shin, J.J., Glickstein, L.J. and Steere, A.C. (2007) High levels of inflammatory chemokines and cytokines in joint fluid and synovial tissue throughout the course of antibiotic-refractory Lyme arthritis. *Arthritis and Rheumatism* 56, 1325–1335.

Shin, J.J., Strle, K., Glickstein, L.J., Luster, A.D. and Steere, A.C. (2010) *Borrelia burgdorferi* stimulation of chemokine secretion by cells of monocyte lineage in patients with Lyme arthritis. *Arthritis Research and Therapy* 12(5), R168. Published online 9 September 2010. DOI: 10.1186/ar3128 PMCID: PMC2990995.

Shoemaker, R.C., Hudnell, H.K., House, D.E., Van Kempen., A., Pakes, G.E. and COL40155 Study Team (2006) Atovaquone plus cholestyramine in patients coinfected with *Babesia microti* and *Borrelia burgdorferi* refractory to other treatment. *Advances in Therapy* 23(1), 1–11.

Sigal, L.H. (1988) Lyme disease: a worldwide borreliosis. *Clinical and Experimental Rheumatology* 6, 411–421.

Sigal, L.H. (1990) Summary of the first one hundred patients seen at a Lyme disease referral center. *American Journal of Medicine* 88, 577–581.

Sigal, L.H. (1993) The flagellin of *Borrelia burgdorferi*, the causative agent of Lyme disease, cross-reacts with a human axonal 64,000 molecular weight protein. *Journal of Infectious Diseases* 167, 1372–1378.

Sigal, L.H. (1994) Persisting complaints attributed to Lyme disease: possible mechanisms and implications for management. *American Journal of Medicine* 96, 365–374.

Sigal, L.H. (1996) The Lyme disease controversy: the social and financial costs of the mismanagement of Lyme disease. *Archives of Internal Medicine* 156, 1493–1500.

Sigal, L.H. (1997) The immunology and potential mechanisms of immunopathogenesis of Lyme disease. *Annual Review of Immunology* 15, 63–92.

Sigal, L.H. (2001) Synovial fluid polymerase chain reaction detection of pathogens: what does it really mean? *Arthritis and Rheumatism* 44, 2463–2467.

Sigal, L.H. and Hassett, A.L. (2002) Contributions of societal and geographical environments to 'Chronic Lyme disease': the psychopathogenesis and aporology of a new 'medically unexplained symptoms' syndrome. *Environmental Health Perspectives – Environmental Factors in Medically Unexplained Physical Symptoms and Related Syndromes* 110(Suppl 4), 607–611.

Sigal, L.H. and Patella, S.J. (1992) Lyme arthritis as the incorrect diagnosis in fibromyalgia in children and adolescents. *Pediatrics* 90, 523–528.

Sigal, L.H. and Tatum, A.H. (1988a) IgM in the serum of patients with Lyme neurologic disease binds to cross-reacting neuronal (NAg) and *Borrelia burgdorferi* (BAg) antigens. *Annals of New York Academy of Sciences* 539, 422–424.

Sigal, L.H. and Tatum, A.H. (1988b) Molecular mimicry in Lyme neurologic disease: cross-reactivity between *Borrelia burgdorferi* and neuronal antigens. *Neurology* 38, 1439–1442.

Sigal, L.H., Steere, A.C. and Dwyer, J.M. (1988) *In vivo* and *in vitro* evidence of B cell hyperactivity during Lyme disease. *Journal of Rheumatology* 15, 648–654.

Singh, S.K. and Girschick, H.J. (2004) Lyme borreliosis: from infection to autoimmunity. *Clinical Microbiology and Infection* 10, 598–614.

Sood, S.K. (2015) Lyme disease in children. *Infectious Disease Clinics of North America* 29(2), 281–294. DOI: 10.1016/j.idc.2015.02.011.

Steere, A.C. (2001) Lyme disease. *New England Journal of Medicine* 345, 115–125.

Steere, A.C. and Angelis, S.M. (2006) Therapy for Lyme arthritis: strategies for the treatment of antibiotic-refractory arthritis. *Arthritis and Rheumatism* 54, 3079–3086.

Steere, A.C., Hardin, J.A. and Malawista, S.E. (1977a) Erythema chronicum migrans and Lyme arthritis: cryoimmunoglobulins and clinical activity of skin and joints. *Science* 196(4294), 1121–1122.

Steere, A.C., Malawista, S.E., Hardin, J.A., Ruddy, S., Askenase, W. and Andiman, W.A. (1977b) Erythema chronicum migrans and Lyme arthritis. The enlarging clinical spectrum. *Annals of Internal Medicine* 86(6), 685–698.

Steere, A.C., Malawista, S.E., Snydman, D.R., Shope, R.E., Andiman, W.A., Ross, M.R. and Steele, F.M. (1977c) Lyme arthritis: an epidemic of oligoarticular arthritis in children and adults in three Connecticut communities. *Arthritis and Rheumatism* 20(1), 7–17.

Steere, A.C., Broderick, T.F. and Malawista, S.E. (1978) Erythema chronicum migrans and Lyme arthritis: epidemiologic evidence for a tick vector. *American Journal of Epidemiology* 108(4), 312–321.

Steere A.C., Hardin, J.A., Ruddy, S., Mummaw, J.G. and Malawista, S.E. (1979) Lyme arthritis: correlation of serum and cryoglobulin IgM with activity, and serum IgG with remission. *Arthritis and Rheumatism* 22(5), 471–483.

Steere, A.C., Malawista, S.E., Newman, J.H., Spieler, P.N. and Bartenhagen, N.H. (1980) Antibiotic therapy in Lyme disease. *Annals of Internal Medicine* 93(1), 1–8.

Steere, A.C., Grodzicki, R.L., Kornblatt, A.N., Craft, J.E., Barbour, A.G., Burgdorfer, W., Schmid, G.P., Johnson, E. and Malawista, S.E. (1983a) The spirochetal etiology of Lyme disease. *New England Journal of Medicine* 308(13), 733–740.

Steere, A.C., Hutchinson, G.J., Rahn, D.W., Sigal, L.H., Craft, J.E., DeSanna, E.T. and Malawista, S.E. (1983b) Treatment of the early manifestations of Lyme disease. *Annals of Internal Medicine* 99(1), 22–26.

Steere, A.C., Green, J., Schoen, R.T., Taylor, E., Hutchinson, G.J., Rahn, D.W. and Malawista, S.E. (1985) Successful parenteral penicillin therapy of established Lyme arthritis. *New England Journal of Medicine* 312(14), 869–874.

Steere, A.C., Schoen, R.T. and Taylor, E. (1987) The clinical evolution of Lyme arthritis. *Annals of Internal Medicine* 107, 725–731.

Steere, A.C., Gross, D., Meyer, A.L. and Huber, B.T. (2001) Autoimmune mechanisms in antibiotic treatment-resistant Lyme arthritis. *Journal of Autoimmunity* 16, 263–268.

Steere, A.C., Falk, B., Drouin, E.E., Baxter-Lowe, L.E., Hammer, J. and Nepom, G.T. (2003) Binding of outer surface protein A and human lymphocyte function-associated antigen 1 peptides to HLA-DR molecules associated with antibiotic treatment-resistant Lyme arthritis. *Arthritis and Rheumatism* 48, 534–540.

Steere, A.C., Drouin, E.E. and Glickstein, L.J. (2011) Relationship between immunity to *Borrelia burgdorferi* outer-surface protein A (OspA) and Lyme arthritis. *Clinical Infectious Diseases* 52(Suppl 3), s259–s265. DOI: 10.1093/cid/ciq117.

Stricker, R.B. (2007) Counterpoint: long-term antibiotic therapy improves persistent symptoms associated with Lyme disease. *Clinical Infectious Diseases* 45(2), 149–157.

Stricker, R.B., Lautin, A. and Burrascano, J.J. (2006) Lyme disease: the quest for magic bullets. *Chemotherapy* 52(2), 53–59. Epub 22 February 2006.

Strle, K., Sulka, K.B., Pianta, A., Crowley, J.T., Arvikar, S.L., Anselmo, A., Sadreyev, R. and Steere, A.C. (2017) T-Helper 17 cell cytokine responses in Lyme disease correlate with *Borrelia burgdorferi* antibodies during early infection and with autoantibodies late in the illness in patients with antibiotic-refractory Lyme arthritis. *Clinical Infectious Diseases* 64(7), 930–938. DOI: 10.1093/cid/cix002.

Taylor, R.S. and Simpson, I.N. (2005) Review of treatment options for Lyme borreliosis. *Journal of Chemotherapy* 17(Suppl 2), 3–16.

Theel, E.S. (2016) The past, present, and (possible) future of serologic testing for Lyme disease. *Journal of Clinical Microbiology* 54(5), 1191–1196. PMC4844714.

Tory, H.O., Zurakowski, D. and Sundel, R.P. (2010) Outcomes of children treated for Lyme arthritis: results of a large pediatric cohort. *Journal of Rheumatology* 37(5), 1049–1055. Epub 1 April 2010.

van Dam, A.P. (2011) Molecular diagnosis of *Borrelia* bacteria for the diagnosis of Lyme disease. *Expert Opinion on Medical Diagnostics* 5(2), 135–149. DOI: 10.1517/17530059.2011.555396. Epub 8 February 2011.

Weiner, Z.P., Crew, R.M., Brandt, K.S., Ullmann, A.J., Schriefer, M.E., Molins, C.R. and Gilmore, R.D. (2015) Evaluation of selected *Borrelia burgdorferi* lp54 plasmid-encoded gene products expressed during mammalian infection as antigens to improve serodiagnostic testing for early Lyme disease. *Clinical and Vaccine Immunology* 22(11), 1176–1186. DOI: 10.1128/CVI.00399-15.

Weyand, C.M. and Goronzy, J.J. (1989) Immune responses to *Borrelia burgdorferi* in patients with reactive arthritis. *Arthritis and Rheumatism* 32(9), 1057–1064.

Whiteside, S.K., Snook, J.P., Ma, Y., Sonderegger, F.L., Fisher, C., Petersen, C., Zachary, J.F., Round, J.L., Williams, M.A. and Weis, J.J. (2018) IL-10 Deficiency reveals a role for TLR2-dependent bystander activation of T-cells in Lyme Arthritis. *Journal of Immunology* 200 (4), 1457–1470. doi: 10.4049/jimmunol.1701248. Epub 12 January 2018.

Wormser, G.P., Dattwyler, R.J., Shapiro, E.D. *et al.*(2006) The clinical assessment, treatment, and prevention of Lyme disease, human granulocytic anaplasmosis, and babesiosis: clinical practice guidelines by the infectious diseases society of America. *Clinical Infectious Diseases* 43(9), 1089–1134. Epub 2 October 2006.

Wormser, G.P., Nadelman, R.B. and Schwartz, I. (2012) The amber theory of Lyme arthritis: initial description and clinical implications. *Clinical Rheumatology* 31(6), 989–994. DOI: 10.1007/s10067-012-1964-x. Epub 12 March 2012.

Wright, W.F. and Oliverio, J.A. (2016) First case of Lyme arthritis involving a prosthetic knee joint. *Open Forum Infectious Diseases* 3(2), ofw096. DOI: 10.1093/ofid/ofw096. eCollection 2016 Apr.

Yssel, H., Shanafelt, M.C., Soderbreg, C., Schneider, P.V., Anzola, J. and Peltz, G. (1991) *Borrelia burgdorferi* activates a T helper cell type-1-like T cell subset in Lyme arthritis. *Journal of Experimental Medicine* 174, 593–601.

13 Nervous System Involvement

John J. Halperin
Overlook Medical Center, Summit, New Jersey and Sidney Kimmel Medical College of Thomas Jefferson University, Philadelphia, Pennsylvania, USA

13.1 Introduction

The earliest descriptions – in both Europe and the United States – of the tick-borne infection now referred to as Lyme disease were of the unusual, slowly expanding erythroderma, erythema migrans (Afzelius, 1910; Scrimenti, 1970). The European and American medical literature then diverged in a critical way. In Europe, the first recognition that this could be associated with systemic disease was Garin and Bujadoux's 1922 report of a striking neurologic disorder (Garin and Bujadoux, 1922), involving meningitis and multifocal painful radiculoneuritis. With the subsequent inclusion of cranial neuritis, this has been felt to constitute the essential triad of the disseminated illness in Europe ever since. Consequently, the European literature, and patient diagnosis and treatment, has dealt with this primarily as a neurologic disorder, with management by physicians with expertise in nervous system diseases. In contrast, in the United States the initial extra-cutaneous focus was on rheumatologic aspects (Steere *et al.*, 1977). Although the same neurologic triad was recognized soon thereafter (Reik *et al.*, 1979; Pachner and Steere, 1984), joint manifestations have dominated the conversation. Few of the leading US voices in the field have had special expertise in the subtleties of what is – and is not – neurologic disease.

Perhaps because of this, much of the debate about Lyme disease has involved symptoms that are primarily neurobehavioral. Logically one might expect this to have been more of an issue in Europe, where nervous system involvement was heavily emphasized for half a century before the term 'Lyme disease' was even coined. However, lay concerns about the potential range of nervous system involvement originated in the United States. If nervous system disease is not more prominent in the United States, this then begs the question of how this concern originated, and why it has grown to be the challenge it is.

The responsibility for this likely rests with both the medical profession and worried patients. Neurologic disease represents a unique challenge. To many patients there is no fate more frightening than being diagnosed with a progressive neurodegenerative disorder. To many physicians, neurology is the area of medicine most challenging to understand; medical illnesses that alter behavior are often incorrectly presumed to do this by damaging the nervous system. When physicians share this misperception with patients, anxiety grows to terror. Neurologists are hardly blameless in this either – our enthusiasm for obscure disorders and mechanisms only serves to amplify other physicians' perception that neurologic disease is incomprehensible.

The goal of this chapter will be to clarify basic neurologic concepts so treating physicians

© CAB International 2018. *Lyme Disease: An Evidence-based Approach*, Second Edition (ed. J.J. Halperin)

can better understand what aspects of this infection truly are neurologic. Hopefully this can then clarify the language of the debate, resulting in lessened patient anxiety about this illness.

13.1.1 What is neurologic disease – phenomenology?

Virtually every behavior that we exhibit is fundamentally dependent on the nervous system – a system that has evolved to allow us to interact successfully with our environment, responding to a broad range of both predictable and unpredictable internal and external stressors. Our behavioral responses to the environment are a combination of hard-wired functions and learned behaviors – dimensions that are remarkably intertwined, in actions ranging from the mechanics of walking to our emotional responses to baseball or opera. Nervous system function is affected by the interplay of at least three different elements (Fig. 13.1): (i) changes in the structure, physiology and biochemistry of the nervous system itself; (ii) changes in its physiologic milieu; and (iii) learned behavioral responses to the broad range of ever-changing external stimuli. Just as the host's immune system's response to external stimuli is impacted by its prior experience and learned responses, so too are neurobehavioral responses heavily dependent on past experiences and learned responses.

As a matter of definition, disorders that we consider neurologic affect – either macroscopically or microscopically – the structure of the nervous system. The physiologic milieu is the province of general medicine. Behaviors not involving the first two dimensions are usually considered psychologic. (Psychiatry encompasses both what are almost certainly biochemical abnormalities of synaptic function such as psychosis, and disorders considered psychologic.) Although the diagnosis of a 'psychologic issue' is viewed by many as pejorative and minimizing of its significance, in fact this means neither

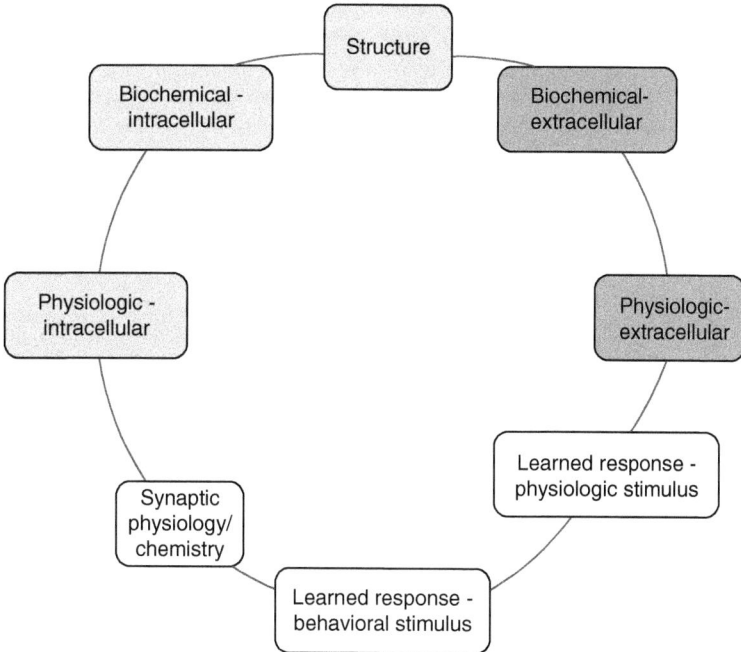

Fig. 13.1. Elements affecting behavior. Disorders due to abnormalities of nervous system structure, cellular physiology or cellular biochemistry (gray background) are generally considered neurologic. Those affecting the extracellular milieu are generally medical (pale background). Those affecting learned responses to stimuli are generally considered psychologic. Psychiatric disorders include psychologic and behavioral disorders presumed to be mediated by altered synaptic physiology.

more nor less than the presence of a learned response to stressors that does not serve the subject well. This should no more be considered a value judgment about neurobehavioral disorders than it would be when an aberrant immune response results in an auto-immune disease.

This 3-fold division is important not just because it defines professional silos but because it defines the appropriate treatment and likely outcome of disease. Disorders that damage the structure of the nervous system are the most difficult to reverse, and therefore the most terrifying to affected patients. Changes in the physiologic milieu are, at least from a neurologic perspective, reversible, assuming the severity and duration of the abnormality is limited (e.g. hypoglycemia or hypoxia). Problems that reflect unhelpful learned behaviors can be challenging to treat, but generally are less daunting than severe neurodegenerative processes. Consequently, when considering a given individual's problem, a key decision point is whether the issue is neurologic, medical or behavioral.

In most instances, differentiating among these is fairly straightforward. Acute focal changes in neurologic function – hemiparesis, visual changes, radiculopathy, etc., are typically fairly obvious. Similarly, significant causes of metabolic encephalopathies – hypoglycemia, renal or hepatic insufficiency, etc. – are fairly straightforward to diagnose. Challenges typically arise with more subtle neurobehavioral disorders in which patients exhibit non-focal changes in behavior and cognitive function. Although these disorders are evidence of aberrant nervous system function, only rarely do they reflect underlying damage to the brain. These non-neurologic disorders generally belong in one of two categories – encephalopathies or psychiatric disease. The term 'encephalopathy' is usually used to denote altered brain function *in the absence* of any underlying brain disease. Encephalopathic patients often have impairment of memory, orientation and other complex cognitive tasks. In contrast, patients with psychiatric disease – who can have remarkably similar subjective perceptions of their difficulties – typically have preservation of these functions but marked impairment of concentration and mental focus. A mini-mental status exam is actually quite effective at differentiating between the two – provided the depressed patient can be cajoled into completing the task, and not 'let off the hook' too easily with protestations that 'I can't do that' – a comment that is actually remarkably uncommon among the neurologically impaired.

13.1.2 What is nervous system disease – patho-anatomy?

Neurologic disease is typically divided into disorders of the peripheral and the central nervous systems. Diseases typically affect one or the other. Some systemic disorders, including inflammatory and infectious diseases, can affect both. The central nervous system (CNS) consists of the brain and spinal cord; the peripheral nervous system (PNS) the nerves that arise from the brainstem and spinal cord, the peripherally located sympathetic, parasympathetic and sensory ganglia, the muscles and sensory end-organs, and the synaptic junctions that allow communication among these different elements.

Medical disorders affecting the CNS can be divided into three broad groups. *Parenchymal damage* can be focal (stroke, trauma, encephalitis, etc.) or cellular (Alzheimer's, Parkinson's, etc.). Other processes can be *extraparenchymal* – involving either inflammation or infiltration of the lining of the brain (meningitis), or alterations in the flow of cerebrospinal fluid (CSF) (hydrocephalus, pseudotumor cerebri) but not the brain itself. Yet others can alter the function of the brain *indirectly* by biochemical or physiologic effects. The latter is by far the most common mechanism, with significant alteration of brain function occurring frequently with numerous metabolic derangements, as well as in non-nervous system infections (pneumonia, sepsis, urinary tract infections, etc.) probably mediated directly by cytokines and indirectly by fever.

The PNS can similarly be affected in a myriad of disorders. Diabetes, the most common cause of neuropathy in the Western world, can cause either diffuse nerve damage or focal damage that can be thought of as 'nerve strokes'. The commonest cause of neuropathy worldwide, leprosy, is an infection that causes multifocal nerve infiltration and inflammation. Metabolic disorders such as renal failure or hypovitaminoses cause fairly diffuse damage. Fluctuating biochemical abnormalities such as uncontrolled hyperglycemia cause transient and reversible changes in nerve function, analogous to a metabolic encephalopathy.

Differentiating neurologic disease from the systemic effects of medical disorders starts with a careful clinical assessment, exploring the wide range of potential contributing medical and other elements. The neurologic exam is designed to detect evidence of structural neurologic disease. If there is a high index of suspicion for neurologic disease, additional testing may be warranted, focusing on the part of the nervous system that appears to be involved. Neurophysiologic testing (nerve conduction studies, electromyography) can be helpful if there is a strong suspicion of peripheral nerve damage. This procedure can differentiate demyelinating from axonal processes, determine if the disorder is focal, multifocal or diffuse, and can quantitate severity. Imaging of the relevant portion of the neuraxis, primarily with magnetic resonance imaging (MRI), can be extremely helpful – if there is reason to suspect CNS involvement. Since MRIs often demonstrate non-specific and irrelevant findings, consistent with Bayes theorem performing this test in an individual with low *a priori* likelihood of disease typically leads only to additional testing, expense and patient stress, without obtaining any information that helps the patient.

In inflammatory disorders of the CNS, examination of CSF can be helpful, primarily in providing evidence of specific infectious or, occasionally, neoplastic disorders, or at a minimum providing objective evidence of brain inflammation that is either acute or chronic. Importantly, bacterial infections of the CNS elicit a local inflammatory response that – virtually without exception – is evidenced in CSF abnormalities.

13.2 Nervous System Disorders in Lyme Disease (Neuroborreliosis)

Nervous system involvement is reported to occur in 12% of confirmed cases of Lyme disease in the US (Bacon *et al.*, 2008). Although neuroborreliosis is sometimes described as protean or mimicking other diseases, this is no more true in neuroborreliosis than it is in any other systemic disorder causing multifocal neurologic damage. Although cerebrovascular disease can affect right arm strength, vision in the left eye, right facial sensation, gait coordination or a myriad of other functions, nobody would call stroke 'the great imitator'. In like manner, *Borreliella burgdorferi* (formerly *Borrelia burgdorferi* sensu stricto) infection causes a small number of pathophysiologic processes. These can affect the nervous system in different locations but the underlying disease process is the same.

Nervous system disorders caused by Lyme disease share one key element with other infectious diseases – involvement is almost certainly due to infiltration of micro-organisms into the nervous system, and the presence of a significant inflammatory response to them. Early in infection, spirochetes invade the subarachnoid space resulting in disseminated infection and inflammation of the meninges – that is, Lyme meningitis (Garin and Bujadoux, 1922; Reik *et al.*, 1979; Pachner and Steere, 1984). In most other instances, neuroborreliosis is due to parenchymal infection and inflammation of peripheral nerve or, very rarely, the CNS. Specific manifestations then depend only on the site of involvement.

The only other form of altered nervous system function seen in Lyme disease is actually quite common but is not caused by nervous system infection or inflammation. Just as in many other systemic infectious or inflammatory diseases (e.g. any febrile illness), patients with active Lyme arthritis or other disseminated forms of infection commonly feel tired and cognitively slowed – probably a result of the CNS actions of a number of circulating cytokines. This entity (Halperin *et al.*, 1988; 1990a) was initially termed 'Lyme encephalopathy' to emphasize that, like most other encephalopathies, it is the remote effect of a systemic process and not evidence of direct CNS involvement. Unfortunately, this point appears not to have been made with sufficient clarity.

These generalizations notwithstanding, there is one clinical syndrome that is quite characteristic of neuroborreliosis – the triad initially described by Garin and Bujadoux and subsequently by Reik. Lymphocytic meningitis, cranial neuritis and painful radiculoneuritis occur alone or in combination in up to 15% of infected individuals – a proportion that is comparable in Europe and in the United States. As summarized in a recent review of European neuroborreliosis: 'the clinical picture of Lyme neuroborreliosis in

North America and Europe seems to be more similar than is often assumed' (Koedel et al., 2015).

13.2.1 Central nervous system involvement

Lymphocytic meningitis occurs as an isolated clinical entity in approximately 2% of confirmed cases of Lyme disease (Bacon et al., 2007). This number is probably an underestimate as symptoms are highly variable. Although often presenting in a manner similar to other forms of 'aseptic meningitis' – i.e. with severe headache, photosensitivity, neck stiffness, fever and other systemic signs – patients with Lyme disease cranial neuritis often have a comparable CSF pleocytosis, without meningitis symptoms. There is good evidence that *B. burgdorferi* penetrates the CSF early (Keller et al., 1992; Logigian and Steere, 1992b; Luft et al., 1992), not consistently accompanied by a vigorous pleocytosis. This suggests that infection of the meninges and subarachnoid space probably occurs more frequently than is clinically recognized or confirmed with a lumbar puncture.

The clinical presentation and seasonal incidence of Lyme meningitis both overlap substantially with viral meningitis. Several algorithms have been published to help differentiate between these two entities (Shah et al., 2005; Garro et al., 2009; Tuerlinckx et al., 2009), important since one requires antibiotic treatment, the other does not. Patients with Lyme meningitis tend to take a little longer to present for medical attention, presumably because the onset of symptoms is less dramatic and symptom severity is less. However, the strongest predictor is the simultaneous occurrence of facial nerve palsy, something that virtually never occurs in viral meningitis.

Particularly among children, there appears to be an association with a pseudotumor cerebri-like (benign intracranial hypertension) syndrome (Jacobson and Frens, 1989; Kan et al., 1998; Zemel, 2000). Affected children develop headaches, raised intracranial pressure, optic disc swelling and potentially visual loss. Most reported cases have had either preceding or concurrent Lyme meningitis, making this more a matter of raised intracranial pressure associated with Lyme meningitis, rather than what is usually considered pseudotumor cerebri. Semantic differences notwithstanding, it is important to recognize this entity, as visual damage and loss have been reported. In addition to treatment of the responsible infection, management of the raised intracranial pressure is important, and may include repeated lumbar puncture, corticosteroids (with and following appropriate antimicrobial therapy), carbonic anhydrase inhibitors, shunting and optic nerve sheath fenestration, as circumstances dictate.

Parenchymal CNS infection is quite rare. Patients with European Lyme radiculitis sometimes develop segmental spinal cord involvement at the affected level (Mygland et al., 2010), something reported anecdotally in the US. Given the infrequent description of Lyme radiculitis in the US, this has not been systematically addressed. Brain involvement is now rarely reported. In the late 1980s and 1990s, when diagnostic tools were still limited and as a result there were patients who went undiagnosed and untreated for a significant period of time, rare cases of Lyme encephalitis were described. At the time the incidence of Lyme encephalitis was estimated at one case per million population at risk per year in both Europe and the US (Halperin et al., 1996). Since then, with widespread early treatment, the disorder is seen rarely, if ever.

In those rare patients with Lyme encephalitis, inflammation appears to affect white matter preferentially (Ackermann et al., 1988; Halperin et al., 1992), perhaps reflecting the spirochetes' demonstrated *in vitro* affinity for oligodendroglia and gangliosides (Garcia-Monco et al., 1989). As a result MRI findings can be confused with demyelinating disease, although the disorders can usually be readily differentiated both by clinical course and by laboratory testing. Unfortunately, because of this rare possibility radiologists often persist in including Lyme disease in the differential diagnosis of any patient with the most trivial white matter abnormality – something that is rarely helpful.

Lyme encephalitis (Ackermann et al., 1988; Halperin et al., 1989; Logigian et al., 1990) can occur in either acute or late disseminated infection. Clinical findings are usually typical of white matter disorders – that is, spasticity, sensory findings, ataxia, etc. Seizures are decidedly uncommon as gray matter is rarely involved. Absent treatment, disease differs from multiple sclerosis in that Lyme disease encephalitis is a monophasic illness without relapses and remissions. Treatment with immunosuppressives in isolation can suppress symptoms, which then recur when treatment is stopped. Treatment with standard courses of antibiotics almost always cures the infection (Halperin et al., 2007; Mygland et al., 2010). Neurologic residua may remain if there has been significant damage but some degree of improvement is the norm and there should be no further loss of function.

In the earliest descriptions of Lyme disease encephalopathy, a few patients were identified who had this as a manifestation of very mild Lyme disease encephalitis (Halperin et al., 1990a). However, this was a rare observation then and in recent experience occurs extremely rarely if ever.

Diagnosis of CNS disease can sometimes be challenging. Lyme disease meningitis (as well as the often co-occurring cranial neuritis and radiculoneuritis) typically occurs very early in infection, occasionally even before there is a measurable antibody response. In such instances if there is likely exposure and the clinical picture is consistent with Lyme disease, empiric antibiotics can be started pending a confirmatory follow-up serology.

CSF findings in Lyme disease meningitis are similar to those in viral meningitis – with a modest lymphocyte-predominant CSF pleocytosis (typically 100s to perhaps low 1000s of cells/mm^3), a mild increase in protein (100–300 mg%) and normal glucose. Culture, in the best of circumstances, is positive in no more than 10–15% of cases of Lyme disease meningitis; clinical laboratories rarely have the necessary specialized medium (BSK-2) or the capabilities to incubate for the requisite prolonged period of time at lower-than-usual temperatures. Unfortunately, even the added technical sensitivity of polymerase chain reaction-based (PCR) techniques has not translated into improved clinical diagnostic sensitivity. It is likely that there are so few spirochetes free in the CSF that any given aliquot may or may not contain one. On the other hand, the presence of organism-specific genomic material does not necessarily imply the presence of viable organisms – PCR positivity has been obtained with long dead organisms (Rovery et al., 2005). Given the additional issue that some laboratories continue to have difficulty performing PCR with sufficient specificity to be certain a reported positive is meaningful, the positive and negative predictive values of this technique are very poor; this test is therefore neither clinically useful nor recommended.

One test that can be useful is measurement of production of specific anti-*B. burgdorferi* antibody in the CSF (intrathecal antibody production, or ITAb) (Henriksson et al., 1986; Wilske et al., 1986; Halperin et al., 1989; Steere et al., 1990). Importantly, this approach is only useful in the presence of CNS infection. CSF examination in patients with purely peripheral nerve disorders would only be expected to be abnormal in individuals who happened to have both peripheral and CNS involvement.

The CNS generally functions as an immunologically distinct compartment. Some immunoglobulin (normally <1%) normally filters in from serum. When an organism invades the CNS and remains for any period of time, reactive lymphocytes migrate in, typically attracted by CXCL13 produced within the CNS in response to the infection (Rupprecht et al., 2009). These B cells then mature and ultimately produce specific antibody locally. When chronic, this can be detected at a superficial level by the detection of oligoclonal bands and an overall increase in IgG synthesis within the CNS – something observed frequently in the European neuroborreliosis literature but less commonly in the US. ITAb measurement can be used to help diagnose a specific infection by measuring the proportion of IgG in the CSF that is specific to the causative organism, comparing that to the corresponding proportion in serum. This can be performed by a number of different techniques. From a technical perspective, capture assays on serum and CSF inherently provide the relevant values (Hansen and Lebech, 1990; Steere et al., 1990). More intuitively understandable is to first measure CSF and serum IgG concentrations, dilute both fluids to the same final IgG concentrations, then perform conventional enzyme linked immunosorbent assays (ELISAs) for the organism in question, comparing the values (Halperin et al., 1989). Because of the non-linear relationship between the optical densities measured by ELISAs and actual antibody concentrations, the approach widely used in Europe – measuring CSF and serum immunoglobulin G (IgG) concentrations, performing CSF and serum ELISAs at standard dilutions, adjusting the ELISA values mathematically for the differing IgG concentrations and calculating an index from those values – is potentially less robust, particularly at low and high antibody concentrations.

Regardless of the technique, it is important to understand that simply performing an anti-B. burgdorferi antibody ELISA in CSF is unhelpful: (i) if there is a significant amount of specific antibody in serum (which then filters into the CSF), giving a 'positive' CSF result; (ii) if there is any blood–brain barrier breakdown, in which case the total concentration of all protein, including IgG, in the CSF is greater than normal, making any measure of a specific antibody artificially high; or (iii) if there is active inflammation in the CNS for another reason, again increasing the total IgG in the CSF, including non-specifically elevating concentrations of unrelated antibodies.

There are three important limitations to this ITAb measurement. First, there is some immune cross-reactivity with other spirochetes, potentially generating false positives. Fortunately, syphilis can usually be differentiated from Lyme disease by measuring reaginic antibodies (e.g. rapid plasma reagin (RPR), Venereal Disease Research Laboratory (VDRL)), which are almost always present in syphilis and rarely present in Lyme disease. Also fortunately, other potentially cross-reacting organisms (such as the relapsing fevers) have little geographic overlap with Lyme disease. Second, the ratio of CSF:-serum antibody may remain elevated long after effective treatment (Hammers Berggren et al., 1993), presumably as antibody production in the two compartments slowly declines in parallel. Consequently, a positive index is indicative of infection, past or present, not necessarily present. Fortunately, just as in neurosyphilis, non-specific markers of CNS inflammation (CSF cell count, protein) provide a reasonable measure of disease activity, as may CXCL13 concentration (Rupprecht et al., 2014; Eckman et al., 2018). Finally, although the specificity of the technique is high, estimates of sensitivity have varied widely, ranging from about 50% (Steere et al., 1990) to over 90% (Blanc et al., 2007; Ljostad et al., 2007; Mygland et al., 2010). This is largely because there is no 'gold standard' diagnostic tool to determine whether or not CNS infection is present and clinical case definitions in published series have varied widely. However, the technique should be nearly 100% sensitive and specific in patients with active CNS infection, particularly those with apparent B cell stimulation as evidenced by overall increases in IgG synthesis and the presence of oligoclonal bands in the CSF. If B cell stimulation in these patients is in response to a specific infecting organism, there should be particularly elevated antibody targeting that organism – that is, this technique should be particularly useful differentiating between neuroborreliosis and multiple sclerosis.

13.2.2 Lyme encephalopathy

In early work with patients with untreated Lyme disease it became apparent that many with active inflammatory arthritis and other non-CNS manifestations described difficulty with memory and information processing – abnormalities which could be confirmed with neuropsychologic testing (Halperin et al., 1988; 1990a; Logigian et al., 1990; Krupp et al., 1991) and which improved after antimicrobial therapy. Subsequent investigations indicated that affected individuals could be divided into two very distinct groups. Starting with the assumption that active CNS Lyme disease – *like every other known CNS bacterial infection* including neurosyphilis – elicits a demonstrable local inflammatory response, a very small subset of these patients, with abnormal CSF (Halperin et al., 1990a; Logigian et al., 1990), was readily identifiable as actually having a very mild form of Lyme encephalomyelitis. These patients generally had abnormal brain MRI scans and significantly abnormal neurologic examinations. *In contrast, the vast majority of patients* with Lyme disease and these cognitive symptoms alone had otherwise normal neurologic examinations, normal imaging and normal CSF. It is this latter group who are most aptly characterized as having 'Lyme encephalopathy', a disorder comparable to the 'toxic-metabolic' encephalopathy seen in myriad other systemic (non-CNS) inflammatory disorders (viral infections, bacterial infections such as pneumonia, systemic lupus, etc.) and almost certainly mediated by the entry of cytokines and other neuro-immunomodulators into the CNS (Halperin and Heyes, 1992).

Unfortunately this entity – named 'Lyme encephalopathy' specifically to differentiate it from a brain infection or encephalitis – has become part of the general folklore about Lyme disease – and is the basis for two particularly important misconceptions. First, when it occurs in the setting of active Lyme disease, it is *not* indicative of nervous system infection. Absent more specific findings, in depth pursuit of a diagnosis of neuroborreliosis – including CSF examination – is rarely if ever informative. More importantly, the symptoms are completely non-specific, occurring in innumerable illnesses, as well as in a significant proportion (2–30%) of the otherwise healthy population (Luo et al., 2005; Blackwell and Clarke, 2013) (Fig. 13.2). Given this background prevalence these symptoms lack any positive predictive value for the diagnosis of Lyme disease – yet are the basis for the diagnoses of 'chronic Lyme disease' and 'post-treatment Lyme disease'. It is particularly important to note that, contrary to the presumed (but inaccurate) relationship of these symptoms to neuroborreliosis, in prospective studies of patients with definite neuroborreliosis, such individuals are the least likely to develop this symptom complex after treatment (Dersch et al., 2016; Wills et al., 2016).

13.2.3 Peripheral nervous system involvement

The assertion that neuroborreliosis has 'protean' manifestations probably derives from the broad range of clinically different PNS phenomena that has been reported. Extensive neurophysiologic evidence indicates that *B. burgdorferi* infection causes just one phenomenon in the PNS – a mononeuropathy multiplex (Halperin et al., 1990b; Logigian and Steere, 1992a; Mygland et al., 2010). This type of disorder, often associated with vasculitic or vasculopathic disorders, causes multifocal peripheral nerve damage. Classically this causes focal damage to one or several large individual nerves. At the other extreme, it can affect innumerable small nerve fascicles, in aggregate mimicking a diffuse polyneuropathy, termed a confluent mononeuropathy multiplex. Early reports describing what was thought to be a diffuse axonal polyneuropathy in patients with more long-standing Lyme disease (Halperin et al., 1987b; Logigian et al., 1990) almost certainly represented examples of this confluent mononeuropathy multiplex, and were analogous to the multifocal neuropathy described earlier in European patients with acrodermatitis atrophicans (Hopf, 1975).

Histologically, mononeuropathy multiplex usually involves vascular changes, often

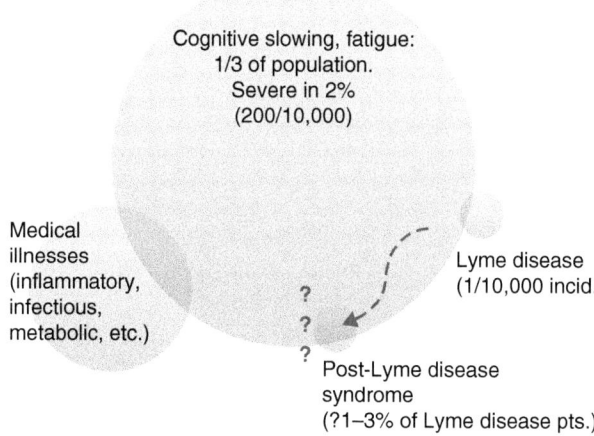

Fig. 13.2. Is it Lyme disease encephalopathy? Subjective symptoms of cognitive slowing (not to scale).

inflammatory, with resultant patchy damage to nerve fascicles – precisely what has been seen in the few published biopsies of human nerves in this disorder (Halperin et al., 1987a; Vallat et al., 1987; Elamin et al., 2009). Importantly, exactly the same neurophysiologic and pathologic changes have been found – with remarkably high frequency – in the only animal model of neuroborreliosis – the rhesus macaque monkey (Roberts et al., 1998).

13.2.3.1 Clinical phenomenology

Cranial neuropathies are the most common peripheral nerve manifestation, occurring in about 8% of confirmed cases (Bacon et al., 2007). In about 80% of these cases, this involves the facial nerve. This can be bilateral in about 20% of these – something quite uncommon otherwise, with other etiologies largely limited to Guillain–Barré syndrome, sarcoidosis, HIV infection and other basilar meningitides. Other cranial nerves can be involved but much less frequently. Of these, nerves to the extra-ocular muscles (III, IV and VI), the trigeminal nerve (V) and the acousticovestibular nerve (VIII) have been reported with some frequency. Very rare cases of optic neuritis (II) have appeared as have rare mentions of the lower cranial nerves. Other than the optic nerve (which is actually a CNS tract) these generally occur as part of a mononeuropathy multiplex. Although it would be reasonable to think these are caused by damage as the nerves pass through the subarachnoid space, not all have simultaneous meningeal inflammation, supporting the notion these are co-occurring but not causally linked phenomena.

The other classically described – and probably significantly under-reported – presentation is the painful radiculoneuritis first described by Garin and Bujadoux. This disorder, documented in about 3% of confirmed US cases (Bacon et al., 2007) presents with symptoms largely indistinguishable from those of a mechanical radiculopathy, with severe dermatomal pain and sensorimotor and reflex changes. Historically the European literature has emphasized that this typically occurs in the limb that was the site of the tick bite; more recent work calls this into question (Ogrinc et al., 2016). No comparable data exist in the United States. Neurophysiologic studies indicate that this, too, is just another presentation of a mononeuropathy multiplex (Halperin et al., 1990b).

Other PNS manifestations include brachial and lumbosacral plexopathies (Wendling et al., 2009) as well as other mononeuropathies. Some patients with long-standing untreated disease have a more diffuse picture, mimicking a diffuse polyneuropathy. Although there have been a few case reports of demyelinating neuropathies (Muley and Parry, 2009) in association with Lyme disease, these are remarkably infrequent and the causal relationship cannot be considered established at this point.

13.3 Pathophysiology

The mechanism underlying these various manifestations remains unclear (Rupprecht et al., 2008). On the one hand, infection seems to play a key role, as antibiotic treatment is curative. On the other, it has been impossible to demonstrate viable spirochetes – or even immunohistochemical or PCR evidence of their presence – in either human biopsies or in realistic animal models. On the one hand, immune amplification clearly plays a role in nerve and brain involvement. On the other it is clear that Lyme disease-associated facial nerve palsy can occur before there has been a measurable antibody response. Molecular mimicry has been suggested but specific targets are limited (Sigal, 1990), disease seems far too restricted in anatomic distribution for such a non-focused mechanism, and both the rapid termination of disease with treatment, as well as the onset before there are demonstrable antibodies render such a mechanism questionable.

With regard to CNS disease, there is evidence that the immune stimulation associated with infection triggers the release of quinolinic acid (Halperin and Heyes, 1992), a tryptophan metabolite that can act as a glutamate receptor agonist, either affecting neuronal function or potentially damaging neurons. In vitro, B. burgdorferi outer-surface protein A (OspA) stimulates monkey astrocytes and microglia to produce TNFα, Il-6 and IL-8, effects that are inhibited by doxycycline and minocycline (Bernardino et al., 2009). Inoculation of B. burgdorferi into the CSF of rhesus monkeys results in early intra-CNS production of IL-6, IL-8, CCL-2 and CXCL13

Table 13.1. Neurologic disorders in Lyme disease, grouped by mechanism.

Peripheral nerve		
	Mononeuropathy multiplex	
		Cranial neuropathy
		Radiculitis
		Brachial plexopathy
		Lumbosacral plexopathy
		Diffuse polyneuropathy
		Motor neuropathy?
		Mononeuropathy +/− multiplex
		'Guillain–Barré-like' (not demyelinating)
Central nervous system		
	Infection in subarachnoid space	
		Lymphocytic meningitis
		Pseudotumor-like presentation in children
	Parenchymal infection	
		Encephalitis ('MS-like' but monophasic)
		Myelitis
	Metabolic encephalopathy	
		Encephalopathy

(markers of the innate immune response), weeks before there is discernible antibody production (Ramesh et al., 2009). In vitro exposure of rhesus brain slices to B. burgdorferi not only results in local production of many of the same cytokines but also triggers some neuronal and oligodendroglial apoptosis (Ramesh et al., 2008). Thus, there are many potential mechanisms by which the immune system and nervous system may be interacting to cause neuroborreliosis – mechanisms that may well inform our understanding of host immune responses in other nervous system infections.

13.4 Treatment

Although treatment is described in detail in Chapter 6 of this volume, it is worthwhile emphasizing several aspects pertaining to nervous system infection. The original rationale for using both high-dose intravenous penicillin (Steere et al., 1983) and then ceftriaxone (Dattwyler et al., 1988) was to obtain good CNS penetration; however, there have now been multiple European studies demonstrating efficacy of oral doxycycline for Lyme disease meningitis, cranial neuritis and radiculoneuritis (Halperin et al., 2007; Mygland et al., 2010), making this an option offered in both US and European nervous system treatment guidelines. Although not proven effective in the US, there is no obvious reason to think efficacy would be different. A reasonable strategy now is to treat orally first, then follow up with parenteral ceftriaxone or other regimen if this should be unsuccessful. As emphasized in Dr Wormser's chapter, treatment for 2–4 weeks with parenteral regimens is reasonable; treatment beyond this duration has not been shown to be efficacious and raises the risk of complications.

There continues to be debate about the role of CSF examination, particularly in patients with facial nerve palsies (Halperin et al., 1996; 2007; Wormser et al., 2006; Rupprecht and Pfister, 2009; Mygland et al., 2010) (and see Chapter 8 in this volume). Although European neuroborreliosis guidelines recommend this, the logic is not necessarily compelling. If oral treatment is almost always effective and will be tried first, the presence or absence of CNS inflammation becomes irrelevant to the treatment strategy and therefore of unclear clinical importance. Greater emphasis on CSF examinations in European patients may well relate to heightened concerns about overdiagnosis and overtreatment, due to the lower specificity of serologic testing there, as the broader range of pathogenic Borreliella in Europe make two-tier testing, with its greater specificity, more challenging. In contrast, CSF examination is clearly important in patients with obvious parenchymal CNS infection, both to prove that this is due to *B. burgdorferi* infection, and to address other potential etiologies.

Finally, over the years there has been concern about the role of corticosteroids, particularly in patients with Lyme-associated facial palsy (LAFP) (Pachner et al., 2001). Steroids are now recommended as effective if given to patients with idiopathic facial nerve palsy within 72 h of onset (Sullivan et al., 2007). In many patients, Lyme serologic test results may not return within this window; in others serology may still be negative. Although several small studies suggest steroids given with antibiotics may be beneficial in LAFP, a recent large retrospective study (Jowett et al., 2016) questioned this approach. Notably, in that study patients with persisting facial paralysis were seen for the first time on average months after symptom onset and the rationale for early use of steroids in some patients but not others was unknown. Patients who had received antibiotics plus steroids were found to have worse outcomes than those just receiving antibiotics. However, given the duration of persisting weakness prior to evaluation, compared to other published information on the rapid expected recovery of LAFP, and the possibility that steroids were used selectively in patients with the most severe weakness, the generalizability of these observations is limited. In contrast, steroids have been shown to be safe and beneficial in painful Lyme radiculitis (Pfister et al., 1988).

Evidence in other bacterial meningitides (Brouwer et al., 2010) and non-systematic evidence in patients with neuroborreliosis suggest that, so long as appropriate antibiotics are also administered at the same time, steroids do not worsen the prognosis and may be considered judiciously in appropriate circumstances. Since even in Lyme disease endemic areas three-quarters of patients with acute facial palsies do not have Lyme disease (Halperin and Golightly, 1992), it would seem prudent to initiate treatment with both steroids and antibiotics in such individuals, adjusting accordingly once the diagnosis has been clarified.

13.5 Summary

Lyme disease affects the nervous system in approximately 12–15% of untreated infected individuals. Patients may develop diffuse meningeal inflammation, multifocal inflammation in peripheral or cranial nerves (mononeuropathy multiplex) or, rarely, in the CNS. The disorder termed Lyme disease encephalopathy is typically an indirect, presumably cytokine-mediated, effect on the brain; rarely is there evidence of CNS infection in these individuals. Treatment with oral doxycycline is probably sufficient for most patients with nervous system Lyme disease not affecting the parenchyma of the brain or spinal cord. In those rare patients with parenchymal CNS infection, parenteral antibiotics are highly effective.

References

Ackermann, R., Rehse, K.B., Gollmer, E. and Schmidt, R. (1988) Chronic neurologic manifestations of erythema migrans borreliosis. *Annals of the New York Academy of Sciences* 539, 16–23.

Afzelius, A. (1910) Verhandlugen der dermatorischen Gesellshaft zu Stockholm. *Archives of Dermatology and Syphilology* 101, 404.

Bacon, R.M., Kugeler, K.J., Griffith, K.S. and Mead, P.S. (2007) Lyme disease – United States, 2003–2005. *Morbidity and Mortality Weekly Report* 56, 573–576.

Bacon, R.M., Kugeler, K.J. and Mead, P.S. (2008) Surveillance for Lyme disease – United States, 1992–2006. *Morbidity and Mortality Weekly Report* 57, 1–9.

Bernardino, A.L., Kaushal, D. and Philipp, M.T. (2009) The antibiotics doxycycline and minocycline inhibit the inflammatory responses to the Lyme disease spirochete *Borrelia burgdorferi*. *Journal of Infectious Diseases* 199, 1379–1388.

Blackwell, D. and Clarke, T.C. (2013) Percentage of adults who often felt very tired or exhausted in the past 3 months, by sex and age group – national health interview survey, United States, 2010–2011. *Morbidity and Mortality Weekly Report* 62, 275.

Blanc, F., Jaulhac, B., Fleury, M., De Seze, J., De Martino, S.J., Remy, V., Blaison, G., Hansmann, Y., Christmann, D. and Tranchant, C. (2007) Relevance of the antibody index to diagnose Lyme neuroborreliosis among seropositive patients. *Neurology* 69, 953–958.

Brouwer, M.C., Mcintyre, P., de Gans, J., Prasad, K. and van de Beek, D. (2010) Corticosteroids for acute bacterial meningitis. *Cochrane Database of Systematic Reviews* CD004405.

Dattwyler, R.J., Halperin, J.J., Volkman, D.J. and Luft, B.J. (1988) Treatment of late Lyme disease. *Lancet*, 1191–1193.

Dersch, R., Sommer, H., Rauer, S. and Meerpohl, J.J. (2016) Prevalence and spectrum of residual symptoms in Lyme neuroborreliosis after pharmacological treatment: a systematic review. *Journal of Neurology* 263, 17–24.

Eckman, E.A., Pacheco-Quinto, J., Herdt, A.R. and Halperin, J.J. (2018) Neuroimmunomodulators in neuroborreliosis and Lyme encephalopathy. *Clinical Infectious Diseases*. DOI: 10.1093/cid/ciy019.

Elamin, M., Alderazi, Y., Mullins, G., Farrell, M.A., O'Connell, S. and Counihan, T.J. (2009) Perineuritis in acute Lyme neuroborreliosis. *Muscle Nerve* 39, 851–854.

Garcia-Monco, J.C., Fernandez-Villar, B. and Benach, J.L. (1989) Adherence of the Lyme disease spirochete to glial cells and cells of glial origin. *Journal of Infectious Diseases* 160, 497–506.

Garin, C. and Bujadoux, A. (1922) Paralysie par les tiques. *Journal De Medecine De Lyon* 71, 765–767.

Garro, A.C., Rutman, M., Simonsen, K., Jaeger, J.L., Chapin, K. and Lockhart, G. (2009) Prospective validation of a clinical prediction model for Lyme meningitis in children. *Pediatrics* 123, e829–e834.

Halperin, J.J. and Golightly, M. (1992) Lyme borreliosis in Bell's palsy. Long Island neuroborreliosis collaborative study group. *Neurology* 42, 1268–1270.

Halperin, J.J. and Heyes, M.P. (1992) Neuroactive kynurenines in Lyme borreliosis. *Neurology* 42, 43–50.

Halperin, J.J., Little, B.W., Coyle, P.K. and Dattwyler, R.J. (1987a) Lyme disease – a treatable cause of peripheral neuropathy. *Neurology* 37, 1700–1706.

Halperin, J.J., Little, B.W., Coyle, P.K. and Dattwyler, R.J. (1987b) Lyme disease: cause of a treatable peripheral neuropathy. *Neurology* 37, 1700–1706.

Halperin, J.J., Pass, H.L., Anand, A.K., Luft, B.J., Volkman, D.J. and Dattwyler, R.J. (1988) Nervous system abnormalities in Lyme disease. *Annals of the New York Academy of Sciences* 539, 24–34.

Halperin, J.J., Luft, B.J., Anand, A.K., Roque, C.T., Alvarez, O., Volkman, D.J. and Dattwyler, R.J. (1989) Lyme neuroborreliosis: central nervous system manifestations. *Neurology* 39, 753–759.

Halperin, J.J., Krupp, L.B., Golightly, M.G. and Volkman, D.J. (1990a) Lyme borreliosis-associated encephalopathy. *Neurology* 40, 1340–1343.

Halperin, J.J., Luft, B.J., Volkman, D.J. and Dattwyler, R.J. (1990b) Lyme neuroborreliosis – peripheral nervous system manifestations. *Brain* 113, 1207–1221.

Halperin, J.J., Rapaport, F., Keller, T. and Whitman, M. (1992) Lyme encephalomyelitis versus multiple sclerosis. *Neurology* 42, 147–148.

Halperin, J., Logigian, E., Finkel, M. and Pearl, R. (1996) Practice parameter for the diagnosis of patients with nervous system Lyme borreliosis (Lyme disease). *Neurology* 46, 619–627.

Halperin, J.J., Shapiro, E.D., Logigian, E.L., Belman, A.L., Dotevall, L., Wormser, G.P., Krupp, L.B., Gronseth, G. and Bever, C. (2007) Practice parameter: treatment of nervous system Lyme disease. *Neurology* 69, 91–102.

Hammers Berggren, S., Hansen, K., Lebech, A.M. and Karlsson, M. (1993) *Borrelia burgdorferi*-specific intrathecal antibody production in neuroborreliosis: a follow-up study. *Neurology* 43, 169–175.

Hansen, K. and Lebech, A.-M. (1990) Intrathecal synthesis of *Borrelia burgdorferi* specific immunoglobulin G, A and M in neuroborreliosis – an antibody capture assay. IV International Conference on Lyme Borreliosis, Stockholm, Sweden, 18–21 June 1990, 144.

Henriksson, A., Link, H., Cruz, M. and Stiernstedt, G. (1986) Immunoglobulin abnormalities in cerebrospinal fluid and blood over the course of lymphocytic meningoradiculitis (Bannwarth's syndrome). *Annals of Neurology* 20, 337–345.

Hopf, H.C. (1975) Peripheral neuropathy in acrodermatitis chronica atrophicans (Herxheimer). *Journal of Neurology, Neurosurgery, and Psychiatry* 38, 452–458.

Jacobson, D.M. and Frens, D.B. (1989) Pseudotumor cerebri syndrome associated with Lyme disease. *American Journal of Ophthalmology* 107, 81–82.

Jowett, N., Gaudin, R.A., Banks, C.A. and Hadlock, T.A. (2016) Steroid use in Lyme disease-associated facial palsy is associated with worse long-term outcomes. *Laryngoscope* 127(6), 1451–1458.

Kan, L., Sood, S.K. and Maytal, J. (1998) Pseudotumor cerebri in Lyme disease: a case report and literature review. *Pediatric Neurology* 18, 439–441.

Keller, T.L., Halperin, J.J. and Whitman, M. (1992) PCR detection of *Borrelia burgdorferi* DNA in cerebrospinal fluid of Lyme neuroborreliosis patients. *Neurology* 42, 32–42.

Koedel, U., Fingerle, V. and Pfister, H.W. (2015) Lyme neuroborreliosis-epidemiology, diagnosis and management. *Nature Reviews Neurology* 11, 446–456.

Krupp, L.B., Masur, D., Schwartz, J., Coyle, P.K., Langenbach, L.J., Fernquist, S., Jandorf, L. and Halperin, J.J. (1991) Cognitive functioning in late Lyme borreliosis. *Archives of Neurology* 48, 1125–1129.

Ljostad, U., Skarpaas, T. and Mygland, A. (2007) Clinical usefulness of intrathecal antibody testing in acute Lyme neuroborreliosis. *European Journal of Neurology* 14, 873–876.

Logigian, E.L. and Steere, A.C. (1992a) Clinical and electrophysiologic findings in chronic neuropathy of Lyme disease. *Neurology* 42, 303–311.

Logigian, E.L. and Steere, A.C. (1992b) Invasion of the central nervous system by *Borrelia burgdorferi* in acute disseminated infection. *Journal of the American Medical Association (JAMA)* 267, 1364–1367.

Logigian, E.L., Kaplan, R.F. and Steere, A.C. (1990) Chronic neurologic manifestations of Lyme disease. *New England Journal of Medicine* 323, 1438–1444.

Luft, B.J., Steinman, C.R., Neimark, H.C., Muralidhar, B., Rush, T., Finkel, M.F., Kunkel, M. and Dattwyler, R.J. (1992) Invasion of the central nervous system by *Borrelia burgdorferi* in acute disseminated infection. *Journal of the American Medical Association* 267, 1364–1367.

Luo, N., Johnson, J., Shaw, J., Feeny, D. and Coons, S. (2005) Self-reported health status of the general adult U.S. population as assessed by the EQ-5D and health utilities index. *Medical Care* 43, 1078–1086.

Muley, S.A. and Parry, G.J. (2009) Antibiotic responsive demyelinating neuropathy related to Lyme disease. *Neurology* 72, 1786–1787.

Mygland, A., Ljostad, U., Fingerle, V., Rupprecht, T., Schmutzhard, E. and Steiner, I. (2010) EFNS guidelines on the diagnosis and management of European Lyme neuroborreliosis. *European Journal of Neurology* 17, 8–16, e1–e4.

Ogrinc, K., Lusa, L., Lotric-Furlan, S., Bogovic, P., Stupica, D., Cerar, T., Ružić-Sabljić, E. and Strle, F. (2016) Course and outcome of early European Lyme neuroborreliosis (Bannwarth syndrome): clinical and laboratory findings. *Clinical Infectious Diseases* 63, 346–353.

Pachner, A.R. and Steere, A.C. (1984) Neurological findings of Lyme disease. *Yale Journal of Biology and Medicine* 57, 481–483.

Pachner, A.R., Amemiya, K., Bartlett, M., Schaefer, H., Reddy, K. and Zhang, W.F. (2001) Lyme borreliosis in rhesus macaques: effects of corticosteroids on spirochetal load and isotype switching of anti-*Borrelia burgdorferi* antibody. *Clinical and Vaccine Immunology* 8, 225–232.

Pfister, H.W., Einhaupl, K.M., Franz, P. and Garner, C. (1988) Corticosteroids for radicular pain in Bannwarth's syndrome: a double blind, randomized, placebo controlled trial. *Annals of the New York Academy of Sciences* 539, 485–487.

Ramesh, G., Borda, J.T., Dufour, J., Kaushal, D., Ramamoorthy, R., Lackner, A.A. and Philipp, M.T. (2008) Interaction of the Lyme disease spirochete *Borrelia burgdorferi* with brain parenchyma elicits inflammatory mediators from glial cells as well as glial and neuronal apoptosis. *American Journal of Pathology* 173, 1415–1427.

Ramesh, G., Borda, J.T., Gill, A., Ribka, E.P., Morici, L.A., Mottram, P., Martin, D.S., Jacobs, M.B., Didier, P.J. and Philipp, M.T. (2009) Possible role of glial cells in the onset and progression of Lyme neuroborreliosis. *Journal of Neuroinflammation* 6, 23.

Reik, L., Steere, A.C., Bartenhagen, N.H., Shope, R.E. and Malawista, S.E. (1979) Neurologic abnormalities of Lyme disease. *Medicine* 58, 281–294.

Roberts, E.D., Bohm Jr, R.P., Lowrie Jr, R.C., Habicht, G., Katona, L., Piesman, J. and Philipp, M.T. (1998) Pathogenesis of Lyme neuroborreliosis in the rhesus monkey: the early disseminated and chronic phases of disease in the peripheral nervous system. *Journal of Infectious Diseases* 178, 722–732.

Rovery, C., Greub, G., Lepidi, H., Casalta, J.-P., Habib, G., Collart, F. and Raoult, D. (2005) PCR detection of bacteria on cardiac valves of patients with treated bacterial endocarditis. *Journal of Clinical Microbiology* 43, 163–167.

Rupprecht, T.A. and Pfister, H.W. (2009) What are the indications for lumbar puncture in patients with Lyme disease? *Current Problems in Dermatology* 37, 200–206.

Rupprecht, T.A., Koedel, U., Fingerle, V. and Pfister, H.-W. (2008) The pathogenesis of Lyme neuroborreliosis: from infection to inflammation. *Molecular Medicine* 14, 205–212.

Rupprecht, T.A., Lechner, C., Tumani, H. and Fingerle, V. (2014) [CXCL13: a biomarker for acute Lyme neuroborreliosis: investigation of the predictive value in the clinical routine]. *Nervenarzt* 85, 459–464.

Rupprecht, T.A., Plate, A., Adam, M., Wick, M., Kastenbauer, S., Schmidt, C., Klein, M., Pfister, H.W. and Koedel, U. (2009) The chemokine CXCL13 is a key regulator of B cell recruitment to the cerebrospinal fluid in acute Lyme neuroborreliosis. *Journal of Neuroinflammation* 6, 42.

Scrimenti, R.J. (1970) Erythema chronicum migrans. *Archives of Dermatology* 102, 104–105.

Shah, S.S., Zaoutis, T.E., Turnquist, J., Hodinka, R.L. and Coffin, S.E. (2005) Early differentiation of Lyme from enteroviral meningitis. *Pediatric Infectious Disease Journal* 24, 542–545.

Sigal, L.H. (1990) Molecular mimicry and Lyme borreliosis [letter]. *Annals of Neurology* 28, 195–196.

Steere, A.C., Malawista, S.E., Hardin, J.A., Ruddy, S., Askenase, W. and Andiman, W.A. (1977) Erythema chronicum migrans and Lyme arthritis. The enlarging clinical spectrum. *Annals of Internal Medicine* 86, 685–698.

Steere, A.C., Pachner, A.R. and Malawista, S.E. (1983) Neurologic abnormalities of Lyme disease: successful treatment with high-dose intravenous penicillin. *Annals of Internal Medicine* 99, 767–772.

Steere, A.C., Berardi, V.P., Weeks, K.E., Logigian, E.L. and Ackermann, R. (1990) Evaluation of the intrathecal antibody response to *Borrelia burgdorferi* as a diagnostic test for Lyme neuroborreliosis. *Journal of Infectious Diseases* 161, 1203–1209.

Sullivan, F.M., Swan, I.R., Donnan, P.T., Morrison, J.M., Smith, B.H., Mckinstry, B., Davenport, R.J., Vale, L.D., Clarkson, J.E., Hammersley, V., Hayavi, S., Mcateer, A., Stewart, K. and Daly, F. (2007) Early treatment with prednisolone or acyclovir in Bell's palsy. *New England Journal of Medicine* 357, 1598–1607.

Tuerlinckx, D., Bodart, E., Jamart, J. and Glupczynski, Y. (2009) Prediction of Lyme meningitis based on a logistic regression model using clinical and cerebrospinal fluid analysis: a European study. *Pediatric Infectious Disease Journal* 28, 394–397.

Vallat, J.M., Hugon, J., Lubeau, M., Leboutet, M.J., Dumas, M. and Desproges-Gotteron, R. (1987) Tick bite meningoradiculoneuritis. *Neurology* 37, 749–753.

Wendling, D., Sevrin, P., Bouchaud-Chabot, A., Chabroux, A., Toussirot, E., Bardin, T. and Michel, F. (2009) Parsonage-Turner syndrome revealing Lyme borreliosis. *Joint Bone Spine* 76, 202–204.

Wills, A.B., Spaulding, A.B., Adjemian, J., Prevots, D.R., Turk, S.P., Williams, C. and Marques, A. (2016) Long-term follow-up of patients with Lyme disease: longitudinal analysis of clinical and quality-of-life measures. *Clinical Infectious Diseases* 62, 1546–1551.

Wilske, B., Schierz, G., Preac-Mursic, V., von Busch, K., Kuhbeck, R., Pfister, H.W. and Einhaupl, K. (1986) Intrathecal production of specific antibodies against *Borrelia burgdorferi* in patients with lymphocytic meningoradiculitis. *Journal of Infectious Diseases* 153, 304–314.

Wormser, G.P., Dattwyler, R.J., Shapiro, E.D., Halperin, J.J., Steere, A.C., Klempner, M.S., Krause, P.J., Bakken, J.S., Strle, F., Stanek, G., Bockenstedt, L., Fish, D., Dumler, J.S. and Nadelman, R.B. (2006) The clinical assessment, treatment, and prevention of Lyme disease, human granulocytic anaplasmosis, and babesiosis: clinical practice guidelines by the Infectious Diseases Society of America. *Clinical Infectious Diseases* 43, 1089–1134.

Zemel, L. (2000) Lyme disease and pseudotumor. *Mayo Clinic Proceedings* 75, 315.

14 Lyme Disease in Children

Eugene D. Shapiro
*Departments of Pediatrics, Epidemiology and Investigative Medicine,
Yale University School of Medicine, New Haven, Connecticut, USA*

14.1 Introduction

Our modern understanding of Lyme disease began when, in the mid-1970s, parents of a cluster of children who lived on a small street in Lyme, Connecticut, with what originally was thought to be juvenile rheumatoid arthritis, reported this 'outbreak' to health authorities. Although we now know that a manifestation of Lyme disease, erythema migrans, was recognized in Scandinavia in the early 20th century (Afzelius, 1921), the expanded spectrum of the manifestations of Lyme disease became apparent when Dr Allen Steere and colleagues investigated this unexplained 'epidemic' of arthritis, which led to the first report of what eventually was recognized as Lyme arthritis (Steere *et al.*, 1977). The illness was characterized by recurrent attacks of asymmetric swelling and pain in a few large joints, particularly the knee. About a quarter of the patients noted an erythematous papule that developed into an expanding, red, annular lesion (now known to be erythema migrans), as much as 50 cm in diameter, that preceded development of the arthritis by weeks to months (Steere *et al.*, 1977). Most of the patients (children and adults) who developed the rash also eventually developed arthritis. While the overall prevalence of the arthritis was <0.5% among residents of the area, 10% of the children who lived on four particular roads developed the illness. From these original observations, the saga of Lyme disease emerged. Within several years, the bacterial etiology of the illness (Burgdorfer *et al.*, 1982; Steere *et al.*, 1983), the fact that the illness is a zoonosis transmitted by ticks, and the effectiveness of antimicrobial treatment of the illness were recognized (Steere *et al.*, 1985).

14.2 Etiology and Epidemiology

The ecology and the epidemiology of Lyme disease is described in Chapters 1 and 5, respectively. Children have the highest incidence of Lyme disease; it is highest in children 5–9 years of age – nearly twice the incidence among adults (Bacon *et al.*, 2008). Updated information about reported cases of Lyme disease is available from the Centers for Disease Control at https://www.cdc.gov/lyme/stats/graphs.html. *Borrelia burgdorferi* is transmitted by ixodid ticks – in the United States, primarily by *Ixodes scapularis*, the deer tick (Lane *et al.*, 1991; Steere *et al.*, 2016). Other vectors include *Ixodes ricinus* (the sheep tick), *Ixodes persulcatus* (the tiaga tick) and *Ixodes pacificus* (the western black-legged tick) in Europe, Asia and the Pacific coast of the United States, respectively. Persons with exposure, either because of where they reside or through occupational or recreational activities, to fields, yards or woodlands in endemic areas that are infested with ticks are at increased risk of developing

Lyme disease. Children may be at increased risk because of their propensity to play in areas in which ticks are found.

14.3 Clinical Manifestations

The clinical manifestations of Lyme disease in children are similar to the manifestations in adults. The manifestations are classified into stages – early localized disease, early disseminated disease and late disease (Shapiro and Gerber, 2000; Shapiro, 2014a; 2014b). In the United States, erythema migrans (single or multiple) is found in 80–90% of patients with Lyme disease (Gerber *et al.*, 1996; Nadelman and Wormser, 1998; Murray and Shapiro, 2010; Steere *et al.*, 2016).

14.3.1 Early localized Lyme disease

Single erythema migrans, the manifestation of early localized disease, appears at the site of the tick bite, 3–30 days (typically within 7–14 days) after the bite. The rash is a result of inflammation at the site of inoculation of the bacteria into the skin by the vector tick. Erythema migrans begins as a red macule and expands, from days to weeks, to form a large, annular, erythematous lesion that is at least 5 cm and as much as 50 cm in diameter (median of 15 cm) (Fig. 14.1). Although erythema migrans commonly is thought of as appearing as a target ('bull's eye') lesion, in the United States it is more common (about two-thirds of the time) for the rash to be uniformly erythematous (Tibbles and Edlow, 2007). However, it may appear as a target lesion with variable degrees of central clearing. It can vary greatly in shape and, occasionally, may have vesicular or necrotic areas in the center. Erythema migrans can develop in any location, but often occurs in the groin or axillary regions. However, in children erythema migrans occurs in the head and neck areas more frequently than it does in adults. Erythema migrans most often is asymptomatic but may be pruritic or painful, and it may be accompanied by systemic findings such as fever, malaise, headache, regional lymphadenopathy, stiff neck, myalgia or arthralgia. Approximately two-thirds of cases of Lyme disease in children present with single erythema migrans (Gerber *et al.*, 1996).

14.3.2 Early disseminated Lyme disease

Early disseminated Lyme disease is a result of dissemination of the bacteria to multiple sites throughout the body via the bloodstream. At this stage of the illness, non-specific systemic manifestations such as fever, headache, fatigue, myalgia and arthralgia are more common than they are with early localized disease. The most common manifestation of early disseminated Lyme disease among children in the United States is multiple erythema migrans (Fig. 14.2) which accounts for 20–25% of cases of Lyme disease overall (Gerber *et al.*, 1996). The secondary skin lesions, which usually appear from 3–5 weeks after initial inoculation of the bacteria, consist of multiple annular erythematous lesions similar to, but usually smaller than, the primary lesion. Sometimes the larger primary lesion is apparent, but multiple erythema migrans may occur without any recognized primary skin lesion.

Neurologic involvement also occurs as a manifestation of early disseminated Lyme disease in children, the most common manifestation of which in the United States is cranial nerve palsy. Palsy of the seventh cranial nerve (facial nerve palsy), which occurs in about 3% of children with Lyme disease in the United States, is most common (Gerber *et al.*, 1996). Involvement is usually unilateral although it can be bilateral, in which case it is virtually pathognomonic for Lyme disease (Skogman *et al.*, 2008).

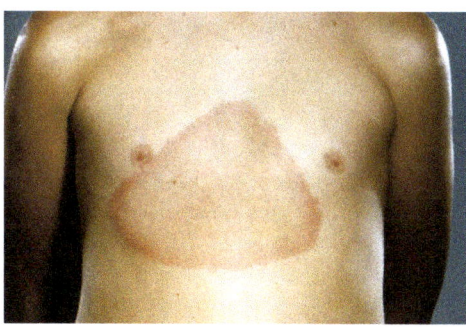

Fig. 14.1. Example of a single erythema migrans on the chest.

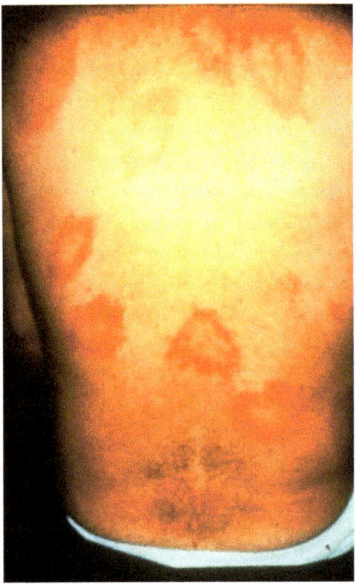

Fig. 14.2. Example of multiple erythema migrans.

About 1–2% of children with Lyme disease in the United States present with meningitis, which manifests like aseptic meningitis, although the duration of symptoms before the patients present is typically longer (days to weeks) than with enteroviral meningitis (Eppes *et al.*, 1999; Tuerlinckx *et al.*, 2003; Shah *et al.*, 2005; Avery *et al.*, 2006). In addition, unlike with most cases of viral meningitis, papilledema and increased intracranial pressure occur in a substantial minority of children with Lyme meningitis (Rothermel *et al.*, 2001; Moses *et al.*, 2003; Shah *et al.*, 2005). Indeed, headache and increased intracranial pressure, which can mimic the presentation of pseudotumor cerebri, can be a prominent feature of Lyme meningitis, and occasionally occurs even in the absence of pleocytosis (Moses *et al.*, 2003).

A rare presentation (<1%) of early disseminated Lyme disease in children is carditis, which usually manifests as complete heart block (Costello *et al.*, 2009). The heart block usually resolves spontaneously within 5–10 days so that only transient artificial pacing of the heart is necessary. Lesser degrees of heart block are more common but usually are asymptomatic. Although it occurs only rarely in the United States, borrelial lymphocytoma, an inflammatory infiltrate that typically occurs in the earlobe or the areola of the breast, is seen with some frequency in patients with Lyme disease in Europe. Likewise, meningoradiculoneuritis (Bannwarth's syndrome), a typically painful radiculopathy due to Lyme disease, is more commonly reported in Europe than in the US (see Chapters 8, 9 and 13).

14.3.3 Late Lyme disease

The manifestation of late Lyme disease in children in the US, which occurs weeks to months after the initial infection, is arthritis, which occurs in about 7% of children with Lyme disease. The arthritis is usually monoarticular or oligoarticular and affects the large joints, particularly the knee. There is a wide spectrum in the mode of presentation of Lyme arthritis (Rose *et al.*, 1994; Gerber *et al.*, 1998; Thompson *et al.*, 2009; Smith *et al.*, 2011). Although the affected joint is typically swollen and somewhat tender, the intense pain associated with a septic arthritis rarely is present. However, Lyme arthritis can occasionally mimic acute septic arthritis. Most often the presentation is subacute. It is not unusual for the patient or the parent to attribute the swelling to an acute event, for example, falling on a knee while playing. If the arthritis is not treated, it usually resolves over the course of 1–2 weeks (though it may persist for many weeks), only to recur in the same or a different joint. Encephalitis, encephalopathy and polyneuropathy are rare manifestations of late Lyme disease in adults, but they virtually never occur among children. Acrodermatitis chronica atrophicans, a chronic sclerosing dermatitis, is an uncommon manifestation of Lyme disease in Europe that has not been described among children in the United States.

14.4 Co-infections

Ixodes ticks may transmit other pathogens in addition to *B. burgdorferi*, including *Babesia*, *Anaplasma*, other *Borreliella* species and viruses (Wormser *et al.*, 2006). These agents may be transmitted either separately from or simultaneously with *B. burgdorferi*. However, the frequency with which co-infection occurs is uncertain and its impact on both the clinical presentation and the response to treatment of Lyme disease is not well defined, especially in children.

14.5 Diagnosis

The diagnosis of Lyme disease, especially if the characteristic rash is not present, may be difficult, since the other clinical manifestations of Lyme disease are not specific. Even the diagnosis of erythema migrans sometimes may be difficult, since the rash initially may be confused with nummular eczema, granuloma annulare, an insect bite, ringworm or cellulitis. The relatively rapid and prolonged (untreated, it lasts for weeks) expansion of erythema migrans helps to distinguish it from these other conditions.

The sensitivity of culture for *B. burgdorferi* is only fair and special media are required; moreover, it is necessary for patients to undergo an invasive procedure to obtain appropriate tissue or fluid for culture. Consequently, such tests are indicated only in rare circumstances. Likewise, diagnostic tests that are based on the identification of antigens of *B. burgdorferi*, including the polymerase chain reaction (PCR) assay, generally are not sufficiently sensitive to be clinically useful because of the small quantity of bacteria present in samples of cerebrospinal fluid (CSF) or of blood. The laboratory confirmation of Lyme disease usually rests on the demonstration of antibodies to *B. burgdorferi*. However, tests for antibodies to *B. burgdorferi* generally are *not* indicated for patients with erythema migrans, both because the rash is usually pathognomonic for Lyme disease and because antibody test results are negative in the majority of patients with erythema migrans since the rash develops sooner than do antibodies. The use of laboratory tests to diagnose Lyme disease is discussed in Chapter 4.

It is critically important to understand that the predictive value of antibody test results, even of very accurate tests, is highly dependent on the prevalence of the infection among patients who are tested. Consequently, tests for antibodies to *B. burgdorferi* should *not* be used as screening tests, especially since many of the non-specific symptoms (e.g. fatigue, headache, arthralgia) that may accompany objective signs of Lyme disease are widely prevalent in the community.

Unfortunately, because many lay persons (as well as physicians) have the erroneous belief that chronic, non-specific symptoms, even in the absence of objective signs of Lyme disease such as erythema migrans, may be manifestations of Lyme disease, parents of children with only non-specific symptoms frequently demand that their child be tested for Lyme disease (and some physicians routinely order tests for Lyme disease on such patients). Even in highly endemic areas, Lyme disease will be the cause of the non-specific symptoms in very few, if any, such children. However, because the specificity of even the best antibody tests for Lyme disease is nowhere near 100%, some of the test results in children without specific clinical evidence of Lyme disease will be positive; the vast majority of these (>95%) will be false positive results (Seltzer and Shapiro, 1996; Tugwell et al., 1997; Lantos et al., 2015a; 2016). Nevertheless, an erroneous diagnosis of Lyme disease, based on the results of these tests, frequently is made and such children often are treated unnecessarily with antimicrobials.

Clinicians should realize that even though a symptomatic patient has a positive serologic test result for antibodies to *B. burgdorferi*, it is possible that Lyme disease is not the cause of that patient's symptoms. First, it may be a false positive result (Seltzer and Shapiro, 1996; Lantos et al., 2016). Or, the patient may have been infected with *B. burgdorferi* previously, and the patient's current symptoms may be unrelated to that previous infection. Once serum antibodies to *B. burgdorferi* do develop, like any other antibodies they (including IgM antibodies) may persist for many years despite adequate treatment and clinical cure of the illness (Feder et al., 1992). In addition, because some who have been infected with *B. burgdorferi* never develop symptoms, some persons will be seropositive from past asymptomatic (and unrecognized) infection. Physicians should not routinely order antibody tests for Lyme disease either for patients who have not been in endemic areas or for patients with only non-specific symptoms (Seltzer and Shapiro, 1996; Lantos et al., 2015a).

On the other hand, in patients with objective signs of early disseminated or of late Lyme disease (e.g. facial nerve palsy or synovitis of the knee) and an epidemiologic history suggestive of Lyme disease, the *a priori* probability of Lyme disease is substantial and the predictive value of a positive serologic test result is high (Seltzer and Shapiro, 1996). By contrast, the results of arthrocentesis usually are not definitive for making a diagnosis of Lyme arthritis (Smith et al., 2011; Deanehan et al., 2014). Testing of synovial fluid for antibodies to B. burgdorferi is not indicated since results have not been shown to be useful. However, testing of CSF for specific antibodies and calculation of a CSF index for these antibodies, which, if positive, suggests intrathecal production of specific antibodies against B. burgdorferi may be informative (see Chapters 8 and 13).

14.6 Treatment

A panel of experts from the Infectious Diseases Society of America has made comprehensive recommendations in a publication that provides practice guidelines for the management of patients with Lyme disease, anaplasmosis and babesiosis (Wormser et al., 2006). These are available on the website of the society (www.idsociety.org) under Practice Guidelines. The American Academy of Neurology has also published evidence-based recommendations for treatment of neuroborreliosis (Halperin et al., 2007) (www.aan.com). Updates of both will be published shortly, and available at the same websites. Recommendations for treatment of Lyme disease in children are shown in Table 14.1a and b. There has been some uncertainty about the need to treat patients with cranial palsies or meningitis due to Lyme disease with intravenously administered antimicrobials. However, the evidence is that orally administered treatment of facial nerve palsy results in excellent outcomes and clinical trials conducted in Europe indicated that treatment of Lyme meningitis with orally administered doxycycline is not inferior to treatment with intravenously administered ceftriaxone (Shapiro and Gerber, 1997; Vazquez et al., 2003; Ljostad et al., 2008; Kowalski et al., 2011).

Occasionally a Jarisch–Herxheimer reaction occurs in the first 24–48 h after treatment is begun. This reaction, usually manifest by increased fever and myalgia, is a response to release of antigens from dying bacteria. Antimicrobial treatment should be continued, the patient should be reassured and treated with non-steroidal anti-inflammatory medications; the reaction usually resolves within a day or two.

14.7 Outcomes

The long-term prognosis for children who are treated with appropriate antimicrobial therapy for Lyme disease, regardless of the stage of the illness, is excellent (Gerber et al., 1996; Seltzer et al., 2000; Vazquez et al., 2003; Wormser et al., 2006). The most common reason for a lack of response to appropriate antimicrobial therapy for Lyme disease is misdiagnosis – that is, the patient actually does not have Lyme disease (Sigal and Patella, 1992; Steere et al., 1993; Seltzer and Shapiro, 1996; Reid et al., 1998; Qureshi et al., 2002). Non-specific symptoms such as fatigue, arthralgia or myalgia occasionally persist for several weeks even in patients with early Lyme disease who are successfully treated; the presence of these non-specific symptoms should not be regarded as an indication for additional treatment with antimicrobials. Such symptoms usually respond to non-steroidal anti-inflammatory agents. Within a few months of completing the initial course of antimicrobial therapy, these non-specific symptoms will usually disappear without additional antimicrobial treatment.

Facial nerve palsy due to Lyme disease usually resolves completely. There is no evidence of residual cognitive neurologic deficits following facial nerve palsy, but a small proportion of children may have persistence of some degree of facial palsy (Vazquez et al., 2003; Skogman et al., 2012). Other manifestations of early disseminated Lyme disease in children, such as Lyme meningitis, also resolve completely (Skogman et al., 2008; 2012). There have been rare reports of patients with papillitis and meningitis in whom increased intracranial pressure persists despite adequate antimicrobial treatment. In such instances, treatment of the increased intracranial pressure is important both for symptomatic relief and to relieve pressure on cranial nerves such as the optic nerve (Rothermel et al., 2001).

Likewise, the long-term outcomes of children with Lyme arthritis also is excellent (Rose et al., 1994; Gerber et al., 1996; Wang et al., 1998). Indeed, long-term follow-up of the original children who developed Lyme arthritis before either the cause of the disease or the appropriate antimicrobial treatment were known revealed that in the overwhelming majority

Table 14.1. Treatment of Lyme disease in children.

(a) Mode and duration of administration

Disease stage	Clinical manifestations	Treatment	Duration
Early localized	Erythema migrans	Oral	10–14 days
Early disseminated	Multiple erythema migrans	Oral	14 days
	Isolated cranial nerve palsy	Oral	14 days
	Meningoradiculoneuritis	Intravenous or oral	14 days
	Meningitis		14 days
	Carditis		
	Ambulatory	Oral	14 days
	Hospitalized	Intravenous[a] followed by oral	14 days
	Borreliellal lymphocytoma	Oral	14–21 days
Late	Arthritis	Oral	28 days
	Recurrent arthritis after oral therapy	Oral or intravenous	28 days / 14 days
	Encephalitis	Intravenous	14–28 days
	Acrodermatitis chronica atrophicans	Oral	14–28 days

[a]At the time of discharge from hospital, the patient may receive oral medication to complete therapy

(b) Dosage of antimicrobials

	Treatment	Adult dose	Pediatric dose[a]
Oral	Doxycycline (patients <8 years of age should not receive for more than 14 days)	100 mg/dose[b] twice a day	4 mg/kg (up to 100 mg/dose[b]) twice a day
	Amoxicillin	500 mg/dose three times/day	50 mg/kg (up to 500 mg/dose) three times/day
	Cefuroxime axetil	500 mg/dose twice a day	30 mg/kg (up to 500 mg/dose) twice a day
Intravenous	Ceftriaxone	2 g once a day	50–75 mg/kg (up to 2 g) once a day
	Cefotaxime	2 g every 8 h	150–200 mg/kg (up to 2 g/dose) every 8 h
	Penicillin G	18–24 million U/day divided every 4 h	200,000–400,000 U/kg divided every 4 h (up to 18–24 million U/day)

[a]Total and maximum daily dosages and frequency of administration/day (divide daily dose by frequency).
[b]Up to 200 mg/dose for neuroborreliosis.

of them symptoms and signs of Lyme disease eventually resolved even though they were not treated with antimicrobials (Szer et al., 1991).

For the rare patients who have persistent symptoms more than 6 months after the completion of antimicrobial therapy, an attempt should be made to determine if these symptoms are the result of a post-infectious phenomenon or of another illness. There is no convincing evidence that 'chronic' Lyme disease (meaning persistent active infection despite treatment with antimicrobials) exists (Feder et al., 2007; Oliveira and Shapiro, 2015). This issue is discussed in Chapters 16 and 17.

14.8 Congenital Lyme Disease

Because Lyme disease is caused by a spirochetal bacterium, there naturally was concern about the possibility that, similar to congenital syphilis (caused by a different spirochetal bacterium), infection of pregnant women with B. burgdorferi could lead to congenital disease. Extensive study has found little or no evidence that congenital Lyme disease is a clinical problem (Silver, 1997). Several studies, designed to assess the potential association between Lyme disease during pregnancy and congenital infection with B. burgdorferi, found no consistent pattern of disease and no clearly documented B. burgdorferi infections of either the fetus or the infant (Strobino et al., 1993; 1999; Williams et al., 1995). In addition, the obstetrical outcomes were similar among women who had documented Lyme disease during their pregnancies and those who did not. Moreover, in a survey of 162 neurologists practicing in areas endemic for Lyme disease, the investigators were unable to identify any well-documented cases of prenatally acquired neuroborreliosis (Gerber and Zalneraitis, 1994). Although there has been a temporal relationship between Lyme disease during pregnancy and adverse outcomes, a causal relationship has not been established. There is no evidence of increased risk of abnormal outcomes with Lyme disease during pregnancy. Transmission of Lyme disease via breast-feeding has not been documented.

14.9 Prevention of Lyme Disease

Reducing the risk of tick bites is one way to prevent Lyme disease. In endemic areas, clearing brush, removing leaf litter, eliminating woodpiles and keeping grass mowed may reduce exposure to ticks. Application of pesticides to residential properties is effective in reducing populations of ticks, but may be harmful both to other wildlife and to people.

Tick and insect repellents that contain n,n-diethylmetatoluamide (DEET) applied to the skin have been shown to provide additional protection (Vazquez et al., 2008), but frequent reapplication may be necessary. Serious neurologic complications have been reported in children from excessive use of DEET-containing repellents, but they are extremely rare and the risk is low when such products are used properly, following instructions on their labels. Use of products with concentrations of DEET greater than 30% is unnecessary and increases the risk of adverse side effects. DEET should be applied sparingly only to exposed skin, but never to a child's face or hands. When the child returns indoors, skin that was treated should be washed with soap and water. Permethrin (a synthetic pyrethroid) is available in a spray for application to clothing only and is highly effective because it kills ticks on contact.

Risk of transmission of Lyme disease is directly related to the duration of feeding by the tick (Nadelman et al., 2001). Because most persons (about 75%) who recognize that they were bitten by a tick remove the tick within 48 h (Falco et al., 1996), the risk of Lyme disease from recognized deer tick bites is low – only 1–3% in areas with a high incidence of Lyme disease. Indeed, the risk of Lyme disease is higher for unrecognized bites (since such ticks will feed for a longer time). Children's bodies and clothing should be inspected daily after possible exposure to ticks. An attached tick should be grasped with fine-tipped tweezers as close to the skin as possible and removed by gently pulling the tick straight out. If some of the mouth parts remain embedded in the skin, they should be left alone, since they usually are extruded spontaneously. Additional attempts to remove them may result in unnecessary damage to the tissue and may increase the risk of local bacterial infection. Analysis of ticks to determine whether they are infected is not indicated because the predictive values of results of such tests for the development of disease in humans is unknown. No vaccine for Lyme disease is at this time available for humans.

A study of antimicrobial prophylaxis for tick bites among persons ≥ 12 years of age found that a single, 200-mg dose of doxycycline was very effective (87%) in preventing Lyme disease, although the 95% confidence interval around this estimate of efficacy was wide – depending on the method used, the lower bound was 25% or less (Nadelman et al., 2001) (see Chapters 6 and 10). In that study, the only persons who went on to develop Lyme disease had been bitten by nymphal stage ticks that were at least partially engorged. The risk of Lyme disease in this group was 9.9% (among recipients of placebo), while it was zero for bites by all larval and adult deer ticks. Unfortunately, the expertise to assess the degree of risk by identifying the species, stage and degree of engorgement of a tick is rarely available to persons who are bitten. After a recognized deer tick bite, the overall risk of Lyme disease, even in highly endemic areas, is low (1–3%). Moreover, the number of patients needed to treat to prevent a single case of Lyme disease in highly endemic areas is high – 50 patients bitten by a tick need to be treated to prevent one case of Lyme disease (Warshafsky et al., 2010). Furthermore, treatment for Lyme disease, if it does develop, is very effective. Consequently, administration of antimicrobial prophylaxis for children is not recommended routinely (Shapiro, 2001).

Serologic testing for Lyme disease after a recognized tick bite also is not recommended. Antibodies to B. burgdorferi that are present at the time that the tick is removed or in the ensuing month or two likely would be due either to a false positive test result or to an earlier infection with B. burgdorferi rather than to a new infection from the recent bite. In this setting, the predictive value of a positive result is very low.

14.10 Fear of Lyme Disease and 'Chronic' Lyme Disease

A panel of experts that developed clinical guidelines for managing patients with Lyme disease for the Infectious Diseases Society of America concluded that there is no such diagnostic entity as 'chronic Lyme disease' (Wormser et al., 2006); more recent studies continue to support this conclusion (Steere et al., 2016). This contention is supported by clinical evidence and by experts from throughout the world (Feder et al., 2007). Nevertheless, there is an extremely media-savvy group of activists, supported by 'Lyme literate' doctors (often reinforced by sensationalized stories in the lay press) that propound that virtually any symptom can be due to Lyme disease and that even serologic test results which are negative in patients with chronic symptoms do not mean that the patient does not have an active infection with B. burgdorferi that requires long-term treatment with antimicrobials. Unvalidated anecdotes on the internet have served to support these misguided notions (Cooper and Feder, 2004).

Some parents whose children have chronic, intractable problems are easy prey for health providers who may profit from these misconceptions. Many unorthodox treatments that are risky, foolish or both may be offered to patients (Lantos et al., 2015b). Long-term treatment with antimicrobials also has been associated with serious, sometimes fatal, adverse effects (Marzec et al., 2017).

The non-specific symptoms sometimes attributed to Lyme disease are highly prevalent in the general population, can be caused by common ailments such as viral illnesses or may be manifestations of either anxiety or depression. In some instances, anxious (often misinformed) parents are driven by the fear that their child's non-specific complaints may be a manifestation of Lyme disease which, if not detected and treated, could lead to serious chronic disability. There is a large body of evidence that Lyme disease rarely causes long-term problems (Feder et al., 2007). Moreover, studies have indicated that the best predictor of the long-term outcome of Lyme disease is the psychological state of the patient before the infection (Solomon et al., 1998). There is a growing body of literature on 'medically unexplained symptoms' that is highly applicable to these situations (Hatcher and Arroll, 2008).

There is absolutely no scientific evidence to support contentions that Lyme disease causes autism, attention deficit/hyperactivity disorder, chronic fatigue syndrome, school phobia or any of the myriad of behavioral problems that some have claimed are caused by Lyme disease. Parents would be well advised to beware of physicians whose practices are primarily focused on treating patients for Lyme disease, as this is likely to be the diagnosis made regardless of the complaint.

On the other hand, academic referral centers where Lyme disease is studied rigorously continue to be deluged by patients who either are thought to have (or who believe they have) 'chronic Lyme disease'. Reports from such centers indicate that in the great majority of instances the patients either never had Lyme disease or the symptoms that led to the referral were not due to Lyme disease (Steere et al., 1993; Seltzer and Shapiro, 1996; Reid et al., 1998; Qureshi et al., 2002; Seriburi et al., 2011). The challenge for clinicians who are faced with such patients (or with the parents of such patients) is to be able to address their concerns without dismissing them. In most instances the patients have (or the parents perceive there is) a problem. Sometimes, a parent's anxiety about a child's behavior can be allayed by reassurance. In other instances, a parent may insist that the child is ill, even though objective signs of organic illness are not present. Helping such patients obtain the type of help they need without alienating both the child and the parents may be difficult. Sometimes this can best be accomplished by affirming the concerns of the parents and explaining that the cause of the problem, while not Lyme disease, may never be known. Instead of focusing on a search for a 'cause' of the symptoms, it is likely that focusing on alleviating the symptoms may be more effective. New approaches to treatment, such as mindfulness-based stress reduction, may be effective (Ali et al., 2017).

14.11 Summary

We now have 40 years of solid, scientific research about Lyme disease, a relatively common, vector-borne illness in parts of the United States and of Europe. Although there is still widespread misunderstanding of and misinformation about the disease among the lay public, its clinical manifestations, as well as how to diagnose and to treat it, are now well understood. In the vast majority of cases of Lyme disease in children, simple treatment with a relatively short course of orally administered antimicrobials results in long-term cure with no adverse sequelae.

References

Afzelius, A. (1921) Erythema chronicum migrans. *Acta Dermato-Venereologica (Stockh)* 2, 120–125.
Ali, A., Weiss, T.R., Dutton, A., McKee, D., Jones, K.D., Kashikar-Zuck, S., Silverman, W.K. and Shapiro, E.D. (2017) Mindfulness-based stress reduction for adolescents with functional somatic syndromes: a pilot cohort study. *Journal of Pediatrics* 183, 184–190.
Avery, R.A., Frank, G., Glutting, J.J. and Eppes, S.C. (2006) Prediction of Lyme meningitis in children from a Lyme disease-endemic region: a logistic-regression model using history, physical, and laboratory findings. *Pediatrics* 117(1), e1–e7.
Bacon, R.M., Kugeler, K.J. and Mead, P.S. (2008) Surveillance for Lyme disease – United States, 1992–2006. *Morbidity and Mortality Weekly Report* 57(SS10), 1–9.
Burgdorfer, W., Barbour, A.G., Hayes, S.F., Benach, J.L., Grunwaldt, E. and Davis, J.P. (1982) Lyme disease: a tick borne spirochetosis? *Science* 216, 1317–1319.
Cooper, J.D. and Feder Jr, H.M. (2004) Inaccurate information about Lyme disease on the internet. *Pediatric Infectious Disease Journal* 23(12), 1105–1108.
Costello, J.M., Alexander, M.E., Greco, K.M., Perez-Atayde, A.R. and Laussen, P.C. (2009) Lyme carditis in children: presentation, predictive factors, and clinical course. *Pediatrics* 123(5), e835–e841.
Deanehan, J.K., Nigrovic, P.A., Milewski, M.D., Tan Tanny, S.P., Kimia, A.A., Smith, B.G. and Nigrovic, L.E. (2014) Synovial fluid findings in children with knee monoarthritis in Lyme disease endemic areas. *Pediatric Emergency Care* 30(1), 16–19.
Eppes, S.C., Nelson, D.K., Lewis, L.L. and Klein, J.D. (1999) Characterization of Lyme meningitis and comparison with viral meningitis in children. *Pediatrics* 103(5 Pt 1), 957–960.
Falco, R.C., Fish, D. and Piesman, J. (1996) Duration of tick bites in a Lyme disease-endemic area. *American Journal of Epidemiology* 143(2), 187–192.
Feder Jr, H.M., Gerber, M.A., Luger, S.W. and Ryan, R.W. (1992) Persistence of serum antibodies to *Borrelia burgdorferi* in patients treated for Lyme disease. *Clinical Infectious Diseases* 15(5), 788–793.
Feder Jr, H.M., Johnson, B.J., O'Connell, S., Shapiro, E.D., Steere, A.C. and Wormser, G.P. (2007) A critical appraisal of 'chronic Lyme disease'. *New England Journal of Medicine* 357(14), 1422–1430.
Gerber, M.A. and Zalneraitis, E.L. (1994) Childhood neurologic disorders and Lyme disease during pregnancy. *Pediatric Neurology* 11(1), 41–43.
Gerber, M.A., Shapiro, E.D., Burke, G.S., Parcells, V.J. and Bell, G.L. (1996) Lyme disease in children in southeastern Connecticut. *New England Journal of Medicine* 335(17), 1270–1274.
Gerber, M.A., Zemel, L.S. and Shapiro, E.D. (1998) Lyme arthritis in children: clinical epidemiology and long-term outcomes. *Pediatrics* 102(4 Pt 1), 905–908.

Halperin, J.J., Shapiro, E.D., Logigian, E.L., Belman, A.L., Dotevall, L., Wormser, G.P., Krupp, L.B., Gronseth, G. and Bever, C. (2007) Practice parameter: treatment of nervous system Lyme disease. *Neurology* 69(1), 91–102.

Hatcher, S. and Arroll, B. (2008) Assessment and management of medically unexplained symptoms. *British Medical Journal* 336(7653), 1124–1128.

Kowalski, T.J., Berth, W.L., Mathiason, M.A. and Agger, W.A. (2011) Oral antibiotic treatment and long-term outcomes of Lyme facial nerve palsy. *Infection* 39(3), 239–245.

Lane, R.S., Piesman, J. and Burgdorfer, W. (1991) Lyme borreliosis: relation of its causative agent to its vectors and hosts in North America and Europe. *Annual Review of Entomology* 36(1), 587–609.

Lantos, P.M., Branda, J.A., Boggan, J.C., Chudgar, S.M., Wilson, E.A., Ruffin, F., Fowler, V., Auwaerter, P.G. and Nigrovic, L.E. (2015a) Poor positive predictive value of Lyme disease serologic testing in an area of low disease incidence. *Clinical Infectious Diseases* 61(9), 1374–1380.

Lantos, P.M., Shapiro, E.D., Auwaerter, P.G., Baker, P.J., Halperin, J.J., McSweegan, E. and Wormser, G.P. (2015b) Unorthodox alternative therapies marketed to treat Lyme disease. *Clinical Infectious Diseases* 60(12), 1776–1782.

Lantos, P.M., Lipsett, S.C. and Nigrovic, L.E. (2016) False positive Lyme disease IgM immunoblots in children. *Journal of Pediatrics* 174, 267–269, e261.

Ljostad, U., Skogvoll, E., Eikeland, R., Midgard, R., Skarpaas, T., Berg, A. and Mygland, A. (2008) Oral doxycycline versus intravenous ceftriaxone for European Lyme neuroborreliosis: a multicentre, non-inferiority, double-blind, randomised trial. *Lancet Neurology* 7(8), 690–695.

Marzec, N.S., Nelson, C., Waldron, P.R., Blackburn, B.G., Hosain, S., Greenhow, T., Green, G.M., Lomen-Hoerth, C., Golden, M. and Mead, P.S. (2017) Serious bacterial infections acquired during treatment of patients given a diagnosis of chronic Lyme disease – United States. *Morbidity and Mortality Weekly Report* 66(23), 607–609.

Moses, J.M., Riseberg, R.S. and Mansbach, J.M. (2003) Lyme disease presenting with persistent headache. *Pediatrics* 112(6 Pt 1), e477–e479.

Murray, T.S. and Shapiro, E.D. (2010) Lyme disease. *Clinics in Laboratory Medicine* 30(1), 311–328.

Nadelman, R.B. and Wormser, G.P. (1998) Lyme borreliosis. *Lancet* 352(9127), 557–565.

Nadelman, R.B., Nowakowski, J., Fish, D. *et al.* (2001) Prophylaxis with single-dose doxycycline for the prevention of Lyme disease after an *Ixodes scapularis* tick bite. *New England Journal of Medicine* 345(2), 79–84.

Oliveira, C.R. and Shapiro, E.D. (2015) Update on persistent symptoms associated with Lyme disease. *Current Opinion in Pediatrics* 27(1), 100–104.

Qureshi, M.Z., New, D., Zulqarni, N.J. and Nachman, S. (2002) Overdiagnosis and overtreatment of Lyme disease in children. *Pediatric Infectious Disease Journal* 21(1), 12–14.

Reid, M.C., Schoen, R.T., Evans, J., Rosenberg, J.C. and Horwitz, R.I. (1998) The consequences of overdiagnosis and overtreatment of Lyme disease. *Annals of Internal Medicine* 128(5), 354–362.

Rose, C.D., Fawcett, P.T., Eppes, S.C., Klein, J.D., Gibney, K. and Doughty, R.A. (1994) Pediatric Lyme arthritis: clinical spectrum and outcome. *Journal of Pediatric Orthopedics* 14(2), 238–241.

Rothermel, H., Hedges, T.R. III and Steere, A.C. (2001) Optic neuropathy in children with Lyme disease. *Pediatrics* 108(2), 477–481.

Seltzer, E.G. and Shapiro, E.D. (1996) Misdiagnosis of Lyme disease: when not to order serologic tests. *Pediatric Infectious Disease Journal* 15(9), 762–763.

Seltzer, E.G., Gerber, M.A., Cartter, M.L., Freudigman, K. and Shapiro, E.D. (2000) Long-term outcomes of persons with Lyme disease. *Journal of the American Medical Association* 283(5), 609–616.

Seriburi, V., Ndukwe, N., Chang, Z., Cox, M.E. and Wormser, G.P. (2011) High frequency of false positive IgM immunoblots for *Borrelia burgdorferi* in clinical practice. *Clinical Microbiology and Infection* 18(12), 1236–1240.

Shah, S.S., Zaoutis, T.E., Turnquist, J., Hodinka, R.L. and Coffin, S.E. (2005) Early differentiation of Lyme from enteroviral meningitis. *Pediatric Infectious Disease Journal* 24(6), 542–545.

Shapiro, E.D. (2001) Doxycycline for tick bites – not for everyone. *New England Journal of Medicine* 345(2), 133–134.

Shapiro, E.D. (2014a) *Borrelia burgdorferi* (Lyme disease). *Pediatrics in Review* 35(12), 500–509.

Shapiro, E.D. (2014b) Lyme disease. *New England Journal of Medicine* 370(18), 1724–1731.

Shapiro, E.D. and Gerber, M.A. (1997) Lyme disease and facial nerve palsy [editorial]. *Archives of Pediatrics and Adolescent Medicine* 151(12), 1183–1184.

Shapiro, E.D. and Gerber, M.A. (2000) Lyme disease. *Clinical Infectious Diseases* 31(2), 533–542.

Sigal, L.H. and Patella, S.J. (1992) Lyme arthritis as the incorrect diagnosis in pediatric and adolescent fibromyalgia. *Pediatrics* 90(4), 523–528.

Silver, H.M. (1997) Lyme disease during pregnancy. *Infectious Disease Clinics of North America* 11(1), 93–97.

Skogman, B.H., Croner, S., Nordwall, M., Eknefelt, M., Ernerudh, J. and Forsberg, P. (2008) Lyme Neuroborreliosis in children; a prospective study of clinical features, prognosis, and outcome. *Pediatric Infectious Disease Journal* 27, 1089–1094.

Skogman, B.H., Glimaker, K., Nordwall, M., Vrethem, M., Odkvist, L. and Forsberg, P. (2012) Long-term clinical outcome after Lyme Neuroborreliosis in childhood. *Pediatrics* 130(2), 262–269.

Smith, B.G., Cruz Jr, A.I., Milewski, M.D. and Shapiro, E.D. (2011) Lyme disease and the orthopaedic implications of Lyme arthritis. *Journal of the American Academy of Orthopaedic Surgeons* 19(2), 91–100.

Solomon, S.P., Hilton, E., Weinschel, B.S., Pollack, S. and Grolnick, E. (1998) Psychological factors in the prediction of Lyme disease course. *Arthritis Care and Research* 11(5), 419–426.

Steere, A.C., Malawista, S.E., Hardin, J.A., Ruddy, S., Askenase, W. and Andiman, W.A. (1977) Erythema chronicum migrans and Lyme arthritis. The enlarging clinical spectrum. *Annals of Internal Medicine* 86(6), 685–698.

Steere, A.C., Grodzicki, R.L., Kornblatt, A.N., Craft, J.E., Barbour, A.G., Burgdorfer, W., Schmid, G.P., Johnson, E. and Malawista, S.E. (1983) The spirochetal etiology of Lyme disease. *New England Journal of Medicine* 308(13), 733–740.

Steere, A.C., Green, J., Schoen, R.T., Taylor, E., Hutchinson, G.J., Rahn, D.W. and Malawista, S.E. (1985) Successful parenteral penicillin therapy of established Lyme arthritis. *New England Journal of Medicine* 312(14), 869–874.

Steere, A.C., Taylor, E., McHugh, G.L. and Logigian, E.L. (1993) The overdiagnosis of Lyme disease. *Journal of the American Medical Association* 269(14), 1812–1816.

Steere, A.C., Strle, F., Wormser, G.P., Hu, L.T., Branda, J.A., Hovius, J.W., Li, X. and Mead, P.S. (2016) Lyme borreliosis. *Nature Reviews Disease Primers* 2, 16090.

Strobino, B.A., Williams, C.L., Abid, S., Chalson, R. and Spierling, P. (1993) Lyme disease and pregnancy outcome: a prospective study of two thousand prenatal patients. *American Journal of Obstetrics and Gynecology* 169, 367–374.

Strobino, B., Abid, S. and Gewitz, M. (1999) Maternal Lyme disease and congenital heart disease: a case-control study in an endemic area. *American Journal of Obstetrics and Gynecology* 180(3 Pt 1), 711–716.

Szer, I.S., Taylor, E. and Steere, A.C. (1991) The long-term course of Lyme arthritis in children. *New England Journal of Medicine* 325(3), 159–163.

Thompson, A., Mannix, R. and Bachur, R. (2009) Acute pediatric monoarticular arthritis: distinguishing Lyme arthritis from other etiologies. *Pediatrics* 123(3), 959–965.

Tibbles, C.D. and Edlow, J.A. (2007) Does this patient have erythema migrans? *Journal of the American Medical Association* 297(23), 2617–2627.

Tuerlinckx, D., Bodart, E., Garrino, M.G. and de Bilderling, G. (2003) Clinical data and cerebrospinal fluid findings in Lyme meningitis versus aseptic meningitis. *European Journal of Pediatrics* 162(3), 150–153.

Tugwell, P., Dennis, D.T., Weinstein, A., Wells, G., Shea, B., Nichol, G., Hayward, R., Lightfoot, R., Baker, P. and Steere, A.C. (1997) Laboratory evaluation in the diagnosis of Lyme disease. *Annals of Internal Medicine* 127(12), 1109–1123.

Vazquez, M., Sparrow, S.S. and Shapiro, E.D. (2003) Long-term neuropsychologic and health outcomes of children with facial nerve palsy attributable to Lyme disease. *Pediatrics* 112(2), e93–e97.

Vazquez, M., Muehlenbein, C., Cartter, M., Hayes, E.B., Ertel, S. and Shapiro, E.D. (2008) Effectiveness of personal protective measures to prevent Lyme disease. *Emerging Infectious Diseases* 14(2), 210–216.

Wang, T.J., Sangha, O., Phillips, C.B., Wright, E.A., Lew, R.A., Fossel, A.H., Fossel, K., Shadick, N.A., Liang, M.H. and Sundel, R.P. (1998) Outcomes of children treated for Lyme disease. *Journal of Rheumatology* 25(11), 2249–2253.

Warshafsky, S., Lee, D.H., Francois, L.K., Nowakowski, J., Nadelman, R.B. and Wormser, G.P. (2010) Efficacy of antibiotic prophylaxis for the prevention of Lyme disease: an updated systematic review and meta-analysis. *Journal of Antimicrobial Chemotherapy* 65(6), 1137–1144.

Williams, C.L., Strobino, B., Weinstein, A., Spierling, P. and Medici, F. (1995) Maternal Lyme disease and congenital malformations: a cord blood serosurvey in endemic and control areas. *Paediatric and Perinatal Epidemiology* 9(3), 320–330.

Wormser, G.P., Dattwyler, R.J., Shapiro, E.D. *et al.* (2006) The clinical assessment, treatment, and prevention of Lyme disease, human granulocytic anaplasmosis, and babesiosis: clinical practice guidelines by the infectious diseases society of America. *Clinical Infectious Diseases* 43, 1089–1134.

15 The Psychology of 'Post-Lyme Disease Syndrome' and 'Not Lyme'

Afton L. Hassett[1] and Leonard H. Sigal[2]

[1]*Chronic Pain and Fatigue Research Center, Department of Anesthesiology, University of Michigan, Ann Arbor, Michigan, USA; [2]Department of Medicine, Division of Rheumatology, RUTGERS – Robert Wood Johnson Medical School, Stockbridge, Massachusetts, USA*

15.1 Introduction

Lyme disease is an infection with the tick-borne organism *Borreliella burgdorferi (B. burgdorferi)*, with a variety of clinical manifestations (Steere, 2001). It is rare for patients treated with adequate antibiotic therapy to manifest objective evidence of ongoing inflammation or organ dysfunction, that is, evidence of persisting infection (Wormser *et al.*, 2006). Yet, in a series of studies 4–40% of adults with Lyme disease previously treated with proper antibiotic regimens report post-antibiotic therapy symptoms that they and their doctors attribute to Lyme disease (Asch *et al.*, 1994; Shadick *et al.*, 1994; Bujak *et al.*, 1996; Dattwyler *et al.*, 1997; Shadick *et al.*, 1999; Seltzer *et al.*, 2000; Smith *et al.*, 2002; Wormser *et al.*, 2003; Hassett *et al.*, 2009). The ongoing controversy over a diagnosis many think does not actually exist continues to rage (Halperin, 2015; Lantos *et al.*, 2015), and has entered the realm of rejection of science and facts by some practitioners, patients and even legislators (Auwaerter and Melia, 2012). The pediatric perspective on this phenomenon was recently reviewed, as well (Oliveira and Shapiro, 2015). These patients often experience ongoing, occasionally severe, disability, with mounting medical bills and toxicities secondary to chronic, often unproven, therapies.

The most common complaints attributed to 'chronic Lyme disease' are 'flu-like' symptoms that can include non-inflammatory musculoskeletal pain, fatigue, cognitive complaints ('brain fog') and mood disturbance (e.g. depression and anxiety). This cluster of symptoms is also consistent with the symptoms of fibromyalgia – the common presence of which in the post-Lyme disease population was first described by our group two decades ago (Sigal, 1990). When depression and anxiety are observed in medical conditions, psychological explanations for these and other coincident symptoms are often sought. This is true for fibromyalgia and for the persistent symptoms attributed to 'chronic Lyme disease'. Herein, we address the psychological aspects of symptom persistence in patients who attribute their ongoing complaints to 'chronic Lyme disease'. It is not our contention that these symptoms are psychiatric in nature. As a matter of fact, our own research has demonstrated that depression and anxiety are present in less than half of Lyme disease specialty center patients and do not predict post-therapy symptom persistence (Hassett *et al.*, 2008a; 2009). Rather, there appears to be a complex interplay among biological, psychological and social factors that might better help understand the problem and explain the pathogenesis of complaints. It is our intention to explore these issues and to suggest potential approaches to treatment that are more likely to decrease pain, suffering and disability, while also decreasing costs related to unnecessary treatments that serve only to increase the likelihood of toxicities and deepen concerns about a purported infection that is stated to be refractory to treatment.

It should be pointed out that the terminology used in describing this 'clinical entity' has been a subject of debate. 'Chronic Lyme disease' implies that there is persistence of infection, a point not generally accepted. Better and less suggestive terms might be 'post-Lyme disease syndrome' (PLDS) or 'post-antibiotic treatment Lyme disease syndrome'. This more correctly defines the persistence of symptoms of Lyme disease (or onset of new symptoms) after the completion of antibiotic therapy. Many patients will have persistence of mild to moderate symptoms of waning intensity for as long as 6 months following appropriate antibiotic therapy (furthermore, it is important to note that inadequate therapy, related to intolerance of the drug used, inattention to completion of prescribed therapy or inappropriate drug or duration of therapy, may result in persistence of infection, but that is not the focus here). When used herein the term 'chronic Lyme disease' does not imply ongoing infection and is used, in large measure, because this is the term many patients use to describe their current predicament.

15.2 The Universe Divided in Three

To lay the groundwork for exploring the relative contributions of psychological factors, our research has shown that patients who ascribe ongoing symptoms to 'chronic Lyme disease' vary in terms of Lyme disease status and commitment to the diagnosis of chronic Lyme disease and can be assigned to one of four groups:

1. Patients who have current Lyme disease (present infection with *B. burgdorferi*): these patients may or may not have been treated with antibiotics previously.
2a. Patients who once had substantiated Lyme disease, but no longer have active infection with *B. burgdorferi* (have a 'post-Lyme disease syndrome').
2b. Patients who once had substantiated Lyme disease, but no longer have active infection with *B. burgdorferi* (have another unrelated medical condition).
3. Patients who never had documentable Lyme disease, but believe, to varying degrees, that Lyme disease is the cause of their ongoing complaints ('Not Lyme').

15.3 Current Infection: is There Such a Thing as 'Antibiotic-Resistant' Lyme Disease

The first and decidedly smallest group we encountered consists of people afflicted with current or persistent infection with *B. burgdorferi*. For some, the diagnosis of Lyme disease may have been missed in its earliest stages. These people may present with later manifestations of the infection, problems often ascribed to other clinical conditions, for example, fibromyalgia, rheumatoid arthritis, multiple sclerosis. Other patients may have been correctly diagnosed, but treated inadequately; the antibiotic used was incorrect, for example, cephalexin, rather than the dependable amoxicillin, doxycycline or cefuroxime axetil; the dosage or duration of an effective antibiotic prescribed was too small or short; the method of therapy was not appropriate to the manifestations, for example, oral antibiotics given for severe carditis or encephalitis; the antibiotic was poorly absorbed; or the patient did not take the proper antibiotic as prescribed (non-compliant). We are unaware of any report of an isolate of *B. burgdorferi* being resistant to the standard antibiotics used.

It has been known for years that some patients will have residual, but self-limited and slowly diminishing, complaints that can last up to 6 months following entirely appropriate treatment for Lyme disease. We know of no prospective markers to reliably predict which patient will experience these lingering complaints, although there has been a suggestion that severity of symptoms at the start of Lyme disease may be predictive of persistence; we do know that further antibiotic therapy will not hasten the resolution of these complaints and may be associated with significant toxicities and comorbidities.

Although there are animal studies demonstrating that viable *B. burgdorferi* can persist after antibiotic therapy (Yrjanainen *et al.*, 2007) there is no convincing evidence that live *B. burgdorferi* persist in humans, for example, as cysts, L-forms or spheroplasts, after appropriate antibiotic therapy (Marques *et al.*, 2000; Klempner,

2002). A set of explanations for the phenomenon of persistence of complaints in patients with Lyme disease despite adequate antibiotic therapy was proposed in 1994 (Table 15.1). Ongoing symptoms are often ascribed to persistent infection, with some medical practitioners hypothesizing antibiotic resistance of the organism or some sort of immune system evasion by the organism, for example, hiding in a dormant and/or intracellular location. There is no evidence that B. burgdorferi produces clinically relevant immunosuppression or that it exports a toxin or other pathogenic product.

There is the theoretical possibility that B. burgdorferi might be resistant to the standard antibiotic agents in use, but as noted, we are unaware of any reports of such isolates. If the organism is capable of causing inflammation, it could not be entirely intracellular at all times and therefore would be susceptible to appropriate antibiotic therapy. Extracellular organisms would then be available to induce an immune response to the organism; thus, ongoing seronegativity in an immunocompetent individual would be implausible (there is no evidence to support the contention that B. burgdorferi has immunosuppressant qualities to interfere with the immune response against itself or induce a state of immune-incompetence in the infected individual). Furthermore, the absence of objective tissue damage or inflammation in almost all of these patients makes persistence of the organism even less likely as an explanation for persistence of symptoms. Although qualitative brain single-photon emission computed tomography (SPECT) scanning has been used to support the presence of brain abnormalities in these patients (Donta et al., 2012) – abnormalities not evident on magnetic resonance imaging (MRI) or even positron emission tomography (PET) scans – this technique is so non-specific that it should not be used. No scientific argument, supported by

Table 15.1. Possible explanations for persistence of complaints. (Adapted from the original that first appeared in Sigal, 1994.)

Unrelated to Lyme disease
   Initial misdiagnosis, never was Lyme disease
   A search for other explanations is necessary
Slowly resolving Lyme disease
   Prior infection, effectively treated, no live organism persists, a long recuperative phase
   No role for further antibiotic therapy
Permanent tissue damage
   Damage from prior infection and associated inflammation, if effectively treated; no persisting live organism
   No role for further antibiotic therapy; need for rehabilitation/compensation strategies
Factors related to chronic illness
   Not specific for Lyme disease
   If there was prior infection with B. burgdorferi it was effectively treated, there are no persisting live organisms and there is no need for further antibiotic therapy
   If there is no compelling objective evidence of prior Lyme disease, a search for other explanations is necessary
True persisting infection with B. burgdorferi
   May never have been treated or was treated inadequately (wrong drug; right drug, inappropriate dose – too short a duration, too low a dose, oral (rather than IV))
   Appropriate antibiotic therapy is called for, with long-term follow-up to determine outcome. Poor outcome is not a mandate to re-treat with antibiotics
Sterile inflammation caused by persisting, poorly degradable dead organism
   Ongoing inflammation not due to persisting infection, possibly due to ongoing release of pro-inflammatory cytokines
Post-Lyme disease syndrome – inflammatory
   Reactive phenomena/immune-mediated symptoms
Post-Lyme disease syndrome – non-inflammatory
   Central augmentation, anxiety/fear of 'chronic Lyme disease', adoption of a 'chronic illness' role, secondary gain

solid data, can be made in favor of the premise that chronic infection is the cause of chronic symptoms.

It is important to note that altered cognition and mood changes/disorders, even in a patient with prior Lyme disease, are not proof of ongoing infection and inflammation in the central nervous system or even elsewhere in the body; the patient's anchoring bias (all too often shared with the healthcare provider making the diagnosis) should not preclude a search for the true explanation of the complaints (Halperin, 2014).

15.4 Post-Lyme Disease Syndrome

PLDS refers to symptoms that continue for at least 6 months following initial diagnosis and appropriate treatment for proven Lyme disease (Wormser et al., 2006). Most patients with Lyme disease have a prompt response to antibiotics although up to 40% may have lingering non-specific complaints for up to 6 months, which resolve thereafter spontaneously (i.e. without further antibiotics); in some these non-specific complaints can last for months or years despite further antibiotic therapy. Our prospective studies of newly infected patients followed over time have shown that between 13 and 32% of patients report ongoing symptoms ascribed to Lyme disease after treatment (Hassett et al., 2008b; 2009). Often these subjective symptoms are not accompanied by objective evidence of organ dysfunction, including absent findings on physical examination or neurocognitive testing (Shadick et al., 1999).

In some cases, organ damage may have occurred that does not heal and resolve even after the infection is eradicated, for example, the rare patients with facial palsies that do not resolve or permanent heart block despite appropriate antibiotic treatment. Inflammation and organ dysfunction may continue after *B. burgdorferi* is killed by antibiotics, as host defenses may still be targeting (and become activated) by residual debris acting as a persisting focus of inflammation (Sigal, 1997; Bockenstedt et al., 2012). Until the residua of the organism are cleared from the site of infection and healing (which makes use of many of the same mechanisms as inflammation) has subsided, there could be active inflammation and damage without active infection, misinterpreted as 'active disease/ongoing infection'. In our experience, far more chronically symptomatic patients have no evidence of inflammation or objective evidence of organ dysfunction; most such patients describe chronic musculoskeletal pain, fatigue, cognitive fogginess, depression and anxiety (Hassett et al., 2008b; 2009), real complaints that simply are not due to ongoing infection.

Although PLDS has been at the center of much debate, to date there is no evidence of persistence of live organisms and no immunopathogenic process has been identified (Sigal, 1997). There has been speculation that immunologic cross-reactivity between the organism and a host component may drive inflammation, but this has not been proven to be of clinical relevance (Sigal, 1997). Instead, about one-third of patients with PLDS meet full criteria for fibromyalgia (Sigal and Patella, 1992; Dinerman and Steere, 1992; Hsu et al., 1993). Fibromyalgia and other similar chronic pain conditions are non-inflammatory conditions and do not respond to antibiotic therapy directed against Lyme disease (Hsu et al., 1993). An immune related activity in patients with cognitive dysfunction has been described, centering on overproduction of alpha interferon in such patients, with frequent significantly elevated antibody response to autoantigens and to specific *borreliellal* proteins; the authors state that this could be due to prolonged exposure to the organism prior to the original diagnosis and delayed treatment. Their data also show that additional β-lactam antibiotic therapy did not alter the described immune activation in affected patients (Jacek et al., 2012).

Nonetheless, many 'chronic Lyme disease' sufferers have been given antibiotics for months, even years, obtaining no lasting relief. Transient 'response' is often interpreted as proof of infection rather than evidence of placebo effect or perhaps an unforeseen immunomodulatory effect of the antimicrobial agent being used, as has been summarized (Sigal, 1999). These illusory improvements often lead to antibiotic-seeking tendencies, sometimes aggressive and/or desperate, on the part of the patient or the parents of younger patients. Oral and intravenous antibiotics, in combinations or sequential cycles, even self-induced malaria (for a pyrexia-induced cure as was used many years ago for neurosyphilis) have been proposed and/or tried.

Cholestyramine has been prescribed for a purported 'toxin' produced by *B. burgdorferi*, although no such toxin has ever been found. Hydroxychloroquine, commonly used in rheumatoid arthritis, has been given to enhance penetration of antibiotics into infected cells. A recent review described over 30 forms of alternative treatments, categorized as: oxygen and reactive oxygen therapies; energy and radiation-based therapies; nutritional therapies; chelation and heavy metal therapies; and biological (including immunoglobulin) and pharmacological therapies, which ranged from the use of a variety of medications without recognized benefit in *B. burgdorferi* infection to stem cell transplantation (Lantos *et al.*, 2012). No benefit has ever been demonstrated in the long-term symptoms following Lyme disease for aggressive and/or long-term antibiotic therapies for PLDS; no benefit for Lyme disease has been demonstrated for antibiotic therapy of any greater intensity than is suggested by the Infectious Disease Society of America guidelines (Wormser *et al.*, 2006). For example, a trial of long-term antibiotics funded by the National Institutes of Health was closed because it failed to show any effect on the symptoms of patients with 'chronic Lyme disease' (Klempner *et al.*, 2001a); another more recent trial also failed to show benefit from longer duration antibiotics in such patients (Berende *et al.*, 2016). The two sides of the debate interpret results differently, each in support of their recommendations for (DeLong *et al.*, 2012; Fallon *et al.*, 2012) and against (Klempner *et al.*, 2013) long-term antibiotic therapy. Nonetheless, it is important to explore explanations for these refractory cases. The antibiotics used for long-term treatment have toxicities, often worse than the patient's original symptoms (Ettestad *et al.*, 1995). Avoiding further iatrogenic damage is critical (Sigal, 1995; Sigal, 1996). Toxicities from both antibiotics and from indwelling catheters have been well described (Marzec *et al.*, 2017). This is in addition to the damage that can be done to patients when their correct underlying diagnosis is missed, for example, malignancies (Nelson *et al.*, 2015).

15.5 Multiple Symptoms Ascribed to Lyme Disease ('Not Lyme')

The third group of 'Lyme disease patients' accounts for well over half of patients evaluated in academic Lyme disease referral centers (Sigal, 1990; Steere *et al.*, 1993; Reid *et al.*, 1998). These patients ascribe multiple, often diffuse symptoms to Lyme disease or 'chronic Lyme disease' but have no objective evidence of infection with *B. burgdorferi* at the time of assessment or objective evidence of prior infection. Some have been previously misdiagnosed by healthcare providers, while others are self-diagnosed (Sigal, 1990; Hsu *et al.*, 1993; Klempner *et al.*, 2001b). Especially in low-prevalence regions, the consulting physician should look carefully at how the initial diagnosis of Lyme disease was made; a study in British Columbia (low prevalence) found that none of the patients in the 'alternatively diagnosed chronic Lyme syndrome (ADCLS)' group had proof of Lyme disease, the diagnosis being made by misinterpretation of alternative laboratory results (Patrick *et al.*, 2015).

Many patients have undergone long-term and/or repeated antibiotic therapy, combination and/or cycling therapies, and treatment with agents previously shown to be ineffective for Lyme disease (Sigal, 1990; Sigal, 1996; Reid *et al.*, 1998; Sigal and Hassett, 2005; Wormser *et al.*, 2006). A number of these patients have utilized considerable healthcare resources, experienced adverse drug reactions and describe high rates of disability (Sigal, 2001). Many present with a multidimensional chronic illness that severely challenges primary care clinicians (Borgermans *et al.*, 2014). The symptoms described are similar to those of PLDS, that is, joint and muscle pain with no evidence of inflammation, fatigue, insomnia, cognitive complaints and mood disturbance (Reid *et al.*, 1998; Sigal and Hassett, 2005); however, we have found that a number of these patients have readily identifiable medical conditions that may or may not have been previously addressed. In our large cross-sectional study, we reported that 53 (22.1%) out of the 240 patients evaluated in our Lyme disease specialty center had an identifiable medical condition, other than fibromyalgia, that accounted for their symptoms. Diagnoses ranged from the benign (e.g. age-related myalgias) to much more threatening conditions (e.g. multiple sclerosis, amyotrophic lateral sclerosis, Parkinson's disease). Of note, Arvikar and colleagues have described patients with autoimmune arthritides following Lyme disease; these are not examples of ongoing infection and are unlikely to be due to a specific immune response elicited by the infection. These are patients who benefit from treatment of their arthritis, not further antibiotic treatment of a prior, resolved infection (Arvikar et al., 2017), for example, tocilizumab for antibiotic-resistant Lyme arthritis (Hirsch et al., 2016).

In our studies we did not study personal attributions; thus, it is not clear how patients arrived at the notion that their symptoms were related to Lyme disease. We speculate that in some cases, patients preferred a diagnosis of Lyme disease to other diagnoses, especially psychiatric diagnoses such as major depressive disorder, or more ominous medical diagnoses without good therapeutic options, for example, amyotrophic lateral sclerosis. In many cases a prior diagnosis of fibromyalgia was rejected and Lyme disease pursued as the cause of the chronic symptoms. In many of these and other cases, certain community physicians (the self-proclaimed 'Lyme literate') misdiagnosed patients and planted the seed of 'chronic Lyme disease' as the cause of their suffering. Some of these doctors prescribed long-term antibiotics and other non-traditional therapies as summarized above. A few marketed therapies in their own offices, for example, vitamins and dietary supplements.

15.6 Commitment to the Diagnosis of 'Chronic Lyme Disease'

'Disease conviction' has been described by Pilowsky and Spence (1983) as the belief that one has a physical illness despite repeated reassurance from physicians to the contrary. We have heard from many patients in our clinic that they are certain ongoing infection with *B. burgdorferi*, *active* Lyme disease, accounts for their symptoms, despite all objective and scientific evidence to the contrary; this belief is often bolstered by material on the internet or local 'Lyme literate' doctors. When a patient has a high level of disease conviction, information is selectively processed: that which supports the belief is accepted, whereas information that refutes the belief is devalued or discarded. A common example of this is when numerous negative laboratory results are dismissed in favor of one equivocal or misinterpreted result (or a result from a non-reputable laboratory) that is taken as proof of active infection. The misnomer that is often attached is 'Lyme disease test' or 'Lyme test', whereas even a documented positive test is not proof of active infection. Moreover, efforts to correct the initial mistaken belief often seem to harden the conviction of the patient and/or family that the diagnosis of Lyme disease is correct. Such efforts are met with anger, resentment or dismissal of the healthcare professional as simply incorrect, obviously not 'Lyme literate'. The level of disease conviction varies among patients: some are reassured when another explanation is found for their symptoms, some are troubled that an incorrect diagnosis of a chronic illness was made and carried for months or even years, while others are incensed that the consulting physician has challenged the standing diagnosis of chronic Lyme disease. When disabused of the diagnosis of 'chronic Lyme disease' many can become beset by doubts, confusion and/or anxiety/fear of the unknown. All share one desire: to have an explanation of their symptoms and establish an approach/treatment that will make the symptoms go away. The phenomenon of Lyme disease conviction is apparently not unique to the United States: Beaman reports a similar disease devotion in Australia, where Lyme disease '…vectors are not found…, and Lyme *Borreliella* has not been found in Australian vectors, animals or patients with autochthonous illnesses' (Beaman, 2016, p. 1370).

15.7 The Psychology of 'Post-Lyme' and 'Not Lyme'

There are very few medical conditions where psychological variables play little or no role in the outcomes of that illness process. The *purely* biomedical model of chronic illness has generally been modified or eschewed in favor of a biopsychosocial approach that takes into consideration the thoughts, affect and behavior of the individual afflicted. In this context, factors such as hostility and depression are seen as important predictors of outcome, for example, having high levels of positive emotions or thoughts (optimism) can be protective in cardiovascular disease (Chida and Steptoe, 2009) and many other conditions including in patients with chronic pain (Cohen et al., 2003; Dockray and Steptoe, 2010; Sin, 2016; Hassett and Finan, 2016). Thus, evaluating the existing research for its role in 'chronic Lyme disease' is not meant to pathologize our patients, but rather to understand their responses and actions more fully, to help chart the course of their disease and their responses to it to obtain a more accurate and holistic approach to their care.

15.8 The Role of Psychiatric Comorbidity

Psychiatric comorbidity is common in nearly all chronic illnesses; having a medical condition that disrupts one's ability to function normally in the physical and social realms of one's life is depressing and/or anxiety-provoking in even the most resilient individuals. This is made even worse by the fear and apprehension that often accompanies a chronic illness that seems to have no cure or effective treatment. Reid and colleagues (1998) were perhaps the first to evaluate the presence of depression in patients presenting for treatment at a Lyme disease specialty clinic. They determined that in 60% of the 209 patients examined at the Yale University Lyme Disease Clinic there was no evidence of current or previous infection with *B. burgdorferi*. However, psychiatric comorbidity was common: 42% reported symptoms of depression, while 16% qualified for a diagnosis of major depressive disorder.

Similarly, early studies in patients with PLDS found that they manifested higher rates of depression than patients who recovered from Lyme disease (Bujak et al., 1996), as well as those with active Lyme disease (Reid et al., 1998). Rates of depression for PLDS have been estimated to be between 23 and 66% (Fallon et al., 1993; Reid et al., 1998). We found over 45% of the PLDS patients evaluated at our academic referral center had a current major depressive episode, using the gold standard Structured Clinical Interview for the Diagnostic and Statistical Manual of Mental Disorders (Hassett et al., 2009). This contrasts with the patients in our 'not Lyme' group (control patients with no evidence of Lyme disease) who had depression at a rate of 26.2%. To provide context, a current major depressive episode occurs in the general population at a 1-year prevalence rate of about 6.7% (Kessler et al., 2005). We found that anxiety disorders occurred in both PLDS and 'not Lyme' patients at a similar elevated rate, 29% and 25.6%, respectively. The 1-year prevalence for any anxiety disorder in the general population is estimated at approximately 18.1% (Kessler et al., 2005). Most striking about our findings was the observation that over 90% of the PLDS patients with one psychiatric disorder qualified for diagnosis of a second psychiatric disorder; depression and anxiety overlapped most frequently.

Consistent with other medical populations, comorbid depression and anxiety were associated with worse outcomes in PLDS. For example, two separate studies reported that the affective symptoms of PLDS patients seemed to predispose them to the perception of cognitive impairment (Barr et al., 1999; Kaplan et al., 1999). Similarly, we found that the presence of clinical disorders such as anxiety and depression in patients seeking care for Lyme disease were predictive of worse functioning scores (Hassett et al., 2009).

Based on the limited research thus far, one cannot say if there is a direct causal relationship between psychiatric comorbidity and PLDS. Few studies have explored this question and the findings have been contradictory, for example, Guadino and colleagues (1997) found that 26% of the PLDS patients evaluated reported having been diagnosed with a psychiatric disorder before Lyme disease. In contrast, findings from our prospective study, described in greater detail later, suggest that psychiatric comorbidity at baseline does not play a role in symptom persistence after treatment for Lyme disease infection (Hassett et al., 2008b).

Bransfield reports a link between 'Lyme and associated diseases' and suicide; were even a small proportion of these patients not to have Lyme disease, sole attention to the misdiagnosis and inattention to the degree of extant depression could be a fatal oversight (Bransfield, 2017).

15.9 The Contribution of Other Psychological Factors

A number of psychological factors can contribute to the behavioral manifestations of PLDS and potentially have a tremendous impact on the patients' subjective experience of illness. For PLDS and 'not Lyme' patients we found several psychological factors including catastrophizing, high levels of negative affect and low levels of positive affect to be associated with poor medical outcomes (Hassett et al., 2008b; 2009). Further, compared to patients with readily identifiable medical conditions, these psychological factors were more pronounced in PLDS and 'not Lyme' and were highly related to poor functioning for all patients (Hassett et al., 2009). However, because of the cross-sectional design of this study, it was not clear if these factors preceded the episode of Lyme disease, were the product of the experience of having a chronic illness or a combination of both.

These cognitive and affective factors seem to be important even in the absence of psychiatric comorbidity. One can have no discernable psychiatric disorder such as depression or anxiety, but still manifest multiple psychological processes that put the patient at risk for poor outcomes. One study found that although most of the individuals in the PLDS group evaluated were not clinically depressed, their low levels of positive affect were associated with the severity of both physical and cognitive symptoms (Elkins et al., 1999). Positive affect refers to having general good feelings, such as interest, enthusiasm and determination and is highly associated with good medical outcomes in other populations including lower levels of pain (Zautra et al., 2005; Hassett et al., 2016) and resistance to viral infection (Cohen et al., 2003; Marsland et al., 2006; Janicki-Deverts et al., 2007). Positive and negative affect are independent constructs, thus having low negative affect (i.e. little or no depression, hostility or anxiety) alone is not sufficient for optimal health outcomes.

The behavior of some patients who present to Lyme disease specialty clinics has been the topic of research and editorials written by healthcare professionals (Sigal and Hassett, 2005; Feder et al., 2007; Halperin, 2008). Lamberg noted that personality disorders are often present in some of the most 'difficult' medical patients seen in many different settings (Lamberg, 2006). We explored this question and did not find antecedent personality disorders to be predictive of PLDS or 'not Lyme'. Patients with PLDS did have slightly elevated rates of these disorders (29% compared to the medical comparison group, 21.1%), but the measurement of personality disorders is a particularly inexact science. Although we used an instrument considered the gold standard for assessment, the Millon Clinical Multiaxial Inventory (MCMI), and used a higher than recommended cut-off score, false positives can still be a problem (Guthrie and Mobley, 1994). This is evidenced by the higher than expected rate of personality disorders in our medical condition comparison group (21.1%); the estimated rate of personality disorder in the general population is approximately 9% (Lenzenweger et al., 2007).

Nearly all the psychosocial risk factors noted above contribute to the general experience of psychological stress and such perceived stress appears to be common in PLDS patients. Reid et al. (1998) reported that 52% of their PLDS group reported high levels of perceived stress. Having a chronic illness can contribute to experiencing high levels of perceived stress, but it is also possible persistent stress could have preceded the infection with B. burgdorferi and represent a risk factor for symptom persistence in PLDS. Stress represents a survival mechanism when there is a target and a defined, short duration. Furthermore, stress in the setting of possible Lyme disease represents a positive feedback loop that does harm, not good. Persistent and intensified activation of the stress response systems results in dysfunctions of these systems. McEwen refers to such 'wear and tear' on the body's organs and systems as 'allostatic load' or the price the body pays for repeatedly responding to excessive stress and/or when the stress response fails to 'turn off' when no longer needed (McEwen, 2007). These changes can affect neuroendocrine processes and may account for the increased levels of pain mediators such as Substance P, glutamate and nerve growth factor observed in chronic pain conditions like fibromyalgia (Clauw, 2009).

Conversely, most PLDS and 'not Lyme' patients do not meet criteria for psychiatric comorbidity, which is consistent with other reports describing subgroups of psychologically healthy fibromyalgia patients who in one study reported lower levels of pain despite increased pain sensitivity (Giesecke et al., 2003). It is quite possible that resilience factors such as positive affect, active coping, social support and self-efficacy could be useful therapeutic targets to consider (Hassett and Finan, 2016). There is growing interest in and evidence to support the notion that identifying and promoting such resilience factors in patients with chronic pain can be quite beneficial (Hausmann et al., 2014; Müller et al., 2015; Peters et al., 2017). A subset of patients with chronic pain tend to function better and report good quality of life despite their pain (Reich et al., 2010; Sturgeon and Zautra, 2010, 2013). Traditionally, resilience has been a concept previously overlooked in favor of focusing on decreasing negative symptoms (e.g. anxiety, depression). Resilience has been defined in a number of ways, including as 'bouncing back' from adversity after an initial emotional setback and decrease in functional status (Rutter, 1987; Smith et al., 2008), maintaining adaptive levels of functioning throughout a period of stress (Bonanno, 2004; Karoly and Ruehlman, 2006; Zautra, 2009), and even flourishing despite adversity (Fredrickson, 2001; Fredrickson and Losada, 2005). Because most resilience interventions (i.e. performing acts of kindness, keeping a gratitude journal, engaging in pleasant activities) largely do not require a healthcare professional to provide the treatment and can be delivered online, as a form of effective treatment they are attractive and highly scalable. Still, prospective studies are required to adequately address the role of such psychological risk and protective factors.

15.10 Is There an Etiological Role for Psychological Factors in Post-Lyme Disease Syndrome?

Whenever depression and anxiety are observed frequently in a medical condition, a causal relationship is hypothesized. However, most studies evaluating psychiatric comorbidity in PLDS and 'not Lyme' patients are cross-sectional so causality cannot be inferred. Only prospective studies in PLDS can begin to answer questions about the true role of psychological factors in symptoms ascribed to Lyme disease. Solomon and colleagues explored the role of psychological factors in Lyme disease and found a strong association between a history of prior psychological trauma and chronic physical symptoms (Solomon et al., 1998), which led them to hypothesize that antecedent traumatic psychological experiences may play an etiologic role in the persistence of PLDS symptoms.

More recently, we tracked 99 patients with newly diagnosed Lyme disease to assess risk factors for persistent symptoms after treatment (Hassett et al., 2008b). Based on the findings of Bujak et al. (2000), who found that the number of symptoms and worse functional status at baseline more than triples the risk of developing chronic symptoms after antibiotic treatment, we assessed patients with documented Lyme disease for these same factors plus depression, anxiety, catastrophizing, somatosensory amplification and affective style (negative affect and positive affect). At 1 year, 32.4% reported chronic symptoms attributed to their previous Lyme disease. Based on the literature and our own research, we predicted that functional status, depression and anxiety at baseline would be strong predictors of later symptomatic status. Much to our surprise we found that only functional status and level of positive affect at baseline were predictive of persistent symptoms. Moreover, level of positive affect was not related to functional status at baseline, which would be the case if symptom severity determined level of positive feelings. Instead, positive affect predicted recovery regardless of symptom severity at baseline. We are not the first to find a protective role for positive affect in infectious disease – the cold studies conducted by Cohen et al. found positive affect to be an even better predictor of catching a cold and cold symptom severity than negative affect (Cohen et al., 2003; Cohen, 2005).

15.11 The Ubiquitous Presence of Fibromyalgia

In a review of the first 100 patients seen at the Lyme Disease Center at Robert Wood Johnson Medical School, only 37% of patients referred had current or preceding Lyme disease as the explanation for their complaints (Sigal, 1990). Instead, in patients where Lyme disease did not explain patient symptoms, close to 40% met the criteria for fibromyalgia. Interestingly, in most of the patients with fibromyalgia, the onset of fibromyalgia was subsequent to Lyme disease as if Lyme disease triggered the fibromyalgia. Steere and his colleagues (1993) confirmed these findings: in the 788 patients evaluated at their clinic, only 23% had active Lyme disease. More than half of these patients appeared never to have had Lyme disease and many qualified for a diagnosis of chronic fatigue syndrome or fibromyalgia. Similarly, Reid et al. (1998) reported that 31% of the patients presenting for evaluation at their academic Lyme disease specialty clinic did not have Lyme disease, but had instead a fibromyalgia-like 'fatigue-arthralgia-myalgia syndrome'.

More recently, we conducted two prospective studies assessing patients with active *B. burgdorferi* infection who received antibiotic treatment. In the first study of 46 patients treated in our own clinic, 13% later met American College of Rheumatology (ACR) criteria for fibromyalgia with many more exhibiting a fibromyalgia-like illness (Hassett et al., 2009). In a separate and more rigorous study of 99 newly diagnosed Lyme disease patients treated and followed for 1 year, 32% developed a fibromyalgia-like syndrome characterized by chronic widespread pain, fatigue, mood disturbance and perceived cognitive dysfunction (Hassett et al., 2008b). This is not to say that there is any clear proof that infection with *B. burgdorferi* causes fibromyalgia or a fibromyalgia-like syndrome. Yet there is good evidence that such syndromes are common after infections with other organisms, including Q fever and other more common infections (Limonard et al., 2016) and could well be at play in fibromyalgia (Buskila et al., 2008).

15.12 Somatization Disorders (It's All in Your Head!)

So, what are the implications for a medical condition that has high rates of psychiatric comorbidity and an overlap with a chronic pain condition like fibromyalgia? Some might argue that PLDS and 'not Lyme', as well as fibromyalgia, should be considered somatization disorders. Escobar and colleagues (1998) defined somatization 'as the presentation of many symptoms suggestive of physical disease, but which remain unexplained after medical and laboratory assessments' (p. 466). Somatization is thought to be the unconscious expression of unacceptable emotions through bodily symptoms, while somatic symptom disorders are psychiatric disorders described in the Diagnostic and Statistical Manual for Mental Disorders Fifth Edition (DSM-5) (American Psychiatric Association, 2013).

Yet, somatization in the classic sense artificially separates bodily and psychological symptoms that patients experience as a whole (Epstein et al., 1999) and entirely connected. Somatization may well have definable neurobiological relationships (Sternberg, 2000). There is overwhelming evidence supporting the hypothesis that humans experience emotions throughout their bodies (Pert, 1997). Neurotransmitters associated with thought and emotion are often the same as those associated with the immune system, stress response systems and pain transmission systems to name only a few (Chrousos and Gold, 1992; Pert, 1997; Sternberg, 2000; Steptoe et al., 2009; Karatsoreos and McEwen, 2011). Although reviewing the evidence for bi-directional relationships between psychological and physiological phenomena is beyond the scope of this chapter, consistent evidence across studies suggests that strong emotions, especially anxiety, hostility and depression, induce or aggravate somatic symptoms (Kellner, 1994). Thus, the concept of the 'psychopathogenesis' of medical illness has increasing relevance today in light of findings from the fields of psychoneuroimmunology and neuroendocrinology.

In some cases, psychological factors appear to play a particularly powerful role in the manifestation and mediation of medical illness. This seems particularly true of chronic pain syndromes like fibromyalgia and perhaps PLDS and 'not Lyme'. In each case, the etiology and pathophysiology of the illness remain unclear, but high rates of clinical overlap between the disorders, including mood and anxiety disorders, suggest a shared pathophysiological basis (Korszun et al., 1998). Wills and colleagues found that pre-existing comorbidities predicted ongoing symptoms and deteriorated quality of life in patients with Lyme disease (Wills et al., 2016); it is possible that coping with one or more pre-existing conditions represents a psychological burden that becomes overwhelming in light of the new infection or that patients seek to offload their explanatory modeling onto the possibility of persisting Lyme disease, which may offer advantages to the patient.

15.13 Centralized Pain Syndromes ('It's All in Your Head (Brain)!')

Over the past decade, research related to the neuroscience of pain has markedly contributed to the understanding of the pathophysiology of chronic pain conditions like fibromyalgia, irritable bowel syndrome (IBS), interstitial cystitis and temporomandibular joint disorder (TMD). This new understanding has had a great impact on how we conceptualize and treat these disorders.

What has become increasingly clear is that pain can be characterized by its underlying mechanisms (Clauw, 2009, 2014). There are at least three distinct mechanisms, that is, peripheral, neuropathic and central, that can in isolation or combination account for the experience of pain. Peripheral pain is primarily caused by inflammation or mechanical damage in the periphery and is observed in conditions like rheumatoid arthritis, osteoarthritis and cancer, as well as physical injury. The second type of pain is neuropathic, which is usually the result of damage or entrapment of peripheral nerves. Examples of neuropathic pain include post-herpetic neuralgia and diabetic neuropathy. Central or non-nociceptive pain is due to a disturbance in the central nervous system that affects the processing of pain and other stimuli. Central pain is observed in conditions like fibromyalgia, TMD and IBS, and there is evidence that it also is present in peripheral pain conditions like osteoarthritis (Clauw and Witter, 2009) and rheumatoid arthritis (Lee et al., 2009). Notably, as many as 25% of patients with autoimmune disease (e.g. systemic lupus erythematosus, rheumatoid arthritis, ankylosing spondylitis) also meet current criteria for the diagnosis of fibromyalgia (Clauw and Katz, 1995), a centralized pain disorder. Of the utmost importance, different pain mechanisms respond to different types of treatment, for example, peripheral pain responds well to non-steroidal anti-inflammatory drugs (NSAIDs), centralized pain responds best to tricyclic antidepressants and other neuromodulators. Neuropathic pain responds to both types of treatment. Psychological and behavioral factors are almost always important in pain, but they appear to play the most prominent role in central pain conditions.

Central nervous system augmentation of the processing of pain and other sensory stimuli has been reliably demonstrated in fibromyalgia, IBS, interstitial cystitis, chronic low back pain and TMD (Naliboff et al., 2001; Gracely et al., 2002; Giesecke et al., 2004a, 2004b), as has attenuated activity of the descending analgesic pathways (Leffler et al., 2002; Julien et al., 2005). These findings have resulted in the more accurate characterization of these conditions as centralized pain syndromes, a phenomenon described in this very patient population (Batheja et al., 2013). Augmented central processing has not explicitly been explored in PLDS, but the common presence of fibromyalgia suggests likely applicability to PLDS patients.

Findings from twin studies suggest that approximately half of the risk of developing chronic widespread pain is genetic, the other half environmental (Kato et al., 2006). Central pain syndromes can be 'triggered' in approximately 5–10% of individuals who experience peripheral pain syndromes (osteoarthritis, rheumatoid arthritis), infections (parvovirus, Epstein–Barr virus, bacterial gastroenteritis, Lyme disease), physical trauma (e.g. automobile accidents) and psychological trauma/distress (Clauw, 2009). Thus, psychological factors can be the result of living with chronic illness, trigger central pain syndromes, influence and predict medical and functional outcomes, contribute to patient suffering and disability, and complicate the clinical picture for healthcare professionals.

15.14 The Concept of 'Chronic Lyme Disease' – Driving and Maintaining Forces

It is one thing to understand the immunopathogenesis of an illness, its manifestations, how to diagnose it, its natural history, how to treat it and its expected response to therapy. It is quite another to understand an illness when it evolves into a movement, as is the case with 'chronic

Lyme disease'. In exploring the psychology of 'not Lyme', it is also important to understand the psychology of a movement that overtook and then supplanted the clinical entity: how anxiety, speculation and empiricism (as well as the self-interest of clinicians and associated groups) overcame logic, objective evidence and scientific study, respectively.

15.15 Pain and Fatigue and the Search for an Explanation – the Patient

Seeking to understand and remedy suffering is part of human nature. Information from our environment and social interactions is processed using filters determined by belief systems (among other influences) established in light of previous experiences. Causative models are shaped and molded by societal norms, then used to make sense of experiences including physical and emotional symptoms. Once an illness model has been established, one that adequately explains the origins of the symptoms, a plan of action is developed that will serve to diminish or eliminate pain, suffering and disability.

Symptoms of pain and fatigue are common complaints that can initiate accessing medical care and embarking upon diagnostic testing; however, 'diagnostic testing' is often not diagnostic. In the case of Lyme disease, the serological tests demonstrate only the presence of circulating antibodies that, *in vitro*, bind to *B. burgdorferi* antigens. A 'positive' result can then be incorrectly interpreted as proof of a diagnosis. Such a result may be the result of prior exposure to *B. burgdorferi* but is often the result of circulating antibodies made in the immune response to other antigens binding in the artificial setting of the test, that is, 'cross-reacting antibodies'. The error of interpreting a 'positive' test result as indicative of a diagnosis of Lyme disease is all too common in primary care, where, similarly, a marginally positive antinuclear antibody test is often incorrectly interpreted as proof of systemic lupus erythematosus. Clinical evaluation by a rheumatologist is usually sufficient to reverse the wrong diagnosis of lupus. The disabusing clinician is not seen as having an ulterior motive, and the patient and the physician making the initial misdiagnosis usually abandon the diagnosis (and the test), neither physician having any personal interest in a specific diagnosis, merely wanting to help the patient as efficiently as possible. There is very rarely a *desire* on the part of clinician or patient to have lupus. However, this is often not how the incorrect diagnosis is greeted in the case of 'chronic Lyme disease'. How then did we come to a circumstance where anger (occasionally quite venomous), is the response to an attempted disabuse of the 'chronic Lyme disease' diagnosis?

15.16 Ranging from Benevolent to Malevolent – the Physician's Role

The practice of medicine in the 21st century should be 'evidence-based', anything else being an abdication of the responsibility of the physician. Diagnostic and therapeutic decisions should be based on facts, derived from scientific study and logical thinking, not speculation and supposition (and perhaps *a priori* bias). Diagnostic criteria should be described and substantiated. Laboratory tests should be used properly, validated as accurate, interpreted correctly and their limitations acknowledged. Therapies should be given that are proven effective, using the correct medications in the correct circumstances at the correct dose and for the correct duration. Physicians who fail at these tasks are failing the responsibility their patients place in them. 'Lyme disease is a clinical diagnosis' is a mantra that has attracted many devotees. The phrase's original intent was to remind physicians that the diagnosis of Lyme disease was not to be made merely based on a blood test result, but should be based on objective clinical criteria. This phrase has been perverted to mean that if Lyme disease is in any way suggested by historical or clinical findings, even the most picayune or tenuous, even if the diagnosis is unlikely (e.g. purported infection acquired in a region where Lyme disease is not known to occur) the diagnosis is assured. Alternative (usually untested and therefore unproven) criteria are applied in the interpretation of validated laboratory tests. Unvalidated tests are used. Many such clinicians eschew laboratory tests entirely, alleging that all techniques are inaccurate and thereby worthless.

The duration, dose and drug of therapeutic choice, some quite novel and dangerous, are based on hearsay and misapplication of scientific facts gleaned from other diseases. 'Innovative' therapies are utilized. Lack of response does not engender reconsideration of the diagnosis, but simply calls forth a redoubling of dubious therapies.

In traditional practice, it is up to the responsible physician to help patients interpret the science and medical jargon so the patient can understand the disease, tests and therapies, and can then be a part of the decision-making process. In the current Lyme disease climate, some physicians are ill-prepared to take on this responsibility. Some are not well informed and willingly study the disease in order to be more responsible clinical care providers. However, others have willingly adopted practices outside the norm, some declaring themselves to be 'Lyme disease experts' or 'Lyme literate' physicians, often holding a view of Lyme disease that can best be called an 'alternative reality', supported by 'alternative facts'. The espoused non-scientifically based views of the organism, the disease and its treatment have formed the justification for a counterculture with new rules of practice.

If the physician views a patient with chronic complaints as having an infectious disease, rather than a centralized pain syndrome, the process of 'medicalization' begins. The former starts with the belief that the physician can cure the condition solely with medication, the latter requires the patient to be a much more active participant in the remedy; the two paths diverge rapidly. In 'chronic Lyme disease' antibiotics are ineffective, but nothing shakes the faith of practitioner and patient in the diagnosis of a chronic, seemingly resistant, infectious disease.

Some physicians are merely following a trend, with no personal interest in the factual vs. the counter-factual view of Lyme disease. Some clearly believe their novel, innovative and daring approaches are in the best interests of their patients. Such true believers are motivated by nothing more than service to their patients in what they interpret as being an uninformed, often hostile, environment. Some, perhaps starting as 'true believers', become aware of benefits other than the satisfaction derived from loyal service, for example, notoriety (a following that may electronically span the globe). These may be powerful motivators and serve to perpetuate practice in the alternative reality of 'chronic Lyme disease'.

15.17 Demands for the 'Cure' – the Activist

In some areas, 'chronic Lyme disease' has become a cultural movement, led by activists working toward the admirable goal of 'proper' care for their followers. Many of these leaders have had family members with supposedly missed diagnoses of Lyme disease, or have suffered because their Lyme disease was 'under-treated', so these leaders have devoted themselves to making sure no one else suffers from lack of knowledge and access to 'Lyme literate' physicians. Some of these leaders have adopted a non-scientific belief system, often with prominent belief in the reality of 'chronic Lyme disease' and the need for aggressive therapy, using unsubstantiated excesses in dose and duration, and alternative unproven approaches. In the past, patients with chronic symptoms but no objective findings of specific disease similarly have promoted 'popular' explanations such as 'chronic candidiasis', 'chronic Epstein–Barr virus infection', 'myalgic encephalitis', 'chronic brucellosis' and many others (Shorter, 1992), all honest attempts to understand and control suffering, but none supported by facts.

The degree of investment in the diagnosis of 'chronic Lyme disease', too often manifested by anger, resentment and suspicion, seems far greater than in any of these antecedent movements (perhaps because antibiotics are effective in true *B. burgdorferi* infection, whereas the others are not so easily treated). These emotional reactions have, on occasion, prevented civil discourse. *Ad hominem* attacks against the disabusing clinician and often academic/research leaders, including allegations of impropriety and self-interest, interfere with their ability to properly practice medicine. No such accusations of possible self-interest brought against 'Lyme literate' physicians are brooked. Such is the desperation that some patients feel any answer, even one that is illogical and leads to no improvement, is better than mystery, confusion and fear. Even a false answer promises a pathway out of one's own personal hell, offers a plan and some sort of action the patient can take. Removing this assurance of a brighter future, replacing it with a darker and less well-defined road, can be devastating. This, even taking into consideration that the purported infection has not responded to prior months, even years, of antibiotics, such is the desire to replace the fear of the unknown with chronic therapeutic failure.

Politicians have identified these activist groups as powerful lobbies, capable of delivering votes, for example, in return for support of legislation that compels insurance in New Jersey to pay for 56 days of intravenous antibiotics as a mandatory minimum duration of therapy, despite the fact that this duration of therapy has never been studied, is not known to be better than standard care or to be 'optimum'. In Connecticut, the attorney general heard the call of these lobbies and demanded the Infectious Diseases Society of America submit its evidence-based criteria to outside analysis – this was done and an impartial review board found the criteria and recommendations to be acceptable as written. We know of no other examples of legislative micro-managing (interfering with) the practice of medicine.

15.18 A Rational Approach to Treatment

When patients and physicians incorrectly attribute symptoms to an infectious disease, unnecessary antibiotic treatment is often given. Almost 68% of the patients in the 'Living with Lyme Disease Study', who had no evidence of Lyme disease, received antibiotic treatment. Nearly 30% received multiple antimicrobials for months or even years. Baker has observed that despite evidence to the contrary, some patients believe that 'chronic Lyme disease' results from ongoing infection with *B. burgdorferi* that requires more than a few months of antibiotic treatment, which is an unprecedented and scientifically unsupported approach for a non-life-threatening disease (Baker, 2008). Further, the judicious use of antibiotics is important from an ecological perspective, as their use affects not only the patient to whom they are prescribed, but future patients through the creation of new antibiotic-resistant strains of bacteria (Schiff *et al.*, 2001; Moellering *et al.*, 2007).

There is evidence that a multidisciplinary approach combining evidence-based pharmacological and non-pharmacological interventions (e.g. including gentle regular exercise and cognitive–behavioral therapies (CBT)) might best address the symptoms and underlying causes of our patients' suffering and debility (Baker, 2012). Thus, medical or drug interventions should focus on symptomatic relief in a manner similar to that recommended for fibromyalgia and other central sensitivity syndromes (Hassett and Gevirtz, 2009; Williams and Clauw, 2009). For a good review of basic pharmacological treatment strategy see the review by Arnold and Clauw (2010). Further, addressing these same symptoms with adjunctive therapies like CBT plus exercise can serve to boost symptomatic and functional improvement. In using this approach, it is critical to avoid suggesting that the symptoms are psychiatric, because they are not. The treatment approaches for many chronic medical conditions (e.g. diabetes, hypertension, cardiovascular disease) rely on a similar integrative approach combining medication with education, exercise, regaining function and managing stress.

Using the principles of comprehensive non-pharmacological pain management represented by the acronym ExPRESS can be quite helpful in organizing the approach to treatment (Hassett and Gevirtz, 2009).

Ex is for Exercise, which refers to the need for regular, low impact exercise.
P is for Psychiatric comorbidity because both depression and anxiety disorders are common in all central sensitivity syndromes and contribute significantly to symptoms and disability.
R stands for Regaining function, which should emphasize the importance of obtainable goals and activity pacing. Too often chronic pain patients do too much on days that they feel good and too little on days that they feel bad.
E is for Education, which reminds the healthcare practitioner that they and patients need to be working from the same illness model. If the patient conceptualizes the symptoms as due to active infection, while the physician views them as due to some other process, treatment adherence will be strongly affected.
S (number one) is for Sleep, which is frequently disturbed and often easily addressed through medication and improving sleep hygiene as

many have developed counter-productive habits that exacerbate sleep disturbance.

Finally, the second S is for Stress and the need for stress management, which can include interventions already employed for addressing other ExPRESS factors, i.e. CBT, relaxation techniques, hydrotherapy and gentle exercise to name just a few.

However, this approach will likely be greeted with resistance by those with high levels of disease conviction. After all, according to their medical model of the illness, a persistent infection underlies the symptoms; thus, a referral to CBT will seem to come out of left field and serve as evidence that the prescribing clinician thinks this is a psychiatric disturbance. Yet, there may be a middle ground – agreeing that the symptoms are real and likely the product of central nervous system dysregulation could begin to pave the way to a détente.

15.19 In Good Faith

Although providing care for these patients can be a frustrating experience for healthcare professionals, it is imperative that these patients, suffering with symptoms and attendant compromised quality of life, not be dismissed. The illness is not 'all in their heads' (the usual meaning of this term being 'psychiatric' as opposed to 'central sensitivity syndrome') but belief in an infectious etiology oftentimes has been implanted in their heads by practitioners of 'chronic Lyme disease' medicine. Equally important is that these patients not be 'medicalized' into believing that only antibiotics hold the promise of symptomatic improvement. It is clear that this experience has adversely affected these patients (Johnson *et al.*, 2014) and there is nothing in the proposed approach that denies this. Patients with unexplained symptoms are in distress (Csallner *et al.*, 2013) and may feel cast adrift by our efforts to make a correct (non-Lyme disease) diagnosis. Lessons we have learned from our experiences with patients with fibromyalgia are applicable to patients with 'chronic Lyme disease'. We must address their pain, fatigue, anxiety and cognitive symptoms, as well as, when present, the psychological and behavioral processes that contribute to their suffering, with compassion and sensitivity to their anxieties, fears and needs. It is wise to remember that these patients are in emotional distress while we attempt to get to the bottom of their ailment and develop a course of (usually prolonged) therapy (Rebman *et al.*, 2015). Education and reassurance have helped some patients abandon their prior belief that they have a chronic incurable infectious disease and allowed them to move forward confidently with the rest of their lives. Patients who believe that chronic Lyme disease explains their current complaints need our respect and support; they should be offered a thorough and complete diagnostic work-up and an honest discussion of how diagnostic decisions are being made (Ljøstad and Mygland, 2013). With further study, we may finally understand all the factors that predispose to this syndrome (neurobiological, genetic, immunological, endocrinological and psychological). We believe these insights will be valuable in understanding and treating this and other forms of central sensitivity syndromes, as well. In the meantime, despite a somewhat hostile environment, we must allow scientific proof and logic to dictate our approach, not speculation, hearsay and baseless beliefs.

References

American Psychiatric Association (2013) *Diagnostic and Statistical Manual of Mental Disorders: DSM-5.* American Psychiatric Association, Washington, DC.

Arnold, L.M. and Clauw, D.J. (2010) Fibromyalgia syndrome: practical strategies for improving diagnosis and patient outcomes. *American Journal of Medicine* 123, S2.

Arvikar, S.L., Crowley, J.T., Sulka, K.B. and Steere, A.C. (2017) Autoimmune arthritides, rheumatoid arthritis, psoriatic arthritis, or peripheral spondyloarthritis following Lyme disease. *Arthritis and Rheumatology* 69(1), 194–202.

Asch, E.S., Bujak, D.I., Weiss, M., Peterson, M.G. and Weinstein, A. (1994) Lyme disease: an infectious and postinfectious syndrome. *Journal of Rheumatology* 21, 454–461.

Auwaerter, P.G. and Melia, M.T. (2012) Bullying *Borrelia*: when the culture of science is under attack. *Transactions of the American Clinical and Climatological Association* 123, 79–89.
Baker, P.J. (2008) Perspectives on 'chronic Lyme disease'. *American Journal of Medicine* 121, 562–564.
Baker, P.J. (2012) The pain of 'chronic Lyme disease': moving the discourse in a different direction. *FASEB Journal* 26(1), 11–12.
Barr, W.B., Rastogi, R., Ravdin, L. and Hilton, E. (1999) Relations among indexes of memory disturbance and depression in patients with Lyme borreliosis. *Applied Neuropsychology* 6, 12–18.
Batheja, S., Nields, J.A., Landa, A. and, Fallon, B.A. (2013) Post-treatment Lyme syndrome and central sensitization. *Journal of Neuropsychiatry and Clinical Neuroscience* 25(3), 176–186.
Beaman, M.H. (2016) Lyme disease: why the controversy? *Internal Medicine Journal* 46(12), 1370–1375.
Berende, A., ter Hofstede, H.J., Vos, F.J., van Middendorp, H., Vogelaar, M.L., Tromp, M., van den Hoogen, F.H., Donders, A.R., Evers, A.W. and Kullberg, B.J. (2016) Randomized trial of longer-term therapy for symptoms attributed to Lyme disease. *New England Journal of Medicine* 374, 1209–1220.
Bockenstedt, L.K., Gonzalez, D.G., Haberman, A.M. and Belperron, A.A. (2012) Spirochete antigens persist near cartilage after murine Lyme borreliosis therapy. *Journal of Clinical Investigation* 122(7), 2652–2660.
Bonanno, G.A. (2004) Loss, trauma, and human resilience: have we underestimated the human capacity to thrive after extremely aversive events? *American Psychologist* 59, 20–28.
Borgermans, L., Goderis, G., Vandevoorde, J. and Devroey, D. (2014) Relevance of chronic Lyme disease to family medicine as a complex multidimensional chronic disease construct: a systematic review. *International Journal of Family Medicine* 2014, 138016.
Bransfield, R.C. (2017) Suicide and Lyme and associated diseases. *Neuropsychiatric Disease and Treatment* 13, 1575–1587.
Bujak, D.I., Weinstein, A. and Dornbush, R.L. (1996) Clinical and neurocognitive features of the post Lyme syndrome. *Journal of Rheumatology* 23, 1392–1397.
Bujak, D.I., Kulsomboon, V. and Handwerger, B.S. (2000) Early Lyme disease patients with elevated Fibromyalgia Impact Questionnaire Scores are at greater risk of developing post Lyme disease syndrome. *Arthritis Care and Research* 13, S17.
Buskila, D., Atzeni, F. and Sarzi-Puttini, P. (2008) Etiology of fibromyalgia: the possible role of infection and vaccination. *Autoimmunity Reviews* 8, 41–43.
Chida, Y. and Steptoe, A. (2009) The association of anger and hostility with future coronary heart disease: a meta-analytic review of prospective evidence. *Journal of the American College of Cardiology* 53, 936–946.
Chrousos, G.P. and Gold, P.W. (1992) The concepts of stress and stress system disorders. Overview of physical and behavioral homeostasis. *Journal of the American Medical Association* 267, 1244–1252.
Clauw, D.J. (2009) Fibromyalgia: an overview. *American Journal of Medicine* 122, S3–S13.
Clauw, D.J. (2014) Fibromyalgia: a clinical review. *Journal of the American Medical Association* 311, 1547–1555.
Clauw, D.J. and Katz, P. (1995) The overlap between fibromyalgia and inflammatory rheumatic disease: when and why does it occur? *Journal of Clinical Rheumatology* 1, 335–342.
Clauw, D.J. and Witter, J. (2009) Pain and rheumatology: thinking outside the joint. *Arthritis and Rheumatism* 60, 321–324.
Cohen, S. (2005) Keynote presentation at the eighth international congress of behavioral medicine: the Pittsburgh common cold studies: psychosocial predictors of susceptibility to respiratory infectious illness. *International Journal of Behavioral Medicine* 12, 123–131.
Cohen, S., Doyle, W.J., Turner, R.B., Alper, C.M. and Skoner, D.P. (2003) Emotional style and susceptibility to the common cold. *Psychosomatic Medicine* 65, 652–657.
Csallner, G., Hofmann, H. and Hausteiner-Wiehle, C. (2013) Patients with 'organically unexplained symptoms' presenting to a borreliosis clinic: clinical and psychobehavioral characteristics and quality of life. *Psychosomatics* 54(4), 359–566.
Dattwyler, R.J., Luft, B.J., Kunkel, M.J. *et al*. (1997) Ceftriaxone compared with doxycycline for the treatment of acute disseminated Lyme disease. *New England Journal of Medicine* 337, 289–294.
DeLong, A.K., Blossom, B., Maloney, E.L. and Phillips, S.E. (2012) Antibiotic retreatment of Lyme disease in patients with persistent symptoms: A biostatistical review of randomized, placebo-controlled, clinical trials. *Contemporary Clinical Trials* 33(6), 1132–1142. DOI:10.1016/j.cct.2012.08.009
Dinerman, H. and Steere, A.C. (1992) Lyme disease associated with fibromyalgia. *Annals of Internal Medicine* 117, 281–285.
Dockray, S. and Steptoe, A. (2010) Positive affect and psychobiological processes. *Neuroscience and Biobehavioral Reviews* 35, 69–75.

Donta, S.T., Noto, R.B. and Vento, J.A. (2012) SPECT brain imaging in chronic Lyme disease. *Clinical Nuclear Medicine* 37(9), e219–e222. DOI: 10.1097/RLU.0b013e318262ad9b.

Elkins, L.E., Pollina, D.A., Scheffer, S.R. and Krupp, L.B. (1999) Psychological states and neuropsychological performances in chronic Lyme disease. *Applied Neuropsychology* 6, 19–26.

Epstein, R.M., Quill, T.E. and McWhinney, I.R. (1999) Somatization reconsidered: incorporating the patient's experience of illness. *Archives of Internal Medicine* 159, 215–222.

Escobar, J.I., Waitzkin, H., Silver, R.C., Gara, M. and Holman, A. (1998) Abridged somatization: a study in primary care. *Psychosomatic Medicine* 60, 466–472.

Ettestad, P.J., Campbell, G.L., Welbel, S.F., Genese, C.A., Spitalny, K.C., Marchetti, C.M. and Dennis, D.T. (1995) Biliary complications in the treatment of unsubstantiated Lyme disease. *Journal of Infectious Diseases* 171, 356–361.

Fallon, B.A., Nields, J.A., Parsons, B., Liebowitz, M.R. and Klein, D.F. (1993) Psychiatric manifestations of Lyme borreliosis. *Journal of Clinical Psychiatry* 54, 263–268.

Fallon, B.A., Petkova, E., Keilp, J.G. and Britton, C.B. (2012) A reappraisal of the U.S. Clinical trials of post-treatment Lyme disease syndrome. *Open Neurology Journal* 6, 79–87.

Feder Jr, H.M., Johnson, B.J., O' Connell, S. *et al.* (2007) A critical appraisal of 'chronic Lyme disease'. *New England Journal of Medicine* 357, 1422–1430.

Fredrickson, B.L. (2001) The role of positive emotions in positive psychology. The broaden-and-build theory of positive emotions. *American Psychologist* 56, 218–226.

Fredrickson, B.L. and Losada, M.F. (2005) Positive affect and the complex dynamics of human flourishing. *American Psychologist* 60, 678–686.

Giesecke, T., Williams, D.A., Harris, R.E., Cupps, T.R., Tian, X., Tian, T.X., Gracely, R.H. and Clauw, D.J. (2003) Subgrouping of fibromyalgia patients on the basis of pressure-pain thresholds and psychological factors. *Arthritis and Rheumatism* 48, 2916–2922.

Giesecke, J., Reed, B.D., Haefner, H.K., Giesecke, T., Clauw, D.J. and Gracely, R.H. (2004a) Quantitative sensory testing in vulvodynia patients and increased peripheral pressure pain sensitivity. *Obstetrics and Gynecology* 104, 126–133.

Giesecke, T., Gracely, R.H., Grant, M.A., Nachemson, A., Petzke, F., Williams, D.A. and Clauw, D.J. (2004b) Evidence of augmented central pain processing in idiopathic chronic low back pain. *Arthritis and Rheumatism* 50, 613–623.

Gracely, R.H., Petzke, F., Wolf, J.M. and Clauw, D.J. (2002) Functional magnetic resonance imaging evidence of augmented pain processing in fibromyalgia. *Arthritis and Rheumatism* 46, 1333–1343.

Guadino, E.A., Coyle, P.K. and Krupp, L.B. (1997) Post-Lyme and chronic fatigue syndrome: neuropsychiatric similarities and differences. *Archives of Neurology* 54, 1372–1376.

Guthrie, P.C. and Mobley, B.D. (1994) A comparison of the differential diagnostic efficiency of three personality disorder inventories. *Journal of Clinical Psychology* 50, 656–665.

Halperin, J.J. (2008) Prolonged Lyme disease treatment: enough is enough. *Neurology* 70, 986–987.

Halperin, J.J. (2014) Lyme disease: neurology, neurobiology, and behavior. *Clinical Infectious Diseases* 58(9), 1267–1272. DOI: 10.1093/cid/ciu106.

Halperin, J.J. (2015) Nervous system Lyme disease. *Clinics in Laboratory Medicine* 35(4), 779–795. DOI: 10.1016/j.cll.2015.07.002.

Hassett, A.L. and Finan, P.H. (2016) The role of resilience in the clinical management of chronic pain. *Current Pain and Headache Reports* 20, 39.

Hassett, A.L. and Gevirtz, R.N. (2009) Nonpharmacologic treatment for fibromyalgia: patient education, cognitive-behavioral therapy, relaxation techniques, and complementary and alternative medicine. *Rheumatic Diseases Clinics of North America* 35, 393–407.

Hassett, A.L., Radvanski, D.C., Buyske, S., Savage, S.V., Gara, M., Escobar, J.I. and Sigal, L.H. (2008a) Role of psychiatric comorbidity in chronic Lyme disease. *Arthritis and Rheumatism* 59, 1742–1749.

Hassett, A.L., Shlimbaum, T., Radvanski, D.C., Herman, D.J., Nahass, R., Buyske, S. and Sigal, L.H. (2008b) Preliminary results from a prospective study assessing psychological factors associated with post-lyme disease syndrome. *Arthritis Rheumatology* 58(9 Suppl), S861.

Hassett, A.L., Radvanski, D.C., Buyske, S., Savage, S.V. and Sigal, L.H. (2009) Psychiatric comorbidity and other psychological factors in patients with 'chronic Lyme disease'. *American Journal of Medicine* 122, 843–850.

Hassett, A.L., Goesling, J., Mathur, S.N., Moser, S.E., Brummett, C.M. and Sibille, K.T. (2016) Affect and Low Back Pain. *The Clinical Journal of Pain* 32(10), 907–914. DOI:10.1097/ajp.0000000000000350

Hausmann, L.R., Parks, A., Youk, A.O. and Kwoh, C.K. (2014) Reduction of bodily pain in response to an online positive activities intervention. *Journal of Pain* 15, 560–567.

Hirsch, J., Rosner, I., Rimar, D., Kaly, L., Rozenbaum, M., Boulman, N. and Slobodin, G. (2016) Tocilizumab efficacy in a patient with positive anti-CCP chronic Lyme arthritis. *North American Journal of Medical Sciences* 8(4), 194–196. DOI: 10.4103/1947-2714.179960.

Hsu, V.M., Patella, S.J. and Sigal, L.H. (1993) 'Chronic Lyme disease' as the incorrect diagnosis in patients with fibromyalgia. *Arthritis and Rheumatism* 36, 1493–1500.

Jacek, E., Fallon, B.A., Chandra, A., Crow, M.K., Wormser, G.P. and Alaedini, A. (2012) Increased IFNα activity and differential antibody response in patients with a history of Lyme disease and persistent cognitive deficits. *Neuroimmunology* 255(1–2), 85–91. DOI: 10.1016/j.jneuroim.2012.10.011.

Janicki-Deverts, D., Cohen, S., Doyle, W.J., Turner, R.B. and Treanor, J.J. (2007) Infection-induced proinflammatory cytokines are associated with decreases in positive affect, but not increases in negative affect. *Brain, Behavior, and Immunity* 21, 301–307.

Johnson, L., Wilcox, S., Mankoff, J. and Stricker, R.B. (2014) Severity of chronic Lyme disease compared to other chronic conditions: a quality of life survey. *PeerJ* March 27(2), e322. DOI: 10.7717/peerj.322. eCollection 2014.

Julien, N., Goffaux, P., Arsenault, P. and Marchand, S. (2005) Widespread pain in fibromyalgia is related to a deficit of endogenous pain inhibition. *Pain* 114, 295–302.

Kaplan, R.F., Jones-Woodward, L., Workman, K., Steere, A.C., Logigian, E.L. and Meadows, M.E. (1999) Neuropsychological deficits in Lyme disease patients with and without other evidence of central nervous system pathology. *Applied Neuropsychology* 6, 3–11.

Karatsoreos, I.N. and McEwen, B.S. (2011) Psychobiological allostasis: resistance, resilience and vulnerability. *Trends in Cognitive Sciences* 15, 576–584.

Karoly, P. and Ruehlman, L.S. (2006) Psychological 'resilience' and its correlates in chronic pain: findings from a national community sample. *Pain* 123, 90–97.

Kato, K., Sullivan, P.F., Evengard, B. and Pedersen, N.L. (2006) Importance of genetic influences on chronic widespread pain. *Arthritis and Rheumatism* 54, 1682–1686.

Kellner, R. (1994) Psychosomatic syndromes, somatization and somatoform disorders. *Psychotherapy and Psychosomatics* 61, 4–24.

Kessler, R.C., Chiu, W.T., Demler, O., Merikangas, K.R. and Walters, E.E. (2005) Prevalence, severity, and comorbidity of 12-month DSM-IV disorders in the National Comorbidity Survey Replication. *Archives of General Psychiatry* 62, 617–627.

Klempner, M.S. (2002) Controlled trials of antibiotic treatment in patients with post-treatment chronic Lyme disease. *Vector Borne and Zoonotic Diseases* 2, 255–263.

Klempner, M.S., Hu, L.T., Evans, J., Schmid, C.H., Johnson, G.M., Trevino, R.P., Norton, D., Levy, L., Wall, D., McCall, J., Kosinski, M. and Weinstein, A. (2001a) Two controlled trials of antibiotic treatment in patients with persistent symptoms and a history of Lyme disease. *New England Journal of Medicine* 345, 85–92.

Klempner, M.S., Schmid, C.H., Hu, L., Steere, A.C., Johnson, G., McCloud, B., Noring, R. and Weinstein, A. (2001b) Intralaboratory reliability of serologic and urine testing for Lyme disease. *American Journal of Medicine* 110, 217–279.

Klempner, M.S., Baker, P.J., Shapiro, E.D., Marques, A., Dattwyler, R.J., Halperin, J.J. and Wormser, G.P. (2013) Treatment trials for post-Lyme disease symptoms revisited. *American Journal of Medicine* 126(8), 665–669.

Korszun, A., Papadopoulos, E., Demitrack, M., Engleberg, C. and Crofford, L. (1998) The relationship between temporomandibular disorders and stress-associated syndromes. *Oral Surgery, Oral Medicine, Oral Pathology, Oral Radiology, and Endodontics* 86, 416–420.

Lamberg, L. (2006) Personality disorder a possibility in 'problem' patients, specialists say. *Journal of the American Medical Association* 296, 1341–1342.

Lantos, P.M., Brinkerhoff, R.J., Wormser, G.P. and Clemen, R. (2012) Empiric antibiotic treatment of erythema migrans-like skin lesions as a function of geography: a clinical and cost effectiveness modeling study. *Vector Borne Zoonotic Diseases* 13(12), 877–883.

Lantos, P.M., Shapiro, E.D., Auwaerter, P.G., Baker, P.J., Halperin, J.J., McSweegan, E. and Wormser, G.P. (2015) Unorthodox alternative therapies marketed to treat Lyme disease. *Clinical Infectious Diseases* 60(12), 1776–1782. DOI: 10.1093/cid/civ186. Epub 2015 Apr 6.

Lee, Y.C., Chibnik, L.B., Lu, B., Wasan, A.D., Edwards, R.R., Fossel, A.H., Helfgott, S.M., Solomon, D.H., Clauw, D.J. and Karlson, E.W. (2009) The relationship between disease activity, sleep, psychiatric distress and pain sensitivity in rheumatoid arthritis: a cross-sectional study. *Arthritis Research and Therapy* 11, R160.

Leffler, A.S., Hansson, P. and Kosek, E. (2002) Somatosensory perception in a remote pain-free area and function of diffuse noxious inhibitory controls (DNIC) in patients suffering from long-term trapezius myalgia. *European Journal of Pain* 6, 149–159.

Lenzenweger, M.F., Lane, M.C., Loranger, A.W. and Kessler, R.C. (2007) DSM-IV personality disorders in the National Comorbidity Survey Replication. *Biological Psychiatry* 62, 553–564.

Limonard, G.J., Peters, J.B., Besselink, R., Groot, C.A., Dekhuijzen, P.N., Vercoulen, J.H. and Nabuurs-Franssen, M.H. (2016) Persistence of impaired health status of Q fever patients 4 years after the first Dutch outbreak. *Epidemiology and Infection* 144(6), 1142–1147.

Ljøstad, U. and Mygland, Å. (2013) Chronic Lyme; diagnostic and therapeutic challenges. *Acta Neurologica Scandinavica* Suppl. 196, 38–47.

Marques, A.R., Stock, F. and Gill, V. (2000) Evaluation of a new culture medium for Borrelia burgdorferi. *Journal of Clinical Microbiology* 38, 4239–4241.

Marsland, A.L., Cohen, S., Rabin, B.S. and Manuck, S.B. (2006) Trait positive affect and antibody response to hepatitis B vaccination. *Brain, Behavior, and Immunity* 20, 261–269.

Marzec, N.S., Nelson, C., Waldron, P.R., Blackburn, B.G., Hosain, S., Greenhow, T., Green, G.M., Lomen-Hoerth, C., Golden, M. and Mead, P.S. (2017) Serious bacterial infections acquired during treatment of patients given a diagnosis of chronic Lyme disease – United States. *Morbidity and Mortality Weekly Report (MMWR)* 66(23), 607–609.

McEwen, B.S. (2007) Physiology and neurobiology of stress and adaptation: central role of the brain. *Physiological Reviews* 87, 873–904.

Moellering Jr, R.C., Graybill, J.R., McGowan Jr, J.E. and Corey, L. (2007) Antimicrobial resistance prevention initiative – an update: proceedings of an expert panel on resistance. *American Journal of Medicine* 120, S4–S25; quiz S26–S28.

Müller, R., Gertz, K.J., Molton, I.R., Terrill, A.L., Bombardier, C.H., Ehde, D.M. and Jensen, M.P. (2015) Effects of a tailored positive psychology intervention on well-being and pain in individuals with chronic pain and a physical disability: a feasibility trial. *Clinical Journal of Pain* 32, 32–44.

Naliboff, B.D., Derbyshire, S.W., Munakata, J., Berman, S., Mandelkern, M., Chang, L. and Mayer, E.A. (2001) Cerebral activation in patients with irritable bowel syndrome and control subjects during rectosigmoid stimulation. *Psychosomatic Medicine* 63, 365–375.

Nelson, C., Elmendorf, S. and Mead, P. (2015) Neoplasms misdiagnosed as 'chronic Lyme disease'. *JAMA Internal Medicine* 175(1), 132–133.

Oliveira, C.R. and Shapiro, E.D. (2015) Update on persistent symptoms associated with Lyme disease. *Current Opinions in Pediatrics* 27(1), 100–104.

Patrick, D.M., Miller, R.R., Gardy, J.L., Parker, S.M., Morshed, M.G., Steiner, T.S., Singer, J., Shojania, K., Tang, P; Complex Chronic Disease Study Group (2015) Lyme disease diagnosed by alternative methods: a phenotype similar to that of chronic fatigue syndrome. *Clinical Infectious Diseases* 61(7), 1084–1091.

Pert, C.B. (1997) *Molecules of Emotion*. Scribner, New York.

Peters, M.L., Smeets, E., Feijge, M., Van Breukelen, G., Andersson, G., Buhrman, M. and Linton, S.J. (2017) Happy despite pain: a randomized controlled trial of an 8-week internet-delivered positive psychology intervention for enhancing well-being in patients with chronic pain. *Clinical Journal of Pain* 33, 962–975.

Pilowsky, I. and Spence, N.D. (1983) *Manual for the IBQ*, 2nd edn. University of Adelaide Press, Adelaide, Australia.

Rebman, W., Aucott, J.N., Weinstein, E.R., Bechtold, K.T., Smith, K.C. and Leonard, L. (2017) Living in limbo: contested narratives of patients with chronic symptoms following Lyme disease. *Qualitative Health Research* 27(4), 534–546.

Reich, J.W., Zautra, A.J. and Hall, J.S. (2010) *Handbook of Adult Resilience*. Guilford Press, New York.

Reid, M.C., Schoen, R.T., Evans, J., Rosenberg, J.C. and Horwitz, R.I. (1998) The consequences of overdiagnosis and overtreatment of Lyme disease: an observational study. *Annals of Internal Medicine* 128, 354–362.

Rutter, M. (1987) Psychosocial resilience and protective mechanisms. *American Journal of Orthopsychiatry* 57, 316–331.

Schiff, G.D., Wisniewski, M., Bult, J., Parada, J.P., Aggarwal, H. and Schwartz, D.N. (2001) Improving inpatient antibiotic prescribing: insights from participation in a national collaborative. *Joint Commission Journal on Quality Improvement* 27, 387–402.

Seltzer, E.G., Gerber, M.A., Cartter, M.L., Freudigman, K. and Shapiro, E.D. (2000) Long-term outcomes of persons with Lyme disease. *Journal of the American Medical Association* 283, 609–616.

Shadick, N.A., Phillips, C.B., Logigian, E.L. et al. (1994) The long-term clinical outcomes of Lyme disease. A population-based retrospective cohort study. *Annals of Internal Medicine* 121, 560–567.

Shadick, N.A., Phillips, C.B., Sangha, O. *et al.* (1999) Musculoskeletal and neurologic outcomes in patients with previously treated Lyme disease. *Annals of Internal Medicine* 131, 919–926.
Shorter, E. (1992) *From Paralysis to Fatigue: A History of Psychosomatic Illness in the Modern Era.* The Free Press, New York.
Sigal, L.H. (1990) Summary of the first 100 patients seen at a Lyme disease referral center. *American Journal of Medicine* 88, 577–581.
Sigal, L.H. (1994) Persisting complaints attributed to Lyme disease: possible mechanisms and implications for management. *American Journal of Medicine* 96(4), 365–374.
Sigal, L.H. (1995) Lyme disease: primum non nocere. *Journal of Infectious Diseases* 171, 423–424.
Sigal, L.H. (1996) The Lyme disease controversy. Social and financial costs of misdiagnosis and mismanagement. *Archives of Internal Medicine* 156, 1493–500.
Sigal, L.H. (1997) The immunology and potential mechanisms of immunopathogenesis of Lyme disease. *Annual Review of Immunology* 15, 63–92.
Sigal, L.H. (1999) Antibiotics for the treatment of rheumatologic syndromes. *Rheumatic Diseases Clinics of North America* 25, 861–881, viii.
Sigal, L.H. (2001) Lyme disease: a clinical update. *Hospital Practice (Minneapolis)* 36, 31–32, 35–37, 41–42, 47.
Sigal, L.H. and Hassett, A.L. (2005) Commentary: 'What's in a name? That which we call a rose by any other name would smell as sweet.' Shakespeare W. Romeo and Juliet, II, ii(47–48) *International Journal of Epidemiology* 34, 1345–1347.
Sigal, L.H. and Patella, S.J. (1992) Lyme arthritis as the incorrect diagnosis in pediatric and adolescent fibromyalgia. *Pediatrics* 90, 523–528.
Sin, N.L. (2016) The protective role of positive well-being in cardiovascular disease: review of current evidence, mechanisms, and clinical implications. *Current Cardiology Reports* 18, 106.
Smith, B.W., Dalen, J., Wiggins, K., Tooley, E., Christopher, P. and Bernard, J. (2008) The brief resilience scale: assessing the ability to bounce back. *International Journal of Behavioral Medicine* 15, 194–200.
Smith, R.P., Schoen, R.T., Rahn, D.W., Sikand, V.K., Nowakowski, J., Parenti, D.L., Holman, M.S., Persing, D.H. and Steere, A.C. (2002) Clinical characteristics and treatment outcome of early Lyme disease in patients with microbiologically confirmed erythema migrans. *Annals of Internal Medicine* 136, 421–428.
Solomon, S.P., Hilton, E., Weinschel, B.S., Pollack, S. and Grolnick, E. (1998) Psychological factors in the prediction of Lyme disease course. *Arthritis Care and Research* 11, 419–426.
Steere, A.C. (2001) Lyme disease. *New England Journal of Medicine* 345, 115–125.
Steere, A.C., Taylor, E., McHugh, G.L. and Logigian, E.L. (1993) The overdiagnosis of Lyme disease. *Journal of the American Medical Association* 269, 1812–1816.
Steptoe, A., Dockray, S. and Wardle, J. (2009) Positive affect and psychobiological processes relevant to health. *Journal of Personality* 77, 1747–1776.
Sternberg, E. (2000) *The Balance Within. The Science of Connecting Health and Emotions.* WH Freeman and Company, New York.
Sturgeon, J.A. and Zautra, A.J. (2010) Resilience: a new paradigm for adaptation to chronic pain. *Current Pain and Headache Reports* 14, 105–112.
Sturgeon, J.A. and Zautra, A.J. (2013) Psychological resilience, pain catastrophizing, and positive emotions: perspectives on comprehensive modeling of individual pain adaptation. *Current Pain and Headache Reports* 17, 317.
Williams, D.A. and Clauw, D.J. (2009) Understanding fibromyalgia: lessons from the broader pain research community. *Journal of Pain* 10, 777–791.
Wills, A.B., Spaulding, A.B., Adjemian, J., Prevots, D.R., Turk, S.P., Williams, C. and Marques, A. (2016) Long-term follow-up of patients with Lyme disease: longitudinal analysis of clinical and quality-of-life measures. *Clinical Infectious Diseases* 62(12), 1546–1551. Doi: 10.1093/cid/ciw189. Epub 2016 Mar 29.
Wormser, G.P., Ramanathan, R., Nowakowski, J., McKenna, D., Holmgren, D., Visintainer, P., Dornbush, R., Singh, B. and Nadelman, R.B. (2003) Duration of antibiotic therapy for early Lyme disease. A randomized, double-blind, placebo-controlled trial. *Annals of Internal Medicine* 138, 697–704.
Wormser, G.P., Dattwyler, R.J., Shapiro, E.D. *et al.* (2006) The clinical assessment, treatment, and prevention of lyme disease, human granulocytic anaplasmosis, and babesiosis: clinical practice guidelines by the Infectious Diseases Society of America. *Clinical Infectious Diseases* 43, 1089–1134.
Yrjanainen, H., Hytonen, J., Song, X.Y., Oksi, J., Hartiala, K. and Viljanen, M.K. (2007) Anti-tumor necrosis factor-alpha treatment activates *Borrelia burgdorferi* spirochetes 4 weeks after ceftriaxone treatment in C3H/He mice. *Journal of Infectious Diseases* 195, 1489–1496.
Zautra, A.J. (2009) Resilience: one part recovery, two parts sustainability. *Journal of Personality* 77, 1935–1943.
Zautra, A.J., Johnson, L.M. and Davis, M.C. (2005) Positive affect as a source of resilience for women in chronic pain. *Journal of Consulting and Clinical Psychology* 73, 212–220.

16 Chronic Lyme Disease

Adriana Marques
Clinical Studies Unit, Laboratory of Clinical Immunology and Microbiology, National Institute of Allergy and Infectious Diseases, National Institutes of Health, Bethesda, Maryland, USA

The real purpose of the scientific method is to make sure that Nature hasn't misled you into thinking you know something you actually don't know.
Robert Pirsig, *Zen and the Art of Motorcycle Maintenance*

16.1 Introduction

Despite being widely used by both the lay and medical communities, chronic Lyme disease (CLD) is a very complicated term (Marques, 2008), used as a label for quite different patient groups. These include patients with late Lyme disease (e.g. arthritis and late neuroborreliosis, addressed in detail in other chapters), as well as patients described as having post-treatment Lyme disease syndrome (PTLDS), and, especially, patients with non-specific complaints of unclear etiology who received this diagnosis based on unproven and non-validated clinical and laboratory criteria. This is a serious problem, as shown by a national survey by the US Centers for Disease Control and Prevention (CDC). In the 2011 survey, participants were asked about CLD; 0.5% said they had CLD and 10.5% said they knew someone else with CLD (Hook *et al.*, 2015).

16.2 Chronic Lyme Disease

Patients diagnosed with CLD have been classified into four categories (Feder *et al.*, 2007; Marques, 2008) (Table 16.1). Patients in Category 1 have unexplained symptoms and lack valid laboratory evidence of *Borreliella* (formerly *Borrelia*) *burgdorferi* infection. Category 2 patients have other diseases and were incorrectly diagnosed with Lyme disease. Patients in Category 3 have symptoms of unknown cause, lack a history consistent with Lyme disease, but have serological evidence of infection with *B. burgdorferi*. Patients in Category 4 fulfill criteria for PTLDS. The majority of patients labeled as having CLD belong to Categories 1 and 2, as shown by how difficult it was to accrue PTLDS patients into the randomized clinical trials of antibiotic treatment, where eligibility varied between 1 and 10% (Marshall, 1999; Krupp *et al.*, 2003; Fallon *et al.*, 2007; Marques, 2008).

Multiple studies have addressed the topic of Lyme disease overdiagnosis. Reports from referral centers describe that Lyme disease was diagnosed in about a quarter to a third of the patients evaluated, while 50 to 60% of the patients had no evidence of the disease (Sigal, 1990; Steere *et al.*, 1993; Rose *et al.*, 1994; Feder and

Table 16.1. Categories of 'chronic Lyme disease'. (Adapted from Feder et al., 2007.)

Category 1	Symptoms of unknown cause, with no evidence of *Borreliella (Borrelia) burgdorferi* infection
Category 2	A well-defined illness unrelated to *B. burgdorferi* infection
Category 3	Symptoms of unknown cause, with antibodies against *B. burgdorferi* but no history of objective clinical findings that are consistent with Lyme disease
Category 4	Post-treatment Lyme disease syndrome

Hunt, 1995; Reid et al., 1998; Qureshi et al., 2002). In a more recent study of 235 patients who had symptoms for more than 12 weeks and were referred for evaluation of possible Lyme disease (Aucott et al., 2012), 128 (54%) had medically unexplained symptoms (MUS) and 15% had another diagnosis. Only 4% fulfilled formal criteria for PTLDS, 11% had post-treatment Lyme disease symptoms, 10% had confirmed late Lyme disease (the majority presenting with Lyme arthritis) and 6% were considered to have probable late Lyme disease.

Patients in Category 1 have non-specific symptoms and are diagnosed using alternative clinical criteria and non-validated laboratory tests and/or interpretation criteria that have been shown to have low specificity (Marques et al., 2009a; Fallon et al., 2014; CDC, 2015). Symptoms attributed to CLD include headaches, neck pain, sleep disturbances, problems with memory, poor concentration, fatigue, irritability and mood swings, depression, anxiety, tremors, low-grade increase of body temperature, night sweats, sore throat, arthralgias, joint stiffness, back pain, muscle pain, chest pain and palpitations, abdominal pain, nausea, constipation, testicular pain, pelvic pain, menstrual irregularities, blurred vision, floaters, photosensitivity, hyperacusis, tinnitus, lightheadedness, dizziness, decreased libido and weight gain. Moreover, 'chronic Lyme disease' has evolved into a 'polymicrobial infectious syndrome' with patients usually being diagnosed with multiple co-infections (*Babesia, Ehrlichia, Anaplasma, Rickettsia, Bartonella, Mycoplasma*), as well as 'metabolic and hormonal imbalances, immune dysfunction, heavy metal toxicity, allergies, damage by toxins, mitochondrial dysfunction and enzyme deficiencies'. Evidence is uncontrolled and based on the clinical experience of the practitioners. The diagnosis is based on 'clinical judgment, tests are not helpful, the disease is difficult to treat, requires prolonged treatment with multiple antibiotics and supplements, usually for months to years and may not be curable' (Alexander, 2009; Auwaerter et al., 2011; Cameron et al., 2014; Lantos and Wormser, 2014; Lantos et al., 2015). There is little formal research performed to evaluate this large, heterogeneous group of patients.

'Alternatively diagnosed chronic Lyme syndrome' (ADCLS) is another term suggested to describe patients in Category 1. A recent study compared patients with ADCLS and patients with myalgic encephalomyelitis/chronic fatigue syndrome (ME/CFS) showed no significant differences between the two groups (Patrick et al., 2015; Bouquet et al., 2017), and that the different label was most likely due to false positive results from alternative laboratory tests. Patients with unexplained persistent physical symptoms are not uncommon in healthcare settings. These patients may fit criteria of specific syndromes such as fibromyalgia (FM), irritable bowel syndrome (IBS) or ME/CFS. Because it has been shown that there is substantial overlap in symptoms between patients (Chalder and Willis, 2017), there has been discussion that these syndromes may not be distinct entities, but a product of medical specialization and differing diagnostic approaches (Wessely et al., 1999).

16.3 Post-Treatment Lyme Disease Syndrome (or Symptoms)

A definition of PTLDS was proposed in 2006 (Box 16.1) to provide a framework for future research. Patients included in this category have had a documented episode of Lyme disease, received treatment with an accepted antibiotic regimen, with improvement or stabilization of objective signs, but continue to have non-specific symptoms for at least a 6-month period, without another cause that could explain these symptoms. The proposed definition requires that the symptom onset be within 6 months of the Lyme disease diagnosis, and that the symptoms be severe enough to cause a substantial decrease in previous levels of activities (Wormser *et al.*, 2006). It must be remembered that this proposed definition is a starting point for future research. For example, one study has focused on a standardized approach to capture symptoms and functional impact, aiming to operationalize the definition of PTLDS (Aucott *et al.*, 2013).

The frequency of subjective symptoms varied between 0 and 23% of patients with early localized Lyme disease (erythema migrans) that were evaluated 6–24 months after completion of therapy (Smith *et al.*, 2002; Nowakowski *et al.*, 2003; Wormser *et al.*, 2003; 2006; Cerar *et al.*, 2010; Kowalski *et al.*, 2010, Tory *et al.*, 2010; Nizic *et al.*, 2012; Stupica *et al.*, 2012; Arnez and Ružić-Sabljić, 2015; Bechtold *et al.*, 2017) (Fig. 16.1). These symptoms were of mild to moderate intensity, and included fatigue, myalgias, arthralgias, headache, paresthesias, neck stiffness, irritability, sleep problems and difficulty with word finding, memory and concentration.

The mechanisms that might underlie PTLDS are not known and it is likely that different factors might play a role in an individual case (Box 16.2). In many patients, the presence of non-specific symptoms represents the natural evolution of improvement after therapy. There is a decrease over time in the numbers of patients reporting symptoms after antibiotic therapy. In one study of patients with erythema migrans, the percentage of symptomatic patients at

---

Box 16.1. Post-treatment Lyme disease syndrome proposed definition. (Adapted from Wormser *et al.*, 2006.)

- Documented Lyme disease.
- Treatment with accepted antibiotic regimen, there is resolution or stabilization of the objective manifestation(s) of Lyme disease.
- Onset of subjective symptoms within 6 months of the diagnosis of Lyme disease, and persistence of continuous or relapsing symptoms for at least a 6-month period after completion of antibiotic therapy:
  - fatigue;
  - widespread musculoskeletal pain;
  - complaints of cognitive difficulties; and
  - no other condition that could explain symptoms.
- Subjective symptoms are of such severity that, when present, they result in substantial reduction in previous levels of occupational, educational, social or personal activities.

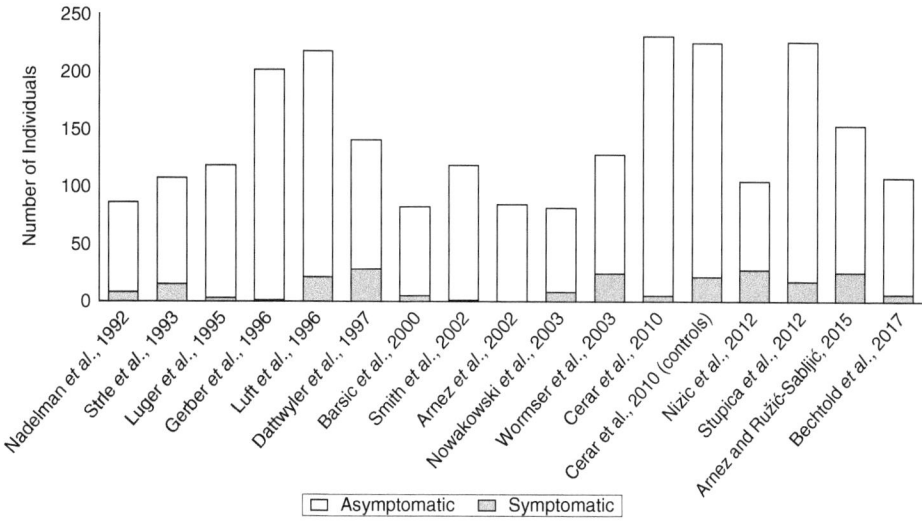

Fig. 16.1. Symptoms 6–24 months after antibiotic therapy in patients with erythema migrans.

Box 16.2. Post-treatment Lyme disease symptoms: possible mechanisms

- Part of the expected resolution of symptoms after treatment.
- Post-infective fatigue syndrome.
- Intercurrent conditions.
- Other tick-borne infections.
- Microbiome changes.
- Host immune response/autoimmune mechanisms.
- Persistence of remnants of spirochetes that cause inflammation.
- Persistent infection with *Borreliella burgdorferi*.

3 weeks, 3 months and 12 months were 34%, 24% and 17%, respectively (Wormser *et al.*, 2003). Patients with late manifestations may have a slower resolution of symptoms after therapy, and recovery can take months in some patients, and can be incomplete due to irreversible damage (e.g. residual weakness after facial nerve palsy) (Dattwyler *et al.*, 1988, 2005; Pfister *et al.*, 1991; Steere *et al.*, 1994; Kalish *et al.*, 2001; Berglund *et al.*, 2002; Kindstrand *et al.*, 2002; Borg *et al.*, 2005; Oksi *et al.*, 2007; Ljostad and Mygland, 2010).

Overall, most patients will have a good health outcome after treatment for Lyme disease. A prospective follow-up study of 101 patients with diverse manifestations of Lyme disease showed that quality of life scores increased to just above the US national average after 3 years of follow-up time, regardless of Lyme disease stage or severity at diagnosis. Patients with disseminated or more severe Lyme disease at diagnosis were not more likely to report long-term symptoms (Wills *et al.*, 2016). Similar results were found in a cross-sectional study where patients with erythema migrans were evaluated for a median of 16 years after initial diagnosis (Wormser *et al.*, 2015a). The only factors significantly associated with long-term symptoms or lower quality of life scores were other comorbid conditions unrelated to Lyme disease; comorbidities should be considered in the evaluation of these patients (Wills *et al.*, 2016).

In other patients, Lyme disease may have triggered a post-infective fatigue syndrome, as can occur with other infections. Fatigue after infections is not uncommon, and in some cases, it can be prolonged and disabling. In a cohort of 250 patients with acute Epstein–Barr virus infection, Q fever and Ross virus infection, fatigue was predicted by the severity of the acute illness, and the incidence after the different infections was similar (Hickie *et al.*, 2006). The case rate for post-infective fatigue syndrome at 6 weeks, 3 months and 12 months was 35%, 27% and 9%, respectively. In another study of 301 adolescents diagnosed with acute mononucleosis, 13% fulfilled criteria for chronic fatigue syndrome at 6 months, 7% at 12 months and 4% at 24 months (Katz *et al.*, 2009). These rates of fatigue are similar to those reported in patients after treatment for erythema migrans (Wormser *et al.*, 2003). But prolonged fatigue attributed to Lyme disease is not common: in a study of 100 patients with erythema migrans evaluated at 11–20 years after presentation, only 3% appeared to have persistent fatigue possibly due to Lyme disease, and the fatigue was not severe or functionally disabling (Wormser *et al.*, 2015b).

It is very important to appreciate that non-specific symptoms attributed to CLD are relatively common in the general population. Musculoskeletal pain is a common complaint, and chronic pain, fatigue and sleep disturbances are often reported together (Rohrbeck *et al.*, 2007). Insomnia is also a common problem, and can be associated with pain, anxiety and depression (Morphy *et al.*, 2007). Surveys have shown that between 5 and 15% of adults report chronic pain, and 8 to 30% report chronic fatigue (Picavet and Schouten, 2003; Aggarwal *et al.*, 2006). There are an estimated 1 million people in the United States who suffer from ME/CFS (Unger *et al.*, 2016). A study of patients with Lyme disease emphasizes the caveats of attributing non-specific symptoms to Lyme disease (Skogman *et al.*, 2008). In this prospective study, patients with erythema migrans were assigned to treatment with doxycycline or cefuroxime for 15 days. Each patient was asked to refer a spouse or family member (within 5 years of age) as a control. Patients and controls were followed for 1 year for the presence of fatigue, headache, myalgias, arthralgias, dizziness, paresthesias, nausea and irritability. At 6 months, there was no difference between patients and controls regarding the presence of new or increased symptoms, and at 12 months, controls were more likely to report new or increased symptoms than patients (Fig. 16.1). These results were repeated in a study of 117 patients with erythema migrans randomized to doxycycline for 10 days vs. 15 days. At 6 months, there was no difference in frequency, number and severity of 14 non-specific symptoms between patients and controls (Stupica et al., 2012). Similar results were found in a study of children with neuroborreliosis. At 6 months, headache and fatigue were less frequently reported among patients than controls, with no difference in the reporting of loss of appetite, neck pain, nausea and vertigo between the two groups (Skogman et al., 2008).

The majority of patients meeting criteria for PTLDS do not have evidence of co-infection with other tick-borne pathogens (Wang et al., 2000; Klempner et al., 2001a; Ramsey et al., 2002; Fallon et al., 2007; Lantos and Wormser, 2014). Although patients with concurrent *Babesia* (untreated) and *B. burgdorferi* infection were more likely to be symptomatic for 3 months or longer (Krause et al., 1996), patients with prior Lyme disease and exposure to *Babesia microti* had similar long-term outcome to patients with only Lyme disease (Wang et al., 2000).

Another possibility, not yet studied in PTLDS patients, is that changes in the microbiome may contribute to disease. The microbiome is a complex microbial ecosystem that has evolved with the human host, and is essential for the maintenance of homeostasis in health and disease (Thomas et al., 2017). Many diseases have been associated with changes in the microbiome, and it is possible that disruptions of the microbiome, maybe due to antibiotic use, could have a significant impact on a susceptible individual, with possible long-lasting effects.

There is evidence that immune dysregulation might play a role in PTLDS. The levels of antibodies against neural proteins was higher in patients with PTLDS than in Lyme disease patients who recovered or in healthy controls (Chandra et al., 2010), while the level of endothelial cell growth factor, an autoantigen target of T and B cell responses in patients with Lyme disease, was not elevated in one study (Tang et al., 2015), but higher in another (Strle et al., 2014). Sera from PTLDS patients showed greater interferon alpha activity (Jacek et al., 2013), and higher TH17-associated immune responses (Strle et al., 2014), and the levels of the chemokine CCL19 after treatment have been associated with later PTLDS (Aucott et al., 2016). There are also higher antibody reactivity frequencies against certain *B. burgdorferi* antigens in PTLDS patients (Chandra et al., 2011a; 2011b). It is possible that characteristics of the strain of *B. burgdorferi* could play a role in PTLDS, as it has been shown that *B. burgdorferi* strains may differ in their inflammatory potential and dissemination capabilities (Wang et al., 2002; Dykhuizen et al., 2008; Strle et al., 2011; Cerar et al., 2016).

In mouse studies, deposits of antigens persisted near the cartilage and within joint entheses, after antibiotic treatment. These deposits have inflammatory potential and can induce tumor necrosis factor production from macrophages (Barbour, 2012; Bockenstedt et al., 2012). It is possible that persistence of remnants of spirochetes could cause inflammation and play a role in PTLDS.

A major concern has been that PTLDS could be due to a persistent infection with *B. burgdorferi*. Some of the confusion dates back to the initial years following the description of Lyme disease and the discovery of *B. burgdorferi* as the cause of the illness. In these early years, non-specific symptoms were categorized as part of 'minor' late manifestations of Lyme disease, to distinguish from the 'major' manifestations, which included meningoencephalitis, carditis and arthritis (Steere et al., 1983; Weber et al., 1988; 1990; Dattwyler et al., 1990). In some instances, non-specific symptoms were classified with facial palsy and short-lived bouts of arthritis (Steere et al., 1983; Dattwyler et al., 1990). Objective manifestations of Lyme disease like facial palsy, meningoencephalitis, carditis and arthritis are clear evidence of treatment failure and require antibiotic therapy (Wormser et al., 2006). On the other hand, there was frequent spontaneous resolution of non-specific symptoms, and further antibiotic therapy did not accelerate this process (Nadelman et al., 1992; Asch et al., 1994). Also, patients with non-specific symptoms did not develop objective manifestations of late Lyme disease (Kalish et al., 2001; Nowakowski et al., 2003). Neurocognitive performance between patients and controls was similar (Shadick et al., 1999), and the frequency of non-specific symptoms was comparable between patients with Lyme disease and age-matched controls (Seltzer et al., 2000; Cerar et al., 2010).

There has been no objective evidence of *B. burgdorferi* infection in PTLDS patients, as evidenced by polymerase chain reaction (PCR) (Klempner et al., 2001a; Fallon et al., 2007) or culture, both in Barbour–Stoenner–Kelly (BSK) II medium (Klempner et al., 2001a; Fallon et al., 2007) and MPM media (Marques et al., 2000; Klempner et al., 2001a; Tilton et al., 2001). However, B. burgdorferi PCR and culture have low sensitivity in most body fluid samples from Lyme disease patients (Marques, 2015). Claims of a high number of positive cultures for B. burgdorferi in CLD and PTLDS patients using different methods have either not been validated (Marques et al., 2000), or are seriously confounded by concerns regarding false positive results due to laboratory contamination (Nelson et al., 2014). Other tests that have not been helpful to evaluate PTLDS patients include changes in C6 antibody levels (Fleming et al., 2004), antibodies in immune complexes (Marques et al., 2005), urinary antigen test results (Klempner et al., 2001b) and the number of CD57 positive cells (Marques et al., 2009a).

Studies in dogs, mice and non-human primates have shown that B. burgdorferi DNA can be detected in tissues for extended periods after antibiotic therapy (Straubinger et al., 1997; 2000; Bockenstedt et al., 2002; 2012; Yrjanainen et al., 2007; Hodzic et al., 2008; 2014; Barthold et al., 2010; Embers et al., 2012). A study suggested that these organisms may be attenuated, non-infectious spirochetes (Bockenstedt et al., 2002); they appear to be non-cultivable (Hodzic et al., 2008; Barthold et al., 2010). There are questions regarding the adequacy of the antibiotic regimens used in these studies (Wormser and Schwartz, 2009). In some studies, the organism could be detected by xenodiagnosis (the use of a natural vector to detect the presence of an organism) and could also be transmitted to immunodeficient mice by the ticks during their next blood meal (Hodzic et al., 2008; 2014). Though positive testing for B. burgdorferi DNA by PCR has been used for diagnosis of the infection (Schwartz et al., 1992; Nowakowski et al., 2001; Liveris et al., 2002; 2012), it must be noted that PCR has the potential to recognize DNA from dead or dying bacteria (Iyer et al., 2013).

A phase 1 study of the use of Ixodes scapularis larva for the xenodiagnosis of B. burgdorferi infection in humans (Marques et al., 2014) showed that the procedure was well tolerated. Although not a primary goal of the phase 1 study, there was one PTLDS participant who tested positive for the presence of B. burgdorferi in the xenodiagnostic ticks by DNA detection. A phase 2 trial is underway to assess whether a positive xenodiagnosis correlates with persistence of symptoms. While xenodiagnosis for Lyme disease is unlikely to be used in clinical practice, it offers researchers a new tool with which to study the mechanisms of disease and develop new biomarkers (Telford et al., 2014).

There have been five randomized, placebo-controlled, double-blind studies of antibiotic treatment in PTLDS and one of patients with symptoms attributed to Lyme disease (Table 16.2). These studies demonstrated that extended antibiotic therapy offers little benefit and can cause serious adverse events. Two studies were published together (Klempner et al., 2001a). These studies included 78 patients who were IgG seropositive for B. burgdorferi at enrollment, and 51 seronegative patients. All patients had well-documented Lyme disease. Pain, fatigue and cognitive changes were the most common complaints. Participants were randomized to receive 30 days of intravenous ceftriaxone, 2 g daily, followed by 60 days of oral doxycycline, 200 mg daily, or matching placebos (intravenous and oral). An improvement in the 36-item Short-Form General Health Survey (SF-36) score on study day 180 was the primary outcome. A planned interim analysis showed that a difference between treatment groups was unlikely to be achieved, and the studies were stopped early. Intention-to-treat analyses between patients in the antibiotic and placebo groups in both studies combined as well as separate had no significant differences in outcome. Approximately one-third of the patients improved, one-third was unchanged and one-third worsened at the end of the intravenous therapy, at the end of the oral treatment and at 3 months after completion of the treatment. There were two serious adverse events associated with treatment.

The third study enrolled 55 PTLDS patients with significant fatigue (Krupp et al., 2003). Twenty-eight patients were randomized to ceftriaxone 2 g and 24 patients to placebo intravenously daily for 28 days. Improvement in fatigue and mental speed at 6 months were the primary clinical endpoints. There was a small improvement of fatigue with ceftriaxone therapy on an intent-to-treat analysis. Results were similar for

Table 16.2. Placebo-controlled, double-blinded randomized treatment studies in post-treatment Lyme disease syndrome and symptoms attributed to Lyme disease.

Reference	Patients	Regimen and primary endpoints	Results	Serious adverse events
Klempner et al., 2001a	Seropositive (78 patients) and seronegative (51 patients) for antibodies to Borreliella burgdorferi at the time of enrollment	IV ceftriaxone (2 g/day) for 30 days, followed by oral doxycycline (200 mg/day) for 60 days (64 patients) or matching IV and oral placebos (65 patients). The primary outcome was improvement on SF-36 score at day 180 of the study	No significant difference was observed between patients who received antibiotic or placebo; approximately one-third of the patients improved, one-third worsened and one-third were unchanged at 30, 90 and 180 days	Two patients had serious adverse events associated with treatment that required hospitalization (IV catheter-related pulmonary embolism and a gastrointestinal bleed)
Krupp et al., 2003	55 patients with persistent severe fatigue post-Lyme disease	28 patients received IV ceftriaxone 2 g/day and 24 patients received IV placebo for 28 days. Primary clinical outcomes were improvement in fatigue score and cognitive function at 6 months	There was improvement on fatigue but no benefit in cognitive function with ceftriaxone treatment	Four patients had serious adverse events associated with treatment that required hospitalization
Fallon et al., 2007	37 seropositive patients with objective memory impairment and at least 3 weeks of previous IV antibiotic therapy	Ceftriaxone 2 g/day IV (23 patients) or IV placebo (14 patients) for 10 weeks. Follow-up was completed in 20 patients in the ceftriaxone group and 12 patients in the placebo group	Using a complex data-driven model for analysis, there was borderline improvement at 12 weeks in the ceftriaxone group. By 24 weeks, both groups had improved similarly from baseline	Nine patients discontinued therapy due to adverse events. One patient on ceftriaxone underwent cholecystectomy at week 16
Sjowall et al., 2012	15 patients with persistent symptoms ≥6 months post-treatment of Lyme neuroborreliosis	Randomized, double-blind, cross-over doxycycline 200 mg once a day vs. placebo for 3 weeks separated by a 6-week wash-out period	There were no differences between the doxycycline and placebo regarding changes in symptom severity, SF-36 scores or cytokine responses	None
Berende et al., 2016	280 patients with symptoms attributed to Lyme disease About 90% of the patients had received previous antibiotic treatment	All patients received open-label IV ceftriaxone 2 g/day for 14 days. Patients were then randomized to a 12-week oral course of doxycycline 100 mg and placebo twice daily, clarithromycin 500 mg and hydroxychloroquine 200 mg twice daily, or two placebos twice daily	There were no differences between the groups at any of the time points (14, 26, 40 and 52 weeks). All groups improved when compared with their baseline scores, but the lack of a IV placebo makes it difficult to assess the significance of these changes	Six patients had a serious adverse event possibly related to treatment 5 during ceftriaxone treatment. A total of 19 patients discontinued treatment due to an adverse event

IV, intravenous; SF-36, Medical Outcomes Study 36-Item Short-Form General Health Survey.

patients who received therapy and who completed follow-up. Mental speed or other neurocognitive measures were not improved. Side effects led to drug discontinuation in three patients in each group. Four patients had to be hospitalized.

The fourth study enrolled PTLDS patients who had objective memory impairment, had received a minimum of 3 weeks of intravenous antibiotic therapy and were seropositive by IgG Western blot (Fallon et al., 2007). This study enrolled only 37 patients. Patients were randomized 2:1 to receive intravenous ceftriaxone (23 patients) or intravenous placebo (14 patients). Duration of treatment was 10 weeks. A complicated model chosen by a data-driven selection process was used as the primary analysis, confusing the interpretation of the results (Marques et al., 2009b). Using this complex model, they reported a borderline improvement in the ceftriaxone group at 12 weeks. However, both groups equally improved from baseline when evaluated at 24 weeks. Side effects led to discontinuation of therapy in nine patients; these side effects were associated with treatment in seven patients.

A small randomized cross-over study evaluated the response of 15 Lyme neuroborreliosis patients with PTLDS who were randomized to receive 200 mg of doxycycline or a placebo for 3 weeks, with a 6-week wash-out period in between treatments (Sjowall et al., 2012). There were no differences in post-treatment symptoms, quality of life or cytokine responses between the groups.

A randomized study of 280 patients with symptoms attributed to Lyme disease was published in 2016 (Berende et al., 2016). The entry criteria for the study included a mixture of patients, including patients with potentially late Lyme disease, patients with PTLDS, and patients with non-specific symptoms and only a positive IgG or IgM immunoblot. Only 96 (34%) of the participants had objective evidence of prior Lyme disease. The median duration of symptoms was more than 2 years. About 90% of the patients had received previous antibiotic treatment. All patients were treated with open-label intravenous ceftriaxone 2 g daily for 14 days. Patients were then randomized to a 12-week oral course of doxycycline 100 mg and placebo twice daily, clarithromycin 500 mg twice daily combined with hydroxychloroquine 200 mg twice daily, or two placebos twice daily. There was no difference in health-related quality of life measurements between the groups at the end of the treatment period (week 14) or at 26, 40 and 52 weeks. All groups improved when compared with their baseline scores, but the lack of a complete placebo arm impedes assessing whether this improvement was an effect of the ceftriaxone therapy or a placebo effect. The improvement in fatigue scores was similar to improvements seen in the intravenous placebo arm in two other studies (Wormser, 2016). The inclusion of a heterogeneous group of patients, some of whom could have untreated late Lyme disease and others who may not have had Lyme disease, further confuses the analysis of the study. But one important point can be taken from these results, which is that prolonged antibiotic therapy offers no benefit (Melia and Auwaerter, 2016).

The randomized trials in PTLDS have been criticized as offering 'too little, too late' and for not 'addressing the range of treatment options in an actual practice' (Cameron, 2006; 2009; Donta, 2007; Stricker, 2007), based on personal opinion and retrospective, open-label case series and case reports that suggested a possible role of prolonged antibiotic therapy in patients diagnosed with CLD (Donta, 1997; 2003). Case series and case reports have the highest risk of bias in the hierarchy of evidence-based medicine (Schunemann et al., 2006). Case series studies have many limitations, the primary one being the lack of a control group. Without a comparison group, it is not possible to know if an outcome is related to an intervention, a placebo effect, time, chance or a biased interpretation of outcomes. Case series studies have a large risk of systematic errors (bias). The lack of blinding can affect outcomes, especially for subjective measures. Due to these limitations, no causal inferences about treatment effect can be made from the results of case series studies. Case series studies are best used to generate hypotheses that can be tested by stronger study designs.

There are serious risks associated with antibiotic therapy, particularly prolonged intravenous therapy. These include death, catheter-related blood stream infections, septic shock, septic thrombophlebitis, osteomyelitis, *Clostridium difficile* colitis, deep venous thrombosis, pulmonary embolism, gastrointestinal bleeding, severe allergic reactions, neutropenia and ceftriaxone-associated biliary complications including cholecystitis leading to cholecystectomy (Ettestad *et al.*, 1995; Reid *et al.*, 1998; Patel *et al.*, 2000; Corapi *et al.*, 2007; Holzbauer *et al.*, 2010; Marks *et al.*, 2016; Marzec *et al.*, 2017). There are also significant psychological, social and financial consequences of such approaches, as well as the risk of delaying the diagnosis of another condition (Nelson *et al.*, 2015).

16.4 Conclusion

At this point, evidence shows that antibiotic therapy, as tested in six randomized placebo-controlled studies, does not offer durable or significant benefit in treating patients with PTLDS and has considerable risk of treatment-related adverse events. In assessing this group of patients, it is important that other comorbid conditions be fully assessed and treated. There is a pressing need of investigations of other approaches that may help these patients. Because of significant placebo effects and the variation in symptom intensity over time seen in such patients, studies evaluating therapeutic options should have a blinded, randomized controlled design. Studies should also have clearly defined target patient populations. Additionally, research to evaluate patients diagnosed with CLD who do not fulfil criteria for PTLDS, focusing on definitional issues and heterogeneity among these individuals, is needed in order to better understand and manage the care of these patients.

Acknowledgments

This research was supported by the Intramural Research Program of the National Institutes of Health (NIH), National Institute of Allergy and Infectious Diseases (NIAID).

The content of this publication does not necessarily reflect the views or policies of the Department of Health and Human Services, nor does mention of trade names, commercial products or organizations imply endorsement by the US Government.

References

Aggarwal, V.R., McBeth, J., Zakrzewska, J.M., Lunt, M. and MacFarlane, G.J. (2006) The epidemiology of chronic syndromes that are frequently unexplained: do they have common associated factors? *International Journal of Epidemiology* 35, 468–476.

Alexander, W. (2009) Integrative healthcare symposium: cancer and chronic Lyme disease. *P T* 34, 202–214.

Arnez, M. and Ružić-Sabljić, E. (2015) Azithromycin is equally effective as amoxicillin in children with solitary erythema migrans. *Pediatric Infectious Disease Journal* 34, 1045–1048.

Arnez, M., Pleterski-Rigler, D., Luznik-Bufon, T., Ruzic-Sabljic, E. and Strle, F. (2002) Solitary erythema migrans in children: comparison of treatment with azithromycin and phenoxymethylpenicillin. *Wiener Klinische Wochenschrift* 114(13–14), 498–504.

Asch, E.S., Bujak, D.I., Weiss, M., Peterson, M.G. and Weinstein, A. (1994) Lyme disease: an infectious and postinfectious syndrome. *Journal of Rheumatology* 21, 454–461.

Aucott, J.N., Seifter, A. and Rebman, A.W. (2012) Probable late Lyme disease: a variant manifestation of untreated *Borrelia burgdorferi* infection. *BMC Infectious Diseases* 12, 173.

Aucott, J.N., Crowder, L.A. and Kortte, K.B. (2013) Development of a foundation for a case definition of post-treatment Lyme disease syndrome. *International Journal of Infectious Diseases* 17, e443–e449.

Aucott, J.N., Soloski, M.J., Rebman, A.W., Crowder, L.A., Lahey, L.J., Wagner, C.A., Robinson, W.H. and Bechtold, K.T. (2016) CCL19 as a chemokine risk factor for posttreatment Lyme disease syndrome: a prospective clinical cohort study. *Clinical Vaccine Immunology* 23, 757–766.

Auwaerter, P.G., Bakken, J.S., Dattwyler, R.J., Dumler, J.S., Halperin, J.J., McSweegan, E., Nadelman, R.B., O'Connell, S., Sood, S.K., Weinstein, A. and Wormser, G.P. (2011) Scientific evidence and best patient care practices should guide the ethics of Lyme disease activism. *Journal of Medical Ethics* 37, 68–73.

Barbour, A. (2012) Remains of infection. *Journal of Clinical Investigation* 122, 2344–2346.

Barsic, B., Maretic, T., Majerus, L. and Strugar, J. (2000) Comparison of Azithromycin and Doxycycline in the Treatment of Erythema migrans. *Infection* 28(3), 153–156.

Barthold, S.W., Hodzic, E., Imai, D.M., Feng, S., Yang, X. and Luft, B.J. (2010) Ineffectiveness of tigecycline against persistent *Borrelia burgdorferi*. *Antimicrobial Agents Chemotherapy* 54, 643–651.

Bechtold, K.T., Rebman, A.W., Crowder, L.A., Johnson-Greene, D. and Aucott, J.N. (2017) Standardized symptom measurement of individuals with early Lyme disease over time. *Archives of Clinical Neuropsychology* 32, 129–141.

Berende, A., Ter Hofstede, H.J., Vos, F.J., Van Middendorp, H., Vogelaar, M.L., Tromp, M., Van Den Hoogen, F.H., Donders, A.R., Evers, A.W. and Kullberg, B.J. (2016) Randomized trial of longer-term therapy for symptoms attributed to Lyme disease. *New England Journal of Medicine* 374, 1209–1220.

Berglund, J., Stjernberg, L., Ornstein, K., Tykesson-Joelsson, K. and Walter, H. (2002) 5-y follow-up study of patients with neuroborreliosis. *Scandinavian Journal of Infectious Diseases* 34, 421–425.

Bockenstedt, L.K., Mao, J., Hodzic, E., Barthold, S.W. and Fish, D. (2002) Detection of attenuated, noninfectious spirochetes in *Borrelia burgdorferi*-infected mice after antibiotic treatment. *Journal of Infectious Diseases* 186, 1430–1437.

Bockenstedt, L.K., Gonzalez, D.G., Haberman, A.M. and Belperron, A.A. (2012) Spirochete antigens persist near cartilage after murine Lyme borreliosis therapy. *Journal of Clinical Investigation* 122, 2652–2660.

Borg, R., Dotevall, L., Hagberg, L., Maraspin, V., Lotric-Furlan, S., Cimperman, J. and Strle, F. (2005) Intravenous ceftriaxone compared with oral doxycycline for the treatment of Lyme neuroborreliosis. *Scandinavian Journal of Infectious Diseases* 37, 449–454.

Bouquet, J., Gardy, J.L., Brown, S. *et al.* (2017) RNA-seq analysis of gene expression, viral pathogen, and B-cell/t-cell receptor signatures in complex chronic disease. *Clinical Infectious Diseases* 64, 476–481.

Cameron, D.J. (2006) Generalizability in two clinical trials of Lyme disease. *Epidemiologic Perspectives Innovations* 3, 12.

Cameron, D.J. (2009) Insufficient evidence to deny antibiotic treatment to chronic Lyme disease patients. *Medical Hypotheses* 72, 688–691.

Cameron, D.J., Johnson, L.B. and Maloney, E.L. (2014) Evidence assessments and guideline recommendations in Lyme disease: the clinical management of known tick bites, erythema migrans rashes and persistent disease. *Expert Review of Anti Infective Therapy* 12, 1103–1135.

CDC (2015) *Laboratory tests that are not recommended* [Online]. Available at: https://www.cdc.gov/lyme/diagnosistesting/labtest/otherlab/index.html (accessed 27 July 2017).

Cerar, D., Cerar, T., Ružić-Sabljić, E., Wormser, G.P. and Strle, F. (2010) Subjective symptoms after treatment of early Lyme disease. *American Journal of Medicine* 123, 79–86.

Cerar, T., Strle, F., Stupica, D., Ružić-Sabljić, E., McHugh, G., Steere, A.C. and Strle, K. (2016) Differences in genotype, clinical features, and inflammatory potential of *Borrelia burgdorferi* sensu stricto strains from Europe and the United States. *Emerging Infectious Diseases* 22, 818–827.

Chalder, T. and Willis, C. (2017) 'Lumping' and 'splitting' medically unexplained symptoms: is there a role for a transdiagnostic approach? *Journal of Mental Health* 26, 187–191.

Chandra, A., Wormser, G.P., Klempner, M.S., Trevino, R.P., Crow, M.K., Latov, N. and Alaedini, A. (2010) Anti-neural antibody reactivity in patients with a history of Lyme borreliosis and persistent symptoms. *Brain Behavior Immunity* 24, 1018–1024.

Chandra, A., Latov, N., Wormser, G.P., Marques, A.R. and Alaedini, A. (2011a) Epitope mapping of antibodies to VlsE protein of *Borrelia burgdorferi* in post-Lyme disease syndrome. *Clinical Immunology* 141, 103–110.

Chandra, A., Wormser, G.P., Marques, A.R., Latov, N. and Alaedini, A. (2011b) Anti-*Borrelia burgdorferi* antibody profile in post-Lyme disease syndrome. *Clinical and Vaccine Immunology* 18, 767–771.

Corapi, K.M., White, M.I., Phillips, C.B., Daltroy, L.H., Shadick, N.A. and Liang, M.H. (2007) Strategies for primary and secondary prevention of Lyme disease. *Nature Clinical Practice Rheumatology* 3, 20–25.

Dattwyler, R.J., Halperin, J.J., Volkman, D.J. and Luft, B.J. (1988) Treatment of late Lyme borreliosis – randomised comparison of ceftriaxone and penicillin. *Lancet* 1, 1191–1194.

Dattwyler, R.J., Volkman, D.J., Conaty, S.M., Platkin, S.P. and Luft, B.J. (1990) Amoxicillin plus probenecid versus doxycycline for treatment of erythema migrans borreliosis. *Lancet* 336, 1404–1406.

Dattwyler, R.J., Luft, B.J., Kunkel, M.J., Finkel, M.F., Wormser, G.P., Rush, T.J., Grunwaldt, E., Agger, W.A., Franklin, M., Oswald, D., Cockey, L. and Maladorno, D. (1997) Ceftriaxone compared with doxycycline for the treatment of acute disseminated Lyme disease. *New England Journal of Medicine* 337(5), 289–294.

Dattwyler, R.J., Wormser, G.P., Rush, T.J., Finkel, M.F., Schoen, R.T., Grunwaldt, E., Franklin, M., Hilton, E., Bryant, G.L., Agger, W.A. and Maladorno, D. (2005) A comparison of two treatment regimens of ceftriaxone in late Lyme disease. *Wiener klinische Wochenschrift* 117, 393–397.

Donta, S.T. (1997) Tetracycline therapy for chronic Lyme disease. *Clinical Infectious Diseases* 25 Suppl 1, S52–S56.

Donta, S.T. (2003) Macrolide therapy of chronic Lyme disease. *Medical Science Monitor* 9, PI136–PI142.

Donta, S.T. (2007) Lyme disease guidelines – it's time to move forward. *Clinical Infectious Diseases* 44, 1134–1135; author reply 1137–1139.

Dykhuizen, D.E., Brisson, D., Sandigursky, S., Wormser, G.P., Nowakowski, J., Nadelman, R.B. and Schwartz, I. (2008) The propensity of different *Borrelia burgdorferi* sensu stricto genotypes to cause disseminated infections in humans. *American Journal of Tropical Medicine Hygiene* 78, 806–810.

Embers, M.E., Barthold, S.W., Borda, J.T. *et al*. (2012) Persistence of *Borrelia burgdorferi* in rhesus macaques following antibiotic treatment of disseminated infection. *PLoS One* 7, e29914.

Ettestad, P.J., Campbell, G.L., Welbel, S.F., Genese, C.A., Spitalny, K.C., Marchetti, C.M. and Dennis, D.T. (1995) Biliary complications in the treatment of unsubstantiated Lyme disease. *Journal of Infectious Diseases* 171, 356–361.

Fallon, B.A., Keilp, J.G., Corbera, K.M., Petkova, E., Britton, C.B., Dwyer, E., Slavov, I., Cheng, J., Dobkin, J., Nelson, D.R. and Sackeim, H.A. (2007) A randomized, placebo-controlled trial of repeated IV antibiotic therapy for Lyme encephalopathy. *Neurology* 70, 992–1003.

Fallon, B.A., Pavlicova, M., Coffino, S.W. and Brenner, C. (2014) A comparison of Lyme disease serologic test results from 4 laboratories in patients with persistent symptoms after antibiotic treatment. *Clinical Infectious Diseases* 59, 1705–1710.

Feder Jr, H.M. and Hunt, M.S. (1995) Pitfalls in the diagnosis and treatment of Lyme disease in children. *Journal of the American Medical Association* 274, 66–68.

Feder Jr, H.M., Johnson, B.J., O'Connell, S. *et al*. (2007) A critical appraisal of 'chronic Lyme disease'. *New England Journal of Medicine* 357, 1422–1430.

Fleming, R.V., Marques, A.R., Klempner, M.S., Schmid, C.H., Dally, L.G., Martin, D.S. and Philipp, M.T. (2004) Pre-treatment and post-treatment assessment of the C(6) test in patients with persistent symptoms and a history of Lyme borreliosis. *European Journal of Clinical Microbiology Infectious Diseases* 23, 615–618.

Gerber, M.A., Shapiro, E.D., Burke, G.S., Parcells, V.J. and Bell, G.L. (1996) Lyme disease in children in southeastern Connecticut. Pediatric Lyme Disease Study Group. *New England Journal of Medicine* 335(17), 1270–1274.

Hickie, I., Davenport, T., Wakefield, D., Vollmer-Conna, U., Cameron, B., Vernon, S.D., Reeves, W.C., Lloyd, A. and Dubbo Infection Outcomes Study (2006) Post-infective and chronic fatigue syndromes precipitated by viral and non-viral pathogens: prospective cohort study. *British Medical Journal* 333, 575.

Hodzic, E., Feng, S., Holden, K., Freet, K.J. and Barthold, S.W. (2008) Persistence of *Borrelia burgdorferi* following antibiotic treatment in mice. *Antimicrobial Agents Chemotherapy* 52, 1728–1736.

Hodzic, E., Imai, D., Feng, S. and Barthold, S.W. (2014) Resurgence of persisting non-cultivable *Borrelia burgdorferi* following antibiotic treatment in mice. *PLoS One* 9, e86907.

Holzbauer, S.M., Kemperman, M.M. and Lynfield, R. (2010) Death due to community-associated *Clostridium difficile* in a woman receiving prolonged antibiotic therapy for suspected Lyme disease. *Clinical Infectious Diseases* 51, 369–370.

Hook, S.A., Nelson, C.A. and Mead, P.S. (2015) U.S. public's experience with ticks and tick-borne diseases: results from national healthstyles surveys. *Ticks and Tick Borne Diseases* 6, 483–488.

Iyer, R., Mukherjee, P., Wang, K., Simons, J., Wormser, G.P. and Schwartz, I. (2013) Detection of *Borrelia burgdorferi* nucleic acids after antibiotic treatment does not confirm viability. *Journal of Clinical Microbiology* 51, 857–862.

Jacek, E., Fallon, B.A., Chandra, A., Crow, M.K., Wormser, G.P. and Alaedini, A. (2013) Increased IFNalpha activity and differential antibody response in patients with a history of Lyme disease and persistent cognitive deficits. *Journal of Neuroimmunology* 255, 85–91.

Kalish, R.A., Kaplan, R.F., Taylor, E., Jones-Woodward, L., Workman, K. and Steere, A.C. (2001) Evaluation of study patients with Lyme disease, 10–20-year follow-up. *Journal of Infectious Diseases* 183, 453–460.

Katz, B.Z., Shiraishi, Y., Mears, C.J., Binns, H.J. and Taylor, R. (2009) Chronic fatigue syndrome after infectious mononucleosis in adolescents. *Pediatrics* 124, 189–193.

Kindstrand, E., Nilsson, B.Y., Hovmark, A., Pirskanen, R. and Asbrink, E. (2002) Peripheral neuropathy in acrodermatitis chronica atrophicans – effect of treatment. *Acta Neurologica Scandinavica* 106, 253–257.

Klempner, M.S., Hu, L.T., Evans, J., Schmid, C.H., Johnson, G.M., Trevino, R.P., Norton, D., Levy, L., Wall, D., McCall, J., Kosinski, M. and Weinstein, A. (2001a) Two controlled trials of antibiotic treatment in patients with persistent symptoms and a history of Lyme disease. *New England Journal of Medicine* 345, 85–92.

Klempner, M.S., Schmid, C.H., Hu, L., Steere, A.C., Johnson, G., McCloud, B., Noring, R. and Weinstein, A. (2001b) Intralaboratory reliability of serologic and urine testing for Lyme disease. *American Journal of Medicine* 110, 217–219.

Kowalski, T.J., Tata, S., Berth, W., Mathiason, M.A. and Agger, W.A (2010) Antibiotic treatment duration and long-term outcomes of patients with early Lyme disease from a Lyme disease-hyperendemic area. *Clinical Infectious Diseases* 50, 512–520.

Krause, P.J., Telford, S.R. III, Spielman, A., Sikand, V., Ryan, R., Christianson, D., Burke, G., Brassard, P., Pollack, R., Peck, J. and Persing, D.H. (1996) Concurrent Lyme disease and babesiosis. Evidence for increased severity and duration of illness. *Journal of the American Medical Association* 275, 1657–1660.

Krupp, L.B., Hyman, L.G., Grimson, R., Coyle, P.K., Melville, P., Ahnn, S., Dattwyler, R. and Chandler, B. (2003) Study and treatment of post Lyme disease (STOP-LD): a randomized double masked clinical trial. *Neurology* 60, 1923–1930.

Lantos, P.M. and Wormser, G.P. (2014) Chronic coinfections in patients diagnosed with chronic Lyme disease: a systematic review. *American Journal of Medicine* 127, 1105–1110.

Lantos, P.M., Shapiro, E.D., Auwaerter, P.G., Baker, P.J., Halperin, J.J., McSweegan, E. and Wormser, G.P. (2015) Unorthodox alternative therapies marketed to treat Lyme disease. *Clinical Infectious Diseases* 60, 1776–1782.

Liveris, D., Wang, G., Girao, G., Byrne, D.W., Nowakowski, J., McKenna, D., Nadelman, R., Wormser, G.P. and Schwartz, I. (2002) Quantitative detection of *Borrelia burgdorferi* in 2-millimeter skin samples of erythema migrans lesions: correlation of results with clinical and laboratory findings. *Journal of Clinical Microbiology* 40, 1249–1253.

Liveris, D., Schwartz, I., McKenna, D., Nowakowski, J., Nadelman, R., Demarco, J., Iyer, R., Bittker, S., Cooper, D., Holmgren, D. and Wormser, G.P. (2012) Comparison of five diagnostic modalities for direct detection of *Borrelia burgdorferi* in patients with early Lyme disease. *Diagnostic Microbiology and Infectious Diseases* 73, 243–245.

Ljostad, U. and Mygland, A. (2010) Remaining complaints 1 year after treatment for acute Lyme neuroborreliosis; frequency, pattern and risk factors. *European Journal of Neurology* 17, 118–123.

Luft, B.J., Dattwyler, R.J., Johnson, R.C., Luger, S.W., Bosler, E.M., Rahn, D.W., Masters, E.J., Grunwaldt, E. and Gadgil, S.D. (1996) Azithromycin compared with amoxicillin in the treatment of erythema migrans. A double-blind, randomized, controlled trial. *Annals of Internal Medicine* 124(9), 785–791.

Luger, S.W., Paparone, P., Wormser, G.P., Nadelman, R.B., Grunwaldt, E., Gomez, G., Wisniewski, M. and Collins, J.J. (1995) Comparison of cefuroxime axetil and doxycycline in treatment of patients with early Lyme disease associated with erythema migrans. *Antimicrobial Agents and Chemotherapy* 39(3), 661–667.

Marks, C.M., Nawn, J.E. and Caplow, J.A. (2016) Antibiotic treatment for chronic Lyme disease-say no to the DRESS. *Journal of the American Medical Association Internal Medicine* 176, 1745–1746.

Marques, A. (2008) Chronic Lyme disease: a review. *Infectious Disease Clinics North America* 22, 341–360, vii–viii.

Marques, A.R. (2015) Laboratory diagnosis of Lyme disease: advances and challenges. *Infectious Disease Clinics North America* 29, 295–307.

Marques, A.R., Stock, F. and Gill, V. (2000) Evaluation of a new culture medium for *Borrelia burgdorferi*. *Journal of Clinical Microbiology* 38, 4239–4241.

Marques, A.R., Hornung, R.L., Dally, L. and Philipp, M.T. (2005) Detection of immune complexes is not independent of detection of antibodies in Lyme disease patients and does not confirm active infection with *Borrelia burgdorferi*. *Clinical and Diagnostic Laboratory Immunology* 12, 1036–1040.

Marques, A., Brown, M.R. and Fleisher, T.A. (2009a) Natural killer cell counts are not different between patients with post-Lyme disease syndrome and controls. *Clinical Vaccine Immunology* 16, 1249–1250.

Marques, A., Shaw, P., Schmid, C.H., Steere, A., Kaplan, R.F., Hassett, A., Shapiro, E. and Wormser, G.P. (2009b) Re: a randomized, placebo-controlled trial of repeated IV antibiotic therapy for Lyme encephalopathy. Prolonged Lyme disease treatment: enough is enough. *Neurology* 72, 383–384, author reply 384.

Marques, A., Telford, S.R. III, Turk, S.P. et al. (2014) Xenodiagnosis to detect *Borrelia burgdorferi* infection: a first-in-human study. *Clinical Infectious Diseases* 58, 937–945.

Marshall, E. (1999) Lyme disease. Patients scarce in test of long-term therapy. *Science* 283, 1431.

Marzec, N.S., Nelson, C., Waldron, P.R., Blackburn, B.G., Hosain, S., Greenhow, T., Green, G.M., Lomen-Hoerth, C., Golden, M. and Mead, P.S. (2017) Serious bacterial infections acquired during treatment of patients given a diagnosis of chronic Lyme disease – United States. *Morbidity and Mortality Weekly Report* 66, 607–609.

Melia, M.T. and Auwaerter, P.G. (2016) Time for a different approach to Lyme disease and long-term symptoms. *New England Journal of Medicine* 374, 1277–1278.

Morphy, H., Dunn, K.M., Lewis, M., Boardman, H.F. and Croft, P.R. (2007) Epidemiology of insomnia: a longitudinal study in a UK population. *Sleep* 30, 274–280.

Nadelman, R.B., Luger, S.W., Frank, E., Wisniewski, M., Collins, J.J. and Wormser, G.P. (1992) Comparison of cefuroxime axetil and doxycycline in the treatment of early Lyme disease. *Annals Internal Medicine* 117, 273–280.

Nelson, C., Hojvat, S., Johnson, B., Petersen, J., Schriefer, M., Beard, C.B., Petersen, L., Mead, P., Centers For Disease and Prevention (2014) Concerns regarding a new culture method for *Borrelia burgdorferi* not approved for the diagnosis of Lyme disease. *Morbidity and Mortality Weekly Report* 63, 333.

Nelson, C., Elmendorf, S. and Mead, P. (2015) Neoplasms misdiagnosed as 'chronic Lyme disease'. *Journal of the American Medical Association Internal Medicine* 175, 132–133.

Nizic, T., Velikanje, E., Ružić-Sabljić, E. and Arnez, M. (2012) Solitary erythema migrans in children: comparison of treatment with clarithromycin and amoxicillin. *Wiener klinische Wochenschrift* 124, 427–433.

Nowakowski, J., Schwartz, I., Liveris, D., Wang, G., Aguero-Rosenfeld, M.E., Girao, G., McKenna, D., Nadelman, R.B., Cavaliere, L.F. and Wormser, G.P. (2001) Laboratory diagnostic techniques for patients with early Lyme disease associated with erythema migrans: a comparison of different techniques. *Clinical Infectious Diseases* 33, 2023–2027.

Nowakowski, J., Nadelman, R.B., Sell, R., McKenna, D., Cavaliere, L.F., Holmgren, D., Gaidici, A. and Wormser, G.P. (2003) Long-term follow-up of patients with culture-confirmed Lyme disease. *American Journal of Medicine* 115, 91–96.

Oksi, J., Nikoskelainen, J., Hiekkanen, H. *et al.* (2007) Duration of antibiotic treatment in disseminated Lyme borreliosis: a double-blind, randomized, placebo-controlled, multicenter clinical study. *European Journal of Clinical Microbiology Infectious Diseases* 26, 571–581.

Patel, R., Grogg, K.L., Edwards, W.D., Wright, A.J. and Schwenk, N.M. (2000) Death from inappropriate therapy for Lyme disease. *Clinical Infectious Diseases* 31, 1107–1109.

Patrick, D.M., Miller, R.R., Gardy, J.L., Parker, S.M., Morshed, M.G., Steiner, T.S., Singer, J., Shojania, K., Tang, P. and Complex Chronic Disease Study (2015) Lyme disease diagnosed by alternative methods: a phenotype similar to that of chronic fatigue syndrome. *Clinical Infectious Diseases* 61, 1084–1091.

Pfister, H.W., Preac-Mursic, V., Wilske, B., Schielke, E., Sorgel, F. and Einhaupl, K.M. (1991) Randomized comparison of ceftriaxone and cefotaxime in Lyme neuroborreliosis. *Journal of Infectious Diseases* 163, 311–318.

Picavet, H.S. and Schouten, J.S. (2003) Musculoskeletal pain in the Netherlands: prevalences, consequences and risk groups, the DMC(3)-study. *Pain* 102, 167–178.

Qureshi, M.Z., New, D., Zulqarni, N.J. and Nachman, S. (2002) Overdiagnosis and overtreatment of Lyme disease in children. *Pediatric Infectious Disease Journal* 21, 12–14.

Ramsey, A.H., Belongia, E.A., Gale, C.M. and Davis, J.P. (2002) Outcomes of treated human granulocytic ehrlichiosis cases. *Emerging Infectious Diseases* 8, 398–401.

Reid, M.C., Schoen, R.T., Evans, J., Rosenberg, J.C. and Horwitz, R.I. (1998) The consequences of overdiagnosis and overtreatment of Lyme disease: an observational study. *Annals of Internal Medicine* 128, 354–362.

Rohrbeck, J., Jordan, K. and Croft, P. (2007) The frequency and characteristics of chronic widespread pain in general practice: a case-control study. *British Journal of General Practice* 57, 109–115.

Rose, C.D., Fawcett, P.T., Gibney, K.M. and Doughty, R.A. (1994) The overdiagnosis of Lyme disease in children residing in an endemic area. *Clinical Pediatrics* 33, 663–668.

Schunemann, H.J., Fretheim, A. and Oxman, A.D. (2006) Improving the use of research evidence in guideline development: 9. Grading evidence and recommendations. *Health Research Policy System* 4, 21.

Schwartz, I., Wormser, G.P., Schwartz, J.J. *et al.* (1992) Diagnosis of early Lyme disease by polymerase chain reaction amplification and culture of skin biopsies from erythema migrans lesions. *Journal of Clinical Microbiology* 30, 3082–3088.

Seltzer, E.G., Gerber, M.A., Cartter, M.L., Freudigman, K. and Shapiro, E.D. (2000) Long-term outcomes of persons with Lyme disease. *Journal of American Medical Association* 283, 609–616.

Shadick, N.A., Phillips, C.B., Sangha, O. *et al.* (1999) Musculoskeletal and neurologic outcomes in patients with previously treated Lyme disease. *Annals of Internal Medicine* 131, 919–926.

Sigal, L.H. (1990) Summary of the first 100 patients seen at a Lyme disease referral center. *American Journal of Medicine* 88, 577–581.

Sjowall, J., Ledel, A., Ernerudh, J., Ekerfelt, C. and Forsberg, P. (2012) Doxycycline-mediated effects on persistent symptoms and systemic cytokine responses post-neuroborreliosis: a randomized, prospective, cross-over study. *BMC Infectious Diseases* 12, 186.

Skogman, B.H., Croner, S., Nordwall, M., Eknefelt, M., Ernerudh, J. and Forsberg, P. (2008) Lyme neuroborreliosis in children: a prospective study of clinical features, prognosis, and outcome. *Pediatric Infectious Disease Journal* 27, 1089–1094.

Smith, R.P., Schoen, R.T., Rahn, D.W., Sikand, V.K., Nowakowski, J., Parenti, D.L., Holman, M.S., Persing, D.H. and Steere, A.C. (2002) Clinical characteristics and treatment outcome of early Lyme disease in patients with microbiologically confirmed erythema migrans. *Annals of Internal Medicine* 136, 421–428.

Steere, A.C., Hutchinson, G.J., Rahn, D.W., Sigal, L.H., Craft, J.E., Desanna, E.T. and Malawista, S.E. (1983) Treatment of the early manifestations of Lyme disease. *Annals of Internal Medicine* 99, 22–26.

Steere, A.C., Taylor, E., McHugh, G.L. and Logigian, E.L. (1993) The overdiagnosis of Lyme disease. *Journal of American Medical Association* 269, 1812–1816.

Steere, A.C., Levin, R.E., Molloy, P.J., Kalish, R.A., Abraham, J.R., Liu, N.Y. and Schmid, C.H. (1994) Treatment of Lyme arthritis. *Arthritis Rheumatism* 37, 878–888.

Straubinger, R.K., Summers, B.A., Chang, Y.F. and Appel, M.J. (1997) Persistence of *Borrelia burgdorferi* in experimentally infected dogs after antibiotic treatment. *Journal of Clinical Microbiology* 35, 111–116.

Straubinger, R.K., Straubinger, A.F., Summers, B.A. and Jacobson, R.H. (2000) Status of *Borrelia burgdorferi* infection after antibiotic treatment and the effects of corticosteroids: an experimental study. *Journal of Infectious Diseases* 181, 1069–1081.

Stricker, R.B. (2007) Counterpoint: long-term antibiotic therapy improves persistent symptoms associated with Lyme disease. *Clinical Infectious Diseases* 45, 149–157.

Strle, F., Cimperman, J., Maraspin, V., Jereb, M., Preac-Mursic, V. and Ružič, E. (1993) Azithromycin versus doxycycline for treatment of erythema migrans: Clinical and microbiological findings. *Infection* 21(2), 83–88.

Strle, K., Jones, K.L., Drouin, E.E., Li, X. and Steere, A.C. (2011) *Borrelia burgdorferi* RST1 (OspC type A) genotype is associated with greater inflammation and more severe Lyme disease. *American Journal of Pathology* 178, 2726–2739.

Strle, K., Stupica, D., Drouin, E.E., Steere, A.C. and Strle, F. (2014) Elevated levels of IL-23 in a subset of patients with post-Lyme disease symptoms following erythema migrans. *Clinical Infectious Diseases* 58, 372–380.

Stupica, D., Lusa, L., Ružić-Sabljić, E., Cerar, T. and Strle, F. (2012) Treatment of erythema migrans with doxycycline for 10 days versus 15 days. *Clinical Infectious Diseases* 55, 343–350.

Tang, K.S., Klempner, M.S., Wormser, G.P., Marques, A.R. and Alaedini, A. (2015) Association of immune response to endothelial cell growth factor with early disseminated and late manifestations of Lyme disease but not posttreatment Lyme disease syndrome. *Clinical Infectious Diseases* 61, 1703–1706.

Telford, S.R. III, Hu, L.T. and Marques, A. (2014) Is there a place for xenodiagnosis in the clinic? *Expert Review of Anti-Infective Therapy* 12, 1307–1310.

Thomas, S., Izard, J., Walsh, E. et al. (2017) The host microbiome regulates and maintains human health: a primer and perspective for non-microbiologists. *Cancer Research* 77, 1783–1812.

Tilton, R.C., Barden, D. and Sand, M. (2001) Culture *Borrelia burgdorferi*. *Journal of Clinical Microbiology* 39, 2747.

Tory, H.O., Zurakowski, D. and Sundel, R.P. (2010) Outcomes of children treated for Lyme arthritis: results of a large pediatric cohort. *Journal of Rheumatology* 37, 1049–1055.

Unger, E.R., Lin, J.S., Brimmer, D.J., Lapp, C.W., Komaroff, A.L., Nath, A., Laird, S. and Iskander, J. (2016) CDC grand rounds: chronic fatigue syndrome – advancing research and clinical education. *Morbidity and Mortality Weekly Report* 65, 1434–1438.

Wang, T.J., Liang, M.H., Sangha, O., Phillips, C.B., Lew, R.A., Wright, E.A., Berardi, V., Fossel, A.H. and Shadick, N.A. (2000) Coexposure to *Borrelia burgdorferi* and *Babesia microti* does not worsen the long-term outcome of Lyme disease. *Clinical Infectious Diseases* 31, 1149–1154.

Wang, G., Ojaimi, C., Wu, H., Saksenberg, V., Iyer, R., Liveris, D., McClain, S.A., Wormser, G.P. and Schwartz, I. (2002) Disease severity in a murine model of Lyme borreliosis is associated with the genotype of the infecting *Borrelia burgdorferi* sensu stricto strain. *Journal of Infectious Diseases* 186, 782–791.

Weber, K., Preac-Mursic, V., Neubert, U., Thurmayr, R., Herzer, P., Wilske, B., Schierz, G. and Marget, W. (1988) Antibiotic therapy of early European Lyme borreliosis and acrodermatitis chronica atrophicans. *Annals New York Academy of Sciences* 539, 324–345.

Weber, K., Preac-Mursic, V., Wilske, B., Thurmayr, R., Neubert, U. and Scherwitz, C. (1990) A randomized trial of ceftriaxone versus oral penicillin for the treatment of early European Lyme borreliosis. *Infection* 18, 91–96.

Wessely, S., Nimnuan, C. and Sharpe, M. (1999) Functional somatic syndromes: one or many? *Lancet* 354, 936–939.

Wills, A.B., Spaulding, A.B., Adjemian, J., Prevots, D.R., Turk, S.P., Williams, C. and Marques, A. (2016) Long-term follow-up of patients with Lyme disease: longitudinal analysis of clinical and quality-of-life measures. *Clinical Infectious Diseases* 62, 1546–1551.

Wormser, G.P. (2016) Longer-term therapy for symptoms attributed to Lyme disease. *New England Journal of Medicine* 375, 997.

Wormser, G.P. and Schwartz, I. (2009) Antibiotic treatment of animals infected with *Borrelia burgdorferi*. *Clinical Microbiology Reviews* 22, 387–395.

Wormser, G.P., Ramanathan, R., Nowakowski, J., McKenna, D., Holmgren, D., Visintainer, P., Dornbush, R., Singh, B. and Nadelman, R.B. (2003) Duration of antibiotic therapy for early Lyme disease. A randomized, double-blind, placebo-controlled trial. *Annals Internal Medicine* 138, 697–704.

Wormser, G.P., Dattwyler, R.J., Shapiro, E.D. *et al.* (2006) The clinical assessment, treatment, and prevention of Lyme disease, human granulocytic anaplasmosis, and babesiosis: clinical practice guidelines by the infectious diseases society of America. *Clinical Infectious Diseases* 43, 1089–1134.

Wormser, G.P., Weitzner, E., McKenna, D., Nadelman, R.B., Scavarda, C., Molla, I., Dornbush, R., Visintainer, P. and Nowakowski, J. (2015a) Long-term assessment of health-related quality of life in patients with culture-confirmed early Lyme disease. *Clinical Infectious Diseases* 61, 244–247.

Wormser, G.P., Weitzner, E., McKenna, D., Nadelman, R.B., Scavarda, C. and Nowakowski, J. (2015b) Long-term assessment of fatigue in patients with culture-confirmed Lyme disease. *American Journal of Medicine* 128, 181–184.

Yrjanainen, H., Hytonen, J., Song, X.Y., Oksi, J., Hartiala, K. and Viljanen, M.K. (2007) Anti-tumor necrosis factor-alpha treatment activates *Borrelia burgdorferi* spirochetes 4 weeks after ceftriaxone treatment in C3H/He mice. *Journal of Infectious Diseases* 195, 1489–1496.

17 Lyme Disease: The Great Controversy

John J. Halperin,[1] Phillip Baker[2] and Gary P. Wormser[3]
[1]Overlook Medical Center, Summit, New Jersey and Sidney Kimmel Medical College of Thomas Jefferson University, Philadelphia, Pennsylvania, USA; [2]American Lyme Disease Foundation, Lyme, Connecticut, USA; [3]New York Medical College, Valhalla, New York, USA

17.1 Background

Once upon a time, a little understood spirochetal infection, known in some circles as 'the French disease' – but more commonly as syphilis – was felt to be responsible for everything from what we now know to be Alzheimer's dementia to myocardial infarctions. In a curious parallel, another spirochetal neuroinfectious disease, regarded by some as first described in France in 1922, is now blamed for everything from dementia to psychiatric disease. The 1922 report, describing a patient who developed a large skin rash, meningitis and painful radiculoneuritis following a tick bite, clearly had features similar to neurologic Lyme disease, although there were several highly atypical features, including a predominance of granulocytes in cerebrospinal fluid (CSF) along with a positive test for syphilis in CSF; thus, it is impossible to know definitively whether the French patient actually had what we now refer to as neuroborreliosis (Wormser and Wormser, 2016). It has been over three decades since the causative spirochete of Lyme disease was first identified, and effective treatment established. The contents of this volume attest to the fact that much has been learned since then about the biology of this infection and the host response to it. Undoubtedly, much more remains to be learned; many aspects continue to be debated. Curiously, though, some elements continue to be debated despite overwhelming scientific evidence supporting only one conclusion.

Several issues are foundational to the persistence of a group of patient advocates and their clinical supporters, and have resulted in the rarely helpful intrusion of politics into medical practice. Such efforts have led to the states of Connecticut, Maryland, Minnesota, Massachusetts, New York, Pennsylvania, Rhode Island and others passing – or considering – legislation or regulations permitting the use of demonstrably ineffective prolonged antibiotic treatment (Klempner et al., 2001, 2013; Krupp et al., 2003; Fallon et al., 2008; Berende et al., 2016) for patients diagnosed with an undefined disorder termed 'chronic Lyme disease'. In 2006 Connecticut's Attorney General opened an investigation of the Infectious Diseases Society of America (IDSA) for issuing evidence-based guidelines for the diagnosis and treatment of Lyme disease, on the legally questionable theory that this clinical guideline represented an antitrust violation. Although this yielded no finding of any antitrust violation, it ultimately cost the IDSA over half a million dollars in legal and other costs (IDSA, personal communication, October, 2010), and resulted in a detailed review of the guidelines by an independent panel that subsequently endorsed the guidelines' original recommendations (Lantos et al., 2010). No other set of guidelines was ever subjected to such thorough scrutiny and review with no substantive changes being recommended or made.

The mutually reinforcing 'alternative facts' underlying this debate are based on misinterpretations centered around three core elements. First, in the early 1980s, using then available – but subsequently shown to be flawed – diagnostic approaches, questions were raised about the sensitivity of serologic testing in established, disseminated Lyme disease. We now know that in patients with *B. burgdorferi* infection of more than 3–6 weeks' duration, two-tier serologic testing is highly sensitive, with more challenges arising from specificity than sensitivity. Second, the presence of some symptoms after completion of standard antimicrobial therapy (as occurs in many other infections) led to questions about the adequacy of the treatment per se. We now know that standard courses of antibiotics are curative in the overwhelming majority of patients with confirmed *B. burgdorferi* infection, and that additional antimicrobial therapy is not only unhelpful but also may present serious risks (Marzec et al., 2017). Third, some interpreted the presence of non-specific symptoms following recommended treatment as evidence of persistent infection. It is now clear that chronic non-specific symptoms following antibiotic therapy known to be effective are not relieved by additional courses of antibiotic therapy, are not associated with nervous system infection, and are unlikely to be due to persistent *B. burgdorferi* infection.

This fascinating story probably relates at least in part to the disease's original characterization in the United States in the early 1970s, when a surprising number of children in Lyme and Old Lyme, Connecticut were diagnosed as having juvenile rheumatoid arthritis. Not satisfied with this diagnosis, mothers of several affected children reached out to Yale and the Centers for Disease Control and Prevention (CDC), ultimately leading to a more detailed investigation. This resulted in the pioneering work of Allen Steere and others (Steere et al., 1977), who identified both the tick vector and the causative bacterial agent, *Borreliella burgdorferi* (formerly *Borrelia burgdorferi* sensu stricto) (Burgdorfer et al., 1982; Benach et al., 1983; Steere et al., 1983). It also resulted in the early creation of multiple patient support and advocacy groups, whose members have been most vocal in advocating strongly for the perceived needs and concerns of patients afflicted – or thought to be afflicted – with this disease (www.lymenet.org). Patient advocacy groups were formed even in areas of the United States where Lyme disease is not endemic, and where there are no ticks that carry and/or transmit Lyme disease. Aided by the internet, these groups have shared information, misinformation, viewpoints and strategies to lobby for their cause, reinforcing each other's perspectives and opinions, thereby setting the stage for much controversy and confusion.

With significant research support and funding from both the National Institutes of Health (NIH) and the CDC, several academic groups – initially primarily those at Yale and the State University of New York at Stony Brook (SUNY-SB) – became actively involved in efforts to better understand the full scope of Lyme disease. The observation in the 1980s that some patients who appeared to have active, disseminated Lyme disease did not have measurable antibody responses as evidenced by the enzyme-linked immunosorbent assays (ELISAs) then in use (Dattwyler et al., 1988) led to the concept of seronegative late Lyme disease – a concept that remains firmly implanted in the consciousness of patients and some healthcare providers, despite the fact that this was almost certainly an artifact of the then available laboratory assays (see Chapter 4 in this volume).

Similarly, in assessing patients in the early 1980s, all with typical signs and symptoms of active Lyme disease, many were noted to have objectively demonstrable cognitive slowing and memory difficulty (Halperin et al., 1988; 1990; Logigian et al., 1990; Krupp et al., 1991) – as do many patients with other active infectious or inflammatory disorders. The observation that some patients with Lyme disease experience cognitive difficulties, chronic pain, and fatigue, in the context of their illness, gave rise to the conclusion – in some circles – that such symptoms are by themselves diagnostic of Lyme disease, even in the absence of more specific clinical findings or positive serologic tests. Since these same symptoms are highly prevalent in the otherwise healthy population (Luo et al., 2005; Kugeler et al., 2011; Blackwell and Clarke, 2013), this logic has indeed been problematic. Annual surveys by the CDC indicate that about 15% of women and 10% of men in the US have felt either exhausted or extremely tired every day or most days of the preceding 3 months (Blackwell and Clarke, 2013). The Institute of Medicine has reported that acute and unspecified chronic pain affects 116 million Americans, about 30% of the general population. Such individuals often go from one physician to another, unable to find anyone who can either identify the cause of their symptoms or suggest a remedy (Institute of Medicine (US) Committee on Advancing Pain Research, Control and Education, 2011). In addition, certain of these symptoms were misinterpreted as evidence of *central nervous system* infection by *B. burgdorferi* – a terrifying prospect for symptomatic individuals – despite the fact that early work clearly showed that the vast majority of Lyme disease patients with cognitive difficulties *did not have active nervous system infection* (Halperin *et al.*, 1992) (see Chapter 13 in this volume). All of these false assumptions set the stage for a medical 'perfect storm'.

Reinforced by information from support groups and the internet, patients with a common – but non-specific – symptom complex became convinced that their difficulties were caused by an infection for which the diagnostic tools were deeply flawed. Even more frightening, they believed that, if left untreated, this infection would result in irreversible brain damage. Not surprisingly, some physicians – who came to be known as 'Lyme literate physicians' or LLMDs – began treating such patients with aggressive courses of antibiotics. When treatment responses were less than satisfactory – and despite the fact that *B. burgdorferi* has never been shown to develop antibiotic resistance – many patients and LLMDs were reluctant to acknowledge that the underlying premises and logic were deeply flawed. Instead, they invoked a series of ever more creative conjectures – substantiated only by inaccurate or misinterpreted snippets of information – as to why this infection was apparently so difficult to treat. These included assertions that *B. burgdorferi* cells adopt a cell wall-free or cyst form (Brorson and Brorson, 1998; 1999; MacDonald, 2006) (and Chapter 2 in this book) and/or that they hide intracellularly. Such assumptions were based primarily on extrapolations from *in vitro* studies, without evidence of any clinical relevance whatsoever (Wormser *et al.*, 2006). The solution they invoked was to extend antibiotic therapy with different antibiotics given singly or in combination until all symptoms disappeared. Such unproven therapeutic approaches were not only without benefit, but also were harmful and administered at great personal costs to the patients who received them.

As many of these LLMDs became increasingly invested in this deeply flawed disease model, the response to treatment became the final element in this self-reinforcing logic. Early work indicated that patients with acute, active early Lyme disease, as indicated by the presence of an erythema migrans skin lesion (when large numbers of spirochetes are presumably present), sometimes exhibited a Jarisch–Herxheimer-like reaction within 24 h after initiation of treatment (Weber *et al.*, 1988; Maloy *et al.*, 1998). This led to the notion that any worsening of symptoms during treatment constituted 'Herxing', regardless of the duration of symptoms or treatment at the time of the worsening. The logical inconsistency of postulating that treatment-resistant disease was due to a small number of undetectable bacteria, while at the same time concluding that symptoms arising or worsening during antibiotic therapy were due to the release of large amounts of pharmacologically active bacterial products, was either discounted or never considered. However, this then completed the very tidy but circular conceptual model. If patients improved even transiently with treatment, this validated the diagnosis and justified further treatment; the possibility of a placebo effect, reported to be as great as 38% in a relatively large antibiotic treatment study (Klempner *et al.*, 2001), or natural fluctuation in symptom severity was either never considered or was completely rejected. If there was no response to therapy, this validated the assumption that this infection is highly resistant to standard antimicrobial therapy, requiring additional treatment. If patients worsened on antibiotic therapy this was thought to be 'Herxing', indicating treatment was effective and more was needed.

At this point, it is informative to examine in more detail some of the key myths that together reinforced this illogical construct (Halperin *et al.*, 2013).

17.2 Laboratory Myths – Seronegative Lyme Disease

17.2.1 Serology

In 1988, using early whole cell sonicate ELISAs for the serodiagnosis of Lyme disease, a group of scientists at SUNY-SB identified 17 patients who had been treated early in the course of Lyme disease, but still had symptoms felt to be indicative of active infection (Dattwyler et al., 1988). Although none of these patients had significant elevations of antibody by ELISA, all had evidence of T cell immunoreactivity against B. burgdorferi, using a T cell proliferation assay now known to be non-specific (Hemmer et al., 1998) and therefore of limited diagnostic value.

To understand how infected individuals with long-standing active infection might be 'seronegative', it is important to understand the process of developing an ELISA for the serodiagnosis of any infection (see Chapter 4 in this volume by Dr. Auwaerter), including an infection caused by B. burgdorferi. Since many bacterial antigens are shared among B. burgdorferi and other groups of microorganisms, there is considerable immunologic cross-reactivity, often leading to false positive serologic results (Magnarelli et al., 1987). Consequently, assays must be designed to balance sensitivity and specificity. With greater sensitivity, it becomes more likely an assay will detect low levels of antibodies specific for Borreliella antigens. However, the same highly sensitive assay will also detect weak cross-reactivities that are not diagnostically significant or meaningful. Such cross-reactivity is more pronounced with IgM antibodies, which have ten binding sites, in comparison to IgG antibodies, which have just two. IgM's additional binding sites enhance its reactivity to minor cross-reacting antigenic determinants from multiple other organisms. Following a CDC-sponsored conference on Lyme disease serodiagnosis, two-tier testing was adopted to address this issue (Dressler et al., 1993; Anonymous, 1995). Screening begins with a sensitive first-tier assay such as an ELISA, realizing that, despite stringent endpoints, this will generate some false positives, particularly with IgM seroreactivity. Samples that demonstrate immunoreactivity (positive or borderline) therefore undergo a second, much more specific test, a Western blot. Moreover, since the early IgM response converts to IgG quite rapidly, after the first 1–2 months of infection, isolated IgM positive seroreactivity will almost certainly be false positive (see Chapter 4). It is likely that the 17 patients included in the above-described SUNY-SB study included some with false negative results who would be positive with current assays, others with post-treatment persistent symptoms and perhaps others who never really had Lyme disease. With the currently recommended two-tier approach, most laboratory experts now conclude that – except in the first 3–6 weeks of infection, before an antibody response has developed sufficiently to be detectable – seronegative Lyme disease is extraordinarily rare.

Although the preceding history explains the origins of the myth of seronegativity in patients with long-standing infection, there is another, often repeated variation of this argument that is more difficult to understand – namely that serologic results become falsely negative *during and because of* antibiotic treatment (Halperin et al., 2013) – that is, the presence of antibiotics in the patient's system in some way interferes with either the production of antibodies at the time, or the assays to detect them. Patients often relate that they were told 'the test was negative because I was on antibiotics'. Not only is there no evidence – or even theoretical rationale – to support such an assertion, there is no precedent for this with reference to any other infectious disease.

These two untenable explanations for 'false negative' serologies are very different from the situation in which a patient is *cured* very early in infection, in which circumstance the rapid removal of *borreliellal* antigens certainly can lead to an aborted or greatly reduced antibody response – because the infecting organisms are not present for long enough to elicit a detectable antibody response. Observations on rabbits experimentally infected with *Treponema pallidum* (syphilis) provide a useful perspective on this point. Rabbits that received penicillin while incubating infection (Hollander et al., 1952, p. 119) were 'either cured or subsequently developed clinically recognizable lesions'. Single subcurative doses of penicillin prolonged the 'incubation period of experimental syphilis … up to a limit of 30–40 days', but when lesions developed, all of the animals became seropositive.

17.2.2 Other diagnostic tests

Because of the technical difficulty of culturing B. burgdorferi using conventional laboratory methods, and because of the presumed small number of organisms present in readily obtainable samples, microbiologic diagnosis of Lyme disease is generally impractical. Even the extremely technically sensitive and specific polymerase chain reaction (PCR), adopted as an alternative to culture, is of remarkably low diagnostic sensitivity with many types of clinical specimens (Lebech et al., 2000; Avery et al., 2005; Roux et al., 2007), presumably because of the low number of microorganisms present. On the other hand, PCR can detect fragments of DNA from long dead organisms. DNA has been detected in tissues as long as 7 years after an infection has been microbiologically cured (Rovery et al., 2005). Thus, although such fragments may be specific for B. burgdorferi, their presence does not prove active infection; it indicates only the presence of Borreliella-specific DNA.

Consequently, the laboratory diagnosis of Lyme disease is antibody-based; that is, the diagnosis relies almost exclusively on demonstrating the presence of a specific host antibody response to the microorganism. However, this too has important limitations. The presence of specific antibody – which commonly persists for long periods of time after infection – indicates past or present exposure to relevant borreliellal antigens, and does not prove active infection (Hammers Berggren et al., 1993). Importantly, for most other infections, serologic testing typically relies on the demonstration of a 4-fold or greater change in antibody titer. In Lyme disease the convention has been to rely on a single serologic determination.

Although the adoption of the two-tier testing strategy has provided a reasonable compromise between sensitivity and specificity, test interpretation requires an appreciation of three key elements. First, the criteria used for the Western blot are only to be applied in patients with positive or borderline ELISAs. In the absence of this much measurable antibody, blots should not even be performed. Second, the IgM criteria are intended for use only in individuals with early infection (Anonymous, 1995). By 4–8 weeks after exposure to B. burgdorferi, the much more specific IgG antibody response should be developing and is of much greater diagnostic value (Wormser et al., 2006). In patients with disease of 1–2 months' duration or longer, isolated IgM responses are far more likely to be unrelated to B. burgdorferi infection. Third, the bands selected for use in the Western blot were not chosen arbitrarily; rather, they were chosen on the basis of *statistical considerations*, which included an analysis of those combinations of bands that provided the best predictive values for well characterized specimens known to have been obtained from individuals with and without Lyme disease (Dressler et al., 1993). Obviously, laboratories using criteria other than these must establish the validity of their own criteria based on equally rigorous scientific assessments (Aguero-Rosenfeld and Wormser, 2015).

Work is in progress to develop simpler, more sensitive and specific diagnostic tests for Lyme disease. The C6 ELISA in particular is increasingly being adopted (Philipp et al., 2003, Vermeersch et al., 2009), and it may be possible to substitute this or other assays for the Western blot in two-tier testing (Branda et al., 2011; Wormser et al., 2013; Lipsett et al., 2016; Branda et al., 2017).

17.3 Clinical Myths: Lyme Disease is a Clinical Diagnosis Based Entirely on Symptomatology

17.3.1 Background

Infectious diseases are associated with a wide array of symptoms. Some are sufficiently unusual outside the context of that particular disease to have a meaningful positive predictive value supporting that diagnosis. Others are common to a broad range of inflammatory disorders and thus have no diagnostic specificity (Halperin et al., 2013). Just as in the interpretation of laboratory results, Bayesian concepts play an important role in determining the diagnostic sensitivity and specificity of clinical signs and symptoms. For the diagnosis of Lyme disease, some findings (e.g. erythema migrans, bilateral facial nerve palsies or childhood facial nerve palsies) are quite unusual, occurring in very few circumstances other than Lyme disease. If these occur in an individual who has been in an endemic area and there is a risk of recent exposure to infected ticks, the probability of the patient having Lyme disease is quite high.

Other signs or symptoms are of intermediate specificity. Unilateral facial nerve palsy in an adult, radicular pain without a mechanical cause, relapsing large joint oligoarthritis and heart block in an otherwise healthy young individual provide clues but are less specific. These are suggestive of the diagnosis and, if there has been potential tick exposure, it is appropriate to consider Lyme disease in the differential diagnosis. Further along the continuum would be lymphocytic meningitis. This can be caused by Lyme disease but there is substantial epidemiologic and symptomatic overlap between this and enteroviral meningitis. Although it would be reasonable to consider Lyme disease in the appropriate context, one must also realize that in many of these patients there will actually be a viral etiology. At the other end of the spectrum are many symptoms (e.g. fatigue, malaise, headaches, diffuse aches and pains, cognitive slowing) that are common to virtually all inflammatory disorders. If these symptoms are present in the absence of more distinctive features, they are of no predictive value for the diagnosis of Lyme disease. In this context even obtaining a serologic test is ill-advised, as a positive result is more likely to be misleading than helpful. In this context, it is worth considering a historic footnote. In the early 1980s, the academic group at SUNY-SB developed a collaboration with several primary care physicians in eastern Long Island, who were seeing many patients with Lyme disease. In an effort to cast a broad net to identify other symptoms that might be related to the infection, they created a database that included a standard review of systems. This completely generic review of systems subsequently became the questionnaire used by many LLMDs as a Lyme-specific symptom inventory.

17.3.2 The assertion that 'Lyme disease is a clinical diagnosis'

Every diagnosis in medicine ultimately relies on an ill-defined process termed 'clinical judgment'. 'Clinical judgment' assumes that an appropriately knowledgeable physician will carefully and correctly gather all relevant clinical, laboratory and epidemiologic data and reach a logical conclusion that is congruous with usual and acceptable medical practice. While King Louis XIV of France famously asserted that he was the law ('Le loi, c'est moi'), diagnoses advanced by physicians are not inherently correct simply because they are asserted by a physician, however well intended.

Diagnosis in any given patient requires the appropriate balancing of several different data elements. For example, a 3-year-old, living in Lyme, Connecticut, with summertime facial nerve palsy, probably has Lyme disease. The child might have a negative serology as this disorder may occur before a measurable antibody response has developed. In this case, the initiation of presumptive treatment might well be reasonable. If that child's father developed acute radicular pain in January after lifting heavy furniture, the probability of the radiculitis being related to Lyme disease is extremely low, even if his serology were positive. If the child's mother has been completely healthy but feeling exhausted and absent-minded ever since the child and her twin sibling were born, it's unlikely that the fatigue and forgetfulness are due to Lyme disease. In this sense, Lyme disease is a clinical diagnosis in which a capable physician will synthesize *all* available data specific to that patient (Halperin *et al.*, 2013). Then, informed by the broader set of evidence-based medical knowledge, that physician will adopt a diagnostic and treatment strategy consistent with current, reasonable medical thinking and practice.

17.4 The Symptom Described as 'Brain Fog'

The central nervous system can be affected in one of three ways in patients with Lyme disease (see Chapters 8 and 13 in this volume). The most common has nothing to do with brain infection. Individuals with systemic inflammatory or infectious disorders commonly feel tired and cognitively slowed, in the absence of any brain infection or direct involvement of any sort – well exemplified by otherwise healthy individuals with a febrile viral upper respiratory infection. Actual central nervous system infection by *B. burgdorferi* almost always includes meningitis. By definition, this disorder consists of inflammation of the lining of the brain, a rather uncomfortable process that is uniformly medically benign. Very rarely, patients develop parenchymal brain or spinal cord involvement, a disorder most accurately termed encephalomyelitis. Patients with encephalomyelitis generally have focally abnormal neurologic examinations, abnormal brain or spinal cord magnetic resonance imaging (MRI) scans and inflammatory CSF. Most will have demonstrable local production of anti-*B. burgdorferi* antibodies in the CSF. Although this encephalomyelitis typically causes focal neurological abnormalities, very rarely it will present only as cognitive difficulty. When cognitive difficulties are substantial, or the brain MRI demonstrates significant and potentially related parenchymal abnormalities, CSF should be examined. Inflammatory changes in the CSF would then lead to the diagnosis of encephalitis and then appropriate antibiotic treatment.

Unfortunately, it has become commonplace for patients and their treating physicians to assume that the first, common disorder (a toxic-metabolic encephalopathy) – often referred to by patients as 'brain fog' – represents evidence of the extremely rare phenomenon of direct brain infection (encephalomyelitis) by *B. burgdorferi*, and that this will progress to severe irreversible brain damage. Multiple studies have now shown that such symptoms following treated Lyme disease occur rarely if ever in patients who have actually had definite central nervous system infection with *B. burgdorferi* (Dersch et al., 2016; Wills et al., 2016). Moreover, Lyme encephalomyelitis can usually be diagnosed quite easily by combining clinical and CSF examinations with MRI imaging (Ljostad and Mygland, 2009). The use of far less accurate diagnostics, particularly qualitative brain single-photon emission computed tomography (SPECT) imaging, has confounded this issue. In many of these patients, SPECT scans are interpreted as showing cerebral vasculitis, despite normal neurologic examinations, laboratory test results on CSF, brain MRI imaging and even brain vascular imaging. Most neurologists find this juxtaposition to be conceptually perplexing, if not frankly illogical. Given this misconception, it should not be surprising that affected patients are so terrified by the misguided fear of a brain-damaging infection that they are willing to undergo extensive and expensive testing and treatment, often at their own expense. Obviously, the key to correct diagnosis is, as always, sound clinical judgment.

17.5 The Assertion that Lyme Disease is a Potentially Lethal Infection

One of the least appreciated aspects of *B. burgdorferi* infection is how benign it actually is. Although heart block and encephalomyelitis could conceivably be lethal, there are only extraordinarily rare cases suggesting Lyme disease was a causative factor in a patient's death. Although advocacy groups occasionally cite examples of patients dying from this infection, the objective data provide little support for such a notion. A few case reports suggest that Lyme carditis might have contributed to the demise of patients (Marcus et al., 1985; Lamaison, 2007; Tavora et al., 2008; Kugeler et al., 2011; CDC, 2013). However, there probably are at least as many case reports of deaths (Patel et al., 2000; Holzbauer et al., 2010) and serious morbidity (Marzec et al., 2017) due to complications of inappropriate antibiotic and other treatments directed at 'chronic Lyme disease'. A group at the CDC reviewed United States death certificate data (Kugeler et al., 2011) from 1999–2003. The diagnosis of Lyme disease was listed on 119 of the reviewed death certificates from this period. However, among these, only one patient had symptoms consistent with Lyme disease. It is important to understand that diagnoses listed on death certificates include previously made diagnoses, often with no independent review or substantiation. In reviewing these data, the authors did not have access to medical records or any information other than the terminal events. If this single patient did die for reasons related to Lyme disease, a comparison to Lyme disease incidence data during the same period would suggest a mortality rate of approximately 1/100,000. If recent suggestions that the real incidence of Lyme disease is actually many times the number of cases meeting the CDC's epidemiologic definition (Nelson et al., 2015), the mortality rate would be even lower. Certainly, in any disease with such extraordinarily low suspected mortality, a causal relationship must be highly suspect.

17.6 Treatment – the Myth That More (and More and More…) is Better

Numerous studies have now shown that Lyme disease – even in the presence of nervous system infection – can be readily treated with fairly short courses of conventional antibiotics (Halperin et al., 2013). Well performed studies have repeatedly demonstrated no meaningful or lasting benefit (Klempner et al., 2001; Krupp et al., 2003; Oksi et al., 2007; Fallon et al., 2008; Berende et al., 2016) of prolonged or extended antibiotic therapy. These findings are completely consistent with what is known of the biology of B. burgdorferi, as well as the cumulative knowledge of treatment effects with innumerable other bacterial infections. Despite this, the notion of a need for treatment of longer duration continues in some circles.

At least three considerations should be kept in mind. First, as already discussed, many patients being treated for 'chronic Lyme disease' do not have evidence indicating an infection with B. burgdorferi – or any other identifiable pathogen. Hence, no amount of antibiotic will alleviate their symptoms.

Second, as is the case for many infections, some or all of a patient's symptoms may continue even after the infection has been microbiologically cured. If a patient has facial nerve palsy, the nerve must still recover from whatever damage it has incurred, even after the precipitating infection has been eliminated. An inflamed knee may continue to be painful and swollen, even after the infection has been eradicated. Many patients with significant infections (e.g. bacterial pneumonia) will continue to feel tired and ill for weeks or months after microbiologic cure. Since symptoms attributed to Lyme disease often do not resolve immediately with treatment and presumed microbiologic cure, one can readily understand why patients might feel that recommended treatment duration is arbitrary and that antibiotic therapy should continue until all symptoms resolve. However, the data for Lyme disease, as in a myriad of other infections, demonstrate that this seemingly logical conclusion is incorrect.

Finally, one very real limitation of our diagnostic technology is that there is no definitive laboratory test that confirms cure of the infection. Since the immune response typically remains demonstrable for an extended period of time after successful treatment, there is an understandable desire for another laboratory test to confirm that the infection is cured. In central nervous system infection, the concentration of CXCL13 – a B cell attracting cytokine – in CSF may provide a sensitive but non-specific marker of active infection (Sillanpaa et al., 2013; Rupprecht et al., 2014; Eckman et al., 2018). Absent a laboratory test that confirms cure, it is easy to understand why a patient with continued symptoms – and who believes those symptoms reflect an unchecked brain-damaging infection – would want to continue antibiotics, regardless of the risk.

17.7 Continuing Non-specific Symptoms – the Myth That Bacteria Must Be Lurking Somewhere... (see Table 17.1)

As in many other infections, non-specific symptoms such as fatigue commonly persist after usually curative antimicrobial therapy for Lyme disease, but gradually disappear over time. The observation that such symptoms appeared to either persist in some cases or develop *de novo* within a few months after treatment led to questions as to whether this constituted a distinct pathophysiologic entity – termed 'chronic Lyme disease' by some who thought it was due to persisting infection, and 'post-treatment Lyme disease syndrome (or symptoms)' (PTLDS) by others who did not. Addressing this, one of the most contentious points in 'the great Lyme disease controversy', requires at least three initial assumptions. First, patients in whom these diagnoses are entertained must have had Lyme disease in the first place. Second, the rare patients who are true microbiologic treatment failures, who present with new inflammatory events, must be excluded. Third, there must be a distinction between symptoms that are purely subjective and objective clinical signs.

This then leads to at least four possible explanations for the clinical observations. First, the late symptoms might be due to low level persisting infection. Second, as in some cases of post-treatment Lyme arthritis, these could represent an aberrant, persisting immune response. Third, this could be a neurobehavioral response to the stressor of an illness. And fourth, this could represent anchoring bias, in which patients who have been given the diagnosis of Lyme disease develop commonplace symptoms

Table 17.1. Hypotheses proposed to explain symptoms following treated Lyme disease.

Pro	Con
Persistence of Borreliella	
Anecdotal reports of improvement with antibiotics	Not responsive to antimicrobial treatment in placebo-controlled treatment trials
Conjecture about bacteria hidden intracellularly or in biofilms	No evidence of residual *Borreliella* found in patients
	If *Borreliella* 'hidden' from the immune system, no immune activation to cause symptoms
	No evidence of a secreted exotoxin to cause symptoms
	Precedent of tuberculosis and other infections with long-standing presence of 'hidden' bacteria but no symptoms
	Good intracellular penetration of tetracyclines
Persisting/aberrant immunologic response	
Evidence of cross-reactive antibodies to neural epitopes, *in vitro* and in serum of patients with persistent symptoms	Syndrome not strongly associated with definite neuroborreliosis, where greatest likelihood of blood–brain barrier penetration by cross-reacting antibodies
	No evidence of central nervous system inflammation in this syndrome, so immune cross-reactivity with neural antigens unlikely to be pathophysiologically relevant
	Quantitative SPECT shows brain hypoperfusion, not the hyperperfusion expected in inflammation
Anchoring bias	
Several controlled trials show same prevalence of these symptoms in post-Lyme disease patients and controls	Observation of persisting symptoms in prospectively identified patients, but most such studies to date have failed to prospectively follow a control group
High prevalence of these symptoms in general population	
PTLDS studies had great difficulty identifying patients meeting criteria	
At risk phenotype	
Precedent of post-infectious arthritis, HLA determined	No evidence of active inflammation in central nervous system in PTLDS, comparable to joint inflammation in post-infectious arthritis
Persisting symptoms if multiple comorbidities	
Persisting symptoms if low positive affect, low resilience	

HLA, human leukocyte antigen; PTLDS, post-treatment Lyme disease syndrome; SPECT, single-photon emission computed tomography.

that they then assume were caused by this infection, but which actually are simply a chance co-occurrence.

The described symptoms are very common – occurring to some extent in up to one-third of the otherwise healthy population, to a degree that disrupts daily activities in 2% (Luo et al., 2005), with an estimated 10–15% of the US population describing themselves as 'often feeling very tired or exhausted' (Blackwell and Clarke, 2013). By comparison, studies to test treatment of PTLDS individuals have had considerable difficulty identifying eligible candidates (Klempner et al., 2001; Krupp et al., 2003; Fallon et al., 2008). Several early population studies may shed some light on the problem. A retrospective study (Shadick et al., 1994) compared 38 patients previously treated for Lyme disease, with a median of 6.2 years follow-up (published prior to the introduction of Western blot confirmation of ELISA testing), to 43 healthy controls; treated patients more frequently described arthralgias, paresthesias, concentration difficulty and fatigue. Importantly, they also more frequently had abnormal joints and objective neurologic abnormalities. In a subsequent larger study (186 patients, 167 controls) of a different population, the same group (Shadick et al., 1999), using current serodiagnostic criteria, found that with a median of 6.0 years follow-up, subjective symptoms but not objective abnormalities were more frequent in patients who had been treated for Lyme disease. Similarly, a population study of 212 Lyme disease patients reported to the Connecticut Department of Health (Seltzer et al., 2000), with mean follow-up of 51 months, found a high frequency of subjective symptoms, but these symptoms consistently occurred more frequently in patients who did not meet the Lyme disease case definition. A more recent analysis (Wills et al., 2016) of a referral population of 101 patients with Lyme disease (mean follow-up 3.9 years) found that, although Lyme disease patients started with low SF36 scores, at follow-up they consistently matched US population norms. Interestingly in this cohort, the only correlate of lower scores at follow-up was the presence of other comorbidities. Finally, an early study of 63 children treated for erythema migrans, with 1 to 6 years of follow-up (Salazar et al., 1993) found no long-term sequelae.

More recently, a number of cohort studies have been performed to address this issue. A Slovenian study, in which patients with erythema migrans were randomized to treatment with doxycycline (145) or cefuroxime axetil (140), and compared to 259 healthy controls, found that at 6 months follow-up 4.6% of treated patients had 'new or increased symptoms' (NOIS), compared to 5.5% of controls. At 12 months 2.2% of treated patients had NOIS vs. 8.0% of controls (Cerar et al., 2010). A more recent study by the same group (Stupica et al., 2018) similarly found non-specific symptoms to be as prevalent in healthy controls as in patients previously treated for erythema migrans. A comparable, controlled US study – including a broader spectrum of patients with Lyme disease, not just erythema migrans – addressing the same question has just been completed, but the results are not yet known. (Arguably inclusion of a second control group consisting of patients with another well-defined acute infectious disease, such as cellulitis, might have been equally or more informative.) A prospective US cohort study provided long-term follow-up of patients with culture-confirmed erythema migrans. One assessed fatigue (Wormser et al., 2015b) in 100 patients at 11–20 years of follow-up (mean 15.4 years) and found only three patients who had fatigue possibly related to Lyme disease; the level of fatigue in these three subjects was not of sufficient severity to be disabling. The second (Wormser et al., 2015a) looked at health-related quality of life in the same 100 subjects at 11–20 years of follow-up; the SF36 scores at follow-up were identical to general population norms.

Finally, since these symptoms are often inappropriately attributed to nervous system Lyme disease, it is helpful to address this subgroup specifically. Most helpful is a meta-analysis (Dersch et al., 2016) of 44 pooled trials, in which patients were stratified by whether or not they met European Federation of Neurological Societies (EFNS) criteria for probable/definite neuroborreliosis (LNB). In this analysis, no patients who had been treated for probable/definite LNB suffered from fatigue. Residual cognitive difficulty was observed in 1.6% of patients with probable/definite LNB but 16.7% with possible LNB, suggesting this was attributable to inaccurate diagnosis (see Chapter 8).

In view of the fact that a symptom complex identical to that of PTLDS occurs very frequently in the general population, perhaps in part due to other infectious and non-infectious stressors, there is the distinct possibility that in some proportion of patients with these symptoms, the association with Lyme disease is by chance – and an example of anchoring bias. With such a large noise to signal ratio, validating the existence of the syndrome in patients is daunting at best. Since it is a question that is widely encountered, it is worthwhile approaching it from a different perspective – biologic plausibility. This requires consideration of possible mechanisms by which it could be related to Lyme disease.

One theory maintains that spirochetes persist in unidentified tissue sites, thereby causing fatigue and other non-specific symptoms. Many theories on the mechanism of persistence assume that *B. burgdorferi* persists intracellularly, protected from extracellular antibiotics. However, tetracyclines readily penetrate cells. If refractory disease and/or continued symptoms were due to spirochetes persisting intracellularly, this would be expected to occur more commonly in beta-lactam-treated patients with Lyme disease than in those treated with tetracycline, which has never been demonstrated (Ljostad et al., 2008). Similarly, the observation that 8 weeks of doxycycline treatment is no more effective than placebo in patients with post-Lyme disease symptoms (Klempner et al., 2001) is difficult to understand if intracellular tetracycline-sensitive organisms are responsible.

Another theory is that *Borreliella* and other spirochetes form cysts that insulate them from both the host's immune defenses and the effects of antibiotic therapy. Interestingly, those who have supported this notion have never defined exactly what is meant by a 'cyst'. Under unfavorable *in vitro* growth conditions and in response to antibiotics, spirochetes often undergo morphological changes and develop a rounded appearance (see Chapter 2 in this volume). Although this is most likely due to the extrusion of cytoplasm due to reverse osmosis in cell wall or membrane deficient forms generated as a result of antibiotic therapy, such rounded forms are assumed to have survival value since they may revert to the original parental cell form within days after antibiotic therapy. In one experiment *B. burgdorferi* that had been cultured in the absence of serum, a necessary ingredient in growth media, survived for 8 days; however, such cultures were no longer viable at 2 weeks (Alban et al., 2000). Even those who previously reported on 'cyst' formation by *Borreliella* have now revised their terminology and refer to this morphological form as 'round bodies', a term apparently intended to encompass and replace prior descriptions such as coccoid bodies, globular bodies, spherical bodies, granules, cysts, L-forms, sphaeroplasts or vesicles (Brorson et al., 2009).

There are at least three fundamental concerns with theories that persistence of symptoms is due to persistence of *Borreliella* cells (Baker and Wormser, 2017). One is that carefully performed microbiologic evaluations have failed to find evidence of *B. burgdorferi* infection in treated patients with persistent subjective symptoms, including studies that have focused on occult central nervous system infection (Klempner, 2002; Kaplan et al., 2003; Krupp et al., 2003; Fallon et al., 2008). The second is that four NIH-sponsored, randomized, placebo-controlled trials of intensive antibiotic retreatment of US patients with persistent symptoms found that additional antibiotic therapy either provided no measurable benefit or a benefit so modest or ambiguous that it was outweighed by the risks associated with the treatment (Klempner et al., 2001; Krupp et al., 2003; Fallon et al., 2008). The third is the absence of a plausible mechanism by which spirochetal persistence, in the absence of a focus of inflammation or elaboration of a toxin, could cause fatigue and other non-specific symptoms. Genome sequencing studies provide no evidence that *Borreliella* sp. possess the genes required to make and secrete an exotoxin. Moreover, there is ample precedent for latent infections to be asymptomatic, as illustrated by the persistence of *Mycobacterium tuberculosis* in one-third of the world's population.

Given the evidence against persistent infection, another plausible mechanism might be the persistence of a triggered immune response, or the presence of an underlying immune phenotype that puts patients at risk – perhaps analogous to post-treatment Lyme arthritis. Evidence in support of the first possibility includes the finding of anti-neural antibodies (Chandra et al., 2010) in patients with post-treatment symptoms, as well as the earlier demonstration of cross-reactivity between antibodies to *B. burgdorferi* and neuronal antigens (Sigal and Tatum, 1988), and evidence of interactions between *B. burgdorferi* spirochetes and nervous system structures (Garcia Monco et al., 1991; 1992). Against this is the abundant evidence that PTLDS is not associated with either nervous system infection (at the outset or when symptoms occur) or inflammation (Ljostad and Mygland, 2009; Eikeland et al., 2013; Dersch et al., 2015; Eckman, 2018).

The third possibility is that PTLDS is a neurobehavioral response to the stressor of the illness, perhaps augmented by common perceptions about this being a common aftereffect. While depression and anxiety disorders occur in only a minority of patients with these symptoms, there is evidence that individuals with lower resilience (Hassett and Sigal, 2011) (see Chapter 15) and greater awareness of and sensitivity to symptoms in general are more likely to experience PTLDS. Such an explanation might well fit with the high prevalence of these symptoms in the population, insofar as they may represent a common response to a myriad of both physical and psychological stressors.

17.8 The State of the Medical Literature – the Assertion of the Controversy

The International Lyme and Associated Diseases Society (ILADS) has published a document titled 'Evidence assessments and guideline recommendations in Lyme disease: the clinical management of known tick bites, erythema migrans rashes and persistent disease' (Cameron et al., 2014). It repeatedly asserts that there is a wealth of information that is being ignored by the medical establishment. However, a detailed review of the ILADS document demonstrates that it references no Class I, Class II or even Class III evidence that rebuts the conclusions of the guidelines for the treatment of Lyme disease developed by the IDSA (Wormser et al., 2006) or the American Academy of Neurology (Halperin et al., 2007). It should be emphasized that the guidelines developed in 2006 by the IDSA are universally accepted and/or recommended by prestigious national and international experts on Lyme disease. This includes: the EFNS (Mygland et al., 2010); the European Union of Concerted Action on Lyme Borreliosis (www.aldf.com/pdf/ECCMID_Poster_4.22.10.pdf); the American Academy of Neurology (Halperin et al., 2007), whose guidelines are almost identical to those of the IDSA; the Canadian Public Health Network (Canadian Public Health Network, 2007); and the German Society for Hygiene and Microbiology (Nau et al., 2009). They also are in agreement with recommendations made by expert panels from at least ten European countries, that is, the Czech Republic, Denmark, Finland, France, the Netherlands, Norway, Poland, Slovenia, Sweden and Switzerland. None of these organizations or expert panels – as well as the NIH or the CDC – recommends extended antibiotic therapy for the treatment of Lyme disease. To date, a recent citation review indicates that the IDSA guidelines have been cited in the medical literature 1,548 times. This further attests to their widespread acceptance and use within the medical community.

In May of 2008, the IDSA entered into an agreement with the Connecticut Attorney General (AG) to voluntarily submit its Lyme disease guidelines to a special expert review panel to determine if they were based on sound medical and scientific evidence, and whether the guidelines should be modified or revised. To avoid conflict of interest issues, all members of the expert panel were selected through an open application process. An ombudsman was jointly selected by the IDSA and the AG to screen all applicants to ensure that each panel member was without any beneficial or financial interests related to Lyme disease, any financial relationship with an entity that has an interest in Lyme disease or any other potential conflict of interest. The chairperson as well as all panel members met the required criteria (Poretz, 2008). After multiple meetings, a public hearing, and extensive review of research and other information, the expert panel concluded in a full report that the recommendations contained in the IDSA guidelines of 2006 were medically and scientifically justified on the basis of all available evidence, and that no changes in the guidelines were warranted (Lantos et al., 2010). Although the IDSA guidelines are currently in the process of being updated to include the results of new or recent research, given currently available high quality studies it is highly unlikely there will be any major revisions.

Although there is no evidence to indicate that the symptoms associated with PTLDS are due to a persistent *Borreliella* infection, they are real and deserving of appropriate attention and care. In a recent report, the Institute of Medicine recommended a broad-based research and educational program that might offer promising solutions applicable to the management of medically unexplained syndromes and perhaps PTLDS (Baker, 2012). If a fraction of the time, money and energy that has been spent on inappropriate care and advocacy had, instead, been invested in scientific studies to better understand the pathophysiology of the disorder referred to as 'chronic Lyme disease' or PTLDS, we all would probably be in a much better position to help those unfortunate individuals whose lives have been severely disrupted by this symptom complex.

References

Aguero-Rosenfeld, M.E. and Wormser, G.P. (2015) Lyme disease: diagnostic issues and controversies. *Expert Review of Molecular Diagnostics* 15, 1–4.

Alban, P.S., Johnson, P.W. and Nelson, D.R. (2000) Serum-starvation-induced changes in protein synthesis and morphology of *Borrelia burgdorferi*. *Microbiology* 146, 119–127.

Anonymous (1995) Recommendations for test performance and interpretation from the second national conference on serologic diagnosis of Lyme disease. *Morbidity and Mortality Weekly Report* 44, 590–591.

Avery, R.A., Frank, G. and Eppes, S.C. (2005) Diagnostic utility of *Borrelia burgdorferi* cerebrospinal fluid polymerase chain reaction in children with Lyme meningitis. *Pediatric Infectious Disease Journal* 24, 705–708.

Baker, P.J. (2012) The pain of 'chronic Lyme disease': moving the discourse in a different direction. *FASEB J* 26, 11–12.

Baker, P.J. and Wormser, G.P. (2017) The clinical relevance of studies on *Borrelia burgdorferi* persisters. *American Journal of Medicine* 130, 1009–1010.

Benach, J.L., Bosler, E.M., Hanrahan, J.P. et al. (1983) Spirochetes isolated from the blood of two patients with Lyme disease. *New England Journal of Medicine* 308, 740–742.

Berende, A., ter Hofstede, H.J., Vos, F.J., van Middendorp, H., Vogelaar, M.L., Tromp, M., van den Hoogen, F.H., Donders, A.R., Evers, A.W. and Kullberg, B.J. (2016) Randomized trial of longer-term therapy for symptoms attributed to Lyme disease. *New England Journal of Medicine* 374, 1209–1220.

Blackwell, D. and Clarke, T.C. (2013) Percentage of adults who often felt very tired or exhausted in the past 3 months, by sex and age group – national health interview survey, United States, 2010–2011. *Morbidity and Mortality Weekly Report* 62, 275.

Branda, J.A., Linskey, K., Kim, Y.A., Steere, A.C. and Ferraro, M.J. (2011) Two-tiered antibody testing for Lyme disease with use of 2 enzyme immunoassays, a whole-cell sonicate enzyme immunoassay followed by a VlsE C6 peptide enzyme immunoassay. *Clinical Infectious Diseases* 53, 541–547.

Branda, J.A., Body, B.A., Boyle, J. et al. (2017) Advances in serodiagnostic testing for Lyme disease are at hand. *Clinical Infectious Diseases*. DOI: 10.1093/cid/cix943.

Brorson, O. and Brorson, S.H. (1998) In vitro conversion of *Borrelia burgdorferi* to cystic forms in spinal fluid, and transformation to mobile spirochetes by incubation in BSK-H medium. *Infection* 26, 144–150.

Brorson, O. and Brorson, S.H. (1999) An in vitro study of the susceptibility of mobile and cystic forms of *Borrelia burgdorferi* to metronidazole. *Apmis* 107, 566–576.

Brorson, Ø., Brorson, S.H., Scythes, J., Macallister, J., Wier, A. and Margulis, L. (2009) Destruction of spirochete *Borrelia burgdorferi* round-body propagules (RBs) by the antibiotic tigecycline. *Proceedings of the National Academy of Sciences of the USA* 106, 18656–18661.

Burgdorfer, W., Barbour, A.G., Hayes, S.F., Benach, J.L., Grunwaldt, E. and Davis, J.P. (1982) Lyme disease: a tick borne spirochetosis? *Science* 216, 1317–1319.

Cameron, D.J., Johnson, L.B. and Maloney, E.L. (2014) Evidence assessments and guideline recommendations in Lyme disease: the clinical management of known tick bites, erythema migrans rashes and persistent disease. *Expert Review of Anti-infective Therapy* 12, 1103–1135.

Canadian Public Health Network (2007) The laboratory diagnosis of Lyme borreliosis: guidelines from the Canadian Public Health Laboratory. In: Laboratory CPH (ed.) *Canadian Public Health Laboratory*, pp. 145–148.

Centers for Disease, Control and Prevention (CDC) (2013) Three sudden cardiac deaths associated with Lyme carditis – United States, November 2012–July 2013. *Morbidity and Mortality Weekly Report* 62, 993–996.

Cerar, D., Cerar, T., Ružić-Sabljić, E., Wormser, G.P. and Strle, F. (2010) Subjective symptoms after treatment of early Lyme disease. *American Journal of Medicine* 123, 79–86.

Chandra, A., Wormser, G.P., Klempner, M.S., Trevino, R.P., Crow, M.K., Latov, N. and Alaedini, A. (2010) Anti-neural antibody reactivity in patients with a history of Lyme borreliosis and persistent symptoms. *Brain, Behavior, and Immunity* 2010, 1018–1024.

Dattwyler, R.J., Volkman, D.J., Luft, B.J., Halperin, J.J., Thomas, J. and Golightly, M.G. (1988) Seronegative Lyme disease. Dissociation of specific T- and B-lymphocyte responses to *Borrelia burgdorferi*. *New England Journal of Medicine* 319, 1441–1446.

Dersch, R., Sarnes, A.A., Maul, M., Hottenrott, T., Baumgartner, A., Rauer, S. and Stich, O. (2015) Quality of life, fatigue, depression and cognitive impairment in Lyme neuroborreliosis. *Journal of Neurology* 262, 2572–2577.

Dersch, R., Sommer, H., Rauer, S. and Meerpohl, J.J. (2016) Prevalence and spectrum of residual symptoms in Lyme neuroborreliosis after pharmacological treatment: a systematic review. *Journal of Neurology* 263, 17–24.

Dressler, F., Whalen, J.A., Reinhardt, B.N. and Steere, A.C. (1993) Western blotting in the serodiagnosis of Lyme disease. *Journal of Infectious Diseases* 167, 392–400.

Eckman, E.A., Pacheco-Quinto, J., Herdt, A.R. and Halperin, J.J. (2018) Neuroimmunomodulators in neuroborreliosis and Lyme encephalopathy. *Clinical Infectious Diseases*. DOI: https://doi.org/10.1093/cid/ciy019.

Eikeland, R., Mygland, A., Herlofson, K. and Ljostad, U. (2013) Risk factors for a non-favorable outcome after treated European neuroborreliosis. *Acta Neurologica Scandinavica* 127, 154–160.

Fallon, B.A., Keilp, J.G., Corbera, K.M., Petkova, E., Britton, C.B., Dwyer, E., Slavov, I., Cheng, J., Dobkin, J., Nelson, D.R. and Sackeim, H.A. (2008) A randomized, placebo-controlled trial of repeated IV antibiotic therapy for Lyme encephalopathy. *Neurology* 70, 992–1003.

Garcia Monco, J.C., Villar, B.F., Szczepanski, A. and Benach, J.L. (1991) Cytotoxicity of *Borrelia burgdorferi* for cultured rat glial cells. *Journal of Infectious Diseases* 163, 1362–1366.

Garcia Monco, J.C., Fernandez, V.B., Rogers, R.C., Szczepanski, A., Wheeler, C.M. and Benach, J.L. (1992) *Borrelia burgdorferi* and other related spirochetes bind to galactocerebroside. *Neurology* 42, 1341–1348.

Halperin, J.J., Pass, H.L., Anand, A.K., Luft, B.J., Volkman, D.J. and Dattwyler, R.J. (1988) Nervous system abnormalities in Lyme disease. *Annals of the New York Academy of Sciences* 539, 24–34.

Halperin, J.J., Krupp, L.B., Golightly, M.G. and Volkman, D.J. (1990) Lyme borreliosis-associated encephalopathy. *Neurology* 40, 1340–1343.

Halperin, J.J., Heyes, M.P., Keller, T.L. and Whitman, M. (1992) Neuroborreliosis – encephalopathy vs encephalitis. *Proceedings of the Vth International Conference on Lyme Borreliosis, Arlington, Virginia, May 1992. Abstr. 1.*, 1.

Halperin, J.J., Baker, P. and Wormser, G.P. (2013) Common misconceptions about Lyme disease. *The American Journal of Medicine* 126, 264.e1-7.

Halperin, J.J., Shapiro, E.D., Logigian, E.L., Belman, A.L., Dotevall, L., Wormser, G.P., Krupp, L.B., Gronseth, G. and Bever, C. (2007) Practice parameter: treatment of nervous system Lyme disease. *Neurology* 69, 91–102.

Hammers Berggren, S., Hansen, K., Lebech, A.M. and Karlsson, M. (1993) *Borrelia burgdorferi*-specific intrathecal antibody production in neuroborreliosis: a follow-up study. *Neurology* 43, 169–175.

Hassett, A.L. and Sigal, L.H. (2011) The psychology of 'post Lyme disease syndrome' and 'not Lyme'. In: Halperin, J.J. (ed.) *Lyme Disease – An Evidence Based Approach*. CAB International, Wallingford, UK, pp. 232–247.

Hemmer, B., Vergelli, M., Pinilla, C., Houghten, R. and Martin, R. (1998) Probing degeneracy in T-cell recognition using peptide combinatorial libraries. *Immunology Today* 19, 163–168.

Hollander, D.H., Turner, T.B. and Nell, E.E. (1952) The effect of long continued subcurative doses of penicillin during the incubation period of experimental syphilis. *Bulletin of the Johns Hopkins Hospital* 90, 105–120.

Holzbauer, S.M., Kemperman, M.M. and Lynfield, R. (2010) Death due to community associated *Clostridium difficile* in a woman receiving prolonged antibiotic therapy for suspected Lyme disease. *Clinical Infectious Diseases* 51, 368–369.

Institute of Medicine (US) Committee on Advancing Pain Research, Control and Education (2011) *Relieving Pain in America: A Blueprint for Transforming Prevention, Care, Education, and Research*. National Academies Press (US), Washington, DC.

Kaplan, R.F., Trevino, R.P., Johnson, G.M., Levy, L., Dornbush, R., Hu, L.T., Evans, J., Weinstein, A., Schmid, C.H. and Klempner, M.S. (2003) Cognitive function in post-treatment Lyme disease: do additional antibiotics help? *Neurology* 60, 1916–1922.

Klempner, M.S. (2002) Controlled trials of antibiotic treatment in patients with post-treatment chronic Lyme disease. *Vector Borne and Zoonotic Diseases* 2, 255–263.

Klempner, M.S., Hu, L.T., Evans, J. et al. (2001) Two controlled trials of antibiotic treatment in patients with persistent symptoms and a history of Lyme disease. *New England Journal of Medicine* 345, 85–92.

Klempner, M.S., Baker, P.J., Shapiro, E.D., Marques, A., Dattwyler, R.J., Halperin, J.J. and Wormser, G.P. (2013) Treatment trials for post-Lyme disease symptoms revisited. *American Journal of Medicine* 126, 665–669.

Krupp, L.B., Masur, D., Schwartz, J., Coyle, P.K., Langenbach, L.J., Fernquist, S., Jandorf, L. and Halperin, J.J. (1991) Cognitive functioning in late Lyme borreliosis. *Archives of Neurology* 48, 1125–1129.

Krupp, L.B., Hyman, L.G., Grimson, R., Coyle, P.K., Melville, P., Ahnn, S., Dattwyler, R. and Chandler, B. (2003) Study and treatment of post Lyme disease (STOP-LD): a randomized double masked clinical trial. *Neurology* 60, 1923–1930.

Kugeler, K.J., Griffith, K.S., Gould, L.H., Kochanek, K., Delorey, M.J., Biggerstaff, B.J. and Mead, P.S. (2011) A review of death certificates listing Lyme disease as a cause of death in the United States. *Clinical Infectious Diseases* 52, 364–367.

Lamaison, D. (2007) Cardiac involvement in Lyme disease. *Médecine et Maladies Infectieuses* 37, 511–517.

Lantos, P.M., Charini, W.A., Medoff, G., Moro, M.H., Mushatt, D.M., Parsonnet, J., Sanders, J.W. and Baker, C.J. (2010) Final report of the Lyme disease review panel of the Infectious Diseases Society of America. *Clinical Infectious Diseases* 51, 1–5.

Lebech, A.M., Hansen, K., Brandrup, F., Clemmensen, O. and Halkier-Sorensen, L. (2000) Diagnostic value of PCR for detection of *Borrelia burgdorferi* DNA in clinical specimens from patients with erythema migrans and Lyme neuroborreliosis. *Molecular Diagnosis* 5, 139–150.

Lipsett, S.C., Branda, J.A., McAdam, A.J., Vernacchio, L., Gordon, C.D., Gordon, C.R. and Nigrovic, L.E. (2016) Evaluation of the C6 Lyme enzyme immunoassay for the diagnosis of Lyme disease in children and adolescents. *Clinical Infectious Diseases* 63, 922–928.

Ljostad, U. and Mygland, A. (2009) Remaining complaints 1 year after treatment for acute Lyme neuroborreliosis; frequency, pattern and risk factors. *European Journal of Neurology* 17, 118–123.

Ljostad, U., Skogvoll, E., Eikeland, R., Midgard, R., Skarpaas, T., Berg, A. and Mygland, A. (2008) Oral doxycycline versus intravenous ceftriaxone for European Lyme neuroborreliosis: a multicentre, non-inferiority, double-blind, randomised trial. *Lancet Neurology* 7, 690–695.

Logigian, E.L., Kaplan, R.F. and Steere, A.C. (1990) Chronic neurologic manifestations of Lyme disease. *New England Journal of Medicine* 323, 1438–1444.

Luo, N., Johnson, J., Shaw, J., Feeny, D. and Coons, S. (2005) Self-reported health status of the general adult U.S. population as assessed by the EQ-5D and Health Utilities Index. *Medical Care* 43, 1078–1086.

MacDonald, A.B. (2006) Spirochetal cyst forms in neurodegenerative disorders, … hiding in plain sight. *Medical Hypotheses* 67, 819–832.

Magnarelli, L.A., Anderson, J. and Johnson, R.C. (1987) Cross reactivity in serologic tests for Lyme disease and other spirochetal infections. *Journal of Infectious Diseases* 156, 183–188.

Maloy, A.L., Black, R.D. and Segurola Jr, R.J. (1998) Lyme disease complicated by the Jarisch-Herxheimer reaction. *Journal of Emergency Medicine* 16, 437–438.

Marcus, L.C., Steere, A.C. and Duray, P.H. (1985) Fatal pancarditis in a patient with coexisting Lyme disease and babesiosis. *Annals of Internal Medicine* 103, 374–376.

Marzec, N.S., Nelson, C., Waldron, P.R., Blackburn, B.G., Hosain, S., Greenhow, T., Green, G.M., Lomen-Hoerth, C., Golden, M. and Mead, P.S. (2017) Serious bacterial infections acquired during treatment of patients given a diagnosis of chronic Lyme disease – United States. *Morbidity and Mortality Weekly Report* 66, 607–609.

Mygland, A., Ljostad, U., Fingerle, V., Rupprecht, T., Schmutzhard, E. and Steiner, I. (2010) EFNS guidelines on the diagnosis and management of European Lyme neuroborreliosis. *European Journal of Neurology* 17, 8–16, e11–e14.

Nau, R., Christen, H.-J. and Eiffert, H. (2009) Lyme disease – current state of knowledge. *Deutsches Ärzteblatt International* 106, 72–82.

Nelson, C.A., Saha, S., Kugeler, K.J., Delorey, M.J., Shankar, M.B., Hinckley, A.F. and Mead, P.S. (2015) Incidence of clinician-diagnosed Lyme disease, United States, 2005–2010. *Emerging Infectious Diseases* 21, 1625–1631.

Oksi, J., Nikoskelainen, J., Hiekkanen, H. *et al.* (2007) Duration of antibiotic treatment in disseminated Lyme borreliosis: a double-blind, randomized, placebo-controlled, multicenter clinical study. *European Journal of Clinical Microbiology and Infectious Diseases* 26, 571–581.

Patel, R., Grogg, K.L., Edwards, W.D., Wright, A.J. and Schwenk, N.M. (2000) Death from inappropriate therapy for Lyme disease. *Clinical Infectious Diseases* 31, 1107–1109.

Philipp, M.T., Marques, A.R., Fawcett, P.T., Dally, L.G. and Martin, D.S. (2003) C6 test as an indicator of therapy outcome for patients with localized or disseminated Lyme borreliosis. *Journal of Clinical Microbiology* 41, 4955–4960.

Poretz, D.M. (2008) Clarification of the Agreement between the Infectious Diseases Society of America and the Attorney General of Connecticut. *Clinical Infectious Diseases* 47, 1200.

Roux, F., Boyer, E., Jaulhac, B., Dernis, E., Closs-Prophette, F. and Puechal, X. (2007) Lyme meningoradiculitis: prospective evaluation of biological diagnosis methods. *European Journal of Clinical Microbiology and Infectious Diseases* 26, 685–693.

Rovery, C., Greub, G., Lepidi, H., Casalta, J.-P., Habib, G., Collart, F. and Raoult, D. (2005) PCR detection of bacteria on cardiac valves of patients with treated bacterial endocarditis. *Journal of Clinical Microbiology* 43, 163–167.

Rupprecht, T.A., Lechner, C., Tumani, H. and Fingerle, V. (2014) [CXCL13: a biomarker for acute Lyme neuroborreliosis : investigation of the predictive value in the clinical routine]. *Nervenarzt* 85, 459–464.

Salazar, J.C., Gerber, M.A. and Goff, C.W. (1993) Long-term outcome of Lyme disease in children given early treatment. *Journal of Pediatrics* 122, 591–593.

Seltzer, E.G., Gerber, M.A., Cartter, M.L., Freudigman, K. and Shapiro, E.D. (2000) Long-term outcomes of persons with Lyme disease. *Journal of the American Medical Association (JAMA)* 283, 609–616.

Shadick, N.A., Phillips, C.B., Logigian, E.L. et al. (1994) The long-term clinical outcomes of Lyme disease. A population-based retrospective cohort study. *Annals of Internal Medicine* 121, 560–567.

Shadick, N.A., Phillips, C.B., Sangha, O. et al. (1999) Musculoskeletal and neurologic outcomes in patients with previously treated Lyme disease. *Annals of Internal Medicine* 131, 919–926.

Sigal, L.H. and Tatum, A.H. (1988) Lyme disease patients' serum contains IgM antibodies to *Borrelia burgdorferi* that cross-react with neuronal antigens. *Neurology* 38, 1439–1442.

Sillanpaa, H., Skogman, B.H., Sarvas, H., Seppala, I.J. and Lahdenne, P. (2013) Cerebrospinal fluid chemokine CXCL13 in the diagnosis of neuroborreliosis in children. *Scandinavian Journal of Infectious Diseases* 45, 526–530.

Steere, A.C., Malawista, S.E., Hardin, J.A., Ruddy, S., Askenase, W. and Andiman, W.A. (1977) Erythema chronicum migrans and Lyme arthritis. The enlarging clinical spectrum. *Annals of Internal Medicine* 86, 685–698.

Steere, A.C., Grodzicki, R.L., Kornblatt, A.N., Craft, J.E., Barbour, A.G., Burgdorfer, W., Schmid, G.P., Johnson, E. and Malawista, S.E. (1983) The spirochetal etiology of Lyme disease. *New England Journal of Medicine* 308, 733–740.

Stupica, D., Veluscek, M., Blagus, R. et al. (2018) Oral doxycycline versus intravenous ceftriaxone for treatment of multiple erythema migrans: an open-label alternate-treatment observational trial. *Journal of Antimicrobial Chemotherapy*. DOI: 10.1093/jac/dkx534.

Tavora, F., Burke, A., Li, L., Franks, T.J. and Virmani, R. (2008) Postmortem confirmation of Lyme carditis with polymerase chain reaction. *Cardiovascular Pathology* 17, 103–107.

Vermeersch, P., Resseler, S., Nackers, E. and Lagrou, K. (2009) The C6 Lyme antibody test has low sensitivity for antibody detection in cerebrospinal fluid. *Diagnostic Microbiology and Infectious Disease* 64, 347–349.

Weber, K., Preac-Mursic, V., Neubert, U., Thurmayr, R., Herzer, P., Wilske, B., Schierz, G. and Marget, W. (1988) Antibiotic therapy of early European Lyme borreliosis and acrodermatitis chronica atrophicans. *Annals of the New York Academy of Sciences* 539, 324–345.

Wills, A.B., Spaulding, A.B., Adjemian, J., Prevots, D.R., Turk, S.P., Williams, C. and Marques, A. (2016) Long-term follow-up of patients with Lyme disease: longitudinal analysis of clinical and quality-of-life measures. *Clinical Infectious Diseases* 62, 1546–1551.

Wormser, G.P. and Wormser, V. (2016) Did Garin and Bujadoux actually report a case of Lyme radiculoneuritis? *Open Forum on Infectious Diseases* 3, ofw085.

Wormser, G.P., Dattwyler, R.J., Shapiro, E.D. et al. (2006) The clinical assessment, treatment, and prevention of Lyme disease, human granulocytic anaplasmosis, and babesiosis: clinical practice guidelines by the infectious diseases society of America. *Clinical Infectious Diseases* 43, 1089–1134.

Wormser, G.P., Schriefer, M., Aguero-Rosenfeld, M.E., Levin, A., Steere, A.C., Nadelman, R.B., Nowakowski, J., Marques, A., Johnson, B.J. and Dumler, J.S. (2013) Single-tier testing with the C6 peptide ELISA kit compared with two-tier testing for Lyme disease. *Diagnostic Microbiology and Infectious Disease* 75, 9–15.

Wormser, G.P., Weitzner, E., McKenna, D., Nadelman, R.B., Scavarda, C., Molla, I., Dornbush, R., Visintainer, P. and Nowakowski, J. (2015a) Long-term assessment of health-related quality of life in patients with culture-confirmed early Lyme disease. *Clinical Infectious Diseases* 61, 244–247.

Wormser, G.P., Weitzner, E., McKenna, D., Nadelman, R.B., Scavarda, C. and Nowakowski, J. (2015b) Long-term assessment of fatigue in patients with culture-confirmed Lyme disease. *American Journal of Medicine* 128, 181–184.

Index

Page numbers in **bold** type refer to figures, tables and boxed text.

acaricides 14–15
acrodermatitis chronica atrophicans (ACA)
    clinical manifestation 111–112
    historical recognition 105
age-related effects
    ACA occurrence 111
    clinical feature frequency 83
    disease incidence 83, **84**, 216–217
agents, Lyme disease 29–30, 32–34, 76–77
aggregates, bacterial **39**, 39–40
'alternatively diagnosed chronic Lyme syndrome'
    (ADCLS) 231, 248
amber hypothesis 188
Amblyomma americanum 150
American College of Rheumatology (ACR) 236
amoxicillin 154, 155
Anaplasma spp. 12
    A. phagocytophilum 97, 98
anchoring bias 230, 269–270, **270**, 271
anti-inflammatory agents 175
antibiotic-refractory arthritis 97, 189, 190–191, 232
antibiotics
    adverse reactions to treatment 175, 254–255
    bacterial persistence 38–39, 99, 188,
        228–229, 252
    demand from patients 230, 269
    extended treatment 130–131, 155, 192–193,
        231, 252–254
    pathogen susceptibility, *in vitro* testing 93–94
    persistence of pain after treatment 186
    recommended for Bb infections 95–97, **96**,
        115, 130, **221**
    recommended for EM treatment 155–156, **156**
    therapy effectiveness 45, 51, 192, 194, 263
    used in prospective treatment trials 153–155
    see also doxycycline
antibodies
    cross-reaction in serological tests 63–64, 265
    immune complexes 182–183
    targets of, epitopes in Bb 48–50
antibody index (AI) 65, 128, 141
antigens
    epitopes for antibody response 48–50
    molecular mimicry 170, 190–191
    recombinant, compared with WCS 129
    used in EIA diagnostic tests 61–62
anxiety disorders 227, 233, 272
arthralgias 157, 181–182, 193
arthritis
    association with Bb infection 83, 114, 185
    in children 218
    clinical signs and symptoms 182–186
    diagnosis using PCR 66, 183
    first identification of Lyme arthritis 106, 180
    following untreated EM 153
    treatment options 97, 191–196
Asia, disease incidence 80
assays
    cellular 50–51
    serological 48–50, 60–66
    see also ELISA
atropine 175
azithromycin 154–155

Babesia spp. 12
babesiosis 98, 150, 152, 251
background seropositivity 64

Bannwarth's syndrome (meningo-polyradiculo-neuritis)
    clinical signs 112–113, 124–125
    first description of 106
    frequency in Europe and USA 109, 205–206,
        210, 218
behaviour, ticks
    feeding 11–12
    host questing 7, 82
beta lactams 96, 98, 130, 272
biofilms 39–40
biogeographical history, ticks 3–5
biological control, ticks 15
birds, as tick hosts 6, 9–10
blood transfusion 85
'*Borrelia burgdorferi* sensu lato' 29, 34
Borrelia miyamotoi (RF pathogen) 12, 31
Borreliella spp.
    B. afzelii 34, 35, 47–48
    B. bavariensis 124
    B. garinii 32, 34, 35
    B. mayonii 32, 35, 147
    B. spielmanii 34, 109, 110, 124
    Lyme disease agents 32–34, 35, 76, 108–109
    no-/low-risk species 34, 76–77
    taxonomy, phylogram 29, **33**
Borreliella burgdorferi (Bb)
    aggregate formation **39**, 39–40
    biological characteristics 30–31, 46
    infection mechanisms 31–32, 187–191
    intracellular viability 32
    laboratory culture 36–37, 66–67
    persistence (antibiotic survival) 38–39, 99,
        271–272
    strains 4, 34, 35–36
borreliosis (Lyme disease, LB)
    description 93
    disease recognition, history 105–107
    historical identification of 107
brain abnormalities 229
'brain fog' 227, 267–268
bridge vectors 3, 11
BSK (Barbour-Stoenner-Kelly) culture medium
    36–37, 150
'bull's eye' rash 142, 145, 217
Burgdorfer, Willy 107

C6 peptide antigen 49, 61–62
cardiac pacing 175, 218
cardiomyopathy, dilated 171–172
carditis
    association with *Borreliella* infection 113–114,
        169–170
    clinical manifestations 170–172
    diagnosis 172–174
    frequency of cases 83, 168–169, 218
    prognosis 175–176
    treatment 174–175, 176

case control studies 126, 254
cefotaxime 97
ceftriaxone
    as parenteral agent 97, 211
    RCT testing fatigue/cognitive improvement
        252, **253**, 254
    treatment trial, compared with doxycycline 154
cefuroxime axetil, compared with doxycycline 154
cellular assays 50–51
cellulitis, bacterial 149
Centers for Disease Control and Prevention (CDC) 45,
    142, 168, 247, 263
centralized pain syndromes 237
cephalosporins 94
cerebral vasculitis 125
cerebrospinal fluid (CSF)
    antibody index 65–66, 128
    clinical signs of LNB 106, 113, 127
    CXCL13 biomarker 66, 128
    pleocytosis 127–128, 206, 207
chemoprophylaxis 94–95, 115, 222–223
children
    antimicrobial treatment recommendations
        156, **156**, 194, 220, **221**
    clinical manifestations **217**, 217–218, **218**
    diagnosis of Lyme disease 219–220, 223–224
    disease incidence 83, 169, 216–217
    earlobe lymphocytoma 110–111, 218
    facial nerve palsy 113, 217, 220
    outcomes, prognosis 220–221
    pseudotumor cerebri-like effects 206, 218
cholestyramine 192, 231
chronic dilated cardiomyopathy 171–172
chronic fatigue syndrome 196, 236, 250
'chronic Lyme disease' (CLD)
    categories of patients 228–232, 247–248, **248**
    concept development 237–241, 262–264
    patient perceptions 232, 247, 264
    types of complaint attributed to CLD 227, 248
    see also post-treatment syndrome (PTLDS)
climate change, and vector expansion 10, 80, 139
'clinical judgement' 267
clinical manifestations
    in children **217**, 217–218, **218**
    epidemiological aspects 83–85, **108**,
        108–109, **169**
    heart 113–114, 170–172
    historical recognition of 105–106
    joints and muscles 114, 181–187
    less common/uncertain manifestations 114
    nervous system 112–113, 205–210, **211**
    skin 109–112, **143**, 144–146, **145**
clothing, protective 15
co-infections 12, 97–98, 150, 152, 218–219
Cochrane Collaboration 126
cognitive impairment 133–135, 204, **209**, 230,
    263–264
    'brain fog' 227, 267–268

cognitive–behavioural therapy (CBT) 240, 241
complement, susceptibility of Bb strains 36, 46
conduction disease 170–171, 175
congenital Lyme disease 158, 222
CRASP lipoproteins 46
'creative' therapies 192
cross-sectional studies 126, 231, 250
crystal-induced arthritic disease 184
cultures, bacterial
    limitations for diagnostic testing 67
    media and methods 36–37, 66–67
'cure,' assessment of success 99, 269
cutaneous lymphoma 112
CXCL13 chemokine 66, 110, 128, 207
cysts, spirochaete (round bodies) 37–38, 272
cytokines, production in immune response 47–48, 50, 170, 188

deaths 85, 171, 268
decorin-binding proteins (Dbp) 31, 49, 51
deer
    population control measures 15
    as tick hosts 5, 6, 8, 9
    white-tailed, populations 4
DEET (N, N-diethyl-meta-toluamide) 15, 222
depression/anxiety 227, 233, 272
dermatological manifestations
    association with *B. afzelii* infection 84
    differential diagnosis 148–150, **149**, **151**
    multiple lesions **144**, 147, 148, 217, **218**
    types 109–112
    see also erythema migrans (EM)
diagnosis
    accuracy improvement, new approaches 52, 67–68
    in children, parental demands 219, 223–224
    culture of pathogen from patient samples 36, 67, 147
    EFNS criteria for neuroborreliosis 112, 126–127, **127**
    incorrect, grounds for suspecting 195, 231–232
    laboratory assays 45–52, 60–66
    PCR, direct pathogen detection 66, 266
    role of 'clinical judgement' 267
    strategies, utility and limitations 58–60, 114–115, **152**, 152–153, 181
differential diagnosis
    grounds for considering Lyme disease 266–267
    musculoskeletal effects 182, 183–184
    neurological features 206
    skin clinical manifestations 148–150, **149**, **151**
disease
    agents 29–30, 32–34, 76–77
    clinical manifestations 83–85, 105–106, 109–114, **169**
    course and prognosis 131–132, 217–218
    incidence 78–83, 108, 216
    patients' subjective experience 234–235, 238
    see also infection; transmission
disease conviction 232
dispersal, ticks 9–10
dogs 78–79
doxycycline
    adverse reactions and contraindications 155
    oral neuroborreliosis treatment 95–96, 130
    prophylactic dose after tick bite 94–95, 222–223
    trials, comparison with alternatives 154, 155

ecology
    human microbiome 251
    microbial, in *I. ricinus* complex 12–13
    and tick population dynamics 8
education
    of patients, and reassurance 241
    of primary care practitioners 148, 273
    tick bite prevention 15, 157
efflux pumps, bacterial 94
electrocardiography (EKG) 172–173, **173**, **174**
ELISA (enzyme-linked immunosorbent assay)
    C6 assay 49, 51, 153, 266
    comparing CSF and serum 207–208
    diagnostic value of tests 264–265
encephalitis, Lyme disease 206–207
encephalitis, tick-borne 10, 12, 150
encephalomyelitis 125, 133, 208, 268
encephalopathy 204, 205, 208–209, **209**
enthesitis 193
entomological risk index 13, 16
enzyme immunoassays (EIA) 60–62
epidemiology
    frequency of clinical features 83–85, **108**, 108–109
    Lyme disease in children 216–217
    regional distribution of cases 78–82, **81–82**, 108
    seasonal variation 82, 107
    see also transmission
epitopes 48–50, 190–191
erythema migrans (EM)
    alternative causes of clinical signs 148–150, **149**, **151**
    frequency of cases 83, 143–144
    historical descriptions of 105–106, 145
    laboratory diagnostic tests **152**, 152–153
    as localized inflammatory response 47, 142, 217
    long-term outcomes 135, 153, 156–158, **249**, 249–250
    recommended antibiotic therapy 95, 155–156, **156**
    repeat episodes 159
    symptoms and clinical diagnosis 110, **143**, 144–148, **145**

Eurasia, distribution of agents/vectors 4, 33–34
Europe
  agent and vector species 107, 108–109
  attention to neurological aspects 202
  disease incidence 80, 108, **125**
European Federation of Neurological Societies (EFNS) 112, 126–127
evidence-based medicine 125–126, 130–131, 196, 238
evolution
  Lyme disease agents (*Borreliella* spp.) 32
  ticks (*Ixodes* spp.) 3–5, 6
eye, involvement in Lyme disease 114, 206, 210

facial nerve palsy 113, 140, 147, 210, 212
false negative results, serology 63, 153, 265
false positive results
  adverse consequences 182
  due to non-standard testing 59, 60, 248, 252
  and 'possible LNB' definition 131–132, **140**, 140–141, 219
  in serology, causes 31, 63–64, 65, 208, 265
fatigue 133, 135, 157, 186, 238
feeding behaviour, ticks 11–12
fibromyalgia 158, 186–187, 196, 230, 235–236
flagellin (Fla) 49, 191
flagging (vegetation sampling) 13
flaviviruses 12

gender-related effects
  carditis frequency 168–169
  clinical feature frequency 84–85
  disease incidence 82–83, **84**
genome characteristics 30, 272
genotypes (RSTs)
  genotyping methods 35
  variation related to reinfections 159
  virulence 36, 147–148
geographic information systems (GIS) 13
geographical distribution
  Borreliella spp. 32–34, 76–77
  Lyme borreliosis cases 78–82, **81–82**
  range expansion of ticks 8–10
  of tick vectors **2**, **77**, 77–78
glucocorticoids 175, 176
gout 184
guidelines
  IDSA recommendations 98–99, **156**, 192, 262, 273
  issued by patient advocacy groups 273
  Lyme neuroborreliosis treatment 130–131

heart
  biopsies 174
  diagnostic imaging methods 172–174, **173**, **174**
  telemetry (cardiac pacing) 175
  tissues infiltrated by Bb 169
  see also carditis
heat shock proteins 191
history, Lyme disease
  Connecticut 'outbreak' 216, 263
  diagnostic strategies 60
  discovery of cause 60, 107, 262
  recognition and early treatments 105–106, 180
hosts (of ticks) 5–6
human granulocytic anaplasmosis (HGA) 97, 98, 150
humans
  B. burgdorferi infection mechanisms 31–32
  behaviour and nervous system function **203**, 203–204
  compared with mouse models 95
  contact with ticks, risks and control 13–16
  disease severity and pathogen strain 36
hydroxychloroquine 192, 195
hyperbaric therapy 192
hypersensitivity reaction, to tick bite **144**, 148–149, **149**

IgG
  in blood/synovial fluid, Lyme arthritis 182
  in CSF, late neuroborreliosis 127, 207
  presence in ACA patients 111
IgM
  intrathecal synthesis in CSF 127
  reliability of immunoblots 64–65
immune complexes, serum 182–183
immune system
  adaptive responses 48–50, 159, 188
  dysregulation 251
  innate responses 46–48, 187
  role in recovery 99
immunoblots
  IgM and IgG, reliability compared 64–65, 265, 266
  role in diagnosis 181
  for second-tier serological testing **62**, 62–63, 64
immunofluorescence assays (IFAs) 60
immunosuppression
  effects of tick saliva 48
  immunocompromised patient outcomes 158–159
  lack of evidence for, in Bb 229
incidence, Lyme disease
  age-/sex-related 82–83, **84**, 168–169, 216
  reasons for underestimates 143–144
  regional analysis 78–82, **81–82**, 108, **125**
  reporting systems 124
  seasonality 82
incubation period 111
infection

management guidelines 98–99
mechanisms in mammals 31–32
pathogenesis and immune responses 187–191, 205, 210–211
prevention strategies 94–95
related to pathogen species and strains 35, 36
stages 45–46
Infectious Diseases Society of America (IDSA) 98–99, **156**, 192, 262, 273
inflammatory response
    anti-inflammatory agents 175
    autonomous (self-perpetuating) 190
    differential diagnosis of causes 183–184
    innate immunity responses 46–48, 187
    maladaptive macrophage activity 169–170
    persistent, due to residual debris 188, 189, 230, 251
    to tick bite, local 142, **144**
interferon (IFN) 47, 51, 230, 251
International Lyme and Associated Diseases Society (ILADS) 130, 273
intrathecal antibody (ITAb) production 207, 208
Ixodes spp.
    I. dammini, taxon status 3–4
    I. pacificus (western black-legged tick) 8, 32, 34
    I. persulcatus (taiga tick) 6, 8, 34
    I. ricinus (sheep tick) 4, 6, 33–34
    I. scapularis (black-legged/deer tick) 1, 4, 32–33
    I. uriae (seabird tick) 3, 34
Ixodes ricinus complex
    guild of associated pathogens 12, 97–98
    life cycles 5–8
    vertebrate hosts 5–6
    see also ticks

Jarisch-Herxheimer-like reaction 95, 153, 175, 220, 264
joints
    non-Lyme causes of pain/swelling 183–184
    patellofemoral, dysfunction 184–186
    sites affected by *Borreliella* infection 114, 182, 185
    symptoms following untreated EM 153, 181–182
    see also arthritis

killing
    complement-mediated 46
    by NKT cells 50
knee
    Lyme arthritis symptoms/diagnosis 182–184
    physical therapy 196
    trauma, injury signs/symptoms 184

laboratory culture of isolates 36–37, 66–67
laboratory-developed tests (LDTs) 37, 59, 63, 238
landscape features, and tick exposure 13–14
legislation 240, 262
leptospirosis 94
LFA-1 (lymphocyte function associated antigen 1) 190–191
life cycles, tick 5–8
lipoproteins
    as antigens, immune response to 46, 47
    see also outer-surface proteins
lizards, as tick hosts 5, 36
LLMDs *see* 'Lyme literate doctors'
lupus erythematosus 182, 186, 195, 238
Lyme disease *see* borreliosis (Lyme disease)
'Lyme literate doctors' (LLMDs)
    and activist/media support 223, 232, 239–240
    diagnostic tests advocated 183
    (mis)use of academic data 267
    therapies suggested 192, 232, 239, 264
    see also 'chronic Lyme disease'
lymphocytic meningitis 206, 267
lymphocytoma, borrelial 106, 110–111, 218

macrophage activity 170
magnetic resonance imaging (MRI) 205, 268
mammals
    B. burgdorferi infection 31–32
    intracellular viability of spirochaetes 32
    tick hosts, types 5, 6
Masters' disease (STARI) 142, 150, **151**
meningitis 125, 206, 218
meningo-(poly)radiculitis *see* Bannwarth's syndrome
meningoencephalitis 106
methotrexate 195
metronidazole 38
mice
    bait boxes, for tick control 14
    immunodeficient 50, 170
    used as models for pathogenesis study 169, 190
microbiome, human 251
migratory polyarthralgias 181, 182
Millon Clinical Multiaxial Inventory (MCMI) 234
minimum bactericidal concentration (MBC) 93–94
MKP (modified Kelly–Pettenkofer) culture medium 36–37
modified two-tier testing (MTTT) 67
molecular biologic therapies 195–196
molecular mimicry 170, 190–191
mono-arthritis 180, 182–184, 185
monoclonal antibodies 107
'Montauk knee' 180
morphological variants, spirochaetes 37–38
mortality 85, 171, 268
multiplex assays 49–50, 52
murine model *see* mice

myalgias 182
myocarditis 171
myths
    continued antibiotic therapy will cure symptoms 268–269
    Lyme disease is lethal 268
    reasons for symptom persistence 269–273, **270**
    seronegative Lyme disease 263, 264–266
    symptoms/clinical diagnosis define Lyme disease 266–267

natural killer T (NKT) cells 50, 170, 189
nervous system
    manifestations of Lyme disease 125, 191, 205–210
    pain processing 237
    peripheral, disorders of 204–205
    symptoms of CNS disorders 133, 204, 267–268
    see also neurologic disease
neuroborreliosis (LNB)
    association with *B. garinii* infection 83–84
    clinical manifestations 112–113, 205–210, **211**
    diagnosis 126–130, **127**, 139, 206–208
    Norwegian case study 139–141, **140**
    oral antibiotic treatment 95–96, 211
    post treatment residual symptoms 131–135, **134**, 209, 271
neurodegenerative disorders 202, 204
neurologic disease
    clinical assessment 205, 208, 233
    medical and psychological aspects **203**, 203–204, 236–237
    patient anxiety about 202–203, 264
'new or increased symptoms' (NOIS) 271
non-pharmacological pain management 240–241
North America
    clinical manifestations compared with Europe **79**, 109, 146–147, 202
    disease incidence 78–80, **79**
    distribution of agents/vectors 1, 32–33, 35
Norway, Lyme neuroborreliosis study 139–141, **140**
'not Lyme' symptoms 231–232
NSAIDs (non-steroidal inflammatory drugs) 97, 193, 220, 237
nymphs, tick 7, 13, 82, 144

Ockham's razor 191
oligoarthritis 185, 189
oral administration, antibiotics 95–96, 174–175
osteoarthritis 184–185, 237
outcomes
    assessment 130–131
    long-term, after EM 156–158
    prognosis for children 220–221
    role of psychological factors 232–235
    special patient groups 158–159
    untreated patients 153
outdoor activities, recreational 13
outer-surface proteins (Osp) 31
    A (OspA) 31, 107, 170, 190–191
    C (OspC) 11, 31, 49
overdiagnosis 247–248

pacemakers 175
pain, chronic 233, 235, 237
parenchymal CNS damage 204, 206
parenteral antibiotic treatment 96–97, 174, 211
patellofemoral joint dysfunction 184–186
pathogen-associated molecular patterns (PAMPs) 46, 47
pathogens
    host responses and pathogenesis 187–191
    interactions with tick vectors 10–13
    tick-borne co-infection 150, 152
patient advocacy groups 130, 240, 262, 263, 273
PCR (polymerase chain reaction)
    genotyping of strains 35
    interpretation of positive/negative results 183, 207, 252
    use in diagnostic testing 34, 58, 66, 266
penicillin 106, 180
pericarditis 171
peripheral nervous system
    common neuropathic disorders 204–205
    Lyme disease involvement 209–210
peripheral pain 237
permethrin 15, 222
persistence
    antibiotic survival by bacteria 38–39, 99, 188, 228–229, 252
    of seropositivity in patients 50, 64, 141
    see also residual symptoms
personality disorders 234
phagocytes 32
phenology, tick life cycles 7–8
phylogenetic analysis
    Borreliella species/strains 4–5, 29, **33**
    ticks 3–5
placebo effect 230, 254, 264
plasmids 30
pleocytosis, CSF 127–128, 206, 207
point-of-care diagnostic testing 67
polyarthritis 185–186
polymerase chain reaction *see* PCR
polymicrobial infectious syndrome 248
population dynamics, ticks 7–8
positive affect 234, 235
post-treatment syndrome (PTLDS)
    definition 228, 248–249, **249**
    encephalopathy 209
    long-term outcomes studies 133–135, **134**, 158, 235, 250

patient perceptions 223–224
possible mechanisms **250**
reported symptoms 46, 98, 133, 139–140, 249
search for evidence 131–132, 230, 250–255, **253**, 270–271
treatments given 230–231
pregnancy 85, 158, 222
prevention strategies 94, 222–223
pro-inflammatory molecules 188–190
proteins
  encoded in Bb 30–31
  salivary, in ticks 11
psoriasis 185
psychiatric disorders 203, **203**, 204, 233
psychological factors 232–233, 234–235
  and physiology (somatization) 236–237
  psychiatric comorbidity 233
PTLDS *see* post-treatment syndrome

quality of life assessment 135, 241, 254
questing behaviour 7, 82
quinolinic acid 210

randomized controlled trials (RCTs) 126, 153–154, 252–254, **253**
rash development, EM **143**, 145–146, 149
reinfection, in endemic areas 159
relapsing fever (RF) 12, 94, 208
repellents, tick 15, 222
reservoir hosts 6, 11, 35
residual symptoms
  perceived severity 131
  possible explanations for 228, **229**, 229–230, **250**, 251
  types and frequency 132, **132**, 133, 228
resilience factors (patients) 235
rheumatoid arthritis 185, 186, 189, 191, 192
Rickettsia spp. 12–13
risk
  factors affecting illness type and severity 83–84, 234, 235
  patient immune phenotype **270**, 272
  tick exposure factors 13–14, 15, 85, 185
rodents, as tick hosts 5, 8, 9
round bodies, spirochaete (cysts) 37–38, 272
roxithromycin 155

saliva, ticks, immunosuppressive properties 11, 48
Salp (salivary) proteins 11
screening
  electrocardiograms, for carditis 172–173, 176
  first-tier serological testing 60–62, 185
seasonality
  disease incidence 82
  tick life cycle phenology 7–8, 107

secondary lesions, EM 147, 153, 217
self-diagnosis 231, 232
septic arthritis 183–184, 194
serology
  diagnostic assays 48–50, 115
  interpretation of results 58, 63–65, 181, 264–266
  sensitivity for EM diagnosis 152–153
  test accuracy, neuroborreliosis diagnosis 129–130, 208
  two-tiered testing 60–63, **61**, 67, 172, 182
  and use of CSF/non-blood fluids 65–66, 129, 207–208
sex-specific incidence *see* gender-related effects
shrubs, tick density 14
skin
  biopsies 110, 111, 152
  inflammatory reaction to tick bite 142, **144**, 148–149, **149**
  scaling 146, 150
  sclerotic lesions 112
  viral lesions 149–150, **151**
  see also dermatological manifestations
sleep disturbance 186, 250
social media influence 141
somatization disorders 236–237
southern hemisphere, incidence 81–82
southern tick-associated rash infection (STARI) 142, 150, **151**
SPECT (single-photon emission computed tomography) 229, 268
spider bite 149, **151**
spirochaetemia (blood sample cultures) 147
spirochaetes
  biological characteristics 30
  morphological variants 37–38, 272
  successful treatments 94
steroid treatments 194, 212
strains, *B. burgdorferi* 34, 35–36, 147–148
stress 234, 241
surveillance
  data interpretation 76, 78
  standardization of definitions 168
symptoms
  'background' (non-specific) 133, 139, 157, 209, 250
  carditis 172
  diagnostic specificity 266–267
  erythema migrans 110, **143**, 144–148, **145**
  multiple, wrongly ascribed to Lyme 231–232, 248
  musculoskeletal dysfunctions 182, 193
  neuroborreliosis 112, 140, 205–206
  residual, frequency and severity 131–132, **132**, 133, 228–230
  response to antibiotic therapy 95, 188
  systemic 95, 98, 146–147, 217

synovial fluid
    diagnostic testing of 66, 183, 184
    isolation of *Borreliella* from 114, 183
    microRNA expression 189
synovitis
    mechanical, due to trauma 184
    persistent, treatment of 97, 186, 194, 195–196
syphilis 94, 128, 186, 208, 262

T-cell activation 50–51
taxonomy
    Ixodes ticks 3–5
    Lyme disease agents 29–30, **33**
tetracyclines 155, 156, 271–272
Th17 cells 189, 190
therapies *see* treatment
tick checks (visual inspection) 15, 94, 222
ticks (*Ixodes* spp.)
    behaviour 7, 11–12, 82
    evolution and biogeography 3–5
    human contact, risks and reduction 9, 13–16, 222
    life cycles 5–8
    population dynamics 8
    range expansion 8–10
    removal methods 115, 222
    transmission of Lyme disease 1, 3, 77
    as vectors of pathogens 10–13, 150, 152
tinea infection 150, **151**
toll like receptors (TLRs) 46–47, 188–189
toxic shock syndrome 189
transmission
    alternative (non-tick) means 85
    related to tick feeding 11–12, 15, 85
    seasonal variation 7, 82
    spirochaete migration 31–32
    tick vectors 1, 3
treatment
    'alternative' therapies 192–193, 231, 239, 264
    duration of **96**, 97, 98, 115
    early chemoprophylaxis 94–95, 115

guidelines for neuroborreliosis 130–131, 211, 220
judgement of success ('cure') 99, 269
of localized infections 95
non-pharmacological pain management 240–241
oral therapies 95–96, 174–175
parenteral therapies 96–97, 174
prospective trials 153–155
untreated patients, outcomes 153
use of (cortico) steroids 194, 212
see also antibiotics
tropical regions, incidence 81–82
two-tiered serological testing 60–63, **61**, 67, 172, 182

vaccines
    anti-tick 12, 16
    Lyme disease, for humans 222
vancomycin 39
vectors
    control strategies 13–16
    geographical distribution **2, 77**, 77–78
    tick–pathogen interactions 10–13
    see also ticks (*Ixodes* spp.)
vertebrate hosts, *Ixodes ricinus* complex 5–6
viral meningitis 206, 207
viral pathogens 152
VlsE protein 31
    see also C6 peptide antigen

web resources
    reported cases, CDC data 216
    'tick-radar Ltd' (Germany) 107
    treatment guidelines 220
Western blots *see* immunoblots
whole cell sonicates (WCS) 61, 129

xenodiagnosis 68, 252

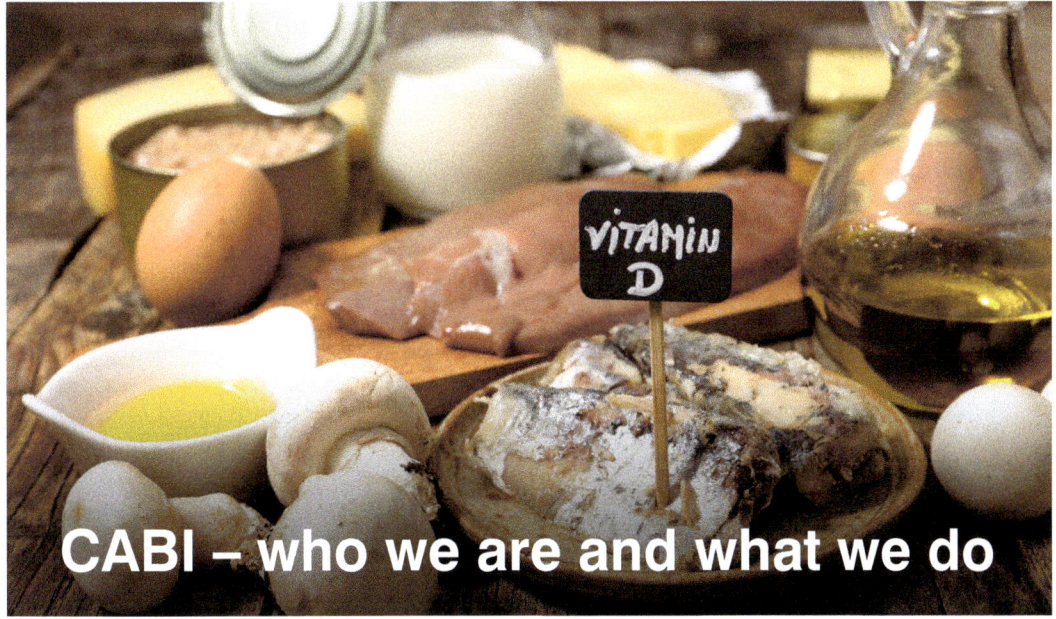

CABI – who we are and what we do

This book is published by **CABI**, an international not-for-profit organisation that improves people's lives worldwide by providing information and applying scientific expertise to solve problems in agriculture and the environment.

CABI is also a global publisher producing key scientific publications, including world renowned databases, as well as compendia, books, ebooks and full text electronic resources. We publish content in a wide range of subject areas including: agriculture and crop science / animal and veterinary sciences / ecology and conservation / environmental science / horticulture and plant sciences / human health, food science and nutrition / international development / leisure and tourism.

The profits from CABI's publishing activities enable us to work with farming communities around the world, supporting them as they battle with poor soil, invasive species and pests and diseases, to improve their livelihoods and help provide food for an ever growing population.

CABI is an international intergovernmental organisation, and we gratefully acknowledge the core financial support from our member countries (and lead agencies) including:

 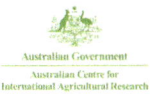 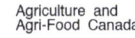 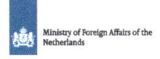 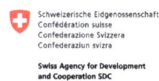

Discover more

To read more about CABI's work, please visit: **www.cabi.org**

Browse our books at: **www.cabi.org/bookshop**,
or explore our online products at: **www.cabi.org/publishing-products**

Interested in writing for CABI? Find our author guidelines here:
www.cabi.org/publishing-products/information-for-authors/